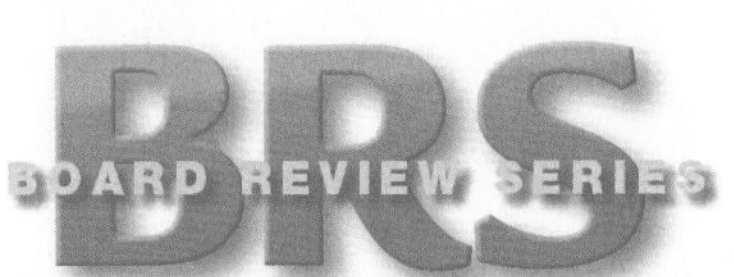

Pharmacology

FIFTH EDITION

Gary C. Rosenfeld, Ph.D.
Professor
Department of Integrated Biology and Pharmacology and
Graduate School of Biomedical Sciences
Assistant Dean for Education Programs
University of Texas Medical School at Houston
Houston, Texas

David S. Loose, Ph.D.
Associate Professor
Department of Integrated Biology and Pharmacology and
Graduate School of Biomedical Sciences
University of Texas Medical School at Houston
Houston, Texas

With special contributions by

Medina Kushen, M.D.
William Beaumont Hospital
Royal Oak, Michigan

Todd A. Swanson, M.D., Ph.D.
William Beaumont Hospital
Royal Oak, Michigan

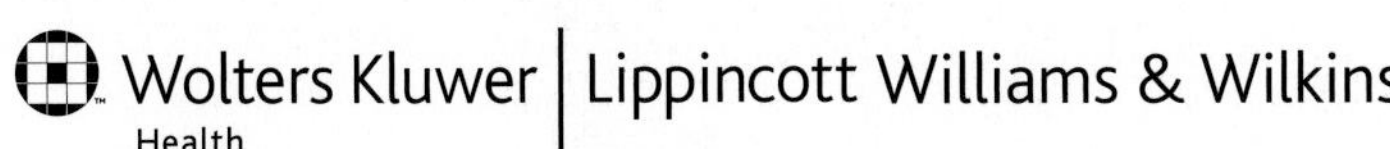

Philadelphia • Baltimore • New York • London
Buenos Aires • Hong Kong • Sydney • Tokyo

Acquisitions Editor: Charles W. Mitchell
Product Manager: Stacey L. Sebring
Marketing Manager: Jennifer Kuklinski
Production Editor: Paula Williams

351 West Camden Street
Baltimore, Maryland 21201-2436 USA

530 Walnut Street
Philadelphia, PA 19106

Printed in China

Library of Congress Cataloging-in-Publication Data

Rosenfeld, Gary C.
Pharmacology / Gary C. Rosenfeld, David S. Loose ; with special contributions by Medina Kushen, Todd A. Swanson. — 5th ed.
p. ; cm. — (Board review series)
Includes index.
ISBN 978-0-7817-8913-4 (soft cover : alk. paper)
1. Pharmacology—Examinations, questions, etc. I. Loose, David S. II. Title. III. Series: Board review series.
[DNLM: 1. Pharmacology—Examination Questions. QV 18.2 R813p 2010]
RM301.13.R67 2010
615′.1076—dc22

2009010547

The publishers have made every effort to trace the copyright holders for borrowed material. If they have inadvertently overlooked any, they will be pleased to make the necessary arrangements at the first opportunity.

We'd like to hear from you! If you have comments or suggestions regarding this Lippincott Williams & Wilkins title, please contact us at the appropriate customer service number listed below, or send correspondence to **book_comments@lww.com.** If possible, please remember to include your mailing address, phone number, and a reference to the book title and author in your message. To purchase additional copies of this book call our customer service department at **(800) 638-3030** or fax orders to **(301) 824-7390.** International customers should call **(301) 714-2324.**

CCS0612

Preface to the Fifth Edition

This concise review of medical pharmacology is designed for medical students, dental students, and others in the health care professions. It is intended primarily to help students prepare for licensing examinations, such as the United States Medical Licensing Examination Step 1 (USMLE) or other similar examinations. This book presents condensed and succinct descriptions of relevant and current Board-driven information pertaining to pharmacology without the usual associated details. It is not meant to be a substitute for the comprehensive presentation of information and difficult concepts found in standard pharmacology texts.

ORGANIZATION

The fifth edition begins with a chapter devoted to the general principles of drug action, followed by chapters concerned with drugs acting on the major body systems. Other chapters discuss autocoids, ergots, anti-inflammatory and immunosuppressive agents, drugs used to treat anemias and disorders of hemostasis, infectious diseases, cancer, and toxicology.

Each chapter includes a presentation of specific drugs with a discussion of their general properties, mechanism of action, pharmacologic effects, therapeutic uses, and adverse effects. A drug list, tables, and figures summarize essential drug information included in all chapters.

Clinically oriented, USMLE-style review questions and answers with explanations follow each chapter to help students assess their understanding of the information. Similarly, a comprehensive examination consisting of USMLE-style questions is included at the end of the book. This examination serves as a self-assessment tool to help students determine their fund of knowledge and diagnose any weaknesses in pharmacology.

Key Features

- Updated with current drug information
- End-of-chapter review tests feature updated USMLE-style questions
- 2-color tables and figures summarize essential information for quick recall
- Updated drug lists for each chapter
- Additional USMLE-style comprehensive examination questions and explanations

Gary C. Rosenfeld, Ph.D.
David S. Loose, Ph.D.

Acknowledgments

The authors acknowledge and thank our colleagues for their support and contributions to this book and our medical students for being our harshest critics.

Contents

12. CANCER CHEMOTHERAPY 287

13. TOXICOLOGY 309

chapter 1

General Principles of Drug Action

I. DOSE–RESPONSE RELATIONSHIPS

A. Drug effects are produced by altering the normal functions of cells and tissues in the body via one of four general mechanisms:

1. *Interaction with receptors,* naturally occurring target macromolecules that mediate the effects of endogenous physiologic substances such as neurotransmitters and hormones

a. Figure 1-1 illustrates the four major classes of drug–receptor interactions, using specific examples of endogenous ligands.

(1) Ligand-activated ion channels. Figure 1-1A illustrates acetylcholine interacting with a nicotinic receptor that is a nonspecific Na^+/K^+ transmembrane ion channel. Interaction of a molecule of acetylcholine with each subunit of the channel produces a conformational change that permits the passage of Na^+ and K^+. Other channels that are targets for various drugs include specific Ca^{2+} and K^+ channels.

(2) G-protein–coupled receptors (Fig. 1-1B–D). G-protein–coupled receptors compose the largest class of receptors. The receptors all have seven transmembrane segments, three intracellular loops, and an intracellular carboxy-terminal tail. The biologic activity of the receptors is mediated via interaction with a number of G (GTP binding)-proteins.

(a) $G\alpha_s$-coupled receptors. Figure 1-1B illustrates a β-adrenoceptor, which when activated by ligand binding (e.g., epinephrine) exchanges GDP for GTP. This facilitates the migration of $G\alpha_s$ ($G\alpha_{stimulatory}$) and its interaction with adenylyl cyclase (AC). $G\alpha_s$-bound AC catalyzes the production of cyclic AMP (cAMP) from adenosine triphosphate (ATP); cAMP activates protein kinase A, which subsequently acts to phosphorylate and activate a number of effector proteins. The βγ dimer may also activate some effectors. Hydrolysis of the guanosine triphoshate (GTP) bound to the Gα to guanosine diphosphate (GDP) terminates the signal.

(b) $G\alpha_i$ ($G_{inhibitory}$)-coupled receptors (Fig. 1-1C). Ligand binding (e.g., somatostatin) to $G\alpha_i$ ($G\alpha_{inhibitory}$)-coupled receptors similarly exchanges GTP for GDP, but $G\alpha_i$ inhibits adenylyl cyclase, leading to reduced cAMP production.

(c) G_q (and G_{11})-coupled receptors (Fig. 1-1D). G_q (and G_{11}) interact with ligand (e.g., serotonin)-activated receptors and increase the activity of phospholipase C (PLC). PLC cleaves the membrane phospholipid phosphatidylinositol 4,5-bisphosphate (PIP_2) to diacylglycerol (DAG) and inositol 1,4,5-triphosphate (IP_3). DAG activates protein kinase C, which can subsequently phosphorylate and activate a number of cellular proteins; IP_3 causes the release of Ca^{2+} from the endoplasmic reticulum into the cytoplasm, where it can activate many cellular processes.

(3) Receptor-activated tyrosine kinases (Fig. 1-1E). Many growth-related signals (e.g., insulin) are mediated via membrane receptors that possess intrinsic tyrosine kinase activity as illustrated for the insulin receptor. Ligand binding causes conformational changes in the receptor; some receptor tyrosine kinases are monomers that dimerize upon ligand binding. The liganded receptors then autophosphorylate tyrosine residues, which recruits cytoplasmic proteins to the plasma membrane where they are also tyrosine phosphorylated and activated.

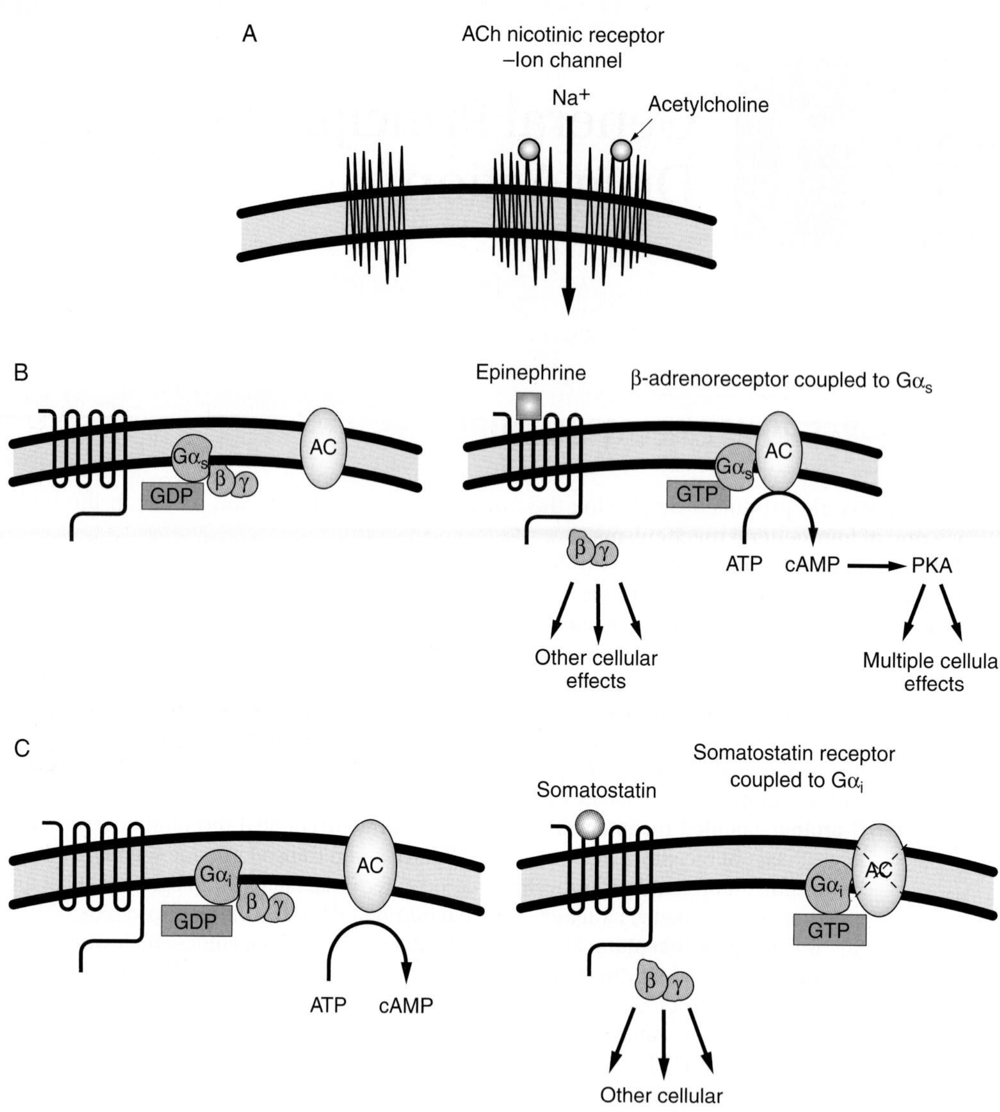

FIGURE 1-1. Four major classes of drug–receptor interactions, with specific examples of endogenous ligands. **A.** Acetylcholine interaction with a nicotinic receptor, a ligand-activated ion channel. **B–D.** G–coupled receptors. **B.** Epinephrine interaction with a $G\alpha_s$-coupled β-adrenoceptor. **C.** Somatostatin interaction with a $G\alpha_i$ ($G_{inhibitory}$)-coupled receptor. **D.** Serotonin interaction with a G_q (and G_{11})-coupled receptor. **E.** Insulin interaction with a receptor-activated tyrosine kinase. **F.** Cortisol interaction with an intracellular nuclear receptor.

(4) **Intracellular nuclear receptors** (Fig. 1-1F). Ligands (e.g., cortisol) for nuclear receptors are lipophilic and can diffuse rapidly through the plasma membrane. In the absence of ligand, nuclear receptors are inactive because of their interaction with chaperone proteins such as heat-shock proteins like HSP-90. Binding of ligand promotes structural changes in the receptor that facilitate dissociation of chaperones, entry of receptors into the nucleus, hetero- or homodimerization of receptors, and high-affinity interaction with the DNA of target genes. DNA-bound nuclear receptors are able to recruit a diverse number of proteins called coactivators, which subsequently act to increase transcription of the target gene.

2. ***Alteration of the activity of enzymes*** by activation or inhibition of the enzyme's catalytic activity
3. ***Antimetabolite action*** in which the drug, acting as a nonfunctional analogue of a naturally occurring metabolite, interferes with normal metabolism

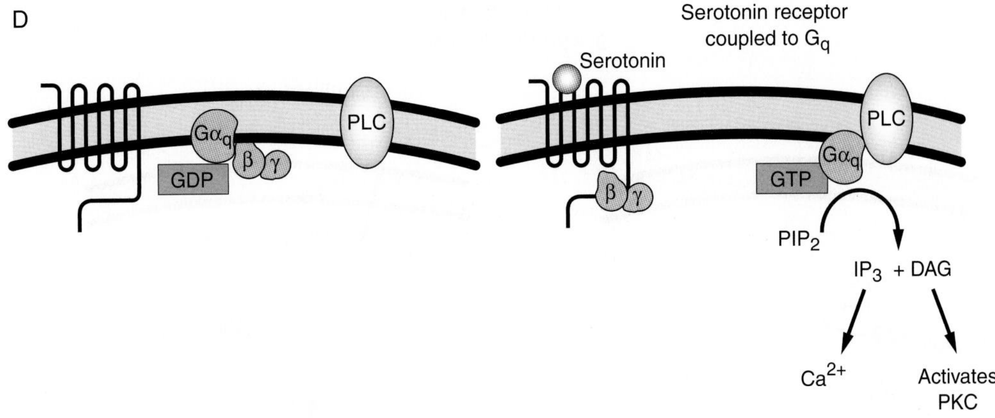

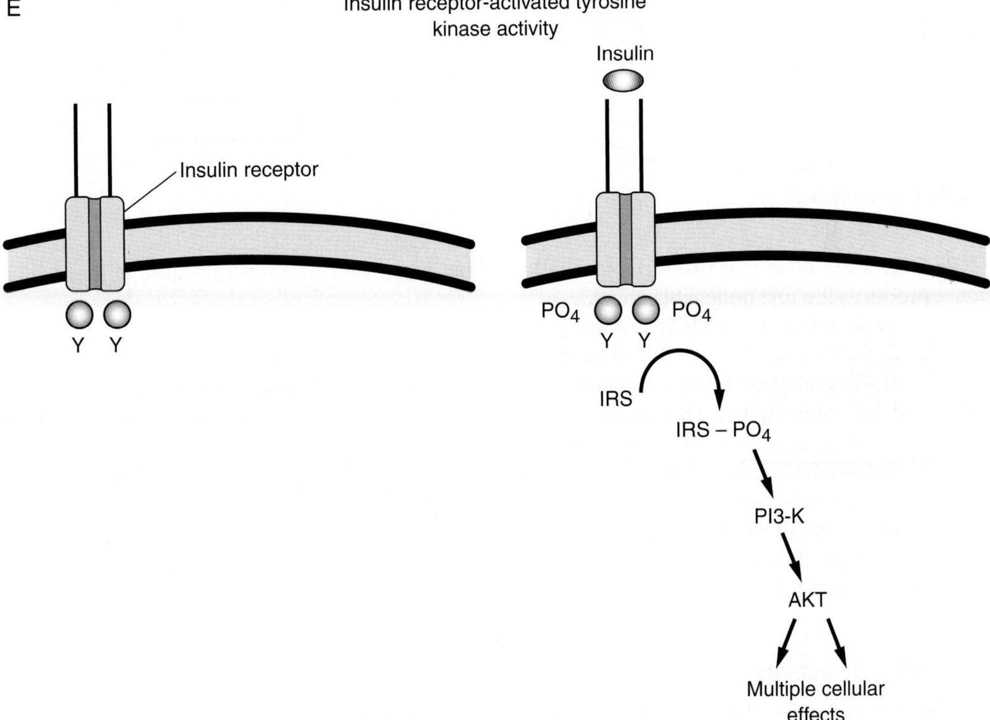

FIGURE 1-1. (*continued*).

4. ***Nonspecific chemical or physical interactions*** such as those caused by antacids, osmotic agents, and chelators

B. **The graded dose–response curve** expresses an individual's response to increasing doses of a given drug. The magnitude of a pharmacologic response is proportional to the number of receptors with which a drug effectively interacts (Fig. 1-2). The graded dose–response curve includes the following parameters:

1. ***Magnitude of response*** is graded; that is, it continuously increases with the dose up to the maximal capacity of the system, and it is often depicted as a function of the logarithm of the dose administered (to see the relationship over a wide range of doses).

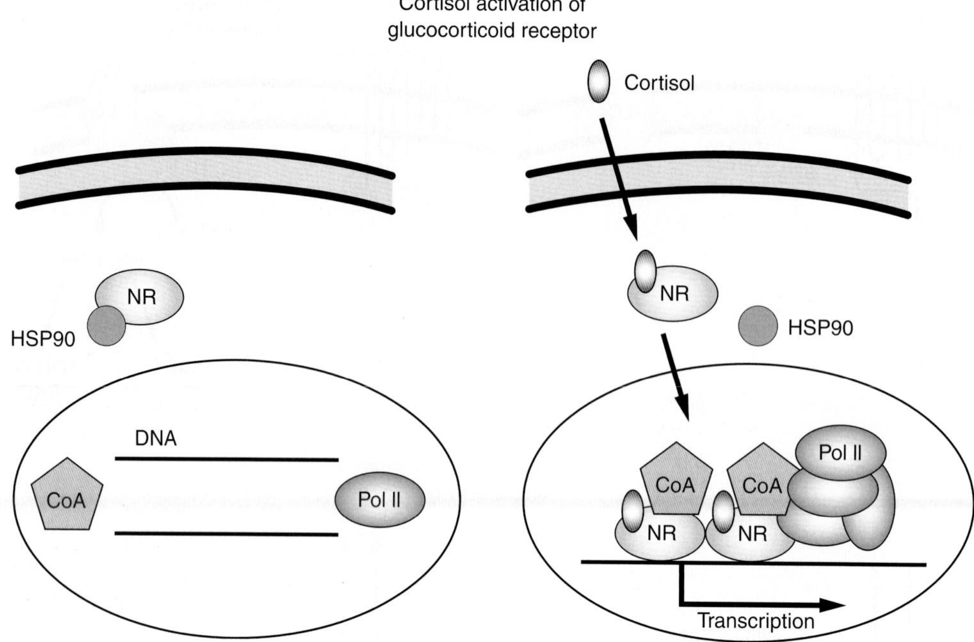

FIGURE 1-1. (*continued*).

2. ***ED_{50}*** is the dose that produces the half-maximal response; the threshold dose is that which produces the first noticeable effect.
3. ***Intrinsic activity*** is the ability of a drug once bound to activate the receptor.
   a. **Agonists** are drugs capable of binding to, and activating, a receptor.
      (1) Full agonists occupy receptors to cause maximal activation; intrinsic activity = 1.
      (2) Partial agonists can occupy receptors but cannot elicit a maximal response. Such drugs have an intrinsic activity of less than 1 (Fig. 1-3; drug C).
   b. **Antagonists** bind to the receptor but do not initiate a response; that is, they block the action of an agonist or endogenous substance that works through the receptor.
      (1) Competitive antagonists combine with the same site on the receptor as the agonist but have little or no efficacy and an intrinsic activity of 0. Competitive antagonists may be reversible or irreversible. Reversible, or equilibrium, competitive antagonists are not

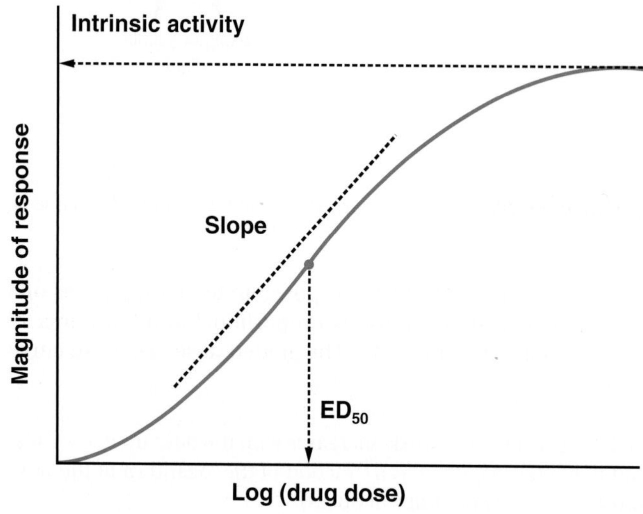

FIGURE 1-2. Graded dose–response curve.

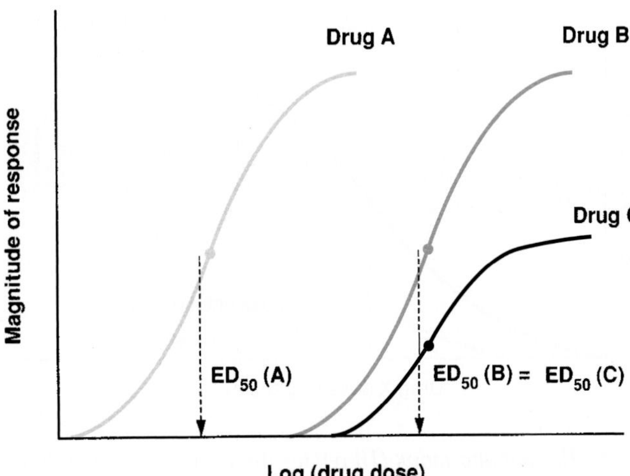

FIGURE 1-3. Graded dose–response curves for two agonists (A and B) and a partial agonist (C).

covalently bound, shift the dose–response curve for the agonist to the right, and increase the ED_{50}; that is, more agonist is required to elicit a response in the presence of the antagonist (Fig. 1-4). Because higher doses of agonist can overcome the inhibition, the maximal response can still be obtained.

(2) Noncompetitive antagonists bind to the receptor at a site other than the agonist-binding site (Fig. 1-5) and either prevent the agonist from binding correctly or prevent it from activating the receptor. Consequently, the effective amount of receptor is reduced. Receptors unoccupied by antagonist retain the same affinity for agonist, and the ED_{50} is unchanged.

4. ***Potency of a drug*** is the relative measure of the amount of a drug required to produce a specified level of response (e.g., 50%) compared to other drugs that produce the same effect via the same receptor mechanism. The potency of a drug is determined by the **affinity** of a drug for its receptor and the amount of administered drug that reaches the receptor site. The relative potency of a drug can be demonstrated by comparing the ED_{50} values of two full agonists; the drug with the lower ED_{50} is more potent. (For example, in Fig. 1-3, drug A is more potent than drug B.)
5. ***The efficacy of a drug*** is the ability of a drug to elicit the pharmacologic response. Efficacy may be affected by such factors as the number of drug–receptor complexes formed, the ability of the drug to activate the receptor once it is bound, and the status of the target organ or cell.
6. ***Slope*** is measured at the midportion of the dose–response curve. The slope varies for different drugs and different responses. Steep dose–response curves indicate that a small change in dose produces a large change in response.
7. ***Variability*** reflects the differences between individuals in response to a given drug.

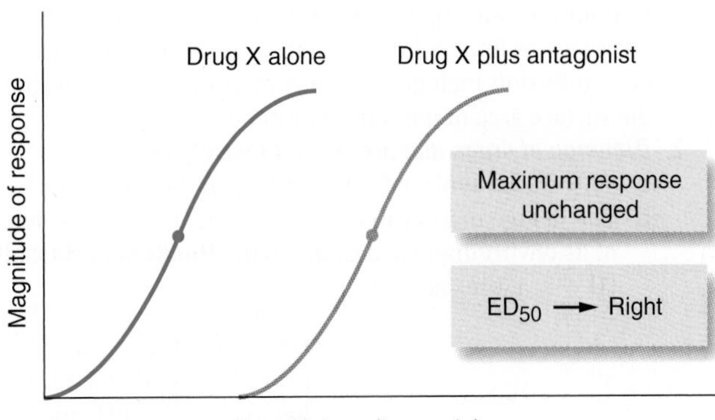

FIGURE 1-4. Graded dose–response curves illustrating the effects of competitive antagonists.

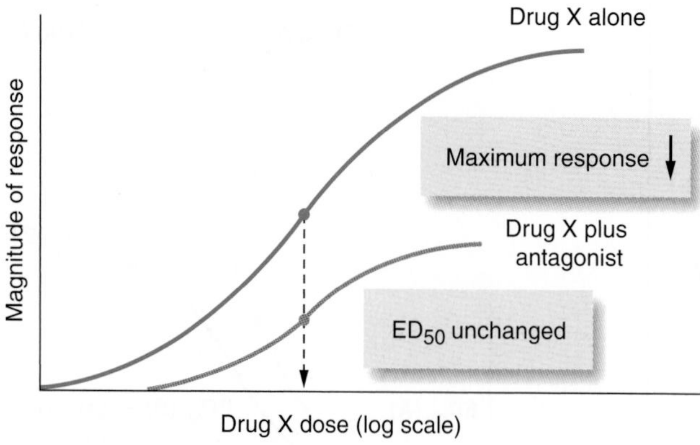

FIGURE 1-5. Graded dose–response curves illustrating the effects of noncompetitive antagonists.

8. ***Therapeutic index (TI)*** relates the desired therapeutic effect to undesired toxicity; it is determined using data provided by the quantal dose-response curve. The therapeutic index is defined as TD_{50}/ED_{50} (i.e., the ratio of the dose that produces a toxic effect in half of the population to the dose that produces the desired effect in half of the population). Note that the therapeutic index should be used with caution in instances when the quantal dose–response curves for the desired and toxic effects are not parallel.

C. **The quantal dose–response curve** (Figs. 1-6A and B) relates the dosage of a drug to the frequency with which a designated response will occur within a population. The response may be an "all-or-none" phenomenon (e.g., individuals either do or do not fall asleep after receiving a sedative) or some predetermined intensity of effect. The quantal dose–response curve is obtained via transformation of the data used for a frequency distribution plot to reflect the cumulative frequency of a response. In the context of the quantal dose–response curve, ED_{50} indicates the dose of drug that produces the response in half of the population. (Note that this differs from the meaning of ED_{50} in a graded dose–response curve.)

II. DRUG ABSORPTION

Drug absorption is the movement of a drug from its site of administration into the bloodstream. In many cases, a drug must be transported across one or more biologic membranes to reach the bloodstream.

A. Drug transport across membranes

1. ***Diffusion of un-ionized drugs*** is the most common and most important mode of traversing biologic membranes; drugs diffuse passively down their concentration gradient. Diffusion can be influenced significantly by the lipid–water **partition coefficient** of the drug, which is the ratio of solubility in an organic solvent to solubility in an aqueous solution. In general, absorption increases as lipid solubility (partition coefficient) increases. Other factors that also can influence diffusion include the concentration gradient of the drug across the cell membrane, and the surface area of the cell membrane.
2. ***Diffusion of drugs that are weak electrolytes***
   a. Only the **un-ionized** form of drug can diffuse across biologic membranes.
   b. The degree of ionization of a weak acid or base is determined by the pK of the drug and pH of its environment according to the **Henderson-Hasselbalch equation.**
      (1) For a weak acid, A,

$$HA \rightleftarrows H^+ + A^-,$$
$$pH = pK + \log[A^-]/[HA], \text{and}$$
$$\log[A^-]/[HA] = pH - pK$$

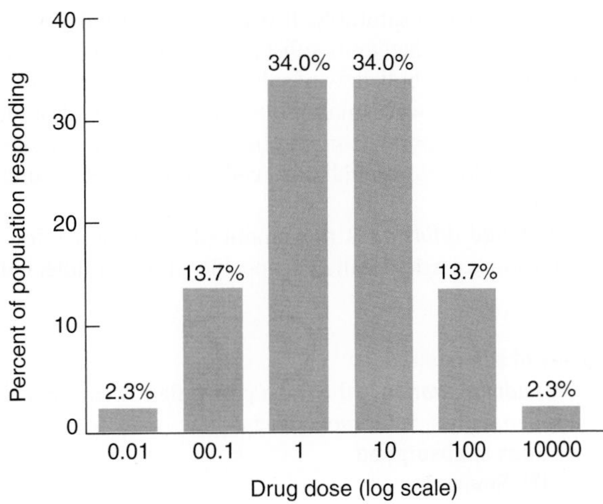

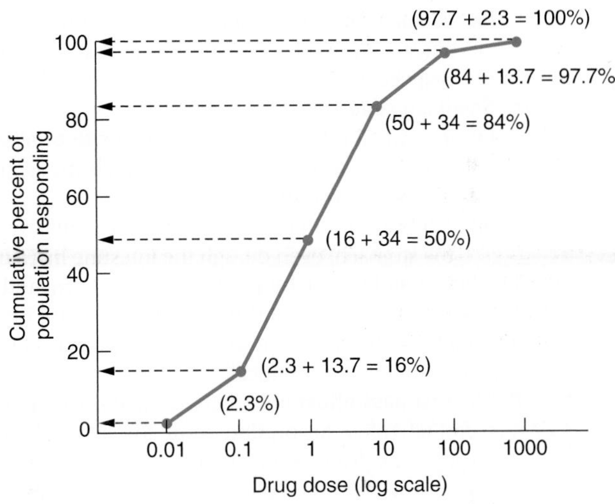

FIGURE 1-6. A. Frequency distribution plot. Number of individuals (as percentage of the population) who require the indicated drug dose to exhibit an identical response. As illustrated, 2.3% of the population require 0.01 units to exhibit the response, 13.7% require 0.1 units, and so on. **B.** Quantal dose–response curve. The cumulative number of individuals (as a percentage of the population) who will respond if the indicated dose of drug is administered to the entire population.

where HA is the concentration of the protonated, or un-ionized, form of the acid and A^- is the concentration of the ionized, or unprotonated, form.

(2) For a weak base, B,

$$BH^+ \rightleftarrows H^+ + B,$$
$$pH = pK + \log[B] / [BH^+], \text{and}$$
$$\log[B] / [BH^+] = pH - pK$$

where BH^+ is the concentration of the protonated form of the base, and B is the concentration of the unprotonated form.

c. When the pK of a drug equals the pH of the surroundings, 50% ionization occurs; that is, equal numbers of ionized and un-ionized species are present. A lower pK reflects a stronger acid; a higher pK corresponds to a stronger base.

d. Drugs with different pK values will diffuse across membranes at different rates.

e. The pH of the biologic fluid in which the drug is dissolved affects the degree of ionization and, therefore, the rate of drug transport.

3. ***Active transport*** is an energy-dependent process that can move drugs against a concentration gradient, as in **protein-mediated transport systems.** Active transport occurs in only one direction and is saturable. It is usually the mode of transport for drugs that resemble actively transported endogenous substances such as sugars, amino acids, and nucleosides.

4. ***Filtration*** is the bulk flow of solvent and solute through channels (pores) in the membrane. Filtration is seen with small molecules (usually with a molecular weight less than 100) that can pass through pores. Some substances of greater molecular weight, such as certain proteins, can be filtered through intercellular channels. Concentration gradients affect the rate of filtration.
5. ***Facilitated diffusion*** is movement of a substance down a concentration gradient. Facilitated diffusion is carrier mediated, specific, and saturable; it does not require energy.

B. Routes of administration

1. ***Oral administration*** is the most convenient, economical, and common route of administration; it is generally safe for most drugs.
   a. **Sites of absorption**
      (1) **Stomach**
         (a) **Lipid-soluble drugs** and **weak acids,** which are normally un-ionized at the low pH (1 to 2) of gastric contents, may be absorbed directly from the stomach.
         (b) **Weak bases** and **strong acids** (pK = 2 to 3) are not normally absorbed from this site since they tend to exist as ions that carry either a positive or negative charge, respectively.
      (2) **Small intestine**
         (a) The small intestine is the **primary site of absorption** of most drugs because of the very large surface area across which drugs, including partially ionized weak acids and bases, may diffuse.
         (b) Acids are normally absorbed more extensively from the small intestine than from the stomach, even though the intestine has a higher pH (approximately 5).
   b. The **bioavailability of a drug** is the fraction of drug (administered by any route) that reaches the bloodstream unaltered (bioavailability = 1 for intravenous administration). Bioequivalence refers to the condition in which the plasma concentration versus time profiles of two drug formulations are identical.
      (1) The **first-pass effect** influences drug absorption by metabolism in the liver or by biliary secretion. After absorption from the stomach or small intestine, a drug must pass through the liver before reaching the general circulation and its target site. If the capacity of liver metabolic enzymes to inactivate the drug is great, only limited amounts of active drug will escape the process. Some drugs are metabolized so extensively as a result of hepatic metabolism during the first pass that it precludes their use.
      (2) **Other factors** that may alter absorption from the stomach or small intestine include the following:
         (a) Gastric emptying time and passage of drug to the intestine may be influenced by **gastric contents** and **intestinal motility.** A decreased emptying time generally decreases the rate of absorption because the intestine is the major absorptive site for most orally administered drugs.
         (b) **Gastrointestinal (GI) blood flow** plays an important role in drug absorption by continuously maintaining the concentration gradient across epithelial membranes. The absorption of small, very lipid-soluble molecules is "blood flow limited," whereas highly polar molecules are "blood flow independent."
         (c) **Stomach acid** and inactivating enzymes may destroy certain drugs. Enteric coating prevents breakdown of tablets by the acid pH of the stomach.
         (d) **Interactions** with food, other drugs, and other constituents of the gastric milieu may influence absorption.
         (e) **Inert ingredients** in oral preparations or the special formulation of those preparations may alter absorption.
2. ***Parenteral administration*** includes three major routes: **intravenous (IV), intramuscular (IM),** and **subcutaneous (SC).** Parenteral administration generally results in more predictable bioavailability than oral administration.

a. With **IV** administration, the drug is injected directly into the bloodstream (100% bioavailable). It represents the most rapid means of introducing drugs into the body and is particularly useful in the treatment of emergencies when absolute control of drug administration is essential.
b. After **IM** and **SC** administration, many drugs can enter the capillaries directly through "pores" between endothelial cells. Depot preparations for sustained release may be administered by IM or SC routes, but some preparations may cause irritation and pain.

3. ***Other routes of administration***
a. **Inhalation** results in **rapid absorption** because of the large surface area and rich blood supply of the alveoli. Inhalation is frequently used for gaseous anesthetics, but it is generally not practical. Inhalation may be useful for drugs that act on the airways, such as epinephrine and glucocorticoids, which are used to treat bronchial asthma.
b. **Sublingual administration** is useful for drugs with **high first-pass metabolism,** such as **nitroglycerin,** since hepatic metabolism is bypassed.
c. **Intrathecal administration** is useful for drugs that do not readily cross the blood–brain barrier.
d. **Rectal administration** minimizes first-pass metabolism and may be used to circumvent the nausea and vomiting that sometimes result from oral administration. Use of rectal administration may be limited by inconvenience or patient noncompliance.
e. **Topical administration** is used widely when a local effect is desired or to **minimize systemic effects,** especially in dermatology and ophthalmology. Preparations must be nonirritating. Note that drugs administered topically may sometimes produce systemic effects.

III. DRUG DISTRIBUTION

Drug distribution is the movement of a drug from the bloodstream to the various tissues of the body.

A. **Distribution of drugs** is the process by which a drug leaves the bloodstream and enters the extracellular fluids and tissues. A drug must diffuse across cellular membranes if its site of action is intracellular. In this case, lipid solubility is important for effective distribution.

1. ***Importance of blood flow***
a. In most tissues, drugs can leave the circulation readily by diffusion across or between capillary endothelial cells. Thus, the **initial rate of distribution** of a drug **depends heavily on blood flow** to various organs (brain, liver, kidney > muscle, skin > fat, bone).
b. At **equilibrium,** or **steady state,** the amount of drug in an organ is related to the mass of the organ and its properties, as well as to the properties of the specific drug.

2. ***Volume of distribution (V_d)*** is the **volume of total body fluid** into which a drug "appears" to distribute after it reaches equilibrium in the body. Volume of distribution is determined by administering a known dose of drug (expressed in units of mass) intravenously and measuring the initial plasma concentration (expressed in units of mass/volume):

$$V_d = \text{amount of drug administered (m/g) / initial plasma concentration (mg/L)}$$

Volume of distribution is expressed in units of volume. In most cases, the "initial" plasma concentration, C_0, is determined by extrapolation from the elimination phase (see VII).
a. **Standard values** of volumes of fluid compartments in an average 70-kg adult are as follows: plasma = 3 liters; extracellular fluid = 12 liters; and total body water = 41 liters.
b. **Features** of volume of distribution:
(1) **V_d values** for most drugs do **not** represent their **actual distribution** in bodily fluids. The use of V_d values is primarily conceptual; that is, drugs that distribute extensively have relatively large V_d values and vice versa.
(2) A very low V_d value may indicate extensive plasma protein binding of the drug. A very high value may indicate that the drug is extensively bound to tissue sites.
(3) Among other variables, V_d may be **influenced by age, sex, weight,** and **disease processes** (e.g., edema, ascites).

3. ***Drug redistribution*** describes when the relative distribution of a drug in the body changes with time. This is usually seen with highly lipophilic drugs such as **thiopental** that initially enter tissues with high blood flow (e.g., the brain) and then quickly redistribute to tissues with lower blood flow (e.g., skeletal muscle and adipose tissue).
4. ***Barriers to drug distribution***
   a. Blood–brain barrier
      (1) Because of the nature of the blood–brain barrier, **ionized** or **polar drugs distribute poorly to the CNS,** including certain chemotherapeutic agents and toxic compounds, because they must pass through, rather than between, endothelial cells.
      (2) **Inflammation,** such as that resulting from meningitis, may increase the ability of ionized, poorly soluble drugs to cross the blood–brain barrier.
      (3) The blood–brain barrier may not be fully developed at the time of birth.
   b. Placental barrier
      (1) **Lipid-soluble drugs** cross the placental barrier more easily than polar drugs; drugs with a molecular weight of less than 600 pass the placental barrier better than larger molecules.
      (2) The possibility that drugs administered to the mother may cross the placenta and reach the fetus is always an important consideration in therapy.
      (3) Drug transporters (e.g., the **P-glycoprotein transporter**) transfer drugs out of the fetus.

B. **Binding of drugs by plasma proteins.** Drugs in the plasma may exist in the free form or may be bound to plasma proteins or other blood components, such as red blood cells.
1. ***General features of plasma protein binding***
   a. The extent of plasma protein binding is **highly variable** and ranges from virtually 0% to more than 99% bound, depending on the specific drug. Binding is generally reversible.
   b. Only the **free drug is small enough to pass through the spaces between the endothelial cells that form the capillaries;** extensive binding retards the rate at which the drug reaches its site of action and may prolong duration of action.
   c. Some plasma proteins bind many different drugs, whereas other proteins bind only one or a limited number. For example, serum albumin tends to bind many acidic drugs, whereas α_1-acid glycoprotein tends to bind many basic drugs.
   d. There are few, if any, documented changes in a drug's effect due to changes in plasma protein binding.

IV. DRUG ELIMINATION AND TERMINATION OF ACTION

A. **Mechanisms of drug elimination and termination of action**
1. In most cases, the action of a drug is terminated by **enzyme-catalyzed conversion** to an inactive (or less active) compound and/or **elimination from the body** via the kidney or other routes.
2. Redistribution of drugs from the site of action may terminate the action of a drug, although this occurs infrequently. For example, the action of the anesthetic **thiopental** is terminated largely by its redistribution from the brain (where it initially accumulates as a result of its high lipid solubility and the high blood flow to that organ) to the more poorly perfused adipose tissue.

B. **Rate of drug elimination from the body**
1. ***First-order elimination.*** The elimination of most drugs at therapeutic doses is "first-order," where **a constant fraction of drug is eliminated per unit time**; that is, the rate of elimination depends on the concentration of drug in the plasma, and is equal to the plasma concentration of the drug multiplied by a **proportionality constant:**

$$\text{Rate of eliminiation from body (mass/time)} = \text{Constant} \times [\text{Drug}]_{\text{plasma}} (\text{mass/vol})$$

Because the rate of elimination is given in units of mass/time and concentration is in units of mass/volume, the units of the constant are volume/time. This constant is referred to as the "clearance" of the drug (see IV C).

2. ***Zero-order kinetics.*** Infrequently, the rate of elimination of a drug is "zero-order," where **a constant amount of drug is eliminated per unit time.** In this case, the mechanism by which the body eliminates the drug (e.g., metabolism by hepatic enzymes, active secretion in the kidney) is saturated. The rate of drug elimination from the body is thus **constant** and does **not depend on plasma concentration.**

C. **Clearance (CL).** Conceptually, clearance is a measure of the capacity of the body to remove a drug. Mathematically, clearance is the proportionality constant that relates the rate of drug elimination to the plasma concentration of the drug. Thus, drugs with "high" clearance are rapidly removed from the body, and drugs with "low" clearance are removed slowly. As noted in IV B, the units of clearance are volume/time.

1. ***Specific organ clearance*** is the capacity of an individual organ to eliminate a drug. Specific organ clearance may be due to metabolism (e.g., "hepatic clearance" by the liver) or excretion (e.g., "renal clearance" by elimination in the urine).

$$\text{Rate of eliminiation by organ} = CL_{\text{organ}} \times [\text{Drug}]_{\text{plasma perfusing organ}}$$

or

$$CL_{\text{organ}} = \text{Rate of elimination by organ}/[\text{Drug}]_{\text{plasma perfusing organ}}$$

2. ***Whole body clearance*** is the capacity of the body to eliminate the drug by all mechanisms. Therefore, whole body clearance is equal to the sum of all of the specific organ clearance mechanisms by which the active drug is eliminated from the body:

$$CL_{\text{whole body}} = CL_{\text{organ 1}} + CL_{\text{organ 2}} + \cdots + CL_{\text{organ N}}$$

The term "clearance" generally refers to whole body clearance unless otherwise specified. In this case,

$$\text{Rate of elimination from body} = CL_{\text{whole body}} \times [\text{Drug}]_{\text{plasma}}$$

and

$$CL = \text{Rate of elimination from body}/[\text{Drug}]_{\text{plasma}}$$

3. ***Plasma clearance*** is numerically the same as whole body clearance, but this terminology is sometimes used because clearance may be viewed as the volume of plasma that contains the amount of drug removed per unit time (recall that the units of clearance are volume/time). If not specified, this term refers to the volume of plasma "cleared" of drug by all bodily mechanisms (i.e., whole body clearance). The term may also be applied to clearance by specific organs; for example, renal plasma clearance is the volume of plasma containing the amount of drug eliminated in the urine per unit time.

V. BIOTRANSFORMATION (METABOLISM) OF DRUGS

A. General properties

1. Biotransformation is a major mechanism for **drug elimination;** most drugs undergo biotransformation, or metabolism, after they enter the body. Biotransformation, which almost always produces metabolites that are more polar than the parent drug, usually terminates the pharmacologic action of the parent drug and, via excretion, increases removal of the drug from the body. However, other consequences are possible, notably after phase I reactions, including similar or different pharmacologic activity, or toxicologic activity.
2. Many drugs undergo several sequential biotransformation reactions. Biotransformation is catalyzed by **specific enzyme systems,** which may also catalyze the metabolism of endogenous substances such as steroid hormones.

3. The liver is the major site of biotransformation, although specific drugs may undergo biotransformation primarily or extensively in other tissues.
4. Biotransformation of drugs is **variable** and can be affected by many parameters, including **prior administration** of the drug in question or of other drugs; **diet; hormonal status; genetics; disease** (e.g., decreased in cardiac and pulmonary disease); **age** and **developmental status** (the very elderly and very young may be more sensitive to drugs, in part, because of decreased or undeveloped levels of drug-metabolizing enzymes); and **liver function** (in cases of severe liver damage, dosage adjustments may be required for drugs eliminated largely via this route).
5. Possible consequences of biotransformation include the production of **inactive metabolites** (most common), metabolites with increased or decreased potencies, metabolites with qualitatively different pharmacologic actions, toxic metabolites, or active metabolites from inactive prodrugs.
6. **Metabolites carry ionizable groups,** and are often **more charged and more polar** than the parent compounds. This increased charge may lead to a more rapid rate of clearance because of possible secretion by acid or base carriers in the kidney; it may also lead to decreased tubular reabsorption.

B. Classification of biotransformation reactions

1. ***Phase I (nonsynthetic) reactions*** involve enzyme-catalyzed biotransformation of the drug without any conjugations. Phase I reactions include **oxidations, reductions,** and **hydrolysis reactions;** they frequently introduce a functional group (e.g., –OH) that serves as the active center for sequential conjugation in a phase II reaction.
2. ***Phase II (synthetic) reactions*** include **conjugation reactions,** which involve the enzyme-catalyzed combination of a drug (or drug metabolite) with an endogenous substance. Phase II reactions require a functional group—an **active center**—as the site of conjugation with the endogenous substance. Phase II reactions require energy indirectly for the synthesis of "activated carriers," the form of the endogenous substance used in the conjugation reaction (e.g., uridine diphosphate [UDP]-glucuronate).

C. Enzymes catalyzing phase I biotransformation reactions include cytochrome P-450, aldehyde and alcohol dehydrogenase, deaminases, esterases, amidases, and epoxide hydratases. **Enzymes catalyzing phase II biotransformation reactions** include glucuronyl transferase (glucuronide conjugation), sulfotransferase (sulfate conjugation), transacylases (amino acid conjugation), acetylases, ethylases, methylases, and glutathione transferase. These enzymes are present in numerous tissues; some are present in plasma. Subcellular locations include cytosol, mitochondria, and endoplasmic reticulum. Only those enzymes located in the endoplasmic reticulum are inducible by drugs.

1. ***Cytochrome P-450 monooxygenase (mixed function oxidase)***
   a. **General features** (Table 1-1)
      (1) Cytochrome P-450 monooxygenase plays a central role in drug biotransformation. A large number of families (at least 18 in mammals) of cytochrome P-450 (abbreviated "CYP") enzymes exists, each member of which catalyzes the biotransformation of a unique spectrum of drugs, with some overlap in the substrate specificities. This enzyme system is the one most frequently involved in **phase I reactions.**
      (2) The cytochrome P-450 families are referred to using an arabic numeral (e.g., CYP1, CYP2, etc.). Each family has a number of subfamilies denoted by an upper case letter (e.g., CYP2A, CYP2B, etc.). The individual enzymes within each subfamily are denoted by another arabic numeral (e.g., CYP3A1, CYP3A2, etc.).
      (3) Cytochrome P-450 catalyzes numerous reactions, including aromatic and aliphatic hydroxylations; dealkylations at nitrogen, sulfur, and oxygen atoms; heteroatom oxidations at nitrogen and sulfur atoms; reductions at nitrogen atoms; and ester and amide hydrolysis.
      (4) The **CYP3A** subfamily is responsible for up to half of the total cytochrome P-450 in the liver and accounts for approximately 50% of the metabolism of clinically important drugs. **CYP3A4** is a particularly abundant enzyme.

table 1-1 Selected Inducers and Inhibitors of Cytochrome P-450 (CYP) Enzymes

Enzyme	Drug Substrate	Inhibitors	Inducers
CYP1A2	Clozapine, imipramine, mexiletine, naproxen, tacrine, sertraline	Cimetidine, fluvoxamine, ticlopidine	Omeprazole, tobacco
CYP2C9	Diclofenac, glipizide, ibuprofen, losartan, naproxen, phenytoin, piroxicam, tamoxifen, tolbutamide, warfarin	Amiodarone, fluconazole, isoniazid	Rifampin
CYP2C19	Amitriptyline, clomipramine, cyclophosphamide, diazepam, omeprazole, phenytoin, progesterone	Fluoxetine, fluvoxamine, ketoconazole, omeprazole, ticlopidine	Rifampin
CYP2D6	**β-blockers:** Metoprolol, propranolol, timolol **Antiarrhythmic agents:** Mexiletine **CNS agents:** Amitriptyline, clomipramine, codeine, desipramine, imipramine, dextromethorphan haloperidol, paroxetine, risperidone, thioridazine	Amiodarone, bupropion, chlorpheniramine, cimetidine, clomipramine, fluoxetine, haloperidol, methadone, paroxetine, quinidine, ritonavir	
CYP3A4,5,7	**Calcium channel blockers:** Diltiazem, felodipine, nifedipine, verapamil **HMG-CoA reductase inhibitors:** Atorvastatin, lovastatin, simvastatin **CNS agents:** Alprazolam, buspirone, diazepam, methadone, midazolam, triazolam **Macrolide antibiotics:** Clarithromycin, erythromycin **Anticancer agents:** Cyclophosphamide, tamoxifen, vinblastine, vincristine **HIV protease inhibitors:** Indinavir, ritonavir, saquinavir **Other:** Chlorpheniramine, cyclosporine, quinidine, tacrolimus	Amiodarone, cimetidine, clarithromycin, diltiazem, erythromycin, fluvoxamine, grapefruit juice, indinavir, imatinib, isoniazid, itraconazole, nefazodone, nelfinavir, ritonavir, verapamil	Carbamazepine, phenobarbital, phenytoin, rifampin, St. John's wort, troglitazone

From www.drug-interactions.com.

b. Localization. The **primary location** of cytochrome P-450 is the **liver,** which has the greatest specific enzymatic activity and the highest total activity; but it is also found in many other tissues, including the adrenals, ovaries and testis, and tissues involved in steroidogenesis and steroid metabolism. The enzyme's subcellular location is the **endoplasmic reticulum.** Lipid membrane location facilitates the metabolism of lipid-soluble drugs.

c. Mechanism of reaction

(1) In the overall reaction, the drug is oxidized and oxygen is reduced to water. Reducing equivalents are provided by **nicotinamide adenine dinucleotide phosphate (NADPH),** and generation of this cofactor is coupled to **cytochrome P-450 reductase.**

(2) The overall reaction for aromatic hydroxylation can be described as

$$\text{Drug} + O_2 + \text{NADPH} + H^+ \rightarrow \text{Drug} - \text{OH} + \text{NADP}^+ + H_2O$$

d. Genetic polymorphism of several clinically important cytochrome P-450s, particularly **CYP2C** and **CYP2D,** is a source of variable metabolism in humans, including differences among racial and ethnic groups. These enzymes have substantially different properties (V_{max} or K_m).

e. Induction (Table 1-1)

(1) Induction is brought about by **drugs** and **endogenous substances,** such as hormones. Any given drug preferentially induces one form of cytochrome P-450 or a particular set of P-450s.

(2) When caused by drugs, induction is pharmacologically important as a major source of **drug interactions.** A drug may induce its own metabolism (metabolic tolerance) and that of other drugs catalyzed by the induced P-450.

(3) Induction can be caused by a wide variety of clinically useful drugs (**drug–drug interactions**), such as **omeprazole, rifampin, carbamazepine,** and **St. John's wort.**

(4) Some of the same drugs that induce CYP3A4 can induce the drug efflux transporter P-glycoprotein (e.g., **rifampin, St. John's wort**).

f. **Inhibition** (Table 1-1)

(1) Competitive or noncompetitive (clinically more likely) inhibition of P-450 enzyme activity can result in the **reduced metabolism** of other drugs or endogenous substrates such as **testosterone.**

(2) Inhibition can be caused by a number of commonly used drugs, including **cimetidine, fluconazole, fluoxetine,** and **erythromycin,** and is another major source of **drug–drug interactions.**

(3) Some of the same drugs that inhibit CYP3A4 can inhibit the drug efflux transporter **P-glycoprotein** (e.g., **amiodarone, clarithromycin, erythromycin, ketoconazole**).

2. ***Glucuronyl transferase***

a. General features

(1) Glucuronyl transferase is a set of enzymes with unique but overlapping specificities that are involved in **phase II reactions.**

(2) It catalyzes the conjugation of glucuronic acid to a variety of active centers, including –OH, –COOH, –SH, and $–NH_2$.

b. Mechanism of reaction

(1) **UDP-glucuronic acid,** the active glucuronide donor, is formed from uridine triphosphate (UTP) and glucose 1-phosphate.

(2) **Glucuronyl transferase** then catalyzes the conjugation to the active center of the drug.

c. Location and induction

(1) Glucuronyl transferase is located in the **endoplasmic reticulum.**

(2) It is the only phase II reaction that is **inducible by drugs** and is a possible site of drug interactions.

D. **Hepatic extraction of drugs.** General extraction by the liver occurs because of the liver's large size (1500 g) and high blood flow (1 mL/g/min).

1. The **extraction ratio** is the amount of drug removed in the liver divided by the amount of drug entering the organ; a drug completely extracted by the liver would have an extraction ratio of 1. Highly extracted drugs can have a hepatic clearance approaching 1500 mL/min.

2. **First-pass effect.** Drugs taken orally pass across membranes of the GI tract into the portal vein and through the liver before entering the general circulation.

a. **Bioavailability** of orally administered drugs is **decreased** by the fraction of drug removed by the first pass through the liver. For example, a drug with a hepatic extraction ratio of 1 would have 0% bioavailability; a drug such as lidocaine, with an extraction ratio of 0.7, would have 30% bioavailability.

b. In the presence of hepatic disease, drugs with a high first-pass extraction may reach the systemic circulation in higher than normal amounts, and dose adjustment may be required.

VI. EXCRETION OF DRUGS

A. **Routes of excretion** may include urine, feces (e.g., unabsorbed drugs and drugs secreted in bile), saliva, sweat, tears, milk (with possible transfer to neonates), and lungs (e.g., alcohols and anesthetics). Any route may be important for a given drug, but the kidney is the major site of excretion for most drugs.

1. Some drugs are secreted by liver cells into the bile, pass into the intestine, and are eliminated in the feces (e.g., **rifampin, indomethacin, estradiol**).

2. Drugs may be also be reabsorbed from the intestine (i.e., **undergo enterohepatic circulation**). In this manner, the persistence of a drug in the body may be prolonged.

B. Net renal excretion of drugs

1. ***Net renal excretion*** of drugs is the result of **three separate processes:** the amount of drug filtered at the glomerulus, plus the amount of drug secreted by active transport mechanisms in the kidney, less the amount of drug passively reabsorbed throughout the tubule.

   a. **Filtration**

      (1) Most drugs have low molecular weights and are thus freely filtered from the plasma at the glomerulus.

      (2) Serum protein binding reduces filtration because plasma proteins are too large to be filtered.

      (3) The glomerular filtration rate is 30%–40% lower during newborns' first year of life than in adults.

   b. **Secretion**

      (1) The kidney proximal tubule contains **two transport systems** that may secrete drugs into the ultrafiltrate, one for **organic acids** and a second for **organic bases.** These systems require energy for active transport against a concentration gradient; they are a site for potential **drug–drug interactions** because drugs may compete with each other for binding to the transporters.

      (2) Plasma protein binding does not normally have a large effect on secretion because the affinity of the transport systems for most drugs is greater than the affinity of plasma binding proteins.

   c. **Reabsorption**

      (1) Reabsorption may occur throughout the tubule; some compounds, including endogenous compounds such as glucose, are actively reabsorbed.

      (2) Reabsorption of the un-ionized form of drugs that are weak acids and bases can occur by simple **passive diffusion,** the rate of which depends on the lipid solubility and pK of the drug and also on the concentration gradient of the drug between the urine and the plasma.

      (3) Reabsorption may be affected by **alterations of urinary pH,** which also affect elimination of weak acids or bases by affecting the degree of ionization. For example, acidification of the urine will result in a higher proportion of the un-ionized form of an acidic drug and will facilitate reabsorption.

2. ***Renal clearance of drugs***

   a. Renal clearance measures the volume of plasma that is cleared of drug per unit time:

$$CL\,(mL/min) = U \times V/P$$

   where **U** = concentration of drug per milliliter of **urine, V** = **volume** of urine excreted per minute, and **P** = concentration of drug per milliliter of **plasma.**

      (1) A drug excreted by **filtration alone** (e.g., insulin) will have a clearance equal to the glomerular filtration rate (GFR; 125–130 mL/min).

      (2) A drug excreted by **filtration and complete secretion** (e.g., *para*-aminohippuric acid) will have a clearance equal to renal plasma clearance (650 mL/min).

      (3) Clearance values between 130 and 650 mL/min suggest that a drug is **filtered, secreted, and partially reabsorbed.**

   b. A variety of factors influence renal clearance, including age (some mechanisms of excretion may not be fully developed at the time of birth), other drugs, and disease.

   c. In the presence of **renal failure,** the clearance of a drug may be reduced significantly, resulting in higher plasma levels. For those drugs with a narrow therapeutic index, dose adjustment may be required.

VII. PHARMACOKINETICS

Pharmacokinetics describes changes in plasma drug concentration over time. Although it is ideal to determine the amount of drug that reaches its site of action as a function of time after administration, it is usually impractical or not feasible. Therefore, the plasma drug concentration is measured. This

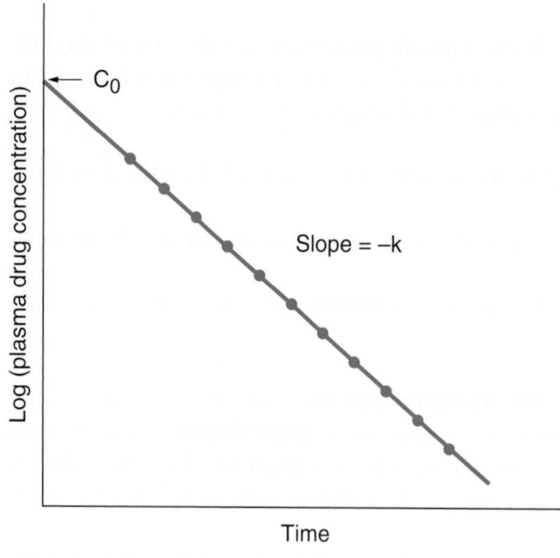

FIGURE 1-7. One-compartment model of drug distribution.

provides useful information, because the amount of drug in the tissues is generally related to plasma concentration.

A. **Distribution and elimination**

1. ***One-compartment model*** (Fig. 1-7)
   a. The drug appears to distribute instantaneously after IV administration of a single dose. If the mechanisms for drug elimination, such as biotransformation by hepatic enzymes and renal secretion, are not saturated following the therapeutic dose, a semilog plot of plasma concentration versus time will be **linear.**
   b. Drug elimination is **first order;** that is, a constant fraction of drug is eliminated per unit time. For example, one-half of the drug is eliminated every 8 hours. Elimination of most drugs is a first-order process.
   c. The slope of the semilog plot is **–k,** where k is the rate constant of elimination and has units of time^{-1}, and the intercept on the *y* axis is C_0 (*Note:* C_0 is used to calculate V_d for drugs that obey a one-compartment model.)
   d. The **plasma drug concentration** (C_t) at any time (t) after administration is given by

$$\ln C_t = \ln C_0 - kt$$

(or $\log C_t = \log C_0 - kt/2.303$, if logs to the base 10 are used rather than natural logs), and the **relationship of the plasma concentrations** at any two points in time is given by

$$\ln C_2 = \ln C_1 - k(t_2 - t_1)$$

or

$$\log C_2 = \log C_1 - k/2.3.03\,(t_2 - t_1)$$

   e. The rate constant of elimination (k), the V_d, and the whole body clearance (CL) are related by the expression

$$CL = k \times V_d$$

2. ***Two-compartment model*** (Fig. 1-8)
   a. The two-compartment model is a more common model for distribution and elimination of drugs. Initial rapid changes in the plasma concentration of a drug are observed because of a **distribution phase,** the time required for the drug to reach an equilibrium distribution

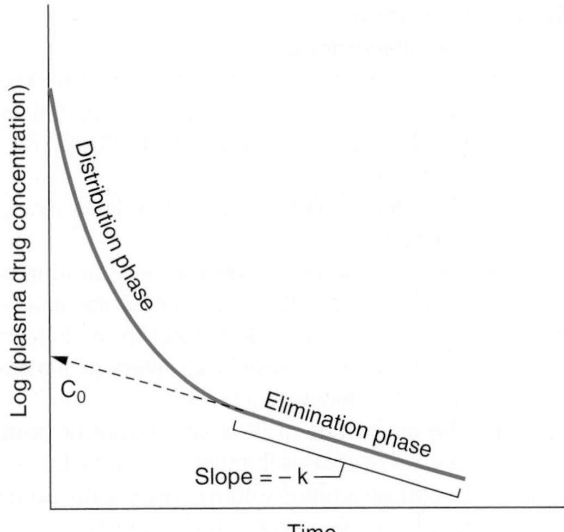

FIGURE 1-8. Two-compartment model of drug distribution.

between a central compartment, such as the plasma space, and a second compartment, such as the aggregate tissues and fluids to which the drug distributes.

b. After distribution, a linear decrease in the log drug concentration is observed if the **elimination phase** is first order.

c. For drugs that obey a two-compartment model, the value of C_0 obtained by extrapolation of the elimination phase is used to calculate V_d, and the elimination rate constant, k, is obtained from the slope of the elimination phase.

d. The expressions for ln C_t and CL shown above for a one-compartment model also apply during the elimination phase for drugs that obey a two-compartment model.

3. ***First-order elimination***

a. First-order elimination accounts for elimination of most drugs. It refers to the elimination of a constant fraction of drug per unit time; that is, the rate of elimination is a **linear function** of the plasma drug concentration.

b. First-order elimination occurs when elimination systems are not saturated by the drug.

4. ***Zero-order elimination***

a. In this model, the plot of the log of the plasma concentration versus time will be concave upward, and a constant amount of drug will be eliminated per unit time (e.g., 10 mg of drug will be eliminated every 8 hours). This is referred to as zero-order elimination, or **zero-order kinetics.** (Note that after an interval of time sufficient to reduce the drug level below the saturation point, first-order elimination occurs.)

b. Zero-order elimination may occur when therapeutic doses of drugs exceed the capacity of elimination mechanisms.

B. Half-life ($t_{1/2}$)

1. Half-life is the time it takes for the plasma drug concentration to be reduced by 50%. This concept applies only to drugs eliminated by **first-order kinetics.**

2. Half-life is determined from the log plasma drug concentration versus time profile for drugs fitting a one-compartment model or from the elimination phase for drugs fitting the two-compartment model. As long as the dose administered does not exceed the capacity of the elimination systems (i.e., the dose does not saturate those systems), the half-life will remain constant.

3. The half-life is related to the **elimination rate constant (k)** by the equation $t_{1/2} = 0.693/k$ and to the **volume of distribution (V_d)** and **clearance (CL)** by the equation $t_{1/2} = 0.693\ V_d/CL$.

4. For all doses in which first-order elimination occurs, >95% of the drug will be eliminated in a time interval equal to five half-lives. This applies for therapeutic doses of most drugs.

C. Multidose kinetics

1. *Repeat administration*

- **a.** If a drug that is eliminated by first-order kinetics is administered repeatedly (e.g., one tablet every 8 hours), the average plasma concentration of the drug will increase until a mean **steady-state** level is reached. (This will not occur for drugs that exhibit zero-order elimination.)
- **b.** The interval of time required to reach steady state is equal to **five half-lives.**

2. *Steady state*

- **a.** Some fluctuation in plasma concentration will occur even at steady state.
- **b.** Levels will be at the high point of the steady state range shortly after a dose is administered; levels will be at the low point immediately before administration of the next dose. Hence, steady state designates an **average plasma concentration** and the range of fluctuations above and below that level.
- **c.** The magnitude of fluctuations can be controlled by the **dosing interval.** A shorter dosing interval decreases fluctuations, and a longer dosing interval increases them. On cessation of multidose administration, >95% of the drug will be eliminated in a time interval equal to five half-lives if first-order kinetics applies.

3. *Maintenance dose rate*

- **a.** Maintenance dose rate is the dose of a drug required per unit time to maintain a desired steady-state level in the plasma to sustain a specific therapeutic effect.
- **b.** To determine the dose rate required to maintain an average steady-state plasma concentration of drug, multiply the desired plasma concentration by the CL:

$$\text{Maintenance dose rate} = \text{Desired } [\text{drug}]_{\text{plasma}} \times \text{Clearance (CL)}$$
$$(\text{amount / time}) = (\text{amount / volume}) \times (\text{volume / time})$$

  This yields dose rate in units of amount per time (e.g., mg/hour). One may understand this fundamental relationship in the following way: To remain at steady state, the **dose rate must equal the elimination rate;** that is, the rate at which the drug is added to the body must equal the rate at which it is eliminated. Recall that the elimination rate = CL $\times$ $[\text{Drug}]_{\text{plasma}}$. Therefore, because the dose rate must equal the elimination rate to be at steady state, dose rate also equals CL $\times$ Desired $[\text{drug}]_{\text{plasma}}$.
- **c.** If one administers a drug at the maintenance dose rate, a steady state plasma concentration of drug will be reached in four to five half-lives. (*Note:* This is four to five half-lives, not four to five doses!)

4. *Loading dose*

- **a.** A large loading dose may be needed initially when the therapeutic concentration of a drug in the plasma must be achieved **rapidly** (e.g., a life-threatening situation in which one cannot wait for 5 half-lives for the drug to reach the desired steady-state level). In this situation one may administer a loading dose.
- **b.** To calculate the loading dose, select the desired plasma concentration of drug and multiply by the V_d:

$$\text{Loading dose} = \text{Desired } [\text{drug}]_{\text{plasma}} \times V_d$$
$$(\text{amount or mass}) = (\text{mass / volume}) \times (\text{volume})$$

- **c.** After administration of the loading dose (which rapidly achieves the desired plasma concentration of drug), one administers the drug at the maintenance dose rate to maintain the drug concentration at the desired steady-state level.

Review Test for Chapter 1

Directions: Each of the numbered items or incomplete statements in this section is followed by answers or by completions of the statement. Select the ONE lettered answer or completion that is BEST in each case.

1. Somatostatin interacts with

(A) G_i-protein–coupled receptor
(B) G_q-protein–coupled receptor
(C) Ligand-activated ion channel
(D) Receptor-activated tyrosine kinase
(E) Intracellular nuclear receptor

2. Cortisol is capable of targeting intranuclear receptors secondary to its ability to

(A) Recruit intracellular kinases
(B) Undergo autophosphorylation
(C) Diffuse through lipid membranes
(D) Interact with G-proteins
(E) Interact with adenylyl cyclase

3. Which of the following parameters is used to indicate the ability of a drug to produce the desired therapeutic effect relative to a toxic effect?

(A) Potency
(B) Intrinsic activity
(C) Therapeutic index
(D) Efficacy
(E) Bioavailability

4. A 64-year-old woman with a history of multiple abdominal surgeries due to Crohn's disease presents to the emergency room with obstipation and feculent emesis. A diagnosis of small bowel obstruction is made, and she is taken to the operating room for lysis of adhesions and resection of stenosed region of small bowel. Postoperatively, the patient is noted to have elevated blood pressure, and oral metoprolol is administered; however, no improvement of hypertension is observed. This is likely due to

(A) The first-pass effect
(B) Decreased passage of drug through intestine
(C) Decreased GI blood flow
(D) Destruction of drug by stomach acid
(E) Increased protein binding of the drug

5. An important feature of congestive heart failure (CHF) regarding drug action is

(A) Impaired blood flow to the intestine
(B) Increased protein binding of various drugs
(C) Increased volume of distribution
(D) Increased drug elimination
(E) Altered drug kinetics

6. Which of the following is the term used to describe the elimination rate via metabolism catalyzed by alcohol dehydrogenase when the enzyme is saturated?

(A) Zero-order kinetics
(B) First-order elimination
(C) Clearance
(D) Biotransformation
(E) Redistribution

7. A 69-year-old woman is being treated in the intensive care unit for presumed staphylococcal sepsis. To avoid problems with possible resistance, she is empirically given IV vancomycin while waiting for the culture results to come back. Vancomycin is a renally excreted drug. The patient's routine laboratory work-up reveals a creatinine value of 3.2, indicating acute renal failure. What specific considerations will have to be made with regard to adjustments of the prescribed medication?

(A) She will have to be switched to an oral (per nasogastric tube) vancomycin preparation
(B) The patient will need to be water restricted to decrease the volume of distribution
(C) No changes to the current regimen will be made because the condition of the patient is life-threatening and the drug needs to be administered regardless
(D) The dose of vancomycin will need to be reduced because of increased accumulation
(E) Dosage adjustments will have to be made because the patient is currently ventilated

8. Glucuronidation reactions

(A) Are considered phase I reactions
(B) Require an active center as the site of conjugation
(C) Include the enzymatic activity of alcohol dehydrogenase
(D) Located in mitochondria are inducible by drugs
(E) Require nicotinamide adenine dinucleotide phosphate (NADPH) for the enzymatic reaction

9. A 38-year-old woman presents to her psychiatrist with a request to try a different antidepressant medication, since she doesn't feel her current medication is helping. She even felt so depressed that she started drinking heavily in the past couple of months. The doctor wants to try imipramine; however, since this drug is known to undergo an extensive first-pass effect, he orders a hepatic function panel before prescribing it, given the patient's recent history of alcohol use. What is the rationale for the doctor's decision?

(A) In the presence of hepatic dysfunction, drugs with a high first-pass metabolism reach high systemic concentrations
(B) The results of the hepatic function panel may reveal a particular susceptibility to the drug
(C) Bioavailability of imipramine is increased by the fraction of drug removed by the first pass
(D) The drug is more rapidly metabolized by the liver when hepatic aminotransferase levels are elevated
(E) Solubility of the drug is affected in the face of hepatic damage

10. A 43-year-old man who was recently fired from a well-paying job decides to commit suicide and ingests a jarful of his antiseizure medication, phenobarbital. His wife finds him at home sleeping, but notices that he has diminished breathing, low body temperature, and skin reddening. She brings him to the ER, where he is appropriately diagnosed with barbiturate overdose. The patient is given bicarbonate to alkalinize his urine. How does alkalinization of urine with bicarbonate help to overcome the toxic effects of phenobarbital in this situation?

(A) It increases glomerular filtration
(B) It decreases proximal tubular secretion
(C) It decreases distal tubular reabsorption
(D) It enhances drug metabolism
(E) It decreases untoward side effects

11. Erythromycin is prescribed "qid," or four times daily, because of its short half-life. The rationale for such a frequent dosing schedule is

(A) To achieve the steady-state plasma concentration of the drug
(B) To avoid the toxicity of the drug because of its low therapeutic index
(C) To aid more complete distribution of the drug
(D) To inhibit the first-pass metabolism of the drug
(E) To ensure that the drug concentration remains constant over time

12. A 13-year-old boy suffers two tonic-clonic seizures within 1 week. He is diagnosed with epilepsy, and phenytoin therapy is started. To achieve proper drug concentrations in plasma, the patient is first given a loading dose, followed by maintenance doses. The blood level of phenytoin is frequently monitored to adjust the maintenance dose as needed. What is the rationale behind such a regimen?

(A) If drug is administered at a maintenance dose rate, steady-state concentration will be reached after two half-lives
(B) A loading dose is administered to achieve the desired plasma concentration rapidly
(C) The maintenance dose rate usually does not equal the elimination rate, which is why the loading dose is required
(D) Loading dose of the drug does not depend on the volume of distribution, whereas the maintenance dose does
(E) The maintenance dose rate does not depend on clearance of the drug, whereas the loading dose does

13. A 78-year-old woman is started on digoxin for her congestive heart failure (CHF). Her initial dose is 0.25 mg. The C_0, obtained by extrapolation of the elimination phase, is determined to be 0.05 mg/L. What is the patient's apparent volume of distribution?

(A) 0.5 L
(B) 0.2 L
(C) 0.0125 L
(D) 1 L
(E) 5 L

14. A drug has a volume of distribution of 50 L and undergoes zero-order elimination at a rate of 2 mg/hour at plasma concentrations greater than 2 mg/L. If a patient is brought to the ER with a plasma concentration of 4 mg/L of the drug, how long will it take (in hours) for the plasma concentration to decrease 50%?

(A) 1
(B) 2
(C) 10
(D) 25
(E) 50

15. You administer a 100 mg tablet of drug X to a patient every 24 hours and achieve an average steady-state plasma concentration of the drug of 10 mg/L. If you change the dose regimen to one 50 mg tablet every 12 hours, what will be the resulting average plasma concentration (in mg/L) of the drug after five half-lives?

(A) 2.5
(B) 5
(C) 10
(D) 20
(E) 40

16. Following IV administration, the initial rates of drug distribution to different tissues depend primarily on which of the following parameters?

(A) Blood flow to the tissues
(B) Fat content of the tissues
(C) Degree of ionization of the drug in the tissues
(D) Active transport of the drug out of different cell types
(E) Specific organ clearances

17. A drug is administered in the form of an inactive pro-drug. The pro-drug increases the expression of a cytochrome P-450 that converts the pro-drug to its active form. With chronic, long-term administration of the pro-drug, which of the following will be observed?

(A) The potency will decrease
(B) The potency will increase
(C) The efficacy will decrease
(D) The efficacy will increase

18. Which subfamily of cytochrome P-450s is responsible for the highest fraction of clinically important drug interactions resulting from metabolism?

(A) CYP1A
(B) CYP2A
(C) CYP3A
(D) CYP4A
(E) CYP5A

19. In most patients, an antibiotic is eliminated 25% by hepatic metabolism, 50% by renal filtration, and 25% by biliary excretion. If the normal maintenance dose rate = 10 mg/hour, what dose rate will you administer to a patient 12 normal with a creatinine clearance that is (assume that hepatic and biliary clearances are normal)?

(A) 2.5 mg/hour
(B) 5.0 mg/hour
(C) 6.0 mg/hour
(D) 7.5 mg/hour
(E) 20 mg/hour

20. If the oral dosing rate of a drug is held constant, what will be the effect of increasing the bioavailability of the preparation?

(A) Increase the half-life for first-order elimination
(B) Decrease the first-order elimination rate constant
(C) Increase the steady-state plasma concentration
(D) Decrease the total body clearance
(E) Increase the volume of distribution

21. You administer to a patient an oral maintenance dose of drug calculated to achieve a steady-state plasma concentration of 5 mcg/L. After dosing the patient for a time sufficient to reach steady state, the average plasma concentration of drug is 10 mcg/L. A decrease in which of the following parameters explains this higher than anticipated plasma drug concentration?

(A) Bioavailability
(B) Volume of distribution
(C) Clearance
(D) Half-life

22. Administration of an IV loading dose to a patient of drug X yields an initial plasma concentration of 100 mcg/L. The table below illustrates the plasma concentration of X as a function of time after the initial loading dose.

Time (hours)	Plasma Conc. (mcg/L)
0	100
1	50
5	25
9	12.5

What is the half-life (in hours) of drug X?

(A) 1
(B) 2
(C) 4
(D) 5
(E) 9

23. Which of the following factors will determine the number of drug–receptor complexes formed?

(A) Efficacy of the drug
(B) Receptor affinity for the drug
(C) Therapeutic index of the drug
(D) Half-life of the drug
(E) Rate of renal secretion

24. Which of the following is an action of a noncompetitive antagonist?

(A) Alters the mechanism of action of an agonist
(B) Alters the potency of an agonist
(C) Shifts the dose–response curve of an agonist to the right
(D) Decreases the maximum response to an agonist
(E) Binds to the same site on the receptor as the agonist

25. The renal clearance of a drug is 10 mL/min. The drug has a molecular weight of 350 and is 20% bound to plasma proteins. It is most likely that renal excretion of this drug involves

(A) Glomerular filtration
(B) Active tubular secretion
(C) Passive tubular reabsorption
(D) Both glomerular filtration and active tubular secretion
(E) Both glomerular filtration and passive tubular reabsorption

Answers and Explanations

1. **The answer is A.** Somatostatin binds to G_i-coupled protein receptor, initiating exchange of GTP for GDP, which inhibits adenylyl cyclase and leads to reduced cAMP production. G_q-protein-coupled receptor is an example of the phospholipase C pathway, in which interaction with the ligand leads to increased phospholipase C activity and eventual activation of protein kinase C via PIP_2 and IP_3 pathway. This is exemplified by interaction of epinephrine with its receptor. Ligand-activated ion channel is an example of interaction of specific ligand with an ion channel, which permits passage of ions through the channel. Acetylcholine is an example of such interaction. Receptor-activated tyrosine kinase is exemplified by insulin, where binding of ligand activates specific tyrosine kinase, leading to a cascade of reactions within the cell. Finally, intracellular nuclear receptor is exemplified by cortisol, which binds to it and exerts its effects on DNA replication.

2. **The answer is C.** The ability to target intracellular receptors depends on the ligand's ability to cross lipid barriers, such as the nuclear envelope. Recruitment of intracellular kinases is characterized by some receptor-activated tyrosine kinases. Autophosphorylation is a feature of many different kinases. Interaction with G-proteins and adenylyl cyclase are characteristics of membrane receptors.

3. **The answer is C.** Lithium is an example of drug with a very low therapeutic index, which requires frequent monitoring of the plasma level to achieve the balance between the desired effect and untoward toxicity. Potency of the drug is the amount of drug needed to produce a given response. Intrinsic activity of the drug is the ability to elicit a response. Efficacy of the drug is the maximal drug effect that can be achieved in a patient under a given set of conditions. Bioavailability of the drug is the fraction of the drug that reaches the bloodstream unaltered.

4. **The answer is B.** Adequate passage of drug through the small intestine is required to observe the effects of the drug, because most of the absorption takes place in the small intestine. After extensive abdominal surgery, especially that involving a resection of a portion of small bowel, the passage may be slowed, or even stopped, for a period of time. Abdominal surgery rarely results in reduced blood flow to the intestine, nor does such an operation influence protein binding, or the first-pass effect. Destruction of drug by stomach acid does not depend on intra-abdominal surgery.

5. **The answer is C.** Because of the patient's edema and ascites, the apparent volume of distribution will be increased, which may require small adjustments in his usual medication doses. Edematous states do not influence GI blood flow, nor do they affect drug–protein interactions. Drug elimination may be slowed with congestive heart failure (CHF) exacerbation, not increased. Drug kinetics are generally not changed by edematous states.

6. **The answer is A.** Alcohol is one of the drugs that follow zero-order kinetics (i.e., higher drug concentrations are not metabolized because the enzyme that is involved in the process is saturable). In first-order elimination, the rate of elimination actually depends on the concentration of the drug, multiplied by proportionality constant. Clearance is a measure of the capacity of the body to remove the drug. Biotransformation simply refers to the general mechanism of a particular drug's elimination. Redistribution is one of the possible fates of a drug, which usually terminates drug action.

7. **The answer is D.** Since vancomycin is cleared by the kidneys, renal functional status needs to be considered when prescribing such a drug, because it may accumulate and produce undesirable toxic side effects. Switching from the vancomycin to an oral preparation will reduce its bioavailability. There is no indication that the patient is in the state of increased volume of distribution (such as edema), and water restriction will not have a noticeable effect on apparent volume of

distribution. Changes to the current regimen are necessary because of the patient's acute renal failure, and this has to be done regardless of the urgency of the situation. The fact that the patient is being ventilated may indicate that she needs extra hydration because of increased insensible losses, but this has nothing to do with her vancomycin dose directly.

8. **The answer is B.** Glucuronidation reactions, which are considered phase II reactions, require an active center (a functional group) as the site of conjugation. Phase I reactions are biotransformation reactions, not conjugation reactions. Alcohol dehydrogenase is an example of a phase I reaction. Phase II reactions' enzymes are located in the endoplasmic reticulum, not mitochondria. Nicotinamide adenine dinucleotide phosphate (NADPH) is required for aromatic hydroxylation, an example of a phase I reaction.

9. **The answer is A.** First-pass metabolism simply means passage through the portal circulation before reaching the systemic circulation. In the face of liver dysfunction, drug levels may reach higher concentrations. A hepatic function panel is generally not used to deduce a patient's susceptibility to the drug. Bioavailability of drugs is decreased, not increased by the fraction removed after the first pass through the liver. Drugs are usually less rapidly metabolized when hepatic enzymes are elevated (which indicates hepatic dysfunction). Solubility of drugs has nothing to do with hepatic damage.

10. **The answer is C.** Alterations of urinary pH affect renal distal tubular reabsorption of drugs by changing the degree of ionization. Glomerular filtration depends mainly on the size of the drug as well as protein binding. Proximal tubular secretion will not be affected by alkalinization of urine. This process depends on the availability of transporters. Drug metabolism is not affected at the levels of the kidney, where most elimination takes place. Alkalinization of urine is unlikely to affect undesirable side effects of the drug.

11. **The answer is A.** Dosing schedules of drugs are adjusted according to their half-lives to achieve steady-state plasma concentration. Attempting to avoid the toxicity of the drug because of its low therapeutic index represents an unlikely scenario, since to reduce toxicity of a drug with a low therapeutic index, one would reduce the dosing schedule, not increase it. Distribution of drug is generally not affected by dosing schedule. Nor is dose scheduling affected by first-pass metabolism. Some fluctuation in plasma concentration occurs even at steady state; it is the average concentration over time that is the goal of steady state.

12. **The answer is B.** The rationale for the loading dose is to give a patient a sufficient dose of a medication to achieve the desired effect quickly, which is necessary in some situation (such as prevention of further seizures). When drug is administered at maintenance rate, steady state is achieved after about five half-lives. The maintenance dose is usually equal to the elimination rate.The loading dose depends on the volume of distribution, whereas the maintenance dose depends on the clearance of the drug.

13. **The answer is E.** To calculate the volume of distribution, use the formula in which the dose of the drug is divided by the plasma concentration. In this case, 0.25 mg is divided by 0.05 mg/L, giving the result of 5 L for volume of distribution.

14. **The answer is E.** For the plasma concentration of drug to decrease by 50%, half the drug present in the body initially must be eliminated. The amount of drug in the body initially is the volume of distribution × the plasma concentration (50 liters × 4 mg/liter = 200 mg). When the plasma concentration falls to 2 mg/liter, the body will contain 100 mg of drug (50 L × 2 mg/L = 100 mg). Since the body eliminates the drug at a rate of 2 mg/hour, it will require 50 hours for 100 mg of the drug to be eliminated.

15. **The answer is C.** A 100 mg tablet every 24 hours is a dose rate of 4.17 mg/hour (100/24 = 4.17), which is the same dose rate as one 50 mg tablet every 12 hours (50/12 = 4.17). Thus, the average plasma concentration will remain the same, but *decreasing both* the dose and the dose interval will decrease the peak to trough variation of plasma concentration.

16. **The answer is A.** The *initial rate* of distribution of a drug to a tissue depends primarily on the rate of blood flow to that tissue. At longer times, however, a drug may undergo redistribution

among various tissues, e.g., a very lipophilic drug may become concentrated in adipose tissue with time.

17. The answer is B. The induction of the cytochrome P-450 following chronic administration will increase the conversion of the inactive pro-drug to the active form. This will shift the dose–response curve of the pro-drug to the left (i.e., increase its potency) without changing its efficacy.

18. The answer is C. The CYP3A subfamily is responsible for roughly 50% of the total cytochrome P450 activity present in the liver and is estimated to be responsible for approximately 12 of all clinically important untoward drug interactions resulting from metabolism.

19. The answer is D. Maintenance dose rate = (clearance) × (desired plasma concentration), and the whole body clearance is the sum of all the individual organ clearances. In most patients the hepatic metabolism, renal filtration, and biliary excretion account for 25%, 50%, and 25% of the whole body clearance, respectively. Since the creatinine clearance in this patient indicates that the renal filtration is only half normal, the renal clearance of the drug will be decreased by 12. This means that the whole body clearance will be 75% of that of normal (25% hepatic, 25% renal, and 25% biliary). Therefore, the dose should also be 75% of the standard dose.

20. The answer is C. If the oral dosing rate is constant but bioavailability increases, the fraction of the administered dose that reaches the general circulation unaltered increases. This, in turn, will increase the steady-state plasma concentration.

21. The answer is C. Steady-state plasma concentration of drug = (dose rate)/(clearance). Thus, a decrease in clearance will increase the plasma drug concentration, whereas an increase in any of the other three parameters will *decrease* the steady state plasma concentration.

22. The answer is C. Inspection of the plasma concentration values indicates that the half-life of drug does not become constant until 1–9 hours after administration. The drug concentration decreases by 12 (from 50 to 25 mcg/L) between 1 and 5 hours (a 4-hour interval) and again decreases by 12 (from 25 to 12.5 mcg/L) between 5 and 9 hours (again, a 4-hour interval). This indicates the half-life of the drug is 4 hours. The rapid decrease in plasma concentration between 0 and 1 hour, followed by a slower decrease thereafter (and the constant half-life thereafter) indicates that this drug obeys a two-compartment model with an initial distribution phase followed by an elimination phase. The half-life is always determined from the elimination phase data.

23. The answer is B. Receptor affinity for the drug will determine the number of drug–receptor complexes formed. Efficacy is the ability of the drug to activate the receptor after binding has occurred. Therapeutic index (TI) is related to safety of the drug. Half-life and secretion are properties of elimination and do not influence formation of drug–receptor complexes.

24. The answer is D. A noncompetitive antagonist decreases the magnitude of the response to an agonist but does not alter the agonist's potency (i.e., the ED_{50} remains unchanged). A competitive antagonist interacts at the agonist binding site.

25. The answer is E. This drug will undergo filtration and passive reabsorption. Because the molecular weight of the drug is small, free drug will be filtered. Because 20% of the drug is bound to plasma proteins, 80% of it is free and available for filtration, which would be at a rate of 100 mL/min (i.e., 0.8 × 125 mL/min; 125 mL/min is the normal glomerular filtration rate [GFR]). A clearance of 10 mL/min must indicate that most of the filtered drug is reabsorbed.

chapter 2

Drugs Acting on the Autonomic Nervous System

I. THE PERIPHERAL EFFERENT NERVOUS SYSTEM

A. The autonomic nervous system (ANS) controls **involuntary activity** (Fig. 2-1, Table 2-1).

1. ***Parasympathetic nervous system (PNS)***
   - **a.** Long preganglionic axons originate from neurons in the cranial and sacral areas of the spinal cord and, with few exceptions, synapse on neurons in ganglia located close to or within the innervated organ.
   - **b.** Short postganglionic axons innervate cardiac muscle, bronchial smooth muscle, and exocrine glands.
   - **c.** Parasympathetic innervation predominates over sympathetic innervation of salivary glands, lacrimal glands, and erectile tissue.
2. ***Sympathetic nervous system (SNS)***
   - **a.** Short preganglionic axons originate from neurons in the thoracic and lumbar areas of the spinal cord and synapse on neurons in ganglia located outside of, but close to, the spinal cord. The adrenal medulla, anatomically considered a modified ganglion, is innervated by sympathetic preganglionic axons.
   - **b.** Long postganglionic axons innervate many of the same tissues and organs as the PNS.
   - **c.** Innervation of **thermoregulatory sweat glands** is anatomically sympathetic, but the postganglionic nerve fibers are cholinergic and release acetylcholine as the neurotransmitter
3. ***Enteric nervous system (ENS)***
   - **a.** Considered a third branch of the ANS
   - **b.** Highly organized, semiautonomous, neural complex localized in the **GI system**
   - **c.** Receives preganglionic axons from the PNS and postganglionic axons from the SNS
   - **d.** Nerve terminals contain peptides and purines as neurotransmitters.

B. The somatic nervous system (Fig. 2-1) controls **voluntary activity.** This system contains long axons that originate in the spinal cord and directly innervate skeletal striated muscle.

C. Neurotransmitters of the autonomic and somatic nervous systems (Fig. 2-1)

1. ***Acetylcholine (ACh)***
   - **a.** ACh is released by exocytosis from nerve terminals.
   - **b.** ACh is the neurotransmitter across synapses at the ganglia of the SNS and PNS and across synapses in tissues innervated by the PNS and the somatic nervous system.
   - **c.** ACh is synthesized in nerve terminals by the cytoplasmic enzyme choline acetyltransferase (ChAT), which catalyzes the transfer of an acetate group from acetyl coenzyme A (acetyl CoA) to choline that has been transported into "cholinergic" neurons by a sodium-dependent membrane carrier. Synthesized ACh is transported from cytoplasm to vesicle-associated transporters (VAT).
   - **d.** ACh is stored in nerve terminal vesicles that, through calcium-dependent exocytosis, are released by nerve action potentials. On release, a step blocked by **botulinum toxin**, ACh is

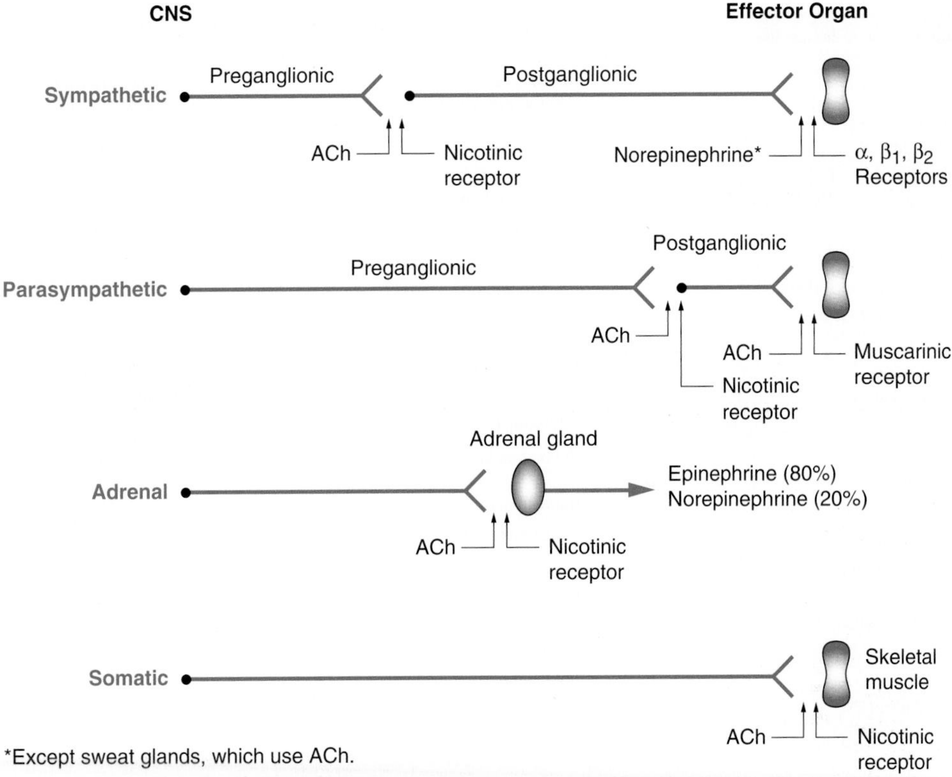

FIGURE 2-1. Organization of the autonomic nervous system.

rapidly hydrolyzed and inactivated by tissue acetylcholinesterase (AChE) and also by nonspecific butyrylcholinesterase (pseudocholinesterase) to choline and acetate.

e. ACh is not administered parenterally for therapeutic purposes because it is hydrolyzed nearly instantly by butyrylcholinesterase.

2. *Norepinephrine and epinephrine* are **catecholamines,** possessing a catechol nucleus and an ethylamine side chain.

a. Storage and release

(1) Norepinephrine is stored in vesicles that, through a calcium-dependent process, release their contents by exocytosis from nerve terminals at postganglionic nerve endings of the SNS (except at thermoregulatory sweat glands, where ACh is the neurotransmitter).

(2) Norepinephrine release can be blocked by such drugs as **bretylium** and **guanethidine.**

(3) Norepinephrine also exists in a nonvesicular cytoplasmic pool that is released by indirectly acting sympathomimetic amines (e.g., **tyramine**, **amphetamine**, **ephedrine**) by a process that is not calcium dependent.

(4) Norepinephrine and some epinephrine are released from adrenergic nerve endings in the brain. In the periphery, epinephrine, along with some norepinephrine, is the major catecholamine released from adrenal medullary chromaffin cells into the general circulation, where they function as hormones.

b. Biosynthesis of catecholamines (Fig. 2-2)

(1) In prejunctional nerve endings, tyrosine is hydroxylated by tyrosine hydroxylase, the rate-limiting enzyme in the synthesis of catecholamines, to form dihydroxyphenylalanine (dopa); dopa is then decarboxylated by dopa decarboxylase to form dopamine.

(2) Dopamine is transported into vesicles, a step blocked by **reserpine**, where it is hydroxylated on the side chain by dopamine β-hydroxylase to form norepinephrine.

(3) In certain areas of the brain and in the adrenal medulla, norepinephrine is methylated on the amine group of the side chain by phenylethanolamine-*N*-methyltransferase (PNMT) to form epinephrine.

table 2-1 Actions of the Autonomic Nervous System on Selected Effector Organs

Effector	Action of Sympathetic (Thoracolumbar) Division	Action of Parasympathetic (Craniosacral) Division
Eye (pupil)	Dilation (ex)	Constriction (ex)
Heart		
Rate	Acceleration (ex)	Slowing (in)
Contractility	Increased (ex)	Decreased (in)
Arterioles		
Skin and most others	Constriction (ex)	—
Skeletal muscle	Dilation (ex)	—
Glands		
Salivary	Viscid secretion (ex)	Watery secretion (ex)
Lacrimal	—	Secretion (ex)
Sweat	Secretion (ex)	—
Bronchial muscle	Relaxation (in)	Contraction (ex)
GI tract		
Muscle wall	Relaxation (in)	Contraction (ex)
Sphincters	Contraction (ex)	Relaxation (in)
Urinary bladder		
Fundus	Relaxation (in)	Contraction (ex)
Trigone; sphincter	Contraction (ex)	Relaxation (in)
Penis	Ejaculation (ex)	Erection (in)
Uterus	Relaxation (in)	—
Metabolism		
Liver	Gluconeogenesis (ex)	—
	Glycogenolysis (ex)	—
Kidney	Renin secretion(ex)	—
Fat Cells	Lipolysis (ex)	

ex, excitatory; in, inhibitory; —, no functionally important innervation.

c. **Termination**

(1) The action of **norepinephrine** is terminated primarily by **active transport** from the cytoplasm into the nerve terminal (**uptake 1**), a process that is inhibited by **cocaine** and tricyclic antidepressant agents such as **imipramine. Norepinephrine** is then transported by a second carrier system into storage vesicles, as is **dopamine** and **serotonin**, a process also blocked by **reserpine**.

(2) Another active transport system (**uptake 2**) is located on glia and smooth muscle cells.

(3) There is also some simple **diffusion** away from the synapse.

(4) **Norepinephrine** and **epinephrine** also are oxidatively deaminated by **mitochondrial monoamine oxidase (MAO)** in nerve terminals and effector cells, notably in the liver and intestine. **Isoforms** of MAO (A and B) have been identified. Dopamine is metabolized primarily by MAO-B.

(5) Nerve cells and effector cells contain **catechol-*O*-methyltransferase (COMT)**, which metabolizes catecholamines. Metabolites, including **3-methoxy-4-hydroxymandelic acid (VMA)**, provide a measure of catecholamine turnover in the body.

D. Receptors of the nervous system

1. *Cholinoceptors*

a. **Nicotinic receptors:** Cholinoceptors that are activated by the alkaloid nicotine (Fig. 2-1)

(1) Nicotinic receptors are localized at myoneural junctions of somatic nerves and skeletal muscle (N_M), autonomic ganglia (N_G), including the adrenal medulla, and certain areas in the brain.

(2) Nicotinic receptors consist of a pentamer of **four protein subunits** in skeletal muscle (e.g., α (2), β, γ, δ) and two protein subunits in neurons (α and β) that form **ligand-gated** (i.e., regulated) ion channel pores in the cell membranes (see Fig. 1-1A).

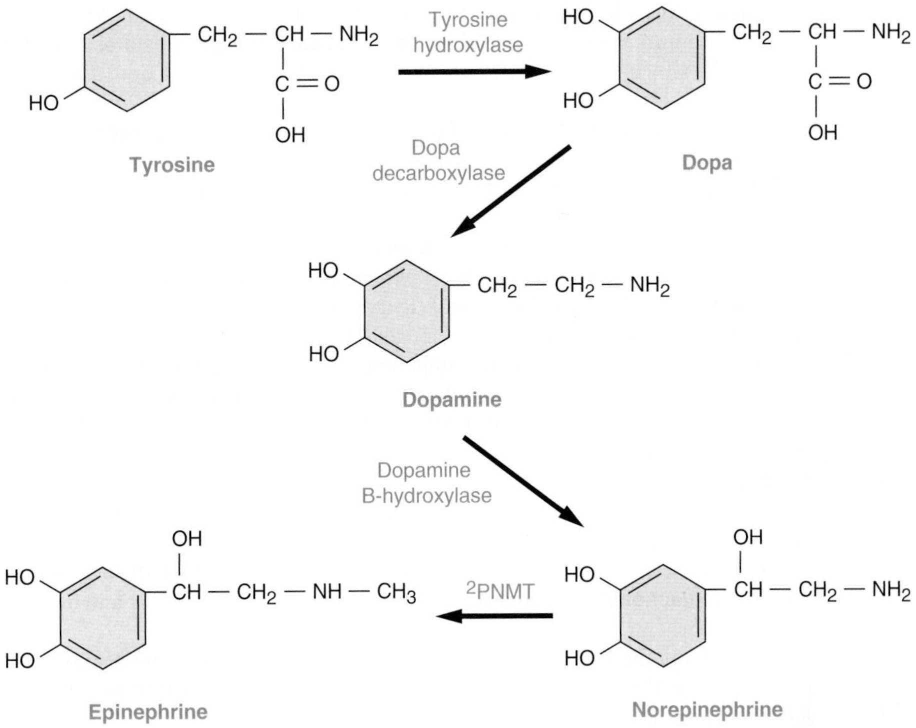

FIGURE 2-2. Biosynthesis of catecholamines.

(3) In skeletal muscle, **ACh interacts with nicotinic receptors** (one molecule of ACh per α subunit) **to open channels that permit passage of ions, mostly Na^+.** The Na^+ current produces membrane depolarization and a propagated action potential through the transverse tubules of skeletal muscle, resulting in the release of Ca^{2+} from the sarcoplasmic reticulum and, through a further series of chemical and mechanical events, **muscle contraction.** Hydrolysis of ACh by AChE results in muscle cell repolarization.

(a) The continued presence of a nicotine agonist, like **succinylcholine**, at nicotinic receptors, or excessive cholinergic stimulation, can lead to a "**depolarizing blockade"** (phase I block), in which normal depolarization is followed by persistent depolarization. During phase I block, skeletal muscle is unresponsive to either neuronal stimulation or direct stimulation.

(b) The selective nicotinic receptor antagonists **tubocurarine** and **trimethaphan** can block the effect of ACh at skeletal muscle and autonomic ganglia, respectively.

b. Muscarinic receptors: Cholinoceptors that are activated by the alkaloid muscarine (Fig. 2-1)

(1) Muscarinic receptors are localized on numerous autonomic effector cells, including cardiac atrial muscle and cells of the sinoatrial (SA) and atrioventricular (AV) nodes, smooth muscle, exocrine glands, and vascular endothelium (mostly arterioles), although the latter does not receive parasympathetic innervation, as well as certain areas in the brain.

(2) Muscarinic receptors consist of at least three **functional receptor subtypes (M_1–M_3).** Muscarinic M_1-receptors are found in sympathetic postganglionic neurons and in CNS neurons; M_2-receptors are found in cardiac and smooth muscle; and M_3-receptors are found in glandular cells (e.g., gastric parietal cells), and the vascular endothelium and vascular smooth muscle. M_2- and M_3-receptors predominate in the urinary bladder. All three subtypes are found in the CNS.

(3) ACh interacts with **M_1 and M_3 muscarinic cholinoceptors** to increase **phosphatidylinositol (PI) turnover** and **Ca^{2+} mobilization** (see Fig. 1-1D).

(a) By activation of **G protein** (G_q), the interaction of ACh with M_1 and M_3 muscarinic cholinoceptors stimulates **polyphosphatidylinositol phosphodiesterase (phospholipase C),** which hydrolyzes PI to **inositol trisphosphate (IP_3)** and **diacylglycerol (DAG).**

(b) **IP_3 mobilizes intracellular Ca^{2+}** from the endoplasmic and sarcoplasmic reticula, and activates Ca^{2+}-regulated enzymes and cell processes.

(c) **Diacylglycerol activates protein kinase C,** which results in phosphorylation of cellular enzymes and other protein substrates and the **influx of extracellular calcium** that results in activation of contractile elements in smooth muscle.

(4) ACh also interacts with **M_2 muscarinic cholinoceptors** to **activate G proteins (G_1),** which leads to **inhibition of adenylyl cyclase** activity with decreased levels of cyclic AMP and to **increased K^+ conductance** with effector cell hyperpolarization.

(5) Cholinergic agonists act on **M_3 muscarinic receptors** of **endothelial cells** to promote the release of **nitric oxide (NO),** which diffuses to the **vascular smooth muscle** to activate guanylyl cyclase and increase cyclic GMP (cGMP) and to produce **relaxation.**

2. ***Adrenoceptors*** (Fig. 2-1)

a. **α-Adrenoceptors**

(1) α-Adrenoceptors are classified into two major receptor subgroups (there are subtypes of each group). **α_1-Receptors** are located in **postjunctional** effector cells, notably vascular smooth muscle, where responses are mainly excitatory; **α_2-receptors** are located primarily in **prejunctional** adrenergic nerve terminals, and also in fat cells and in beta cells of the pancreas.

(2) α-Adrenoceptors mediate vasoconstriction (α_1), GI relaxation (α_1), mydriasis (α_1), prejunctional inhibition of release of norepinephrine and other neurotransmitters (α_2), inhibition of insulin release (α_2), and inhibition of lipolysis (α_2).

(3) α-Adrenoceptors are distinguished from β-adrenoceptors by their interaction (in descending order of potency), with the adrenergic agonists **epinephrine = norepinephrine ≫ isoproterenol,** and by their interaction with relatively selective antagonists such as **phentolamine.**

(4) **α_1-Receptors,** like muscarinic M_1 and M_3 cholinoceptors, **activate guanine nucleotide-binding proteins (Gq)** in many cells, which results in activation of **phospholipase C** and stimulation of phosphoinositide (PI) hydrolysis that leads to increased formation of **inositol trisphosphate (IP_3)** and mobilization of intracellular stores of Ca^{2+} and to increased **diacylglycerol (DAG)** and activation of protein kinase C.

(5) **α_2-Receptors,** like muscarinic M_2-cholinoceptors, **activate inhibitory guanine nucleotide-binding proteins (G_i), inhibit adenylyl cyclase** activity, and decrease intracellular cyclic AMP (cAMP) levels and the activity of cAMP-dependent protein kinases (see Fig. 1-1C).

b. **β-Adrenoceptors** (Fig. 2-1)

(1) β-Adrenoceptors, located mostly in postjunctional effector cells, are classified into two major receptor subtypes, β_1-receptors (primarily excitatory) and β_2-receptors (primarily inhibitory).

(a) **β_1-Receptor subtype**

(i) β_1-Receptors mediate increased contractility and conduction velocity, and renin secretion in the kidney (β_3-receptors mediate activation of fat cell lipolysis).

(ii) The β_1-receptor subtype is defined by its interaction (in descending order of potency) with the adrenergic agonists **isoproterenol > epinephrine = norepinephrine** and by its interaction with relatively selective antagonists such as **atenolol.**

(b) **β_2-Receptor subtype**

(i) β_2-Receptors mediate vasodilation and intestinal, bronchial, and uterine smooth muscle relaxation.

(ii) The β_2-receptor subtype is defined by its interaction (in descending order of potency) with the adrenergic agonists **isoproterenol = epinephrine ≫ norepinephrine.**

(2) **β-Receptor activation**

(a) β-Receptors activate **guanine nucleotide-binding proteins** (G_s; see Fig. 1-1B).

(b) Activation **stimulates adenylate cyclase** activity and increases intracellular cAMP levels and the activity of cAMP-dependent protein kinases. Adrenoceptor-mediated changes in the activity of protein kinases (and also levels of intracellular Ca^{2+}) bring about changes in the activity of specific enzymes and structural and regulatory proteins, resulting in modification of cell and organ activity.

II. PARASYMPATHOMIMETIC DRUGS

A. Direct-acting muscarinic cholinoceptor agonists

1. *Action and chemical structure*

a. Direct-acting parasympathomimetic drugs act at muscarinic cholinoceptors to mimic many of the physiologic effects that result from stimulation of the parasympathetic division of the autonomic nervous system (see Fig. 2-1).

b. **Bethanechol** (Urecholine) and **carbachol** are choline esters with a quaternary ammonium group that are structurally similar to acetylcholine but more resistant to hydrolysis by acetylcholinesterase. The β-methyl group of bethanechol substantially reduces its activity at nicotinic receptors.

c. **Pilocarpine** is a tertiary amine alkaloid.

2. *Pharmacologic effects* (Tables 2-2 and 2-3)

a. Eye

(1) Direct-acting muscarinic cholinoceptor agonists contract the circular smooth muscle fibers of the ciliary muscle and iris to produce, respectively, a spasm of accommodation and an increased outflow of aqueous humor into the canal of Schlemm, resulting in a **reduction in intraocular pressure.**

(2) These drugs contract the smooth muscle of the iris sphincter to cause **miosis.**

b. Cardiovascular system

(1) Direct-acting muscarinic cholinoceptor agonists produce a **negative chronotropic effect** (reduced SA node activity).

(2) These drugs **decrease conduction velocity** through the AV node.

(3) These drugs have no effect on force of contraction because there are no muscarinic receptors on, or parasympathetic innervation of, ventricles.

(4) Direct-acting muscarinic cholinoceptor agonists produce **vasodilation** that results primarily from their action on endothelial cells to promote the release of **nitric oxide (NO),** which diffuses to the vascular smooth muscle and produces relaxation. Vascular smooth muscle has muscarinic receptors but no parasympathetic innervation. The resulting

table 2-2 Actions of Direct-Acting Cholinoceptor Agonists

Effector	Effects of Muscarinic Agonists
Heart (rate, conduction velocity)[a]	Decrease
Arterioles (tone)	Decrease
Blood pressure	Decrease
Pupil size	Decrease
Salivation	Increase
Lacrimation	Increase
Bronchial tone	Increase
Intestine (motility)	Increase
GI secretions	Increase
Urinary bladder	
Body (tone)	Increase
Sphincter	Decrease

[a]Responses (e.g., heart rate) may be affected by reflexes.

table 2-3 Effects of Muscarinic Cholinoceptor and Adrenoceptor Agonists on Smooth Muscles of the Eye

Type of Drug	Muscle	Effect	Result
Muscarinic agonist	Iris circular (constrictor)	Contraction	Miosis
	Ciliary circular	Contraction	Accommodation
Muscarinic antagonist	Iris circular (constrictor)	Relaxation	Mydriasis
	Ciliary circular	Relaxation	Cycloplegia
α-Adrenergic agonist	Iris radial (dilator)	Contraction	Mydriasis
	Ciliary circular	None	None

decrease in blood pressure can result in a reflex increase in heart rate. (Intravenous infusion of low doses of ACh causes a reflex sympathetic-stimulated increase in heart rate; higher doses directly inhibit heart rate.)

c. **GI tract**
   (1) Direct-acting muscarinic cholinoceptor agonists increase smooth muscle contractions and tone, with increased **peristaltic activity and motility.**
   (2) These drugs increase salivation and acid secretion.

d. **Urinary tract**
   (1) Direct-acting muscarinic cholinoceptor agonists **increase contraction of the ureter and bladder smooth muscle.**
   (2) These drugs increase **sphincter relaxation.**

e. **Respiratory system** effects of direct-acting muscarinic cholinoceptor agonists include **bronchoconstriction** with increased resistance and increased bronchial secretions.

f. **Other effects**
   (1) These drugs increase the secretion of tears from lacrimal glands and increase sweat gland secretion.
   (2) These drugs produce tremor and ataxia.

3. ***Specific drugs and their therapeutic uses.*** These drugs are used primarily for diseases of the eye, GI tract, urinary tract, the neuromuscular junction, and the heart (Table 2-4).

   a. **Bethanechol** (Urecholine)
      (1) Bethanechol is used to stimulate smooth muscle motor activity of the urinary tract to **prevent urine retention.**
      (2) It is used occasionally to stimulate GI smooth muscle motor activity for **postoperative abdominal distention** and for **gastric atony** following bilateral vagotomy (in the absence of obstruction).
      (3) Bethanechol is administered PO or SC, not by IV or IM route, because parenteral administration may cause cardiac arrest.
      (4) This drug has low lipid solubility and is poorly absorbed from the GI tract. When given orally, GI effects predominate, and there are relatively minor cardiovascular effects.
      (5) Bethanechol has limited distribution to the CNS.
      (6) It is resistant to hydrolysis by AChE and plasma cholinesterase and thus has a longer duration of action than ACh (2–3 hours).

table 2-4 Selected Therapeutic Uses of Selected Direct-Acting Cholinoceptor Agonists

Agent	Conditions/Disorders
Bethanechol	Prevents urine retention; postoperative abdominal distension; gastric atony
Methacholine	Diagnostic for bronchial hypersensitivity
Pilocarpine	Open-angle glaucoma; acute narrow-angle glaucoma; Sjögren syndrome

b. **Methacholine** (Mecholyl) is occasionally used **to diagnose bronchial hypersensitivity.** Patients with no clinically apparent asthma are more sensitive to methacholine-induced bronchoconstriction than normal patients.

c. **Pilocarpine**

(1) Pilocarpine is occasionally used topically for **open-angle glaucoma,** either as eyedrops or as a sustained-release ocular insert (Ocusert). β-Adrenergic receptor antagonists such as **timolol** and **betaxolol** and prostaglandin analogues such as **latanoprost** are the drugs of choice to treat open-angle glaucoma. Other drug classes used include α-adrenergic receptor agonists such as **epinephrine** and diuretics such as **acetazolamide.**

(2) When used before surgery to treat **acute narrow-angle glaucoma** (a medical emergency), pilocarpine is often given in combination with an indirectly acting muscarinic agonist such as **physostigmine.**

(3) Pilocarpine and **cevimeline** (Evoxac), a newer muscarinic receptor agonist, increase salivary secretion. They are used to treat **Sjögren syndrome.**

(4) Pilocarpine is a tertiary amine that is well absorbed from the GI tract and enters the CNS.

d. **Carbachol** is rarely used except if pilocarpine is ineffective as a treatment for open-angle glaucoma.

e. **Cevimelene** (Evoxac) is used to treat **Sjögren syndrome**–associated dry mouth.

f. **Varenicline** (Chantix), a direct-acting nicotinic receptor agonist, is approved for use in smoking cessation (Chapter 5 X D 2).

4. ***Adverse effects and contraindications***

a. The **adverse effects** associated with direct-acting muscarinic cholinoceptor agonists are extensions of their pharmacologic activity. The most serious include **nausea, vomiting, sweating, salivation, bronchoconstriction, decreased blood pressure, and diarrhea,** all of which can be blocked or reversed by atropine. Systemic effects are minimal for drugs applied topically to the eye.

b. These drugs are contraindicated in the presence of **peptic ulcer** (because they increase acid secretion), **asthma, cardiac disease, and Parkinson disease.** They are not recommended in hyperthyroidism because they predispose to arrhythmia; they are also not recommended when there is mechanical obstruction of the GI or urinary tract.

B. Indirect-acting parasympathomimetic agents

1. ***Chemical structure***

a. **Edrophonium** is an alcohol with a quaternary ammonium group.

b. **Neostigmine** and **physostigmine** are examples of carbamic acid esters of alcohols (carbamates) with either quaternary or tertiary ammonium groups.

c. **Echothiophate** and **isoflurophate** are examples of organic derivatives of phosphoric acid.

2. ***Mechanism of action*** (Fig. 2-3A and B)

a. Indirect-acting parasympathomimetic agents **inhibit AChE** and **increase ACh levels** at both muscarinic and nicotinic cholinoceptors to mimic many of the physiologic effects that result from increased ACh in the synaptic junction and stimulation of cholinoceptors of the parasympathetic division of the ANS.

b. **ACh interacts with AChE at two sites:** The N^+ of choline (ionic bond) binds to the **anionic site,** and the acetyl ester binds to the **esteratic site** (serine residue). As ACh is hydrolyzed, the serine-OH side chain is acetylated and free choline is released. Acetyl-serine is hydrolyzed to serine and acetate. The half-life ($t_{1/2}$) of acetylserine hydrolysis is 100–150 microseconds.

c. **Edrophonium** (Tensilon) acts at the same sites of AChE to competitively inhibit ACh hydrolysis by the following processes:

(1) N^+ of edrophonium binds the anionic site.

(2) Phenolic hydroxyl of edrophonium interacts with histidine imidazolium N^+ of the esteratic site.

(3) Edrophonium has a short duration of action (5–15 min).

d. **Neostigmine** (Prostigmin), **physostigmine** (Eserine, Antilirium), and **demecarium** (Humorsol), like ACh, interact with AChE and undergo a two-step hydrolysis. However, the serine

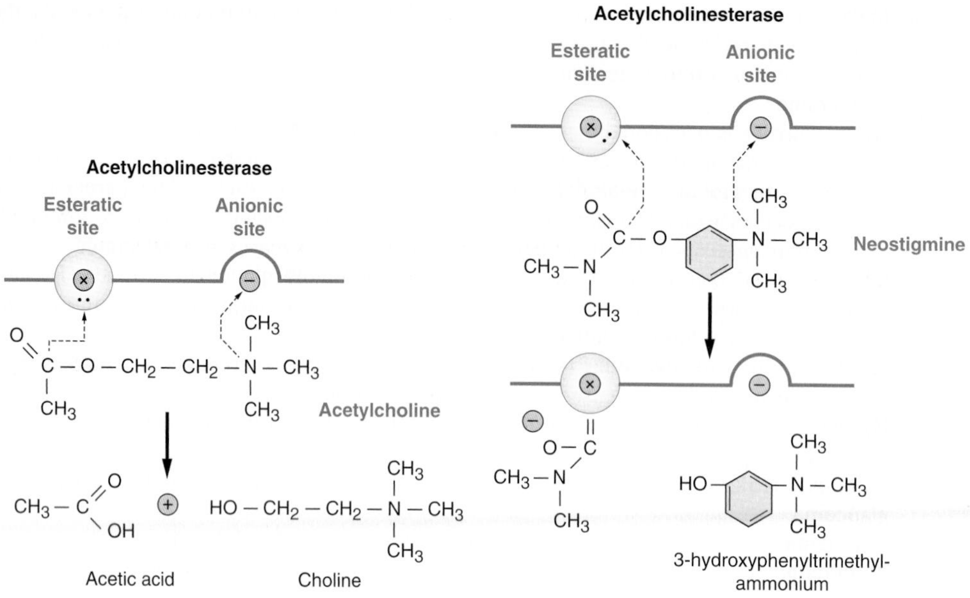

FIGURE 2-3. **A.** Hydrolysis of acetylcholine by acetylcholinesterase. **B.** Interaction of neostigmine with acetylcholinesterase.

residue of the enzyme is covalently carbamylated rather than acetylated. Hydrolysis of the carbamylserine residue is much slower than that of acetylserine (30 min–6 h).

(1) Neostigmine, physostigmine, and demecarium also have direct agonist action at skeletal muscle nicotinic cholinoceptors.

(2) These drugs differ in absorption as follows:

(a) Because of its quaternary ammonium structure, **neostigmine** is **poorly absorbed** from the GI tract and has negligible distribution into the CNS.

(b) **Physostigmine** is **well absorbed** after oral administration, and it enters the CNS.

e. **Echothiophate** (Phospholine) and **isoflurophate** (Floropryl), irreversible and toxic organophosphate cholinesterase inhibitors, result in **phosphorylation of AChE** rather than acetylation. With time, the strength of the bond increases ("aging"), and AChE becomes irreversibly inhibited. The enzyme can be reactivated within the first 30 minutes by **pralidoxime.** Hydrolysis of the covalent alkylphosphoryl–serine bond takes days.

(1) **Echothiophate** is poorly absorbed from the GI tract and has negligible distribution into the CNS.

(2) **Isoflurophate** is highly lipid soluble and is well absorbed across all membranes, including skin.

f. **Pralidoxime** (Protopam)

(1) Pralidoxime is an **AChE reactivator** that must be administered IV within minutes of exposure to an AChE inhibitor because it is effective only prior to "aging."

(2) Pralidoxime acts as an **antidote for organophosphorus insecticide and nerve gas poisoning.** It binds the anionic site and undergoes a nucleophilic reaction with P=O group of alkylphosphorylated serine to cause hydrolysis of the phosphoserine bond that is at least 10^6 times faster than that occurring in water.

(3) This drug is most effective at the neuromuscular junction. It is ineffective in the CNS and against carbamylated AChE.

(4) Pralidoxime produces few adverse effects in normal doses.

3. ***Pharmacologic effects*** (Table 2-2)

a. With the major exception of arteriole tone and blood pressure, where their effects are less pronounced, the pharmacologic effects of indirect-acting parasympathomimetic agents are similar to those of direct-acting muscarinic cholinoceptor agonists.

b. By increasing ACh at the neuromuscular junction, these drugs increase the contraction strength of skeletal muscle. The effect is more pronounced if muscle contraction is already weak, as occurs in **myasthenia gravis.**

4. *Therapeutic uses*

a. Glaucoma

(1) Physostigmine is often used concurrently with **pilocarpine** for maximum effect in the treatment of **acute angle-closure glaucoma,** a medical emergency.

(2) Physostigmine, demecarium, echothiophate, and other cholinesterase inhibitors have been largely replaced for the treatment of chronic **open-angle glaucoma** by topical β-adrenergic receptor antagonists such as **timolol** and **betaxolol,** and by prostaglandin analogues such as **latanoprost.** They are used when other drugs are ineffective. Prolonged use may increase the possibility of cataracts.

b. GI and urinary tract atony can be treated with **neostigmine,** which is used much like bethanechol.

c. Myasthenia gravis

(1) Myasthenia gravis is an **autoimmune disease** in which antibodies complex with nicotinic receptors at the neuromuscular junction to cause skeletal muscle weakness and fatigue. **Neostigmine,** or the related AChE inhibitors **pyridostigmine** (Mestinon, Regonol) or **ambenonium** (Mytelase), is used to increase ACh levels at the neuromuscular junction to activate fully the remaining receptors.

(2) Myasthenia gravis can be diagnosed using the **Tensilon test,** which can also assess the adequacy of treatment with AChE inhibitors. Small doses of **edrophonium** improve muscle strength in untreated patients with myasthenia or in treated patients in whom AChE inhibition is inadequate. If there is no effect, or if muscle weakness increases, the dose of the AChE inhibitor is too high (excessive ACh stimulation at the neuromuscular junction results in a depolarizing blockade).

(3) Atropine can be used to control excessive muscarinic stimulation by AChE inhibitors.

(4) Tolerance may develop to long-term use of the AChE inhibitors.

d. Alzheimer disease: Donepezil (Aricept), **galantamine** (Reminyl), **rivastigmine** (Exelon), and **tacrine** (Cognex) are AChE inhibitors used to ameliorate the cognitive deficit associated with Alzheimer disease (see Chapter 5 VI E).

e. Neostigmine or **edrophonium** can be used following surgery to **reverse neuromuscular blockade** and paralysis resulting from adjunct use of nondepolarizing agents.

f. Atropine and **scopolamine poisoning** can be treated with **physostigmine,** which reverses the central and (to some extent) the peripheral effects of competitive muscarinic antagonists.

5. *Adverse effects and toxicity*

a. The adverse effects associated with indirect-acting sympathomimetic agents are an extension of pharmacologic activity and arise from **excessive cholinergic stimulation.**

b. Adverse effects include muscarinic effects similar to those of direct-acting cholinergic drugs and nicotinic effects such as **muscle weakness, cramps and fasciculations, excessive bronchial secretions, convulsions, coma, cardiovascular collapse,** and **respiratory failure.**

c. Many lipid-soluble organophosphates are used as insecticides (e.g., malathion) or nerve gases (e.g., sarin) and may be absorbed in sufficient quantities from the skin or lungs to cause cholinergic intoxication. Treatment includes the following steps:

(1) Maintain respiration and decontaminate to prevent further absorption.

(2) Administer **atropine** parenterally to inhibit muscarinic effects.

(3) Administer **pralidoxime** within minutes of exposure.

III. MUSCARINIC-RECEPTOR ANTAGONISTS

A. Mechanism and chemical structure (Table 2-5)

1. Muscarinic-receptor antagonists are competitive antagonists of ACh at all muscarinic cholinoceptors.

table 2-5 Properties of Some Cholinoceptor Blocking Agents

Agent	Action	Receptors: Muscarinic	Receptors: Nicotinic	Comments
Atropine	Competitive antagonist	+		Prototype muscarinic cholinoceptor blocking agent
Scopolamine	Competitive antagonist	+		Actions similar to those of atropine
Propantheline	Competitive antagonist	+		Peripheral-acting cholinoceptor blocking agent
Trimethaphan	Competitive, nondepolarizing antagonist		+	Peripheral-acting ganglionic blocking agent
Cisatracurium	Competitive, nondepolarizing antagonist at motor endplate		+	Neuromuscular junction blocking agent
Succinylcholine	Depolarizing agonist at motor endplate		+	Neuromuscular junction blocking agent

2. Muscarinic-receptor antagonists are either tertiary amine alkaloids (e.g., **atropine, scopolamine, tropicamide)** or quaternary amines (e.g., **propantheline [Pro-Banthine], ipratropium [Atrovent]**).
3. **Tertiary amines** are often used for their effects on the **CNS. Quaternary amines**, which have minimal CNS actions, are often used for their effects on **peripheral systems.**

B. Pharmacologic effects

1. ***Eye*** (Table 2-3)
   a. Muscarinic-receptor antagonists produce **cycloplegia** by blocking parasympathetic tone, leading to paralysis of the ciliary muscle and loss of accommodation.
   b. These drugs produce **mydriasis** by blocking parasympathetic tone to the iris circular (constrictor) muscle. Unopposed sympathetic stimulation of the radial muscle results in dilation of the pupil.
2. ***Cardiovascular system***
   a. Muscarinic-receptor antagonists **increase heart rate** due to cholinergic blockade at the SA node.
   b. These drugs dilate blood vessels in facial blush area (atropine flush), which is not related to the antagonist action.
3. ***GI tract***
   a. Muscarinic-receptor antagonists **decrease salivation.**
   b. These drugs **reduce peristalsis,** resulting in prolonged gastric emptying and intestinal transit.
   c. They also reduce gastric acid secretion.
4. ***Other effects***
   a. Muscarinic-receptor antagonists produce some **bronchodilation** and decrease mucus secretion.
   b. These drugs relax the ureters and bladder in the urinary tract and constrict the urinary sphincter.
   c. Tertiary amines can produce restlessness, headache, excitement, hallucinations, and delirium.
   d. These drugs produce **anhidrosis** and dry skin because of the inhibition of sympathetic cholinergic innervation of the sweat glands.

C. Pharmacologic properties

1. Unlike quaternary ammonium drugs (10%–30% absorption), most tertiary muscarinic-receptor antagonists are well absorbed across the GI tract or mucosal surfaces and distribute throughout the body, including the brain.
2. **Atropine** and **scopolamine** have relatively long durations of action.

table 2-6 Selected Therapeutic Use of Muscarinic Cholinoceptor Antagonists

Organ/System	Therapeutic Use
Eye	Refractive measurement; ophthalmologic examination, uveitis and iritis
Heart	Acute myocardial infarction
Bladder	Urinary urgency
Lung	Surgical anesthesia to suppress secretions
CNS	Motion sickness (scopolamine); Parkinson disease
Multiple organs/systems	Cholinergic poisoning

D. Therapeutic uses (Table 2-6)

1. ***Eye***
   a. Shorter-acting muscarinic-receptor antagonists (e.g., **homatropine**, **cyclopentolate** [Cyclogyl], **tropicamide**) are administered topically as eyedrops or as ointments for **refractive measurements** and for **ophthalmoscopic examination** of the retina and other structures of the eye (α-adrenoceptor agonists, such as **phenylephrine**, are used for simple funduscopic examination without cycloplegia).
   b. Longer-acting muscarinic-receptor antagonists (such as **homatropine**) are generally preferred as adjuncts to **phenylephrine** to prevent synechia formation in **anterior uveitis and iritis.**
2. ***Cardiovascular system*** uses are limited and include the administration of these drugs as a treatment for **acute myocardial infarction** with accompanying bradycardia and hypotension or arrhythmias (e.g., **atropine**).
3. ***Urinary tract*** uses of **atropine** and other muscarinic-receptor antagonists include the administration of these drugs for symptomatic treatment of **urinary urgency** in inflammatory bladder disorder. **Oxybutynin** (Ditropan), a selective muscarinc M_2-receptor antagonist, **tolterodine** (Detrol), a selective muscarinic M_3-receptor antagonist, and **trospium** (Spas Max), are additional agents in this class used to treat certain urinary disorders.
4. ***Central nervous system***
   a. Antimuscarinic drugs, **benztropine, biperiden, trihexyphenidyl,** and others, are used as adjunct to levodopa therapy for some patients with **Parkinson disease** (see Chapter 5).
   b. **Scopolamine** (used orally, intravenously, or transdermally) prevents motion sickness by blocking muscarinic receptors in the vestibular system and in the CNS (see Chapter 8).
5. ***Respiratory system***
   a. **Atropine** and **scopolamine** can be used to suppress bronchiolar secretions during **surgical and spinal anesthesia** and to prevent the muscarinic effects of AChE inhibitors used to reverse muscle paralysis at the end of surgery. **Scopolamine** also has additional amnestic and sedative properties.
   b. **Ipratropium** is used as an inhalant to treat reactive airway disease such as asthma and chronic obstructive pulmonary disease (COPD).
6. ***Other uses:*** Tertiary agents such as **atropine** are used to block peripheral and CNS effects due to cholinergic excess, especially those caused by poisoning with AChE inhibitor-containing insecticides and muscarine-containing mushrooms.

E. Adverse effects and contraindications

1. ***The adverse effects*** of muscarinic-receptor antagonists are extensions of pharmacologic activity and include **mydriasis, cycloplegia, dry eyes, tachycardia, dry mouth, elevated temperature, dry skin, urine retention, agitation, hallucinations, and delirium** ("hot as a hare, dry as a bone, red as a beet, blind as a bat, mad as a hatter"). **Physostigmine** administration for treatment of tertiary amine overdose is not recommended. Rather, treatment is symptomatic. **Neostigmine** is used to treat poisoning with quaternary muscarinic-receptor antagonists.
2. ***Contraindications (relative)*** are **glaucoma,** particularly angle-closure glaucoma, **GI and urinary tract obstruction** (e.g., prostatic hypertrophy), and **gastric ulcer.**

3. ***Drug interactions*** of muscarinic-receptor antagonists include the production of additive effects when administered with other drugs with muscarinic-receptor antagonist activity (certain antidepressants, antipsychotics, and antihistamines).

IV. GANGLION-BLOCKING DRUGS

A. **Mechanism and therapeutic uses** (see Table 2-5)
   1. ***Ganglion-blocking drugs***
      a. **Trimethaphan** (Arfonad) and **mecamylamine** (Inversine) inhibit the effect of ACh at nicotinic receptors by acting competitively (**nondepolarizing blockade**) at both sympathetic and parasympathetic autonomic ganglia.
      b. Because of a lack of selectivity and numerous adverse effects, they are **used rarely in the clinical setting** (hypertensive emergencies).

V. SKELETAL MUSCLE RELAXANTS

A. **Classification and structure**
   1. ***Neuromuscular junction-blocking drugs*** (see Table 2-5)
      a. Classified as either **nondepolarizing or depolarizing** types, neuromuscular junction-blocking drugs cause neuromuscular paralysis. They are structurally similar to ACh.
      b. These drugs contain one or two **quarternary nitrogens** that limits their entry into the CNS.
      c. Nondepolarizing neuromuscular junction-blocking drugs, the prototype is **tubocurarine,** are arranged in a bulky, rigid conformation.
      d. Depolarizing neuromuscular junction-blocking drugs have a linear structure. **Succinylcholine,** the only one used clinically, is composed of two ACh molecules linked end to end.
   2. ***Spasmolytic drugs*** act to reduce abnormal muscle tone without paralysis. These drugs increase or mimic the activity of **γ-aminobutyric acid (GABA)** in the spinal cord and brain or interfere with the release of calcium in skeletal muscle.

B. **Nondepolarizing agents**
   1. ***Mechanism***
      a. Nondepolarizing agents **competitively inhibit the effect of ACh** at the postjunctional membrane nicotinic receptor of the neuromuscular junction. There is some prejunctional inhibition of ACh release.
      b. These agents prevent depolarization of the muscle and propagation of the action potential.
   2. ***Pharmacologic properties***
      a. Nondepolarizing agents are administered parenterally and are generally used for long-term motor paralysis. Paralysis and muscle relaxation occur within 2–5 minutes.
      b. Nondepolarizing agents have durations of action that range from 20–90 minutes, which can be extended by supplemental fractional dosing and is increased by larger initial doses (although this also increases the likelihood of adverse effects).
      c. Most nondepolarizing agents are metabolized by the liver or are excreted unchanged. The duration of action may be prolonged by hepatic or renal disease.
      d. Intermediate-acting steroid muscle relaxing agents (e.g., **rocuronium** [Zemuron], **vecuronium** [Norcuron]) are more commonly used than long-acting agents.
   3. ***Specific drugs*** (Table 2-7)
      a. **Tubocurarine** (prototype), an isoquinoline derivative, is seldom used clinically at this time.
      b. **Metocurine** (Metubine) is a derivative of tubocurarine. It has the same properties, but with less histamine release and thus less hypotension and bronchoconstriction. Metocurine has a long duration of action (>40 min).

table 2-7 Properties of Some Skeletal Muscle Relaxants

Nondepolarizing Agent	Duration of Action	Ganglion Blockade	Histamine Release	Cardiac Muscarinic Receptors	Comments
Tubocurarine[a]	Long	+	++	—	Prototype
Metocurine[a]	Long	+	+	—	Less hypotension and bronchoconstriction than tubocurarine
Atracurium[a]	Intermediate	—	+	—	Inactivated spontaneously in plasma; laudanosine, a breakdown product, may cause seizures.
Cisatracurium[a]	Intermediate	—	—	—	Less laudanosine formed than atracurium.
Mivacurium[a]	Short	—	++	—	Hydrolyzed by plasma cholinesterase.
Pancuronium[b]	Long	—	—	++	Increased heart rate
Vecuronium[b]	Intermediate	—	—	—	Metabolized by liver
Depolarizing Agent					
Succinylcholine	Very short	++	+	++	Hydrolyzed by cholinesterase; malignant hyperthermia is a rare, potentially fatal complication

[a]Isoquinoline derivative.
[b]Steroid derivative.

c. **Atracurium** (Tracrium)
   (1) Atracurium causes some histamine release. It is **inactivated spontaneously in plasma** by nonenzymatic hydrolysis that is delayed by acidosis. Its duration of action is reduced by hyperventilation-induced respiratory alkalosis. **Laudanosine,** a breakdown product of atracurium, may accumulate to cause **seizures.**
   (2) **Cisatracurium** (Nimbex) is a stereoisomer of atracurium that releases less histamine and forms less laudanosine. It has **replaced atracurium** use in clinical practice.

d. Other available isoquinoline derivatives similar to atracurium include short-acting (10–20 min) **mivacurium** (Mivacron), which is rapidly hydrolyzed by plasma cholinesterase (pseudocholinesterase), has a short duration of action, and produces moderate histamine release at high doses, and **doxacurium** (Nuromax), which is stable in plasma, has a long duration of action (90–120 min), is excreted unchanged, and is devoid of vagolytic activity.

e. **Pancuronium** (Pavulon)
   (1) Pancuronium has a steroid nucleus with two attached quaternary amine groups.
   (2) This drug has a long duration of action (120–180 min).
   (3) Pancuronium produces **no histamine release or ganglia blockade.**
   (4) Pancuronium causes a moderate **tachycardia,** primarily due to cardiac muscarinic receptor blockade.
   (5) This drug is excreted by the kidney with only minimal hepatic metabolism.

f. **Vecuronium** (Norcuron)
   (1) Vecuronium is a steroid derivative that has an intermediate duration of action (30–40 min).
   (2) Vecuronium has **little vagolytic, histaminic, or ganglion-blocking activity.**
   (3) This drug is primarily metabolized by the liver.

g. **Rocuronium** (Zemuron) is a derivative of vecuronium with an intermediate duration of action (30–40 min) that undergoes primarily hepatic clearance (75%–90%).

h. **Pipecuronium** (Arduan) has a long duration of action (80–100 min) and undergoes both renal (60%) and hepatic clearance.

4. ***Therapeutic uses***
   a. Nondepolarizing agents are used during surgery as adjuncts to general anesthetics to induce muscle paralysis and muscle relaxation. The order of muscle paralysis is small, rapidly contracting muscles (e.g., extrinsic muscles of the eye) before slower contracting muscle groups (e.g., face and extremities), followed by intercostal muscles, and then the

diaphragm. Recovery of muscle function is in reverse order, and respiration often must be assisted.

b. These agents are also used for muscle paralysis in patients when it is critical to control ventilation, and they are used to control muscle contractions during **electroconvulsive therapy.**

5. *Reversal of nondepolarizing drug blockade:* AChE inhibitors, such as **neostigmine,** are administered for pharmacologic antagonism to reverse residual postsurgical muscarinic receptor blockade and avoid inadvertent hypoxia or apnea.

6. *Adverse effects and contraindications* (Table 2-7)

a. Cardiovascular system

(1) Nondepolarizing agents that are **isoquinoline derivatives** may produce **hypotension** due to histamine release and ganglionic-blocking activity.

(2) Nondepolarizing agents that are **steroid derivatives** may produce **tachycardia** due to vagolytic activity, leading to potential arrhythmias. These drugs should be used cautiously in patients with cardiovascular disease.

b. Respiratory system: Some nondepolarizing agents that are **isoquinoline derivatives** can produce **bronchospasm** in sensitive individuals due to histamine release. Agents that release histamine are contraindicated for asthmatic patients and patients with a history of anaphylactic reactions.

7. *Drug interactions*

a. General inhalation anesthetics, particularly **isoflurane,** increase the neuromuscular blocking action of nondepolarizing agents. The dose of the neuromuscular junction-blocking drug may have to be reduced.

b. Aminoglycoside antibiotics, among others, inhibit prejunctional ACh release and potentiate the effect of nondepolarizing and depolarizing neuromuscular junction-blocking drugs.

C. Depolarizing agents (Table 2-7) include **succinylcholine** (Anectine), the only depolarizing drug of clinical importance.

1. *Mechanism of action*

a. Succinylcholine is a **nicotinic receptor agonist** that acts at the motor endplate of the neuromuscular junction to produce **persistent stimulation and depolarization of the muscle,** thus preventing stimulation of contraction by ACh.

b. After a single IV injection and depolarization of the muscle, there are initial muscle contractions or **fasciculations** (in the first 30–60 s) that may be masked by general anesthetics. Because succinylcholine is metabolized more slowly than ACh at the neuromuscular junction, the muscle cells remain depolarized **(depolarizing or phase I block)** and unresponsive to further stimulation, resulting in a **flaccid paralysis** (5–10 min).

c. With continuous long-term exposure (45–60 min), the muscle cells repolarize. However, they cannot depolarize again while succinylcholine is present and, therefore, remain unresponsive to ACh **(desensitizing or phase II block).**

d. AChE inhibition will enhance the initial phase I block by succinylcholine, but can reverse phase II block.

2. *Pharmacologic properties*

a. Succinylcholine has a rapid onset and short duration of action. Action is rapidly terminated (5–10 min) by **hydrolysis by plasma and liver cholinesterase.**

b. Reduced plasma cholinesterase synthesis in end-stage hepatic disease or reduced activity following the use of irreversible AChE inhibitors may increase the duration of action.

3. *Therapeutic uses* of succinylcholine include the administration of the drug to induce brief **paralysis in short surgical procedures** such as tracheal intubation or in electroconvulsive shock therapy.

4. *Adverse effects*

a. Postoperative muscle pain at higher doses

b. Hyperkalemia

(1) Hyperkalemia results from loss of tissue potassium during depolarization.

(2) Risk of hyperkalemia is enhanced in patients with burns, muscle trauma, or spinal cord transections.

(3) Hyperkalemia can be life-threatening, leading to **cardiac arrest** and circulatory collapse.

c. **Malignant hyperthermia**
   (1) Malignant hyperthermia is a rare but often fatal complication in susceptible patients that results from a rapid increase in muscle metabolism. About 50% of patients are genetically predisposed, with mutations in the skeletal muscle Ca^{2+}-release channel of the sarcoplasmic reticulum (ryanodine receptor, RYR1).
   (2) Malignant hyperthermia is most likely to occur when succinylcholine is used with the general anesthetic **halothane.**
   (3) It is characterized by tachycardia and, among other manifestations, intense **muscle spasm** that results in a rapid and profound **hyperthermia.**
   (4) Drug treatment is with **dantrolene** (see following).

d. **Prolonged paralysis** may result in apnea (lasting 1–4 h) in a small percentage of patients (1/10,000) with **genetically atypical or low levels of plasma cholinesterase.** Mechanical ventilation is necessary.

e. **Bradycardia** from direct stimulation of muscarinic cholinoceptor stimulation is prevented by atropine

f. **Increased intraocular pressure** may result from extraocular muscle contractions; use of succinylcholine may be contraindicated for penetrating eye injuries.

g. Succinylcholine produces increased intragastric pressure, which may result in fasciculations of abdominal muscles and a danger of aspiration.

D. Spasmolytic drugs

1. ***These muscle relaxants* reduce increased muscle tone** associated with a variety of nervous system disorders (e.g., **cerebral palsy, multiple sclerosis, spinal cord injury, and stroke**) that result in loss of supraspinal control and hyperexcitability of α- and γ-motoneurons in the spinal cord, causing abnormal skeletal muscle, bowel, and bladder function.

2. ***Selected drugs***
   a. **Dantrolene** (Dantrium)
      (1) Dantrolene acts directly on muscle to reduce skeletal muscle contractions.
      (2) Dantrolene is also used to treat **malignant hyperthermia.**
      (3) This drug interferes with Ca^{2+} release from the sarcoplasmic reticulum; benefit may not be apparent for a week or more.
      (4) The major adverse effects of dantrolene are **muscle weakness,** which may limit therapy, and sedation. Long-term use can result in hepatotoxicity that may be fatal. Hepatic function should be monitored during treatment.
   b. **Baclofen** (Lioresal)
      (1) Baclofen is an analogue of GABA. It is a $GABA_B$-receptor agonist that hyperpolarizes neurons to inhibit synaptic transmission in the spinal cord.
      (2) Adverse effects include some drowsiness and an increased frequency of seizures in epileptic patients.
   c. **Benzodiazepines** (see Chapter 5)
      (1) Benzodiazepines such as **diazepam** act on the spinal cord and CNS to facilitate GABA activity.
      (2) The major adverse effect is **sedation.**

3. **Botulinum toxin (Botox)**
   a. Botulinum toxin acts by **inhibiting the release of ACh from motor nerve terminals.**
   b. **Botulinum toxin** is used to treat local muscle spasms associated with **cervical dystonia** and blepharospasm- and strabismus-associated dystonia. It is also used for cosmetic reduction of **facial wrinkles.**

VI. SYMPATHOMIMETIC DRUGS

A. Action and chemical structure

1. These drugs act either **directly** or **indirectly** to **activate** postjunctional and prejunctional **adrenoceptors** to **mimic** the effects of **endogenous catecholamines** such as norepinephrine and

epinephrine. Their actions can generally be predicted from the type and location of the receptors with which they interact and whether or not they cross the blood–brain barrier to enter the CNS.

2. Indirectly acting agents either act within nerve endings to **increase the release of stored catecholamines** or at the prejunctional membrane to **block the reuptake of catecholamines** that have been released from nerve endings.
3. Sympathomimetic agents are usually derived from the parent compound β-phenylethylamine. Chemical modifications of the side chain or the catechol nucleus can markedly alter their relative selectivity and intrinsic activity at α- and β-receptors, their disposition, and their metabolism.

B. Pharmacologic effects (Table 2-8)

1. ***Cardiovascular system***
   a. **β_1-Receptor agonists** increase the rate (chronotropic effect) and force (inotropic effect) of myocardial contraction and increase the conduction velocity through the AV node, with a decrease in the refractory period.
   b. **β_2-Receptor agonists** cause relaxation of vascular smooth muscle that may invoke a reflex increase in heart rate.
   c. **α_1-Receptor agonists** constrict smooth muscle of resistance blood vessels (e.g., in the skin and splanchnic beds), causing increased peripheral resistance and venous return. In normotensive patients (less effect in those with hypotension), the increased blood pressure may invoke a reflex baroreceptor vagal discharge and a slowing of the heart, with or without an accompanying change in cardiac output.
   d. **α_2-Receptor agonists** reduce blood pressure by a prejunctional action on neurons in the CNS to inhibit sympathetic outflow.
2. ***Eye*** (see Table 2-3)
   a. **α-Receptor agonists** contract the radial muscle of the iris and dilate the pupil (mydriasis). These drugs also increase outflow of aqueous humor from the eye.
   b. **β-Receptor antagonists** decrease the production of aqueous humor.
3. ***Respiratory system effects*** include **β_2-receptor agonist**-induced relaxation of bronchial smooth muscle and decreased airway resistance.

table 2-8 Direct Effects of Adrenoceptor Agonists

Effector	α_1	α_2	β_1	β_2
Heart				
Rate			Increase	
Force			Increase	
Arterioles (most)	Constrict			Dilate
Blood pressure	Increase			Decrease
Intestine				
Wall	Relax	Relax		Relax
Sphincters	Contract			
Salivation				
Volume	Increase			
Amylase			Increase	
Pupil	Dilate			
Bronchial smooth muscle				Relax
Urinary bladder				
Body	Constrict			Relax
Sphincter	Constrict			
Release of NE from nerves		Decrease		

4. ***GI tract***
   a. **α-Receptor and β-receptor** agonists relax GI smooth muscle. α-Receptor agonists reduce the release of ACh and other transmitters from intramural nerves by a prejunctional action; β-receptors are located directly on smooth muscle.
   b. **α_1-Receptor agonists** contract GI sphincters.
5. ***Metabolic and endocrine effects***
   a. **β-Receptor agonists** increase liver and skeletal muscle glycogenolysis and increase lipolysis in fat cells (β_3).
   b. **β-Receptor agonists** increase, and **α_2-receptor agonists** decrease, insulin secretion.
6. ***Genitourinary tract effects*** include **β_2-receptor agonist**–induced relaxation of uterine smooth muscle and the bladder wall. **α-Receptor agonists** constrict the bladder wall (α_1).

C. **Specific sympathomimetic drugs** are selected for use depending on the duration of action, route of administration, and also the specific effect on a particular tissue, which in turn depends on the tissue population of adrenoceptor subtypes.

1. ***Epinephrine and norepinephrine***
   a. Epinephrine and norepinephrine are poorly absorbed from the GI tract and do not enter the CNS to any appreciable extent. Absorption of epinephrine from subcutaneous sites is slow because of local vasoconstriction. Although rarely used, nebulized and inhaled solutions and topical preparations of epinephrine are available. Epinephrine and norepinephrine are most often **administered IV** (with caution to avoid cardiac arrhythmias or local tissue necrosis).
   b. These drugs are metabolized extensively by enzymes in the liver. **COMT** methylates the *meta*-hydroxyl group of the catechol, and **MAO** removes the amine group of the side chain. Metabolites are excreted by the kidney.
   c. Epinephrine and norepinephrine actions at neuroeffector junctions are terminated primarily by **simple diffusion** away from the receptor site and by **active uptake** into sympathetic nerve terminals and subsequent active transport into storage vesicles. Actions are also partially terminated at neuroeffector junctions by metabolism by extraneuronal COMT and intraneuronal MAO.
      (1) Epinephrine
         (a) Epinephrine activates β_1-, β_2-, and α-adrenoceptors.
         (b) Epinephrine administration in humans **increases systolic pressure** as a result of positive inotropic and chronotropic effects on the heart (β_1-receptor activation) and generally results in **decreased total peripheral resistance** and **decreased diastolic pressure due to vasodilation** in the vascular bed of skeletal muscle (β_2-receptor activation) that overcomes the vasoconstriction produced in most other vascular beds, including the kidney (α-receptor activation). The mean arterial pressure may increase slightly, decrease, or remain unchanged, depending on the balance of effects on systolic and diastolic pressure.
         (c) At high doses, epinephrine causes vasoconstriction in the vascular bed of skeletal muscle (α-receptor activation).
         (d) Epinephrine **increases coronary blood flow** as a result of increased cardiac workload; it may precipitate **angina** in patients with coronary insufficiency.
         (e) Epinephrine **increases the drainage of aqueous humor** (α-receptor activation) and reduces pressure in **open-angle glaucoma.** It **dilates the pupil** (mydriasis) by contraction of the radial muscle of the eye (α-receptor activation).
         (f) Epinephrine **relaxes bronchial smooth muscle** (β_2-receptor activation).
      (2) Norepinephrine
         (a) Norepinephrine **activates β_1-receptors** (it is equipotent to epinephrine) and **α-receptors** (it is slightly less potent than epinephrine). It has little activity at β_2-receptors.
         (b) Norepinephrine **increases total peripheral resistance** and **diastolic blood pressure** to a greater extent than epinephrine because of its vasoconstrictor activity and lack of effect on β_2-receptors in the skeletal muscle vascular bed.
         (c) Norepinephrine increases systolic blood pressure and mean arterial pressure.

(d) It has a direct stimulant effect on heart rate, but this is overcome by reflex baroreceptor-mediated vagal bradycardia.
(e) Norepinephrine is rarely used therapeutically.

2. ***Dopamine*** (Intropin)
   a. Dopamine activates peripheral **β_1-adrenoceptors** to increase heart rate and contractility.
   b. Dopamine **activates** prejunctional and postjunctional dopamine **D_1-receptors** in the renal, coronary, and splanchnic vessels to reduce arterial resistance and increase blood flow. Prejunctionally, dopamine inhibits norepinephrine release.
   c. At **low doses,** dopamine has a positive inotropic effect and increases systolic pressure, with little effect on diastolic pressure or mean blood pressure.
   d. At **higher doses,** dopamine activates α-receptors and causes vasoconstriction, with a reflex decrease in heart rate.
3. ***β-Adrenoceptor agonists***
   a. **Dobutamine**
      (1) Dobutamine is a **synthetic catecholamine** that is related to **dopamine.**
      (2) Dobutamine has a relatively selective effect on **β_1-receptors** and no effect on dopamine receptors.
      (3) This drug increases cardiac output with limited vasodilating activity and reflex tachycardia.
      (4) Dobutamine is administered by **IV infusion** because of its short half-life ($t_{1/2} = 2$ min).
   b. **Terbutaline** (Brethine, Bricanyl), **albuterol** (Proventil, Ventolin), **metaproterenol** (Alupent), **pirbuterol** (Maxair), **levalbuterol** (Xopenex), **bitolterol** (Tornalate), **salmeterol** (Serevent), and **formoterol** (Foradil)
      (1) These drugs are more **selective β_2-receptor agonists** that **relax bronchial smooth muscle** with fewer cardiac effects and longer duration of action than epinephrine.
      (2) Selectivity is lost at high concentrations.
   c. **Isoproterenol** (Isuprel)
      (1) Isoproterenol **activates β-receptors** with little activity on α-receptors.
      (2) Isoproterenol **dilates bronchial smooth muscle.**
      (3) This drug **increases heart rate and contractility** and causes **vasodilation** in skeletal muscle vascular beds with decreased total peripheral resistance and decreased diastolic blood pressure.
      (4) It is infrequently used because of the availability of selective β_2-adrenoceptor agonists.
4. ***α-Adrenoceptor agonists***
   a. **Phenylephrine, methoxamine** (Vasoxyl), and **metaraminol** (Aramine)
      (1) These drugs produce effects primarily by **direct α_1-receptor stimulation** that results in vasoconstriction, increased total peripheral resistance, and increased systolic and diastolic pressure. **Metaraminol** also has **indirect activity;** it is taken up and released at sympathetic nerve endings, where it acts as a false neurotransmitter. It also releases epinephrine.
      (2) Because they are not metabolized by COMT, these drugs are less potent but have longer durations of action than catecholamines.
   b. **Xylometazoline** (Otrivin) and **oxymetazoline** (Afrin)
      (1) These drugs have selective action at α-receptors.
      (2) At **high doses,** these drugs may cause **clonidine-like effects** because of their action in the CNS.
   c. **Clonidine** (Catapres), **methyldopa** (Aldomet), **guanabenz** (Wytensin), and **guanfacine** (Tenex)
      (1) These antihypertensive agents directly or indirectly activate prejunctional and, probably, postjunctional **α_2-receptors** in the **vasomotor center** of the medulla to **reduce sympathetic tone.**
      (2) These drugs reduce **blood pressure,** with a decrease in total peripheral resistance and minimal long-term effects on cardiac output and heart rate.
      (3) **Methyldopa** is a **prodrug** that is metabolized to the active agent **α-methylnorepinephrine** (and α-methyldopamine) in nerve endings. It **lowers blood pressure by reducing peripheral vascular resistance.** At higher, nontherapeutic doses, it activates peripheral α-receptors to cause vasoconstriction.

5. ***Other adrenoceptor agonists***
   a. **Ephedrine** and **mephenteramine**
      (1) These drugs act indirectly to release norepinephrine from nerve terminals and have some direct action on adrenoceptors.
      (2) Ephedrine and mephenteramine have effects similar to those of **epinephrine,** but they are less potent; they have a longer duration of action because they are resistant to metabolism by COMT and MAO.
      (3) These drugs are effective orally and, unlike catecholamines, penetrate the brain and can produce CNS stimulation.
      (4) **Ephedrine** is found in the herbal medication **ma huang.**
      (5) **Pseudoephedrine** (Sudafed) is an isomer of ephedrine.
      (6) After continued use, **tachyphylaxis** may develop due to their peripheral effects.
   b. **Amphetamine, dextroamphetamine** (Dexedrine), **methamphetamine** (Desoxyn), **phendimetrazine** (Preludin), **modafinil** (Provigil), **methylphenidate** (Ritalin), and **hydroxyamphetamine** (Paredrine) (see Chapter 5)
      (1) These drugs produce effects similar to those of **ephedrine,** with indirect and some direct activity.
      (2) **Dextroamphetamine** has more CNS-stimulatory activity than the *levo* isomer, which has more cardiovascular activity.
      (3) These drugs are well absorbed and, except for **hydroxyamphetamine,** enter the CNS readily and have marked stimulant activity.

D. **Therapeutic uses** (Table 2-9)
1. ***Cardiovascular system***
   a. **Phenylephrine, methoxamine, norepinephrine,** and other direct-acting α-receptor sympathomimetic drugs are used for **short-term hypotensive emergencies** when there is inadequate perfusion of the heart and brain such as during severe hemorrhage.
   b. **Ephedrine and midodrine** (Pro-Amatine), prodrug that are hydrolyzed to the **α_1-adrenoceptor agonist desglymidodrine,** to treat **chronic orthostatic hypotension**.
   c. **The use of sympathomimetic agents in most forms of shock is controversial and should be avoided. Further vasoconstriction may be harmful.**
      (1) Low-to-moderate doses of **dobutamine** or **dopamine** may be useful in cases of **cardiogenic or septic shock** because they increase cardiac output with minimal vasoconstrictive effect on the peripheral vasculature.
      (2) **Epinephrine** is used to reverse hypotension and angioedema associated with **anaphylactic shock.**
   d. **Dobutamine** is used to treat **congestive heart failure.**
   e. **Methyldopa** is used to treat **hypertension.**
   f. **Fenoldopam** (Corlopam) is a selective dopamine **D_1-receptor agonist** used to treat severe hypertension.

table 2-9 Selected Therapeutic Uses of Adrenoceptor Agonists

Clinical Condition/Application	Agonist	Receptor
Hypotensive emergency	Phenylephrine; methoxamine; norepinephrine	α_1
Orthostatic hypotension	Ephedrine; midodrine	α_1
Anaphylactic shock	Epinephrine	α and β
Heart block, cardiac arrest	Isoproterenol; epinephrine	β_1
Congestive heart failure	Dobutamine	β_1
Infiltration nerve block	Epinephrine	α_1
Hay fever and rhinitis	Phenylephrine; OTC[a]	α_1
Asthma	Metaproterenol; terbutaline; albuterol	β_2

[a]Over-the-counter preparations.

g. **Isoproterenol** and **epinephrine** have been used for temporary emergency treatment of **cardiac arrest** and **heart block** because they increase ventricular automaticity and rate and increase AV conduction.

h. **Epinephrine** is commonly used in combination with local anesthetics (1:200,000) during infiltration block to reduce blood flow. α-Receptor agonist activity causes local vasoconstriction, which **prolongs local anesthetic action** and allows the use of lower doses with reduced chance of toxicity. **Phenylephrine** and **norepinephrine** have also been used.

i. **Epinephrine** is used during **spinal anesthesia** to maintain blood pressure, as is **phenylephrine,** and topically to reduce superficial bleeding.

2. ***Respiratory system***

a. **Phenylephrine** and other short- and longer acting **α-adrenoceptor agonists,** including **oxymetazoline, xylometazoline, tetrahydrozoline** (Tyzine), ephedrine, and pseudoephedrine, are used for symptomatic relief of **hay fever and rhinitis** of the common cold. Long-term use may result in ischemia and rebound hyperemia, with development of chronic rhinitis and congestion.

b. **Metaproterenol, terbutaline, albuterol, bitolterol,** and other β_2-adrenoceptor agonists are preferred for treating **asthma. Epinephrine** is also used for management of acute **bronchospasm.**

c. **Epinephrine** is administered IM to treat bronchospasm, congestion, angioedema, and cardiovascular collapse of **anaphylaxis.**

3. ***Eye***

a. **Phenylephrine** facilitates **examination of the retina** because of its mydriatic effect. It is also used for minor allergic hyperemia of the conjunctiva.

b. **α_2-Receptor agonists** (**apraclonidine** [Lopidine] and **brimonidine** [Alphagan]) that lower intraocular pressure by increasing aqueous outflow (**epinephrine and dipivefrin** [Propine] are rarely used) have been largely **supplanted by β-adrenoceptor blockers and prostaglandin analogues** for treatment of **chronic open-angle glaucoma.**

4. ***CNS***

a. **Amphetamine** and related analogues (e.g., **modafinil**) are used to treat **narcolepsy** (controversial) because of their arousal effects and their ability to increase the attention span; as occasional adjunct therapy for obesity because of their anorexiant effects; and to treat **attention-deficit hyperactivity disorder** in children (e.g., **methylphenidate**).

b. **Hydroxyamphetamine** and **phenylephrine** are used for the **diagnosis of Horner syndrome.**

c. **Dexmedetomidine** (Precedex), a novel selective **α_2-adrenoceptor agonist** that acts centrally, is used intravenously as a **sedative** in patients hospitalized in intensive care settings.

5. ***Other uses*** include **ritodrine** and **terbutaline** to **suppress premature labor** by relaxing the uterus, although the efficacy of these drugs is controversial.

E. Adverse effects and toxicity

1. The adverse effects of sympathomimetic drugs are generally extensions of their pharmacologic activity.
2. Overdose with **epinephrine** or **norepinephrine** or other pressor agents may result in **severe hypertension,** with possible **cerebral hemorrhage, pulmonary edema,** and **cardiac arrhythmia.** Milder effects include headache, dizziness, and tremor. Increased cardiac workload may result in angina or myocardial infarction in patients with coronary insufficiency.
3. Phenylephrine should not be used to treat closed-angle glaucoma before iridectomy as it may cause **increased intraocular pressure.**
4. Sudden discontinuation of an **α_2-adrenoceptor agonist** may cause **withdrawal symptoms** that include headache, tachycardia, and a rebound rise in blood pressure.
5. Drug abuse may occur with amphetamine and amphetamine-like drugs.
6. Drug interactions

a. **Tricyclic antidepressants** block catecholamine reuptake and may potentiate the effects of norepinephrine and epinephrine.

b. Some **halogenated anesthetic agents** and **digitalis** may sensitize the heart to β-receptor stimulants, resulting in ventricular arrhythmias.

VII. ADRENERGIC RECEPTOR ANTAGONISTS

These drugs interact with either α- or β-adrenoceptors to prevent or reverse the actions of endogenously released norepinephrine or epinephrine or exogenously administered sympathomimetic agents.

A. α-Adrenoceptor antagonists

1. ***Pharmacologic effects***
   a. The pharmacologic effects of α-adrenoceptor antagonists are predominantly cardiovascular and include **lowered peripheral vascular resistance and blood pressure.** These agents prevent pressor effects of α-receptor agonists.
   b. α-Adrenoceptor antagonists convert the pressor action of sympathomimetic agents with both α- and β-adrenoceptor agonist activity to a depressor response; this is referred to as **epinephrine reversal.**
2. ***Specific drugs*** (Table 2-10)
   a. **Phentolamine** (Regitine) is an intravenously administered, short-acting competitive antagonist at both α_1- and α_2-receptors. It reduces peripheral resistance and decreases blood pressure. **Tolazoline** (Priscoline), a drug similar to phentolamine, is rarely used.

table 2-10 Therapeutic Uses of Selected Adrenoceptor Antagonists

Drug	Receptor	Features	Major Uses
Phentolamine[a]	α_1 and α_2	Short duration of action (1–2 h)	Hypertension of pheochromocytoma
Phenoxybenzamine[a]		Long duration of action (15–50 h)	Hypertension of pheochromocytoma
Prazosin[a]	α_1	Minimal reflex tachycardia	Mild-to-moderate hypertension (often with a diuretic or a β-adrenoceptor antagonist); severe congestive heart failure (with a cardiac glycoside and a diuretic)
Terazosin			Mild-to-moderate hypertension
Doxazosin			Mild-to-moderate hypertension
Propranolol[a]	β_1 and β_2	Local anesthetic activity	Hypertension; angina; pheochromocytoma, cardiac arrhythmias; migraine headache; hypertrophic subaortic stenosis
Timolol			Hypertension; glaucoma
Metipranolol			Glaucoma
Levobunolol			Glaucoma
Nadolol		Long duration of action (15–25 h)	Hypertension; angina
Pindolol		Partial β_2-receptor agonist activity[b]	Hypertension; angina
Penbutolol		Partial β_2-receptor agonist activity[b]; mild-to-moderate hypertension	Hypertension; angina
Carteolol		Partial β_2-receptor agonist activity[b]; excreted unchanged	Hypertension; angina; glaucoma
Metoprolol[a]	$\beta_1 > \beta_2$	Patient bioavailability is variable; extended release form available	Hypertension; angina
Atenolol		Eliminated by the kidney	Hypertension; angina
Esmolol		Ultrashort acting (10 min)	Supraventricular tachycardia
Betaxolol		Long duration of action (15–25 h)	Glaucoma; hypertension
Acebutolol		Partial agonist[b]	Hypertension; ventricular arrhythmias
Labetalol[a]	β_1, β_2, and α_1	Partial agonist[b]; rapid blood pressure reduction; local anesthetic activity	Mild-to-severe hypertension; hypertensive emergencies

[a]Drugs listed in **boldface type** are considered prototype drugs.
[b]Lower blood pressure without significant reduction in cardiac output or resting heart rate; also do not elevate triglyceride levels or decrease high-density lipoprotein cholesterol.

b. **Prazosin** (Minipress)

(1) Prazosin is the prototype of competitive antagonists selective for α_1-receptors. Others include **terazosin** (Hytrin), **doxazosin** (Cardura), **tamsulosin** (Flomax), and **alfuzosin** (Uroxatral).

(2) Prazosin reduces peripheral resistance and blood pressure.

(3) This drug is administered orally. Prazosin has a **slow onset** (2–4 h) and a **long duration of action** (10 h) and is extensively metabolized by the liver (50% during first pass).

c. **Labetalol** (Normodyne and Trandate)

(1) Labetalol is a **competitive antagonist** (partial agonist) that is relatively selective for α_1-receptors and also blocks β-receptors.

(2) Labetalol reduces heart rate and myocardial contractility, decreases total peripheral resistance, and lowers blood pressure.

(3) This drug is administered **orally** or **intravenously** and undergoes extensive first-pass metabolism.

d. **Phenoxybenzamine** (Dibenzyline)

(1) Phenoxybenzamine is a noncompetitive, irreversible α_1-receptor antagonist.

(2) Phenoxybenzamine binds covalently, resulting in a long-lasting (15–50 h) blockade.

3. ***Therapeutic uses*** (Table 2-10)

a. Overview

(1) α_1-Adrenoceptor antagonists are used most often to treat hypertension and urinary obstruction of benign prostatic hypertrophy.

(2) α_2-Adrenoceptor antagonists have no important therapeutic uses.

b. **Pheochromocytoma**

(1) Pheochromocytoma is a **tumor** of the **adrenal medulla** that secretes excessive amounts of catecholamines. Symptoms include hypertension, tachycardia, and arrhythmias.

(2) **Phentolamine** and **phenoxybenzamine** are used to treat the tumor in the preoperative stage; they also are used for long-term management of inoperable tumors.

(3) β-Receptor antagonists are often used to prevent the cardiac effects of excessive catecholamines after an α-receptor blockade is established.

c. Adrenoceptor antagonists, particularly **labetalol,** are occasionally used to **reverse hypertensive crisis** due to sudden increase in α-receptor stimulation (e.g., with a pheochromocytoma or with an overdose of a sympathomimetic agonist).

d. **Prazosin** and **labetalol** are used to treat **essential hypertension.**

e. α_1-Adrenoceptor antagonists, such as **prazosin, terazosin, doxazosin,** and **alfuzosin,** are used to treat urinary obstruction of **benign prostatic hypertrophy** (BPH). **Tamsulosin** may have greater efficacy due to its selective action at **α_{1A}-receptors.**

f. Other uses of α-adrenoceptor antagonists (e.g., **phentolamine**) include reversible peripheral vasospasm like **Raynaud syndrome,** and **erectile dysfunction** (in combination with **papaverine**).

4. ***Adverse effects***

a. Adverse effects of **phentolamine** include postural hypotension, reflex tachycardia, arrhythmia, angina, and diarrhea. This drug should be used cautiously in patients with a peptic ulcer or with coronary artery disease.

b. **Prazosin, terazosin,** and **doxazosin** produce postural hypotension and bradycardia on initial administration; these drugs produce no significant tachycardia.

c. Adverse effects of **labetalol** include postural hypotension and GI disturbances. Bradycardia occurs with overdose. Labetalol produces fewer adverse effects on the bronchi and cardiovascular system than selective β-receptor antagonists.

B. β-Adrenoreceptor antagonists

1. ***Pharmacologic effects***

a. **Cardiovascular system**

(1) β-Adrenoreceptor antagonists **lower blood pressure,** possibly because of their combined effects on the heart, the renin–angiotensin system, and the CNS.

(2) These drugs **reduce** sympathetic-stimulated increases in **heart rate** and **contractility** and **cardiac output.**

(3) β-Adrenoreceptor antagonists **lengthen AV conduction time and refractoriness and suppress automaticity.**

(4) Initially, they may increase peripheral resistance. However, long-term administration results in decreased peripheral resistance in patients with hypertension.
(5) β-Adrenoreceptor antagonists reduce renin release.

b. **Respiratory system**
(1) β-Adrenoreceptor antagonists **increase airway resistance** as a result of β_2-receptor blockade.
(2) This respiratory effect is more pronounced in asthmatics because of unopposed, compensatory, reflex sympathomimetic α-receptor activity resulting from decreased cardiac output.

c. **Eye**
(1) β-Adrenoreceptor antagonists decrease the production of aqueous humor, resulting in **reduced intraocular pressure.**

d. **Other activities**
(1) β-Adrenoreceptor antagonists **inhibit lipolysis** (β_3).
(2) These drugs **inhibit glycogenolysis** (β_2) in the liver (they may impede recovery from the hypoglycemic effect of insulin).
(3) These drugs decrease high-density lipoprotein (HDL) levels.
(4) Some β-adrenoceptor antagonists have local anesthetic action, including **propranolol** and **labetalol.**

2. ***Specific drugs*** (Table 2-10)

a. **Overview**
(1) **Propranolol** is the **prototype** β-adrenoreceptor antagonist.
(2) These drugs have an **antihypertensive effect** that is slow to develop (the mechanism is unclear).
(3) β-Adrenoreceptor antagonists are absorbed well after oral administration. Including **propranolol,** many have **low bioavailability** (<50%) because of extensive first-pass metabolism; marked interpatient variability is seen, particularly with **metoprolol.**
(4) With the exceptions of **esmolol** (10 min) and **nadolol** and **betaxolol** (15–25 h), most have a $t_{1/2}$ of 3–12 hours.

b. **Propranolol** (Inderal)
(1) Propranolol is a competitive antagonist at β_1- and β_2-receptors.
(2) Propranolol is used in **long-term treatment of hypertension,** but it is not useful for hypertensive crisis.
(3) This drug is used to treat **supraventricular and ventricular arrhythmias** and is administered IV for the emergency treatment of arrhythmias.
(4) Propranolol is 90% bound to plasma proteins.
(5) This drug is cleared by hepatic metabolism and, therefore, has prolonged action in the presence of liver disease.
(6) Propranolol is also available in sustained-release preparation.

c. **Metoprolol** (Lopressor), **betaxolol** (Betoptic), **bisoprolol** (Zebeta), **atenolol** (Tenormin), **acebutolol** (Sectral), and **esmolol** (Brevibloc)
(1) These drugs are somewhat selective **β_1-receptor antagonists** that may offer some advantage over nonselective β-adrenoceptor antagonists to treat cardiovascular disease in asthmatic patients, although cautious use is still warranted.
(2) **Atenolol** is **eliminated** primarily by the **kidney** and undergoes little hepatic metabolism; it has little local anesthetic activity; it enters the CNS poorly.
(3) **Acebutolol** has partial agonist activity.
(4) **Betaxolol** is used topically for chronic **open-angle glaucoma.**
(5) **Esmolol** is **ultrashort acting** ($t_{1/2}$ = 10 min) because of extensive plasma hydrolysis by esterases; it is administered by **IV infusion.**
(6) **Metoprolol** is also available in sustained-release preparation.

d. **Labetalol** (Normodyne and Trandate), **Carvedilol** (Coreg)
(1) Labetalol is a partial agonist that blocks β-receptors and α_1-receptors (3:1 to 7:1 ratio). Carvedilol also has mixed activity but is equiactive at β-receptors and α_1-receptors.
(2) Labetalol reduces heart rate and myocardial contractility, decreases total peripheral resistance, and lowers blood pressure.
(3) This drug is administered PO or IV and undergoes extensive first-pass metabolism.

e. **Timolol** (Blocadren), **levobunolol** (Betagan), **nadolol** (Corgard), and **sotalol** (Betapace)
   (1) These drugs are **nonselective β-receptor antagonists.**
   (2) **Timolol and levobunolol** have excellent **ocular effects** when applied **topically for glaucoma.** Like propranolol, these drugs have no local anesthetic activity. **Metipranolol** (OptiPranolol) is also used to treat glaucoma.
   (3) **Sotalol** additionally prolongs the cardiac action potential and is used to treat **arrhythmias.**

f. **Pindolol** (Visken), **carteolol** (Cartrol), and **penbutolol** (Levatol) are nonselective antagonists with partial β_2-receptor agonist activity.
   (1) **Carteolol** is used topically to treat **open-angle glaucoma.** It is **excreted unchanged.**

3. ***Therapeutic uses*** (see Table 2-10)
   a. **Cardiovascular system** (see also Chapter 4)
      (1) β-Adrenoreceptor antagonists are used to treat **hypertension,** often in combination with a diuretic or vasodilator.
      (2) These drugs reduce incidence of **myocardial infarction.**
      (3) These drugs provide prophylaxis for **supraventricular and ventricular arrhythmias.**
      (4) β-Adrenoreceptor antagonists provide prophylaxis for **angina pectoris.** Long-term use of **timolol, propranolol,** and **metoprolol** may prolong survival after myocardial infarction.
      (5) **Propranolol** relieves angina, palpitations, dyspnea, and syncope in **obstructive cardiomyopathy.** This effect is thought to be related to the slowing of ventricular ejection and decreased resistance to outflow.
   b. **Eye**
      (1) Topical application of **timolol, betaxolol, levobunolol,** and **carteolol** reduces intraocular pressure in **glaucoma.**
      (2) Sufficient **timolol** can be absorbed after topical application to increase airway resistance and decrease heart rate and contractility.
   c. **Other uses**
      (1) **Propranolol** is used to control clinical symptoms of sympathetic overactivity in **hyperthyroidism** by an unknown mechanism, perhaps by inhibiting conversion of thyroxine to triiodothyronine.
      (2) **Propranolol** and others may be beneficial in the prophylaxis of **migraine headache** by an unknown mechanism.
      (3) **Propranolol** relieves acute **anxiety** and panic symptoms by inhibiting overactivity of the SNS.

4. ***Adverse effects and contraindications***
   a. **All agents**
      (1) β-Adrenoreceptor antagonists should be administered with extreme caution in patients with preexisting compromised cardiac function because they can precipitate **heart failure** or heart block.
      (2) These drugs may augment insulin action in diabetics and **mask tachycardia** associated with hypoglycemia.
      (3) β-Adrenoreceptor antagonists may **mask** the signs of developing **hyperthyroidism.**
      (4) After abrupt withdrawal, adrenoceptor "supersensitivity" and increased risk of **angina** and **arrhythmias** may occur. **Tapered withdrawal** is recommended.
   b. **Nonselective adrenoceptor antagonists**
      (1) These drugs may cause **bronchoconstriction,** and thus they are contraindicated for asthmatics. Patients with chronic obstructive lung disease are particularly susceptible.
      (2) These drugs should be used cautiously in patients with **peripheral vascular disease.**
      (3) β_1-Selective antagonists should also be used cautiously to treat asthmatics and patients with peripheral vascular disease because they have some β_2-receptor antagonist activity.
   c. **Propranolol,** and other β-receptor blockers, cause **sedation, sleep disturbances, and depression.**

DRUG SUMMARY TABLE

Direct-Acting Cholinoceptor Agonists
Acetylcholine (Miochol-E)
Bethanechol (Urecholine)
Carbachol (generic)
Cevimeline (Evoxac)
Methacholine (Mecholyl)
Pilocarpine (generic)
Varenicline (Chantix)

Indirect-Acting Cholinoceptor Agonists
Ambenonium (Mytelase)
Demecarium (Humorsol)
Donepezil (Aricept)
Echothiophate (Phospholine)
Edrophonium (Tensilon)
Galantamine (Reminyl)
Neostigmine (Prostigmin)
Physostigmine (Eserine, Antilirium)
Pyridostigmine (Mestinon, Regonol)
Rivastigmine (Exelon)
Tacrine (Cognex)

Cholinesterase Regenerator
Pralidoxime (Protopam)

Muscarinic Cholinoceptor Antagonists
Atropine (generic)
Clidinium (Quarzan)
Cyclopentolate (Cyclogyl)
Darifenacin (Enablex)
Dicyclomine (Bentyl)
Flavoxate (Uripas)
Glycopyrrolate (Robinul)
Homatropine (generic)
Ipratropium (Atrovent)
Mepenzolate (Cantil)
Methantheline (Banthine)
Oxybutynin (Ditropan)
Propantheline (Pro-Banthine)
Scopolamine (generic)
Solifenacin (Vesicare)
Tiotropium (Spiriva)
Tolterodine (Detrol)
Tridihexethyl (Pathilon)
Tropicamide (generic)
Trospium (Spasmex)

Ganglion Blocking Drugs
Mecamylamine (Inversine)
Trimethaphan (Arfonad)

Skeletal Muscle Relaxants
Neuromuscular Blocking Drugs
Atracurium (generic)
Cisatracurium (Nimbex)
Doxacurium (Nuromax)
Metocurine (Metubine)
Mivacurium (Mivacron)
Pancuronium (Pavulon)
Pipecuronium (Arduan)
Rocuronium (Zemuron)
Succinylcholine (Anectine)
Tubocurarine (generic)
Vecuronium (Norcuron)
Spasmolytic Drugs
Baclofen (Lioresal)
Botulinum toxin-type A (Botox)
Botulinum toxin-type B (Myobloc)
Dantrolene (Dantrium)

Sympathomimetic Drugs
Albuterol (Proventil, Ventolin)
Amphetamine (generic)
Apraclonidine (Lopidine)
Bitolterol (Tornalate)
Brimonidine (Alphagan)
Clonidine (Catapres)
Dexmedetomidine (Precedex)
Dextroamphetamine (Dexedrine)
Dipivefrin (Propine)
Dobutamine (Dobutrex)
Dopamine (Intropin)
Ephedrine (generic)
Epinephrine (generic)
Fenoldopam (Corlopam)
Formoterol (Foradil)
Guanabenz (Wytensin)
Guanfacine (Tenex)
Hydroxyamphetamine (Paredrine)
Isoproterenol (Isuprel)
Levalbuterol (Xopenex)
Mephenteramine (Wyamine)
Metaproterenol (Alupent)
Metaraminol (Aramine)
Methamphetamine (Desoxyn)
Methoxamine (Vasoxyl)
Methyldopa (Aldomet)
Methylphenidate (Ritalin)
Midodrine (ProAmatine)
Modafinil (Provigil)
Naphazoline (Privine)
Norepinephrine (generic)
Oxymetazoline (Afrin, Visine)
Phenylephrine (Neo-Synephrine)
Pirbuterol (Maxair)
Pseudoephedrine (Sudafed)
Salmeterol (Serevent)
Terbutaline (Brethine, Bricanyl)
Tetrahydrozoline (Tyzine)
Xylometazoline (Otrivin)

Adrenergic Receptor Antagonists
Alpha-Receptor Blockers
Alfuzosin (Uroxatral)
Doxazosin (Cardura)
Phenoxybenzamine (Dibenzyline)
Phentolamine (Regitine)
Prazosin (Minipress)
Tamsulosin (Flomax)
Terazosin (Hytrin)
Tolazoline (Priscoline)
Beta-Receptor Blockers
Acebutolol (Sectral)
Atenolol (Tenormin)
Betaxolol (Betoptic)
Bisoprolol (Zebeta)
Carteolol (Cartrol)
Carvedilol (Coreg)
Esmolol (Brevibloc)
Labetalol (Normodyne, Trandate)
Levobunolol (Betagan)
Metipranolol (OptiPranolol)
Metoprolol (Lopressor)
Nadolol (Corgard)
Penbutolol (Levatol)
Pindolol (Visken)
Propranolol (generic)
Sotalol (Betapace)
Timolol (Blocadren)

Review Test for Chapter 2

Directions: Each of the numbered items or incomplete statements in this section is followed by answers or by completions of the statement. Select the ONE lettered answer or completion that is BEST in each case.

1. Botulinum toxin causes paralysis by

(A) Inhibiting choline acetyltransferase
(B) Blocking transport of choline into neurons
(C) Blocking release of acetylcholine from storage vesicles
(D) Inhibiting acetylcholinesterase
(E) Blocking the synapse at ganglia

2. Which of the following neurotransmitters interacts with guanethidine?

(A) Acetylcholine
(B) Epinephrine
(C) Dopamine
(D) Norepinephrine
(E) Serotonin

3. What is the mechanism of action of cocaine?

(A) Propagation of action of norepinephrine by inhibiting its active transport from the synapse
(B) Oxidative deamination of norepinephrine in nerve terminals and the effector cells
(C) Inhibition of metabolism of norepinephrine in nerve terminals
(D) Potentiation of tyrosine hydroxylase, the rate-limiting enzyme in the synthesis of norepinephrine
(E) Promotion of release of norepinephrine from adrenergic nerve endings

4. What intracellular effect does albuterol, a β_2-agonist, produce?

(A) Allows passage of sodium through a ligand-gated ion channel
(B) Activates G_s-protein, resulting in stimulation of adenylyl cyclase
(C) Activates G_q-protein, resulting in increase of phosphatidylinositol and calcium mobilization
(D) Activates G_i-protein, resulting in inhibition of adenylyl cyclase
(E) Binds to μ-receptors in the specific areas of the brain

5. What class of medications does bethanechol belong to?

(A) Nicotinic blockers
(B) α-Agonists
(C) β_1-Blockers
(D) β_2-Blockers
(E) Muscarinic agonists

6. A 38-year-old farmer is brought to the ER by his wife with symptoms of sudden difficulty breathing, sweatiness, and anxiety. He was spraying insecticide when this happened. It has been 25 minutes since the symptoms started. The patient is emergently intubated and given atropine and another medication that acts to reactivate acetylcholinesterase. What medication is it?

(A) Physostigmine
(B) Propranolol
(C) Pralidoxime
(D) Phenylephrine
(E) Pancuronium

7. Oxybutynin works by

(A) Inhibiting acetylcholinesterase at muscarinic and nicotinic receptors
(B) Causing a neuromuscular blockade
(C) Antagonizing α_1-adrenoceptors
(D) Binding to muscarinic receptors
(E) Activating β_2-adrenoceptors

8. A 78-year-old man with Parkinson disease experiences worsening of his symptoms. He is already taking levodopa. Since the disease is characterized by degeneration of dopaminergic neurons, leading to the lack of inhibition of cholinergic neurons, the addition of which medication is likely to help alleviate the patient's symptoms?

(A) Benztropine
(B) Reserpine
(C) Doxazocin
(D) Timolol
(E) Tubocurarine

9. A 66-year-old woman with a long history of heavy smoking presents to her doctor with complaints of shortness of breath and chronic coughing that has been present for about 2 years and has been worsening in frequency. The doctor decides to prescribe a bronchodilator agent that has minimal cardiac side effects, since the patient also has an extensive cardiac history. Which medication did the doctor likely prescribe?

(A) Albuterol
(B) Prazosin
(C) Atenolol
(D) Ipratropium
(E) Pseudoephedrine

10. From the list below, choose the depolarizing neuromuscular blocker most likely to be used in "rapid sequence intubation," a procedure that is done when the stomach contents have a high risk of refluxing and causing aspiration.

(A) Baclofen
(B) Succinylcholine
(C) Neostigmine
(D) Homatropine
(E) Pralidoxime

11. Ephedra (ephedrine) causes increased blood pressure by

(A) Indirect action on cholinergic receptors
(B) Blockade of adrenergic receptors
(C) Stimulation of release of epinephrine
(D) Inhibition of reuptake of catecholamines
(E) Direct action on dopamine receptors

12. A 34-year-old carpenter presents to the ER after an accident in which he inadvertently chopped off the tip his index finger. He is taken to the OR for reattachment of the digit, and after sedation, a local anesthetic is administered around the site of the injury. The local anesthetic used in the procedure did not contain any epinephrine, as it usually does for most surgical procedures. The reason for this is

(A) Epinephrine causes increased blood loss during delicate surgery
(B) Epinephrine causes swelling of the tissues, making surgery more challenging
(C) Epinephrine is contraindicated in emergency surgery
(D) Epinephrine causes vasoconstriction, which can lead to vascular ischemia in digits
(E) Epinephrine can cause hypotension when administered with sedative agents

13. A 7-year-old boy is brought in by his parents for complaints of hyperactivity at school. He is also inattentive and impulsive at home. After a detailed interview, the physician decides to give the boy amphetamine-containing medication for presumed attention hyperactivity disorder. Amphetamine

(A) Inhibits epinephrine reuptake
(B) Indirectly acts on norepinephrine receptors
(C) Blocks effects of norepinephrine
(D) Directly acts on cholinoreceptors
(E) Inhibits serotonin reuptake

14. Which of the following medications is used to prevent premature labor?

(A) Tamsulosin
(B) Cevimeline
(C) Atracurium
(D) Tolterodine
(E) Terbutaline

15. What significant side effect of terazosin should the doctor warn a 69-year-old patient about?

(A) Bronchospasm
(B) Postural hypotension
(C) Heart failure
(D) Sedation
(E) Drug abuse

16. A floor nurse pages you about a patient who is having chest pain. You order an electrocardiogram and rush to see the patient. He describes the pain as tight pressure and is demonstrably sweating and gasping for air. The ECG comes back with acute ST-segment elevations in inferior leads, and you diagnose a myocardial infarction. You start giving the patient oxygen and give him sublingual nitroglycerin and morphine for pain. You also give him another medication, which you have read may prolong his survival in this dire situation. What class of medication is it?

(A) β-Blocker
(B) α-Agonist
(C) Muscarinic agonist
(D) Neuromuscular blocker
(E) Dopamine agonist

17. A 35-year-old woman presents to your office for a regular check-up. Her only complaint is recurrent migraine headaches, which have increased in frequency over the years. On examination, her blood pressure is elevated at

150/70. You decide to start her on antihypertensive therapy that is also used for prophylaxis of migraines. Which medication is it?

(A) Clonidine
(B) Prazosin
(C) Hydrochlorothiazide
(D) Propranolol
(E) Verapamil

18. In contrast to propranolol, metoprolol

(A) Is used for the management of hypertension
(B) Has greater selectivity for β_2-adrenoceptors
(C) May be beneficial for the acute treatment of migraine headache
(D) Is less likely to precipitate bronchoconstriction in patients with asthma

19. Intravenous administration of epinephrine to a patient results in a severe decrease in diastolic pressure and an increase in cardiac output. Which of the following drugs might the patient have previously taken that could account for this unexpected effect?

(A) Propanolol
(B) Atropine
(C) Phenylephrine
(D) Prazosin

20. Which of the following drugs is used to diagnose myasthenia gravis?

(A) Atropine
(B) Neostigmine
(C) Bethanechol
(D) Edrophonium
(E) Pralidoxime

21. Pilocarpine reduces intraocular pressure in patients with glaucoma because it

(A) Activates nicotinic cholinoceptors
(B) Blocks muscarinic cholinoceptors
(C) Selectively inhibits peripheral activity of sympathetic ganglia
(D) Inhibits acetylcholinesterase

22. Prolonged apnea may occur following administration of succinylcholine to a patient with a hereditary deficiency of which of the following enzymes?

(A) Glucose-6-phosphate dehydrogenase
(B) Plasma cholinesterase
(C) Monoamine oxidase
(D) Cytochrome $P450_{3A}$
(E) Acetylcholinesterase

23. Dantrolene is the drug of choice to treat malignant hyperthermia caused by succinylcholine because dantrolene

(A) Blocks Ca^2 release from sarcoplasmic reticulum
(B) Induces contraction of skeletal muscle
(C) Increases the rate of succinylcholine metabolism
(D) Inhibits succinylcholine binding to nicotinic receptors
(E) Acts centrally to reduce fever

24. A drug that acts at prejunctional α_2-adrenoceptors and is used to treat hypertension is

(A) Clonidine
(B) Methoxamine
(C) Metaproterenol
(D) Dobutamine
(E) Dopamine

25. Drug X causes an increase in blood pressure and a decrease in heart rate when administered to a patient intravenously. If an antagonist at ganglionic nicotinic receptors is administered first, drug X causes an increase in blood pressure and an increase in heart rate. Drug X most likely is

(A) Propranolol
(B) Norepinephrine
(C) Isoproterenol
(D) Terbutaline
(E) Curare

26. Poisoning with an insecticide containing an acetylcholinesterase inhibitor is best managed by administration of which one of the following agents?

(A) Physostigmine
(B) Bethanechol
(C) Propranolol
(D) Pilocarpine
(E) Atropine

27. Receptor actions of acetylcholine are mimicked by nicotine at which one of the following sites?

(A) Adrenal medullary chromaffin cells
(B) Urinary bladder smooth muscle cells
(C) Iris circular (constrictor) muscle
(D) Heart sinoatrial pacemaker cells

28. Muscarinic cholinoceptor agonists may cause vasodilation through the release of endothelial

(A) Histamine
(B) Norepinephrine
(C) Acetylcholine
(D) Nitric oxide

29. Emergency treatment of acute heart failure is best managed with which of the following drugs?

(A) Metaproterenol
(B) Phenylephrine
(C) Dobutamine
(D) Norepinephrine
(E) Isoproterenol

30. Which one of the following agents, when applied topically to the eye, would cause both mydriasis and cycloplegia?

(A) Phenylephrine
(B) Carbachol
(C) Prazosin
(D) Atropine

31. Neostigmine would be expected to reverse which one of the following conditions?

(A) Paralysis of skeletal muscle induced by a competitive, nondepolarizing muscle relaxant
(B) Paralysis of skeletal muscle induced by a depolarizing muscle relaxant
(C) Cardiac slowing induced by stimulation of the vagus nerve
(D) Miosis induced by bright light

32. The direct cardiac effects of dobutamine would be blocked by which one of the following agents?

(A) Prazosin
(B) Metoprolol
(C) Clonidine
(D) Isoproterenol

33. Topical application of timolol to the eye would be expected to induce which of the following?

(A) Miosis
(B) Mydriasis
(C) Decreased formation of aqueous humor
(D) Increased outflow of aqueous humor

34. Phenylephrine is used to treat patients with nasal mucosa stuffiness because it causes vasoconstriction by

(A) Blocking nicotinic cholinoceptors
(B) Blocking β-adrenoceptors
(C) Stimulating α-adrenoceptors
(D) Stimulating muscarinic cholinoceptors

Answers and Explanations

1. **The answer is C.** Botulinum toxin blocks calcium-dependent exocytosis of acetylcholine from storage vesicles, producing paralysis. Common sources of botulinum toxin include canned home goods and, in cases of infant botulism, honey. The condition is life threatening, and urgent care is necessary. Choline acetyltransferase is an enzyme catalyzing synthesis of acetylcholine from an acetate and choline. Sodium-dependent transport of choline can be blocked by hemicholinium. Enzyme acetylcholinesterase is responsible for catalyzing hydrolysis of acetylcholine. Acetylcholine synapses at the ganglia of many neurons and tissues, and this step is not blocked by botulinum toxin.

2. **The answer is D.** Guanethidine blocks the release of norepinephrine from storage vesicles into the nerve terminals. Acetylcholine release can be blocked by botulinum toxin. Epinephrine, dopamine, and serotonin release can be blocked by other agents (beyond the scope of this chapter), but not by guanethidine.

3. **The answer is A.** Cocaine is a potent inhibitor of norepinephrine uptake, a process that normally terminates norepinephrine's action. Oxidative deamination of norepinephrine in nerve terminals and the effector cells describes the action of monoamine oxidase, which is targeted by certain antidepressant medications. Inhibition of metabolism of norepinephrine in nerve terminals describes catechol-*O*-methyltransferase, which is found in nerve and other effector cells. Potentiation of tyrosine dehydroxylase would, in fact, cause excessive amounts of norepinephrine to accumulate; however, this enzyme is not affected by cocaine. Norepinephrine release can be blocked, not promoted, by agents such as bretylium and guanethidine.

4. **The answer is B.** β_2-agonists, like albuterol, activate G_s-protein, which results in stimulation of adenylyl cyclase, with subsequent increase in intracellular cAMP. Passage of sodium via ligand-gated ion channel is manifested by nicotinic acetylcholine receptors. Activation of G_q-protein resulting in increase of phosphatidylinositol and calcium mobilization refers to the mechanism of action of muscarinic receptors type M_1 and M_3, as well as α_1-adrenoceptors. Activation of G_q-protein resulting in increase of phosphatidylinositol and calcium mobilization refers to mechanism of action of M_2-cholinoceptors and α_2-adrenoceptors. Finally, binding to μ-receptors in the specific areas of the brain describes the action of opioid agents.

5. **The answer is E.** Bethanechol is a type of muscarinic receptor agonist that is used clinically to ameliorate urinary retention. Nicotinic blockers such as trimethaphan are rarely used in clinical practice because of the lack of selectivity. α-Agonists such as epinephrine can be used in management of acute bronchospasm (anaphylaxis). β_1-Blockers do not have direct effects on bronchial smooth muscle. β_2-Agonists such as albuterol are used for treatment of asthma.

6. **The answer is C.** Acetylcholinesterase reactivator pralidoxime has to be given within 30 minutes of exposure to insecticide because of the effects of "aging" (i.e., strengthening of the alkylphosphoryl-serine bond formed between AChE and organophosphate). Physostigmine is a cholinesterase inhibitor that is occasionally used in atropine or scopolamine poisoning. Propranolol is a β-blocker used for hypertension as well as other indications. Phenylephrine is an α-agonist used for hypotensive emergencies. Pancuronium is a nondepolarizing inhibitor of acetylcholine that is used for muscle paralysis.

7. **The answer is D.** Oxybutynin acts by binding to muscarinic receptors located on the detrusor muscle of the bladder, suppressing involuntary contraction of the muscle. Acetylcholinesterase inhibitors such as edrophonium are used for myasthenia gravis. Neuromuscular blockers such as succinylcholine are used for anesthesia. α_1-Antagonists such as terazosin are used for benign prostatic hypertrophy. β_2-Agonists such as terbutaline can be used to suppress premature labor.

8. **The answer is A.** Benztropine, an antimuscarinic agent, is used as an adjunct for treatment of Parkinson disease. Reserpine is a norepinephrine uptake inhibitor occasionally used for treatment of hypertension. Doxazocin, an α-blocker, is used for benign prostatic hyperplasia. Timolol is a β-blocker used for glaucoma. Tubocurarine is a neuromuscular blocker used in anesthesia.

9. **The answer is D.** Ipratropium bromide is used extensively for chronic obstructive pulmonary disease (COPD), which is the most likely diagnosis in this case. It acts by antagonizing muscarinic receptors in bronchial smooth muscle, thereby causing bronchodilation. Albuterol is also used for treatment of COPD; however, it can cause adverse cardiac effects such as tachycardia and is not recommended in this case. Prazosin is an α-blocker used for benign prostatic hypertrophy (BPH). Atenolol is a β-blocker used for hypertension. Pseudoephedrine is an α-agonist used for nasal congestion.

10. **The answer is B.** Succinylcholine is a depolarizing neuromuscular blocker that is used in rapid-sequence intubation, as well as other procedures. It quickly relaxes all muscles in the body, allowing a prompt intubation to prevent the reflux of gastric contents into the trachea. Baclofen is a centrally acting skeletal muscle relaxant used for spasticity. Neostigmine is an indirect-acting cholinergic agonist used for treatment of myasthenia gravis and reversal of neuromuscular blockade. Homatropine is an antimuscarinic agent used for induction of mydriasis for ophthalmologic examinations. Pralidoxime is an acetylcholinesterase reactivator used for organophosphate poisoning.

11. **The answer is C.** Ephedrine acts indirectly to release norepinephrine from nerve terminals, causing effects similar to those of catecholamines, including elevated blood pressure. This potentially dangerous agent has been removed from the OTC market because of an increasing number of deaths being reported as caused by this agent. An example of an indirect-acting cholinergic agonist is edrophonium, which is used for diagnosis of myasthenia gravis. Some adrenoceptor blockers, such as atenolol, are used for treatment of hypertension. Catecholamine reuptake inhibition is a property of some antidepressant medications. Dopamine receptor agonists are used in treatment of Parkinson disease.

12. **The answer is D.** Epinephrine is contraindicated as an anesthetic adjuvant for surgeries involving most facial structures, digits, and the penis, because of the risk of vascular compromise. This agent causes decreased blood loss for most other surgeries because of vasoconstriction. Although local anesthetic agents such as Marcaine or Xylocaine can cause mild local tissue swelling, epinephrine does not; either way, it is not a contraindication for hand surgery. Epinephrine causes elevated blood pressure when administered systemically; however, it has no systemic side effects when administered locally.

13. **The answer is B.** Amphetamine and similar compounds are stimulants used for treatment of attention-deficit/hyperactivity disorder (ADHD) in which they are thought to act centrally to increase attention span. Currently there is no medication on the U.S. market that inhibits reuptake of epinephrine. Blocking of the effects of norepinephrine will not alleviate symptoms of ADHD. Direct-acting cholinoceptor agonists are not used in treatment of ADHD. Serotonin reuptake inhibitors are used for depression and some other conditions.

14. **The answer is E.** Terbutaline, a β_2-agonist, is used to suppress premature labor because of its ability to stop uterine contractions. Tamsulosin, an α_1-blocker, is used for benign prostatic hypertrophy. Cevimeline, a cholinergic agonist, is used for Sjögren syndrome. Atracurium a non-depolarizing muscular blocker, is used for anesthesia. Tolterodine, a muscarinic blocker, is used for urinary incontinence.

15. **The answer is B.** α_1-Adrenoceptor agonists such as terazosin may cause significant postural hypotension, and should be prescribed carefully in the elderly population. Bronchospasm is a possible side effect of β-blockers. β-Blockers can also produce heart failure in some patients. Sedation is common with the use of some agents such as propranolol. Drug abuse can be observed in patients using centrally acting adrenoreceptor agonists such as amphetamine.

16. **The answer is A.** β-Blockers such as atenolol are now part of management of acute myocardial infarction, along with oxygen, nitroglycerin, and morphine. They reduce sympathetic activity and heart contractility, thereby reducing the oxygen demand. α-Agonists such as phenylephrine are used in management of hypotension due to shock. Muscarinic agonists such as pilocarpine can be used in management of glaucoma. Neuromuscular blockers such as atracuronium are used in anesthesia. Dopamine agonists are used in management of Parkinson disease.

17. **The answer is D.** The β-blocker propranolol is a good choice for an antihypertensive medication; however, it is also successfully used for other indications, such as prophylaxis of migraine headaches, situational anxiety, and hyperthyroidism-induced palpitations. The other choices are all acceptable antihypertensive medications, but from this list, only propranolol is used for migraine prophylaxis.

18. **The answer is D.** Metoprolol is more selective at β_1-adrenoceptors, which are more abundant in the heart than in the lungs. Like propranolol, it may be beneficial in the prophylaxis of migraine.

19. **The answer is D.** Prazosin is the only drug listed that blocks postjunctional α_1-adrenoceptors and inhibits epinephrine-mediated vasoconstriction.

20. **The answer is D.** Edrophonium, which will increase muscle strength in untreated myasthenic patients, is the preferred acetylcholinesterase inhibitor (Tensilon test) because it has a short duration of action.

21. **The answer is B.** Pilocarpine is a muscarinic cholinoceptor agonist.

22. **The answer is B.** Plasma cholinesterase is responsible for the rapid inactivation of succinylcholine.

23. **The answer is A.** In patients with malignant hyperthermia, a rare hereditary disorder, an impaired sarcoplasmic reticulum is unable to sequester calcium. The sudden release of calcium results in extensive muscle contraction that can be reduced with dantrolene.

24. **The answer is A.** Clonidine acts at prejunctional α_2-adrenoceptors and is used to treat hypertension. Methoxamine is a non-selective α-adrenoceptor agonist. Metaproterenol is a selective β_2-adrenoceptor agonist. Dobutamine is a relatively selective β_1-adrenoceptor agonist. Dopamine activates both pre-junctional and postjunctional dopamine receptors and also β_1-adrenoceptor.

25. **The answer is B.** In the absence of a nicotinic receptor antagonist, norepinephrine may result in a reflex baroreceptor-mediated increase in vagal activity. The presence of such an agent unmasks the direct stimulant effect of norepinephrine on heart rate.

26. **The answer is E.** Atropine blocks the effects of increased acetylcholine resulting from cholinesterase inhibition. Physostigmine indirectly activates cholinoceptors; bethanechol and pilocarpine directly activate cholinoceptors. Propanolol is a β-adrenoceptor antagonist.

27. **The answer is A.** Nicotinic cholinoceptors are found in adrenal medullary chromaffin cells. At the other sites, acetylcholine activates muscarinic cholinoceptors.

28. **The answer is D.** The release of nitric oxide activates guanylate cyclase, increasing guanosine 3′,5′-monophosphate (cyclic GMP) and sequestering calcium. This leads to a relaxation of vascular smooth muscle.

29. **The answer is C.** Dobutamine, a relatively selective β_1-adrenoceptor agonist, increases cardiac output and lowers peripheral resistance. Metaproterenol has a relatively more selective action on the respiratory system than the cardiovascular system. Phenylephrine and norepinephrine increase peripheral resistance. Isoproterenol increases heart rate.

30. **The answer is D.** Atropine produces both mydriasis and cycloplegia (the inability to accommodate for near vision). Phenylephrine causes mydriasis without cycloplegia. Carbachol causes pupillary constriction. Prazosin is an α-adrenoceptor antagonist.

31. **The answer is A.** Acetylcholine accumulation due to neostigmine inhibition of cholinesterase will reverse the action of the competitive neuromuscular blocking agents.

32. **The answer is B.** The β_1-adrenoceptor antagonist metoprolol blocks the β_1-adrenoceptor activity of dobutamine.

33. **The answer is C.** β-Adrenoceptor blocking agents such as timolol reduce aqueous humor formation.

34. **The answer is C.** Phenylephrine activates α-adrenoceptors, producing vasoconstriction.

chapter 3

Drugs Acting on the Renal System

I. DIURETICS

A. Introduction

1. ***Function.*** Diuretics **increase urine production** by acting on the kidney (Fig. 3-1). Most agents affect water balance indirectly by altering electrolyte reabsorption or secretion. Osmotic agents affect water balance directly.
2. ***Effects.*** Natriuretic diuretics produce **diuresis,** associated with increased sodium (Na^+) excretion, which results in a concomitant loss of water and a reduction of extracellular volume.
3. ***Therapeutic uses.*** Diuretic agents are generally used for the management of edema, hypertension, **congestive heart failure (CHF),** and abnormalities in body fluid distribution.
4. ***Side effects.*** Diuretics can cause electrolyte imbalances such as hypokalemia, hyponatremia, and hypochloremia and disturbances in acid–base balance.

B. Thiazide diuretics

1. ***Mechanism.*** Thiazide diuretics are **absorbed from the gastrointestinal (GI) tract** and produce diuresis within 1–2 hours. They are **secreted into the lumen** of the proximal tubule via an organic acid carrier. They exert effects only after reaching the lumen.
   - a. These agents inhibit active reabsorption of sodium chloride (NaCl) in the distal convoluted tubule by interfering with Na^+–Cl^- cotransporter (NCC), a specific Na^+/Cl^- transport protein (Fig. 3-2), resulting in the net excretion of Na^+ and an accompanying volume of water.
     - **(1)** These agents increase excretion of Cl^-, Na^+, potassium (K^+), and, at high doses, HCO_3^-.
     - **(2)** They reduce excretion of calcium (Ca^{2+}).
   - b. Thiazide diuretics can be derivatives of sulfonamides (sulfonamide diuretics). Many also **inhibit carbonic anhydrase,** resulting in diminished bicarbonate (HCO_3^-) reabsorption by the proximal tubule.
2. ***Specific agents***
   - a. **Prototype drugs** include **chlorothiazide** and **hydrochlorothiazide.** Other agents include methyclothiazide. Chlorothiazide is the only thiazide available for parenteral use.
   - b. **Thiazide-like drugs. Quinazolinones** (e.g., **metolazone, chlorthalidone**) and **indolines** (e.g., **indapamide**) have properties generally similar to those of the thiazide diuretics (Table 3-1). However, unlike thiazides, these agents may be effective in the presence of some renal impairment. Indapamide has proven especially useful in diabetic patients with hypertension, where it reduces the risk of cardiovascular disease.
3. ***Therapeutic uses***
   - a. Thiazide diuretics are the preferred class of diuretic for treatment of **hypertension** when renal function is normal; they are often used in combination with other antihypertensive agents to enhance their blood pressure-lowering effects.
   - b. These agents reduce the formation of new calcium stones in **idiopathic hypercalciuria.**
   - c. Thiazide diuretics may be useful in patients with diabetes insipidus that is not responsive to antidiuretic hormone (ADH).

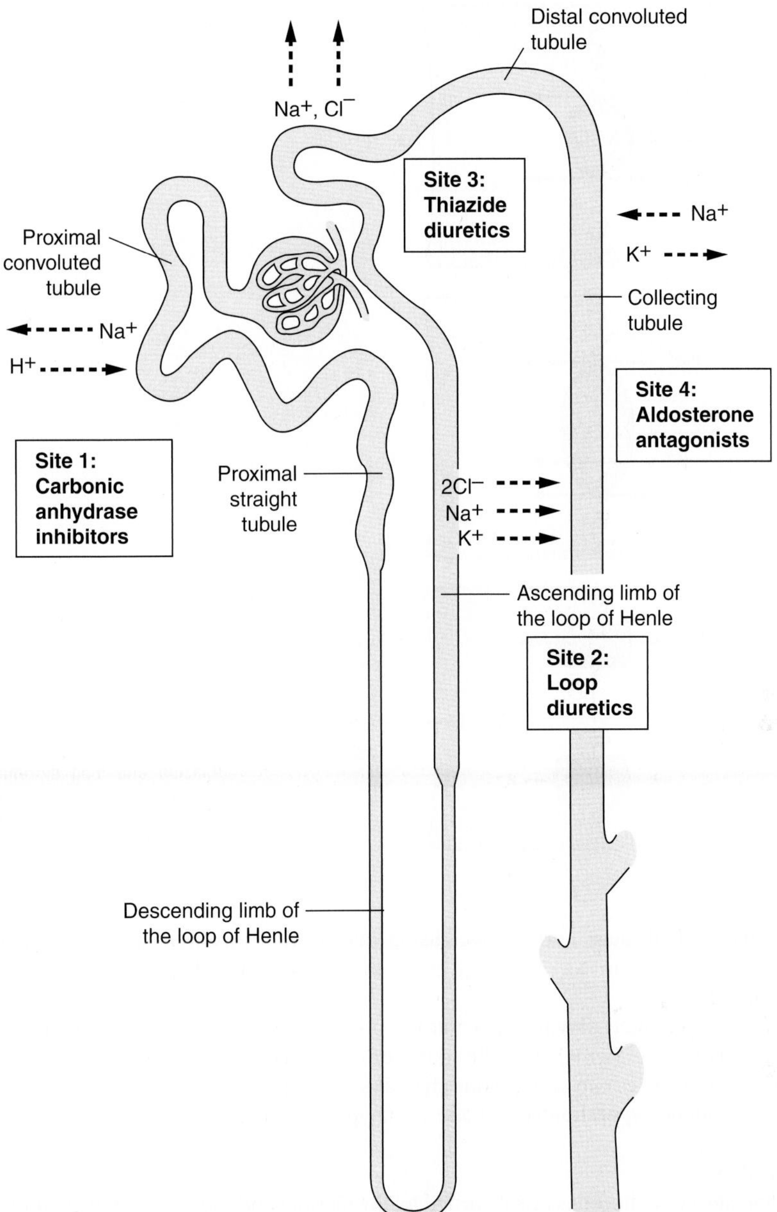

FIGURE 3-1. The nephron can be divided into four sites anatomically and pharmacologically. Site 1 is the proximal tubule, site of action of carbonic anhydrase inhibitors. Site 2 is the ascending limb of the loop of Henle, site of action of the loop diuretics. Site 3 is the distal convoluted tubule, site of action of the thiazides. Site 4 is the collecting tubule, site of action of aldosterone antagonists. Cl^-, chloride; H^+, hydrogen; K^+, potassium; Na^+, sodium.

d. These agents are often used in combination with a potassium-sparing diuretic to manage **mild cardiac edema, cirrhotic** or **nephrotic edema,** and **edema produced by hormone imbalances.** They are frequently used in the treatment of **Ménière disease.**

4. ***Adverse effects and contraindications.*** Thiazide diuretics should be used cautiously in the presence of renal or hepatic diseases such as cirrhosis, and they should be used only as an ancillary treatment in nephrotic syndrome.

a. Thiazide diuretics produce electrolyte imbalances such as **hypokalemia, hyponatremia,** and **hypochloremic alkalosis.** These imbalances are often accompanied by central nervous system (CNS) disturbances, including dizziness, confusion, and irritability; muscle weakness;

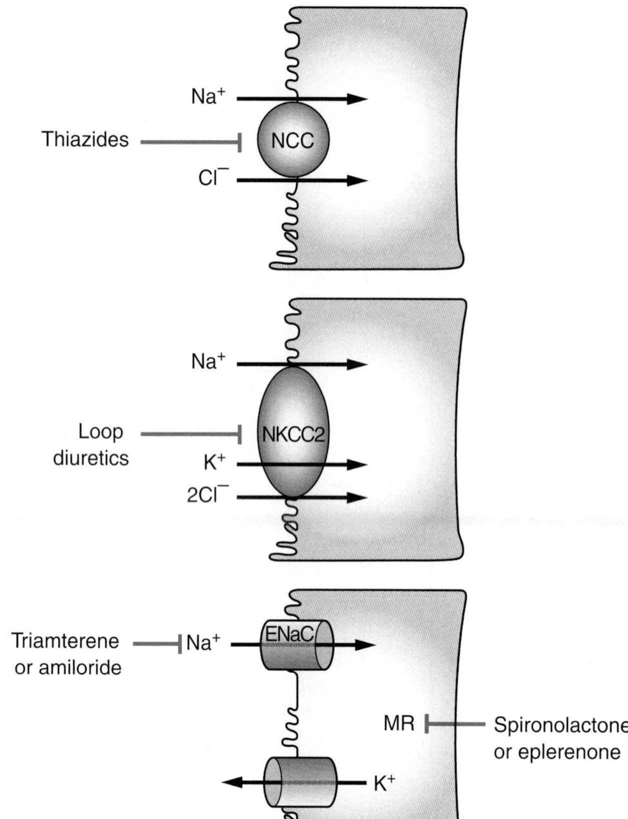

FIGURE 3-2. The molecular targets of thiazide and loop diuretics are transmembrane cotransporter channels, whereas the molecular target of amiloride is a specific Na^+ channel.

cardiac arrhythmias; and by decreasing plasma K^+, increased sensitivity to digitalis-like drugs. Diets low in Na^+ and high in K^+ are recommended; K^+ supplementation may be required.

b. These agents often **elevate serum urate,** presumably as a result of competition for the organic acid carrier (which also eliminates uric acid). Goutlike symptoms may appear.

c. Thiazide diuretics can cause **hyperglycemia** (especially in patients with diabetes)**, hypertriglyceridemia, hypercholesterolemia**, and hypersensitivity reactions.

C. Loop diuretics

1. *Mechanism.* Loop diuretics are absorbed by the GI tract and are eliminated by filtration and tubular secretion; some elimination occurs via the hepatic–biliary route. They are administered either orally or parenterally. Diuresis occurs within 5 minutes of intravenous (IV) administration and within 30 minutes of oral administration.

table 3-1 Thiazide Diuretics and Related Agents

Drug	Chemical Class	Potency	Half-Life (h)
Chlorothiazide	Benzothiadiazide	0.1	2
Hydrochlorothiazide	Benzothiadiazide	1.0	3
Metolazone	Quinazoline	5	5
Chlorthalidone	Quinazoline	10	26
Indapamide	Indoline	20	16

a. Loop diuretics inhibit active NaCl reabsorption in the thick ascending limb of the loop of Henle by inhibiting NKCC2, a specific $Na^+/K^+/2Cl^-$ cotransporter. Because of the high capacity for NaCl reabsorption in this segment, agents active at this site markedly increase water and electrolyte excretion and are referred to as **high-ceiling diuretics.**

b. Loop diuretics cause increased renal prostaglandin production, which accounts for some of their activity

c. These agents reduce reabsorption of Cl^- and Na^+; they increase K^+, magnesium (Mg^{2+}), and Ca^{2+} excretion.

2. ***Specific agents.*** Prototype drugs include furosemide and its derivatives piretanide and bumetanide, as well as ethacrynic acid and torsemide.

3. ***Therapeutic uses***

a. Loop diuretics are used in the treatment of **CHF** by reducing **acute pulmonary edema** and edema refractory to other agents. They are synergistic with thiazide diuretics when coadministered.

b. These agents are used to treat **hypertension,** especially in individuals with diminished renal function.

c. They are also used to treat acute **hypercalcemia** and **halide poisoning.**

d. These drugs are often effective in producing diuresis in patients responding maximally to other types of diuretics.

4. ***Adverse effects and contraindications***

a. Loop diuretics produce **hypotension** and **volume depletion,** as well as **hypokalemia,** because of enhanced secretion of K^+. They may also produce **alkalosis** due to enhanced H^+ secretion. **Mg^{2+} wasting** can also occur; therapy is often instituted gradually to minimize electrolyte imbalances and volume depletion.

b. Loop diuretics can cause dose-related **ototoxicity,** more often in individuals with renal impairment. These effects are more pronounced with ethacrynic acid than with furosemide. These agents should be administered cautiously in the presence of renal disease or with use of other ototoxic agents such as **aminoglycosides.**

c. These agents can cause hypersensitivity reactions. Ethacrynic acid produces GI disturbances.

D. Potassium-sparing diuretics

1. ***Mechanism***

a. Potassium-sparing diuretics reduce **Na^+ reabsorption** and reduce **K^+ secretion** in the distal part of the nephron (collecting tubule).

b. These are not potent diuretics when used alone; they are primarily used in combination with other diuretics.

2. ***Selected drugs***

a. **Antagonists of the mineralocorticoid** (aldosterone) **receptor** include **eplerenone,** which is highly receptor selective, and **spironolactone,** which binds to other nuclear receptors such as the androgen receptor.

(1) Mechanism. These agents inhibit the action of aldosterone by competitively binding to the mineralocorticoid receptor and preventing subsequent cellular events that regulate K^+ and H^+ secretion and Na^+ reabsorption. An important action is a reduction in the biosynthesis of ENaC, the Na^+ channel in principal cells of the collecting duct.

(a) These agents are active only when endogenous mineralocorticoid is present; effects are enhanced when hormone levels are elevated.

(b) These agents are **absorbed** from the **GI tract** and are **metabolized** in the **liver;** therapeutic effects are achieved only after several days.

(2) **Therapeutic uses.** These drugs are generally used in combination with a thiazide or loop diuretic to treat **hypertension, CHF,** and **refractory edema.** They are also used to induce diuresis in clinical situations associated with hyperaldosteronism, such as in **adrenal hyperplasia** and in the presence of **aldosterone-producing adenomas** when surgery is not feasible.

(3) Adverse effects and contraindications
(a) These agents can cause **hyperkalemia, hyperchloremic metabolic acidosis,** and arrhythmias. Spironolactone is associated with **gynecomastia** and can also cause menstrual abnormalities in women.
(b) These drugs are **contraindicated in renal insufficiency,** especially in diabetic patients. They must be used cautiously in the presence of liver disease. They are contraindicated in the presence of other potassium-sparing diuretics and should be used with extreme **caution** in individuals taking an **angiotensin-converting enzyme (ACE) inhibitor.**

b. **Amiloride and triamterene**
(1) **Mechanism.** Amiloride and triamterene bind to and block ENaC and thereby decrease absorption of Na^+ and excretion of K^+ in the cortical collecting tubule, independent of the presence of mineralocorticoids.
(a) These drugs produce diuretic effects 2–4 hours after oral administration.
(b) **Triamterene** increases urinary excretion of Mg^{2+}; amiloride does not; triamterene and amiloride are metabolized in the liver. Both drugs are **secreted** in the **proximal tubule.**
(2) **Therapeutic uses.** These agents are used to manage **CHF, cirrhosis,** and **edema** caused by secondary hyperaldosteronism. They are available in combination products containing thiazide or loop diuretics (e.g., triamterene/hydrochlorothiazide, amiloride/hydrochlorothiazide) to treat hypertension.
(3) **Adverse effects and contraindications.** Amiloride and triamterene produce **hyperkalemia,** the most common adverse effect, and ventricular arrhythmias. Dietary potassium intake should be reduced. Minor adverse effects include nausea and vomiting. Use of these drugs is contraindicated in the presence of diminished renal function.

E. Carbonic anhydrase inhibitors

1. ***Mechanism.*** Carbonic anhydrase inhibitors inhibit carbonic anhydrase in all parts of the body. In the kidney, the effects are predominantly in the proximal tubule.
   a. These drugs reduce HCO_3^- reabsorption and concomitant Na^+ uptake. They also inhibit excretion of hydrogen (H^+) and coupled Na^+ uptake.
   b. Carbonic anhydrase inhibitors are **absorbed** from the **GI tract** and are **secreted** by the **proximal tubule.** Urine pH changes are observed within 30 minutes.
2. ***Prototype drugs*** include **acetazolamide** and **methazolamide.** These agents are **sulfonamide derivatives,** forerunners of thiazide diuretics. (Thiazides separate natriuresis from carbonic anhydrase inhibition.)
3. ***Therapeutic uses.*** Carbonic anhydrase inhibitors are rarely used as diuretics.
   a. These drugs are most useful in the treatment of **glaucoma.** They serve to decrease the rate of HCO_3^- formation in the aqueous humor and consequently reduce ocular pressure.
   b. Carbonic anhydrase inhibitors are sometimes used as adjuvants for the treatment of **seizure disorder,** but the development of tolerance limits their use.
   c. These agents may be used to produce a desired alkalinization of urine to **enhance renal secretion of uric acid and cysteine.**
   d. They may be used for prophylaxis and treatment of **acute mountain sickness.**
4. ***Adverse reactions and contraindications***
   a. Adverse reactions include **metabolic acidosis** due to reduction in bicarbonate stores. Urine alkalinity decreases the solubility of calcium salts and increases the propensity for renal calculi formation. **Potassium wasting** may be severe.
   b. Following large doses, carbonic anhydrase inhibitors commonly produce drowsiness and paresthesias.
   c. Use of these drugs is **contraindicated** in the presence of **hepatic cirrhosis.**

F. Agents influencing water excretion

1. ***Osmotic agents*** include **mannitol, glycerin, urea, and hypertonic saline.** These agents are easily filtered, poorly reabsorbable solutes that alter the diffusion of water relative to sodium by "binding" water. As a result, net reabsorption of Na^+ is reduced.

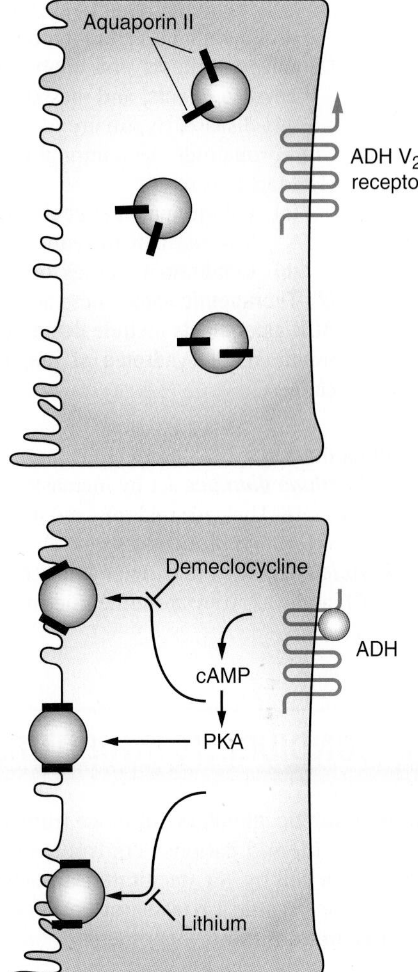

FIGURE 3-3. The mechanism of action of ADH includes ligand binding to the V_2 receptor, which is coupled to increased cAMP production. This ultimately causes an increase in the insertion of the water-specific transporter aquaporin II into the apical plasma membrane.

a. **Mannitol** and **urea** are administered intravenously.
   (1) Therapeutic uses
      (a) **Mannitol** is used in **prophylaxis of acute renal failure** resulting from physical trauma or surgery. Even when filtration is reduced, sufficient mannitol usually enters the tubule to promote urine output.
      (b) **Mannitol** may also be useful for reducing cerebral edema and intraocular pressure.
      (c) Parenteral **urea** is approved for the reduction of intracranial and intraocular pressure.
   (2) **Adverse effects and contraindications.** Because the osmotic forces that reduce intracellular volume ultimately expand extracellular volume, serious adverse effects may occur in patients with CHF. Minor adverse effects include headache and nausea.
b. **Glycerin** is administered orally. This drug is used primarily for **ophthalmic procedures.** Topical anhydrous glycerin is useful for **corneal edema.**

2. ***Agents that influence the action of ADH (vasopressin)*** influence the permeability of the luminal surface of the medullary collecting duct to water by causing water-specific water channels called aquaporin II to be inserted into the plasma membrane (Fig. 3-3). Under conditions of dehydration, ADH levels increase to conserve body water. Agents that **elevate** or mimic ADH are **antidiuretic;** agents that **lower** or antagonize ADH action are **diuretic.**
   a. Vasopressin or analogues
      (1) **Therapeutic uses.** These agents are useful in the management of ADH-sensitive **diabetes insipidus. Desmopressin** (DDAVP), one of the most useful analogues, is also used to

treat **nocturnal enuresis.** Studies have suggested that vasopressin and its analogues are useful to maintain blood pressure in patients with **septic shock.**

(2) **Adverse effects and contraindications.** These drugs produce serious **cardiac-related adverse effects,** and they should be used with caution in individuals with coronary artery disease. Hyponatremia occurs in ~5% of patients.

b. Chlorpropamide, acetaminophen, indomethacin, and clofibrate

(1) Mechanisms

(a) **Chlorpropamide, acetaminophen,** and **indomethacin** enhance the action of ADH, at least partially by reducing production of prostaglandins in the kidney.

(b) **Clofibrate** increases the release of ADH centrally.

(2) **Therapeutic uses.** These agents are useful as antidiuretics in diabetic patients.

c. **ADH antagonists** include **demeclocycline** and **lithium carbonate.** They may be useful in the treatment of **syndrome of inappropriate ADH (SIADH)** secretion as seen in some lung cancers.

G. Other diuretics

1. ***Xanthine diuretics*** act by increasing cardiac output and promoting a higher glomerular filtration rate. They are seldom used as diuretics, but diuresis occurs under other clinical applications (e.g., for bronchodilatation).
2. ***Acidifying salts*** (e.g., **ammonium chloride**) lower pH and increase luminal concentrations of Cl^- and Na^+. They are sometimes used in combination with high-ceiling diuretics to counteract alkalosis.

II. NONDIURETIC INHIBITORS OF TUBULAR TRANSPORT

A. Nondiuretic inhibitors influence transport of organic anions, including the endogenous anion uric acid, and cations. Transport takes place in the proximal tubule; organic compounds enter a cell by Na^+-facilitated diffusion and are excreted from the cell into the lumen by a specific organic ion transporter. ***Para*-aminohippurate,** not used clinically, is a classic compound used to study these phenomena.

B. Uricosuric agents

1. ***Mechanism.*** Uricosuric agents **increase excretion of uric acid.** Paradoxically, because of the balance among uptake into a cell, excretion from the cell, and reabsorption from the lumen, low doses of these agents often decrease excretion, whereas high doses increase excretion.
2. ***Therapeutic uses.*** These drugs are often used in the treatment of gout.
3. ***Selected drugs***

a. Probenecid

(1) Mechanism. Probenecid is absorbed from the GI tract and is secreted by the proximal tubule.

(a) Probenecid **inhibits secretion of organic acids** (e.g., from the plasma to the tubular lumen). Probenecid was developed to **decrease secretion of penicillin** (an organic acid) and thus prolong elimination of this antibiotic. Other drugs whose secretion is inhibited by probenecid include **indomethacin** and **methotrexate.**

(b) At higher doses, probenecid also **decreases reabsorption of uric acid by inhibiting URAT1, a urate transport protein.** This results in a net increase in urate excretion and accounts for the drug's usefulness in treating gout.

(2) **Therapeutic uses.** Probenecid is used to prevent **gout** in individuals with normal renal function. It is also used as an **adjuvant to penicillin therapy** when prolonged serum levels following a single dose are required or to enhance antibiotic concentrations in the CNS.

(3) **Adverse effects and contraindications.** The most common adverse effects of probenecid are hypersensitivity reactions and gastric irritation.

b. Allopurinol

(1) Mechanism. Allopurinol is not a uricosuric agent. It **inhibits xanthine oxidase,** which is involved in the synthesis of uric acid. Allopurinol is metabolized by xanthine oxidase to produce **alloxanthine,** which has long-lasting inhibitory effects on the enzyme; the net result is **decreased production of uric acid.**

(2) Therapeutic uses. Allopurinol is used in the treatment of **gout.**

DRUG SUMMARY TABLE

Diuretics—Thiazides
Chlorothiazide (Diuril, generic)
Hydrochlorothiazide (Esidrix, Oretic, others)
Methyclothiazide (Aquatensin, Enduron)
Polythiazide (Renese)

Diuretics—Thiazide-like
Metolazone (Zaroxolyn)
Chlorthalidone (Hydone, Thalitone)
Indapamide (Lozol)

Diuretics—Loop
Furosemide (Lasix, Delone, generic)
Bumetanide (Bumex)
Ethacrynic acid (Edecrin)
Torsemide (Demadex, generic)

Diuretics—Potassium Sparing
Spirolactone (Aldactone, generic)
Amiloride (Midamor, generic)
Triamterene (Dyrenium)
Eplerenone (Inspra)

Carbonic Anhydrase Inhibitors
Acetazolamide (Diamox)
Methazolamide (GlaucTabs)
Dichlorphenamide (Daranide)

Osmotic Diuretics
Mannitol (Osmitrol)
Urea (generic)
Glycerin (generic)

Antidiuretic Hormone Agonists
Desmopressin (DDAVP)
Lysine vasopressin (generic)
Vasopressin (Pitressin)

Antidiuretic Antagonists
Demeclocycline (Declomycin)
Lithium carbonate (generic)

Uricosuric Agents
Probenecid (generic)

Urate Synthesis Inhibitors
Allopurinol (Aloprim, Zyloprim)

Other Antigout Agents
Colchicine (generic)

Review Test for Chapter 3

Directions: Each of the numbered items or incomplete statements in this section is followed by answers or by completions of the statement. Select the ONE lettered answer or completion that is BEST in each case.

1. A 35-year-old woman presents to your office for a regular check-up. She has no complaints. On examination, her blood pressure is slightly elevated at 145/85. She is physically fit and follows a healthy diet. You decide to start her on antihypertensive therapy and prescribe hydrochlorothiazide. How does this agent work?

(A) Inhibits reabsorption of sodium chloride in the early distal convoluted tubule
(B) Decreases net excretion of chloride, sodium, and potassium
(C) Increases excretion of calcium
(D) Inhibits reabsorption of sodium chloride in the thick ascending limb of the loop of Henle
(E) Interferes with potassium secretion

2. A 7-year-old boy is brought to the clinic by his mother. He complains of sharp pain in his flanks, as well as dysuria and frequency. The doctor orders a 24-hour urine calcium test, and the results come back abnormal. After additional work-up, the child is diagnosed with idiopathic hypercalciuria. What is a common type of medication used for this aliment?

(A) Loop diuretics
(B) Carbonic anhydrase inhibitors
(C) Thiazide diuretics
(D) Potassium-sparing diuretics
(E) Osmotic diuretics

3. A 45-year-old man with a history of medication-controlled hypertension presents to your office with complaints of a painful, swollen big toe on the left foot. You suspect gout and check his uric acid levels, which are elevated. From looking at the list of the medications the patient is taking, you realize that one of the medications may be the cause of his current symptoms. Which medication might that be?

(A) Acetazolamide
(B) Amiloride
(C) Spironolactone
(D) Hydrochlorothiazide
(E) Mannitol

4. A 57-year-old man with a history of heavy alcohol use is being admitted for a first episode of congestive heart failure (CHF), which likely resulted from untreated alcoholic cardiomyopathy. The cardiologist decides to start the patient on diuretic therapy. Which class of diuretics is preferred in this scenario?

(A) Loop diuretics, because they exert their action at the distal convoluted tubule
(B) Loop diuretics, because the thick ascending limb is an area of high capacity for NaCl reabsorption
(C) Thiazide diuretics, because they exert their action at the thick ascending limb of the loop of Henle
(D) Thiazide diuretics, because they increase cardiac output
(E) Thiazide diuretics, because they increase peripheral vascular resistance

5. A 66-year-old woman suffers a myocardial infarction while in the hospital and immediately goes into respiratory distress. On examination you realize the patient has flash pulmonary edema as a result of her infarction. Along with the management of the myocardial infarction, you start the patient on furosemide therapy to treat pulmonary edema. What is the mechanism of action of this agent?

(A) Inhibition of action of aldosterone by binding to its receptor in principal cells of the collecting duct
(B) Reduction of bicarbonate reabsorption and concomitant sodium uptake
(C) Inhibition of active reabsorption of sodium chloride at the distal convoluted tubule
(D) Alteration of the diffusion of water relative to sodium, thereby reducing sodium reabsorption
(E) Inhibition of active reabsorption of sodium chloride at the thick ascending limb of the loop of Henle

6. An 87-year-old woman who is taking multiple medications for her "heart disease" is prescribed gentamicin for diverticulitis. After a few days of taking the antibiotic, she complains of dizziness and tinnitus. What "heart medication" might she be on?

(A) Spironolactone
(B) Hydrochlorothiazide
(C) Mannitol
(D) Ethacrynic acid
(E) Urea

7. A 54-year-old man develops congestive heart failure (CHF) after suffering his second myocardial infarction. His physician puts him on a regimen of several medications, including furosemide. On follow-up, the patient is found to have hypokalemia, likely secondary to furosemide use. The addition of which medication would likely resolve the problem of hypokalemia, while helping to treat the underlying condition, CHF?

(A) Allopurinol
(B) Hydrochlorothiazide
(C) Spironolactone
(D) Acetazolamide
(E) Ethacrynic acid

8. A 60-year-old previously healthy fit man presents to your office with new-onset hypertension. Since this is an unusual age to present with essential hypertension, you order an extensive work-up. The results show low levels of potassium, high levels of aldosterone, and low levels of renin. The patient is diagnosed with Conn syndrome, or hyperaldosteronism. A computed tomographic (CT) scan of the abdomen reveals bilateral adrenal hyperplasia, which renders this patient inoperable. You decide to start the patient on spironolactone therapy. How does this medication work?

(A) It is an agonist of the mineralocorticoid receptor
(B) It interferes with the action of the mineralocorticoid receptor
(C) It promotes sodium reabsorption
(D) It increases the synthesis of sodium channels in the principal cells
(E) It is only active when endogenous mineralocorticoids are absent

9. A 45-year-old woman with a long history of alcohol abuse is being treated for cirrhosis-associated ascites. Her internist decided to give her amiloride, a diuretic helpful in edema caused by cirrhosis. What common side effect should be monitored in this patient?

(A) Hypernatremia
(B) Hypocalcemia
(C) Hyperphosphatemia
(D) Hypermagnesemia
(E) Hyperkalemia

10. A 57-year-old man develops progressive vision loss with a sensation of pressure behind his eyes. His ophthalmologist diagnoses the patient with glaucoma. To prevent further progression of the disease and to alleviate current symptoms, the physician starts the patient on acetazolamide therapy. What is the mechanism of action of this medication?

(A) Potentiates carbonic anhydrase in all parts of the body
(B) Reduces reabsorption of bicarbonate
(C) Increases excretion of hydrogen
(D) Increases rate of formation of bicarbonate in the aqueous humor
(E) Increases uptake of sodium in the proximal tubule

Answers and Explanations

1. **The answer is A.** Thiazide diuretics inhibit active reabsorption of sodium chloride in the early distal convoluted tubule of the nephron by interfering with the Na/Cl cotransporter, resulting in net excretion of sodium and water. These agents increase net excretion of chloride, sodium, and potassium. They decrease excretion of calcium. Inhibiting reabsorption of sodium chloride in the thick ascending limb of the loop of Henle describes the mechanism of action of loop diuretics. Interfering with potassium secretion refers to mechanism of action of potassium-sparing diuretics.

2. **The answer is C.** Thiazide diuretics decrease excretion of calcium and thus can be used for idiopathic hypercalciuria. Loop diuretics stimulate tubular calcium excretion and can thus be used to treat hypercalcemia. Carbonic anhydrase inhibitors, potassium-sparing diuretics, and osmotic diuretics do not have a significant impact on net calcium balance.

3. **The answer is D.** Hydrochlorothiazide, a thiazide diuretic, can precipitate a gouty attack in predisposed individuals. This is because these agents increase serum uric acid as a result of competition for the organic acid carrier. Loop diuretics can have this effect too. Acetazolamide is a carbonic anhydrase inhibitor; this agent does not have a significant impact on the levels of uric acid. Amiloride and spironolactone are potassium-sparing diuretics, and they do not have a significant impact on the levels of uric acid either. The same is true for mannitol, an osmotic diuretic.

4. **The answer is B.** Loop diuretics are used in cases of congestive heart failure (CHF) and pulmonary edema because they result in fast and significant diuresis. These agents exert their action at the thick ascending limb of the loop of Henle, which is the area of highest capacity for NaCl reabsorption. Thiazide diuretics actually decrease cardiac output initially, because of decrease blood volume. As well, thiazides decrease peripheral vascular resistance, because they relax arteriolar smooth muscle.

5. **The answer is E.** Loop diuretics inhibit active NaCl reabsorption in the thick ascending limb of the loop of Henle by inhibiting a specific $Na^+/K^+/2\ Cl^-$ cotransporter. Inhibition of action of aldosterone by binding to its receptor in principal cells of the collecting duct describes the mechanism of action of potassium-sparing diuretics. Reduction of bicarbonate reabsorption and concomitant sodium uptake refers to carbonic anhydrase inhibitors. Inhibition of active reabsorption of sodium chloride at the distal convoluted tubule describes thiazide diuretics. Finally, alteration of the diffusion of water relative to sodium, thereby reducing sodium reabsorption, refers to osmotic diuretics.

6. **The answer is D.** Ototoxicity, as demonstrated by tinnitus and dizziness, is a common side effect of loop diuretics, especially ethacrynic acid. This effect is magnified when aminoglycoside antibiotics are added to the regimen. A common side effect of spironolactone is gynecomastia. Hydrochlorothiazide can cause gout in susceptible individuals. Mannitol and urea are osmotic diuretics and are not indicated in patients with heart disease, especially congestive heart failure (CHF).

7. **The answer is C.** Spironolactone is commonly added to the regimen of anti-congestive heart failure (CHF) medications, since it counteracts the loss of potassium caused by the loop diuretics such as furosemide. This agent is also effective in reducing the symptoms of refractory edema. Allopurinol is not used to treat CHF. Hydrochlorothiazide will exacerbate hypokalemia caused by the loop diuretics. Acetozolomide will not counteract hypokalemia. Ethacrynic acid is an example of another loop diuretic.

8. **The answer is B.** Sprironolactone interferes with the action of the mineralocorticoid receptor. Spironolactone prevents cellular events that regulate potassium and hydrogen secretion and sodium reabsorption. Spironolactone is an antagonist of mineralocorticoid receptors. It decreases

the synthesis of sodium channels in the principal cells of the collecting ducts. This agent is only active when endogenous mineralocorticoids are present.

9. **The answer is E.** Hyperkalemia, a potentially life-threatening side effect, should be recognized as a possible result of amiloride use. Hyponatremia, not hypernatremia, can be observed with amiloride. This agent does not affect calcium or phosphorus balance to a significant degree. Triamterene, another potassium-sparing diuretic, can cause increased urinary excretion of magnesium; amiloride is not known to produce this effect.

10. **The answer is B.** Acetazolamide belongs to a class of medications termed carbonic anhydrase inhibitors. These agents reduce bicarbonate reabsorption in the proximal tubule. They inhibit carbonic anhydrase in all parts of the body, including the aqueous humor, which makes these agents very useful in treatment of glaucoma. Acetazolamide inhibits excretion of hydrogen and concomitant sodium uptake.

chapter 4

Drugs Acting on the Cardiovascular System

I. AGENTS USED TO TREAT CONGESTIVE HEART FAILURE (CHF)

A. Overview

1. ***CHF*** results when the output of the heart is insufficient to supply adequate levels of oxygen for the body. Impaired contractility and circulatory congestion are both components of failure. Compensatory elevation in angiotensin II production results in sodium retention and vasoconstriction and increases both matrix formation and remodeling.
2. ***Therapeutic agents*** (Fig. 4-1)
   a. Increase cardiac contractility
   b. Reduce preload (left ventricular filling pressure) and aortic impedance (systemic vascular resistance)
   c. Normalize heart rate and rhythm

B. Drugs That Inhibit the Activity of the Renin–Angiotensin System

1. ***Overview***
   a. **Drugs that either interfere with the biosynthesis of angiotensin II (angiotensin converting enzyme [ACE] inhibitors),** or act as antagonists of angiotensin receptors (**angiotensin receptor blockers [ARBs]**), are indicated in all patients with left ventricular (LV) dysfunction, whether symptomatic or asymptomatic. ACE inhibitors are becoming increasingly important in the treatment of CHF and have been shown to prevent or slow the progression of heart failure in patients with ventricular dysfunction. Agents that inhibit **renin activity** are useful for treating hypertension.
   b. Principles of the renin–angiotensin system (Fig. 4-2)
2. Several parameters regulate the **release of renin** from the kidney cortex. Reduced arterial pressure, decreased sodium delivery to the cortex, increased sodium at the distal tubule, and stimulation of sympathetic activity all increase renin release.
3. Renin cleaves the protein angiotensinogen and **releases the decapeptide angiotensin I.** Angiotensin I is converted enzymatically (mostly in the lung) to an octapeptide, **angiotensin II** (**AgII** or Ag1-8), by the activity of **ACE;** further metabolism produces the heptapeptide **angiotensin III (Ag2-8).** Both angiotensin II and angiotensin III stimulate the **release of aldosterone.** Angiotensin I can also be metabolized by **ACE2 to Ag1-7. The actions of Ag1-7 oppose those of AgII.**
4. Angiotensin II is a vasoconstricting agent and **causes sodium retention via release of aldosterone;** angiotensin III is less active as a vasoconstricting agent than angiotensin II.
5. The actions of angiotensin II are mediated by AT1, AT2, and AT4 receptors located in most tissues. The pressor actions of angiotensin II are mediated by AT1 receptors. Ag1-7 acts via the MARS receptor.
6. Angiotensin II can be produced locally (e.g., in the myocardium, kidney, adrenals, or in vessel walls by the action of non-ACE pathways) by the action of chymases and cathepsins.
7. Because angiotensin I is produced via pathways other than the ACE pathway, angiotensin II receptor antagonists may be more effective and specific in reducing angiotensin II actions.

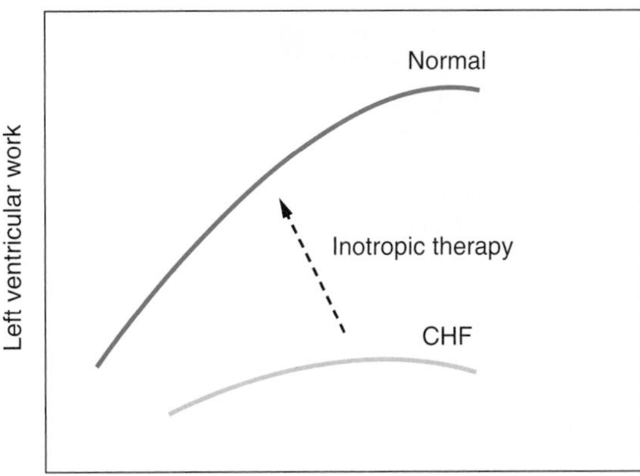

FIGURE 4-1. Pharmacologic goal in treating heart failure.

C. ACE inhibitors

1. ***Mechanism.*** ACE inhibitors inhibit the production of angiotensin II from angiotensin I (see Fig. 4-2).
   a. These agents **counteract** elevated peripheral vascular resistance and sodium and water retention resulting from angiotensin II and aldosterone.
   b. ACE inhibitors are becoming increasingly important in the treatment of CHF and have been shown to prevent or slow the progression of heart failure in patients with ventricular dysfunction.
   c. ACE inhibitors increase cardiac output and induce systemic arteriolar dilation (reduce afterload).
   d. ACE inhibitors **cause venodilation** and **induce natriuresis,** thereby reducing preload.
   e. These drugs are especially useful for **long-term therapy.**

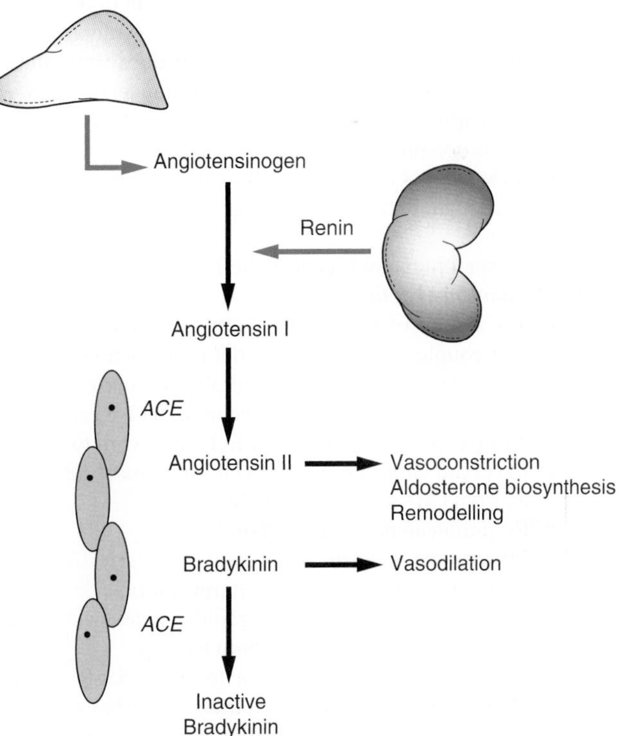

FIGURE 4-2.

table 4-1 Commonly Used ACE Inhibitors and ARBs

ACE Inhibitors	ARBs	AT1/AT2 Affinity
Captopril	Losartan (p)[a]	1,000
Enalapril (p)	Valsartan	20,000
Fosinopril (p)	Irbesartan	8,500
Lisinopril	Candesartan (p)	10,000
Quinapril (p)	Telmisartan	3,000
Benazepril (p)	Eprosartan	1,000
Moexipril (p)	Olmesartan (p)	12,500
Perindopril (p)		
Ramipril (p)		
Trandolapril (p)		

[a]p denotes prodrug, active metabolite produced by deesterification.

2. ***Therapeutic uses.*** ACE inhibitors are very useful in the treatment of **CHF, reducing risk of recurrent post-myocardial infarction (MI),** and treating **hypertension.** These agents have the advantage of producing minimal electrolyte disturbances and fewer adverse effects than many other agents used to treat hypertension.
3. ***Selected drugs*** (See Table 4-1 for a complete listing)
   a. **Enalapril** is a prodrug that is deesterified in the liver to produce **enalaprilat,** which inhibits ACE.
      (1) **Therapeutic uses.** Enalapril is a first-line drug in the treatment of CHF and is used to treat mild-to-severe hypertension. Diuretics enhance its activity. ACE inhibitors are also used to slow the progression of renal disease, **especially in diabetic patients.**
      (2) **Adverse effects and contraindications.** Blood dyscrasias and aplastic anemia are rare but serious adverse effects of enalapril. Renal function may be impaired.
   b. Captopril, the first ACE inhibitor and the only sulfur-containing ACE inhibitor, is absorbed from the gastrointestinal (GI) tract and is metabolized to disulfide conjugates. Drug absorption is decreased ~30% by food. It does not enter the CNS. Captopril produces adverse effects that include rash, taste disturbance, pruritus, weight loss, and anorexia.
   c. **Lisinopril** is an ACE inhibitor that permits once-a-day dosing. The bioavailability of lisinopril is not affected by food.
4. ***Adverse effects*** common to all ACE inhibitors include a dry cough and, rarely, angioedema (both thought to be due to increased bradykinin levels), hypotension, and hyperkalemia.

D. Angiotensin II receptor blockers (ARBs)

1. ***Mechanism of action***
   a. The actions of angiotensin II are mediated by receptors that are 7-transmembrane proteins that couple to numerous signal transduction pathways. AT1 receptors are responsible for the pressor actions, increased aldosterone biosynthesis, and the proliferative and fibrotic actions of angiotensin II. In general, AT2 receptors antagonize the action of AT1 receptors. AT4 receptors bind angiotensin IV and seem to be involved in memory and learning.
   b. In several clinical trials ARBs have proved as effective as ACE inhibitors in reducing mortality from CHF or following an MI.
2. ***ARBs: prototype drug—valsartan***
   a. **Mechanism.** Valsartan is an imidazole derivative with high affinity for AT1 receptors (about 20,000-fold higher than for AT2 receptors).
      (1) Oral doses are absorbed rapidly. Peak levels of the drug are obtained in about 3 hours, and it has a half-life of about 6 hours.
      (2) Valsartan is excreted in the feces, probably via biliary excretion.
   b. **Therapeutic uses.** In clinical trials, valsartan was about as effective as captopril in patients with left ventricular dysfunction following an MI. Valsartan is as effective as ACE inhibitors

in reducing blood pressure and is available in combination with hydrochlorothiazide for patients refractory to monotherapy.

c. **Adverse effects and contraindications. Dizziness and hyperkalemia** can occur with valsartan. Since ARBs do not lead to accumulation of kinins, the incidence of both the nonproductive cough and angioedema associated with ACE inhibitors is reduced.

d. Other ARBs (see Table 4-1) all have the same mechanism of action and adverse effect profile but have subtle pharmacokinetic differences. They vary markedly in their relative affinity for AT1 and AT2 receptors.

3. ***Renin inhibitors—Aliskiren*** is a small molecule inhibitor of renin. It is administered orally and is eliminated mostly unchanged in the urine. Clinical trials suggest it is about as effective as ACE inhibitors or ARBs for reducing blood pressure. Diarrhea, angioedema, and hyperkalemia have been reported. The incidence of cough is reduced compared to ACE inhibitors.

E. Cardiac glycosides

1. ***Cardiac glycosides*** are used for treatment of **CHF** and **certain arrhythmias** (atrial fibrillation and flutter and paroxysmal atrial tachycardias). However, their use overall has diminished in the absence of data supporting a reduction in mortality.
2. ***The most common*** cardiac glycosides are **digoxin** and **digitoxin** (discontinued in the United States), the major active ingredients found in digitalis plants, which are collectively referred to as **digitalis.** (**Ouabain** is another plant glycoside that is currently not used clinically.)
3. ***Structure.*** Cardiac glycosides are cardenolides that contain a lactone ring and a steroid (aglycone) moiety attached to sugar molecules.
4. ***Mechanism***
   a. Cardiac glycosides **inhibit Na^+/K^+-ATPase,** resulting in increased intracellular Na^+ and decreased intracellular K^+. Increased Na^+ reduces the normal exchange of intracellular Ca^{2+} for extracellular Na^+ and yields somewhat elevated intracellular Ca^{2+} (Fig. 4-3).
   b. There are **multiple isoforms** of Na^+/K^+-ATPase; the cardiac **isoform** has the highest affinity for digitalis.
   c. Following treatment, each action potential produces a greater release of Ca^{2+} to activate the contractile process. The net result is a **positive inotropic effect.**
5. ***Effects.*** Cardiac glycosides have both direct effects on the heart and indirect effects mediated by an increase in vagal tone.

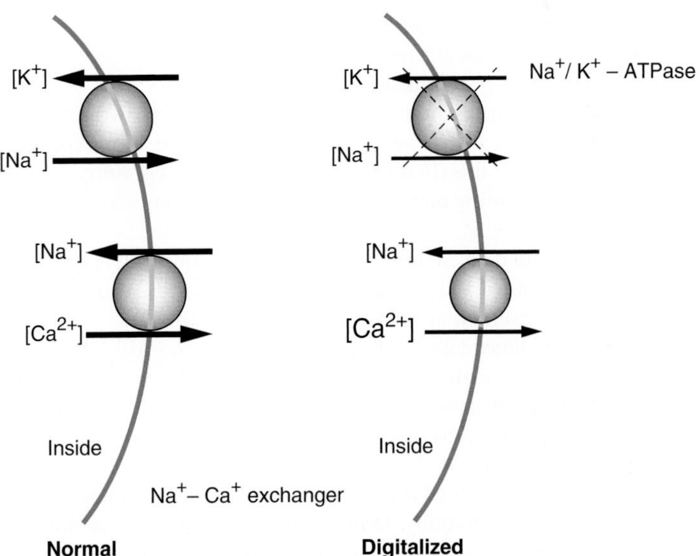

FIGURE 4-3. Changes in myocardial ion concentration following digitalis treatment.

a. Cardiac effects
  (1) Under normal cardiac conditions, digitalis treatment results in an increase in systemic vascular resistance and the constriction of smooth muscles in veins (cardiac output may decrease).
  (2) In the failing heart, the capacity to develop force during systole is compromised, and increased end-diastolic volume is required to achieve the same amount of work. Heart rate, ventricular volume, and pressure are elevated, whereas stroke volume is diminished.
    (a) Under these conditions, cardiac glycosides **increase stroke volume** and **enhance cardiac output.** Concomitantly, blood volume, venous pressure, and end-diastolic volume decrease.
    (b) The congested heart becomes smaller with treatment, and efficiency of contraction is increased (restored toward normal). **Improved circulation** reduces sympathetic activity and permits further improvement in cardiac function as a result of decreased systemic arterial resistance and venous tone.
  (3) Improved renal blood flow augments the elimination of Na^+ and water.

b. Neural effects
  (1) Cardiac glycosides **increase vagal activity,** resulting in inhibition of the sinoatrial (SA) node and delayed conduction through the atrioventricular (AV) node.
  (2) Cardiac glycosides decrease sympathetic tone.

6. ***Pharmacologic properties***

a. Only **digoxin** (Lanoxin) is available in the U.S. market. Digoxin distributes to most body tissues and **accumulates in cardiac tissue.** The concentration of the drug in the heart is twice that in skeletal muscle and at least 15 times that in plasma.

b. The **dose** of digoxin must be **individualized.** The initial loading (digitalizing) dose is often selected from prior estimates and adjusted for the patient's condition. The **maintenance dose** is based on the daily loss of the drug.

c. Dosing levels for the treatment of CHF are generally lower than those required to decrease the ventricular response in atrial fibrillation.

d. Digoxin has somewhat variable oral absorption; it can be given **orally** or **intravenously.** The peak effect after an intravenous (IV) dose occurs in 1.5–2 hours; the half-life ($t_{1/2}$) of digoxin is approximately 1.5 days. The maintenance dose of digoxin is approximately 35% of the loading dose.

e. Digoxin produces a therapeutic effect (and its toxic effects disappear) more rapidly than digitoxin. However, because of a relatively rapid clearance, lack of compliance may diminish the therapeutic effects.

f. Digoxin is **eliminated** by the **renal route;** the $t_{1/2}$ is prolonged in individuals with impaired renal function. Digoxin dosage can be adjusted on the basis of creatinine clearance.

7. ***Adverse effects and toxicity***

a. Narrow therapeutic index
  (1) Cardiac glycosides can cause fatal adverse effects.
  (2) These drugs induce virtually every type of arrhythmia.
  (3) Digoxin affects all excitable tissues; the most common site of action outside the heart is the GI tract (anorexia, nausea, vomiting, and diarrhea can occur), resulting either from direct action or through stimulation of the chemoreceptor trigger zone (CTZ).
  (4) Use of digoxin may result in disorientation and visual disturbances.

b. Toxicity is treated primarily by discontinuing the drug.
  (1) Potassium may help in alleviating arrhythmias.
  (2) Antidigoxin antibodies (digoxin immune FAB) (Digibind) or hemoperfusion are useful in acute toxicity.
  (3) Antiarrhythmic agents such as phenytoin and lidocaine may be helpful in treating acute digoxin-induced arrhythmias.

c. Drug interactions
  (1) Drugs that bind digitalis compounds, such as cholestyramine and neomycin, may interfere with therapy. Drugs that enhance hepatic metabolizing enzymes, such as phenobarbital, may lower concentrations of the active drug.

(2) The risk of toxicity is increased by the following:
 (a) Hypokalemia
  (i) Reduced K^+ results in increased phosphorylation of the Na^+/K^+-ATPase, and this **increases digoxin binding.** Thus, hypokalemia enhances the effects of these drugs and greatly increases the risk of toxicity. Hypokalemia may be seen with **thiazide** or other potassium-lowering diuretics.
  (ii) Hypokalemia **increases** the **therapeutic effects** of cardiac glycosides.
 (b) Hypercalcemia and calcium channel-blocking agents (e.g., verapamil)
  (i) Calcium channel-blocking agents cause toxicity by adding to the drug effects on Ca^{2+} stores.
  (ii) Hypocalcemia renders digitalis less effective.
 (c) **Quinidine** displaces digoxin from tissue-binding sites. The $t_{1/2}$ of digoxin is prolonged because of decreased renal elimination.

F. Other inotropic agents

1. ***Inamrinone lactate (formerly known as amrinone) and milrinone, the "inodilators"***
   a. These drugs are bipyridine derivatives related to the anticholinergic agent **biperiden.**
   b. Inamrinone lactate and milrinone reduce left ventricular filling pressure and vascular resistance and enhance cardiac output.
   c. These drugs inhibit cardiac phosphodiesterases, especially PDE type 3.
   d. Inamrinone lactate and milrinone act by inhibiting phosphodiesterases in cardiac and vascular muscle, thereby increasing cyclic AMP (cAMP); this leads to elevated intracellular Ca^{2+} levels and excitation contraction.
   e. These drugs are used in patients who do not respond to digitalis; they are most effective in individuals with elevated left ventricular filling pressure.
   f. Inamrinone lactate and milrinone produce considerable **toxicity on extended administration;** they are administered intravenously only for short-term therapy. The most common **adverse effects** are transient thrombocytopenia and **hypotension.** Fever and GI disturbances occur occasionally.
   g. Fewer and **less severe adverse effects** are seen with **milrinone** than with inamrinone
2. ***Dobutamine*** hydrochloride is a **synthetic catecholamine** derivative that increases contractility; it acts primarily on myocardial β_1-adrenoceptors with lesser effects on β_2- and α-adrenoceptors. Dobutamine hydrochloride increases cAMP-mediated phosphorylation and the activity of Ca^{2+} channels.
   a. Moderate doses of dobutamine hydrochloride do not increase heart rate.
   b. Dobutamine hydrochloride does not activate dopamine receptors.
   c. This drug is administered only by the IV route.
   d. Dobutamine hydrochloride is used in **short-term therapy** in individuals with **severe chronic cardiac failure** and for inotropic support after an MI and cardiac surgery. It does not substantially increase peripheral resistance and, thus, is not useful in cardiac shock with severe hypotension.
   e. Combined infusion therapy with **nitroprusside** or **nitroglycerin** may improve cardiac performance in patients with advanced heart failure.
   f. Dobutamine hydrochloride produces tachycardia and hypertension, but it is less arrhythmogenic than **isoproterenol.**
3. ***Dopamine*** is a neurotransmitter and a metabolic precursor of the catecholamines. It can increase myocardial contractility and renal blood flow.
4. ***Nesiritide (Natrecor)***
   a. Nesiritide is a recombinant B-type natriuretic peptide approved for short-term use for acute decompensated heart failure.
   b. Nesiritide increases cGMP and thereby produces vasodilation. It reduces pulmonary capillary wedge pressure and increases stroke volume.
   c. Nesiritide is a peptide that must be given parenterally.
   d. Adverse effects include headache, nausea, and hypotension.
   e. Data supporting a reduction in mortality with nesiritide are lacking.

G. **Diuretics** (See Chapter 3)

1. Diuretics reduce left ventricular filling pressure and decrease left ventricular volume and myocardial wall tension (lower oxygen demand).
2. Diuretics are frequently combined with an ACE inhibitor in **mild CHF;** they also are used for **acute pulmonary edema.**

H. **Vasodilators**

1. ***Cardiac effects.*** Vasodilators reduce arterial resistance or increase venous capacitance; the net effect is a reduction in vascular pressure. In response to failures of pump function, sympathetic tone increases during the resting state, causing excessive venoconstriction and ultimately reducing cardiac output. Thus, vasodilators can be effective in CHF, and they are particularly useful when heart failure is associated with hypertension, congestive cardiomyopathy, mitral or aortic insufficiency, or ischemia.
2. ***Therapeutic use***
   a. Vasodilators are used to treat **severe, decompensated CHF** refractory to diuretics and digitalis.
   b. Agents used in **short-term therapy** include **nitroprusside,** which has a direct balanced effect on arterial and venous beds, and **nitroglycerin,** which has more effect on venous beds than on arterial beds. Nitroglycerin is not as effective as nitroprusside in enhancing cardiac output.
   c. Agents used in **long-term therapy** include the direct-acting vasodilators **isosorbide** and **hydralazine,** and **prazosin,** an α_1-adrenergic blocking agent that produces arterial and minor venous dilation. **Carvedilol,** a combined α- and nonselective β-adrenoreceptor antagonist, has been shown in several clinical trials to reduce morbidity and mortality in mild-to-severe heart failure.

II. ANTIARRHYTHMIC DRUGS

A. **Causes of arrhythmias.** Arrhythmias may be due to both improper impulse generation and impulse conduction. These manifest as abnormalities of rate or regularity or as disturbances in the normal sequence of activation of atria and ventricles.

1. ***Altered automaticity.*** Altered automaticity can arise from the following:
   a. **Sinus node (sinus tachycardia and bradycardia). Increased vagal activity** can impair nodal pacemaker cells by elevating K^+ conductance, leading to hyperpolarization. **Increased sympathetic activity** increases the rate of phase 4 depolarization. Intrinsic disease can produce faulty pacemaker activity **(sick sinus syndrome).**
   b. **Ectopic foci** are areas within the conduction system that may, in the diseased state, develop high rates of intrinsic activity and function as pacemakers.
   c. **Triggered automaticity** results from delayed after-polarizations that reach threshold and are capable of initiating an impulse.
2. ***Abnormal impulse conduction in conduction pathways***
   a. Heart blocks may produce **bradyarrhythmias.**
   b. Reentry circus conduction may produce **tachyarrhythmias.**

B. **Goals of therapy** (Table 4-2)

a. Therapy aims to restore normal pacemaker activity and modify impaired conduction that leads to arrhythmias.
b. Therapeutic effects are achieved by sodium- or calcium-channel blockade, prolongation of effective refractory period, or blockade of sympathetic effects on the heart. Many antiarrhythmic drugs affect depolarized tissue to a greater extent than they affect normally polarized tissue.

C. **Treatment of tachyarrhythmias: Class I drugs**

1. ***Mechanism.*** Class I drugs block fast Na^+ channels, thereby reducing the rate of phase 0 depolarization, prolonging the effective refractory period, increasing the threshold of excitability, and reducing phase 4 depolarization. These drugs also have local anesthetic properties.

table 4-2 Some Antiarrhythmic Drugs

Group	Prototype Drug	Mechanism	Uses
Class Ia	Quinidine Procainamide Disopyramide	Moderate block of Na^+ channels; prolong action potentials	Suppress ventricular arrhythmias
Class Ib	Lidocaine Mexiletine	Weakly block Na^+ channels; shorten action potentials	Suppress ventricular arrhythmias
Class Ic	Flecainide	Strongly blocks Na^+ and K^+ channels	Treat severe ventricular tachyarrhythmias
Class II	Propranolol Atenolol Nadolol	Blocks β-adrenoceptors	Suppress some ventricular arrhythmias; inhibit AV node
Class III	Amiodarone	Prolongs refractory period	Suppress ventricular arrhythmias
Class IV	Verapamil	Blocks Ca^+ channel	Treat reentrant supraventricular tachycardia; suppress AV node conduction
Class V	Adenosin	Muscarinic antagonist	Treat paroxysmal atrial tachycardia
Others			
Atropine	Atropine	Increases vagal tone	Increase heart rate in bradycardia and heart blocks
Digitalis	Digoxin	P_1-receptor antagonist	Inhibit AV node; treat atrial fibrillation

a. **Class IA drugs** prolong the refractory period and slow conduction.
b. **Class IB agents** shorten the duration of the refractory period.
c. **Class IC drugs** slow conduction.

2. ***Class IA***
   a. Quinidine (Quinidex, Duraquin, Cardioquin)
      (1) Effects and pharmacologic properties
         (a) At therapeutic levels, direct **electrophysiologic effects** predominate, including depression of the pacemaker rate and depressed conduction and excitability, prolongation of Q-T interval, and heart block. At low doses, **anticholinergic** (vagolytic) **effects** predominate; they may increase conduction velocity in the AV node and accelerate heart rate.
         (b) Quinidine is administered **orally** and is rapidly absorbed from the **GI tract.**
         (c) Quinidine is **hydroxylated in the liver** and has a $t_{1/2}$ of approximately 5–12 hours, which is longer in hepatic or renal disease and in heart failure.
      (2) Therapeutic uses
         (a) Quinidine is used for **supraventricular and ventricular arrhythmias,** especially if caused by ectopia, and it is used to maintain **sinus rhythm** after conversion of atrial flutter or fibrillation by **digoxin, propranolol,** or **verapamil.**
         (b) Quinidine is used to prevent frequent premature ventricular complexes and ventricular tachycardia. Paradoxical tachycardia may be seen.
         (c) As the dextrorotary isomer of **quinine,** quinidine also exhibits antimalarial, antipyretic, and oxytocic actions.
      (3) Adverse effects
         (a) Quinidine depresses all muscles, which can lead to skeletal muscle weakness, especially in individuals with myasthenia gravis.
         (b) Quinidine can produce severe hypotension and shock after rapid infusion.
         (c) This drug can produce **cinchonism** (ringing of the ears and dizziness) and diarrhea.
         (d) Quinidine may induce thrombocytopenia, most probably as a result of platelet-destroying antibodies developed in response to the circulating protein–quinidine complexes.
         (e) Quinidine can cause ventricular arrhythmias. **Quinidine syncope** (dizziness and fainting) may occur as a result of ventricular tachycardia; this condition is associated with a prolonged Q-T interval.

(f) GI disturbances including abdominal pain, diarrhea, nausea, and esophagitis are common with quinidine

(4) Drug interactions

(a) Quinidine increases digoxin plasma levels and the risk of **digitalis toxicity.**

(b) The $t_{1/2}$ of quinidine is reduced by agents that induce drug-metabolizing enzymes **(phenobarbital, phenytoin).**

(c) Quinidine may enhance the activity of **coumarin** anticoagulants and other drugs metabolized by hepatic microsomal enzymes.

(d) The cardiotoxic effects of quinidine are exacerbated by hyperkalemia.

b. Procainamide (Pronestyl, Procan)

(1) Procainamide has actions similar to those of quinidine, but it is safer to use intravenously and produces fewer adverse GI effects.

(2) Procainamide is acetylated in the liver to N-acetylprocainamide (NAPA) at a genetically determined rate. "Slow acetylators" have earlier onset and a greater prevalence of drug-induced lupuslike syndrome than "fast acetylators." NAPA is also active as an antiarrhythmic.

(3) Procainamide is eliminated by the kidney; its $t_{1/2}$ is approximately 3–4 hours. Dose reduction is required in renal failure.

(4) Procainamide has a high incidence of adverse effects with long-term use. It is more likely than quinidine to produce severe or irreversible heart failure.

(5) Procainamide often causes drug-induced lupuslike syndrome (with symptoms resembling systemic lupus erythematosus).

c. Disopyramide (Norpace)

(1) Disopyramide has action similar to that of quinidine, but has the longest $T_{1/2}$ of its class.

(2) Disopyramide is approved for the treatment of ventricular arrhythmias; it is generally reserved for cases refractory or intolerant to quinidine or procainamide.

(3) Disopyramide produces pronounced anticholinergic effects, including dry mouth, blurred vision, constipation, urine retention, and (rarely) acute angle-closure glaucoma. It may worsen heart block and adversely affect sinus node function.

3. ***Class IB***

a. Lidocaine (Xylocaine)

(1) Lidocaine acts exclusively on the sodium channel (both activated and inactivated), and it is highly selective for damaged tissues.

(2) Lidocaine is a second-line choice (behind amiodarone, see following) for treatment of ventricular arrhythmias; it is ineffective in the prevention of arrhythmias subsequent to MI. It does not slow conduction and, thus, has little effect on atrial function.

(3) Lidocaine undergoes a large first-pass effect. It is administered via the IV or IM route, and its $t_{1/2}$ is approximately 1.5–2 hours.

(4) Lidocaine is administered in a loading dose followed by infusion. The dose must be adjusted in CHF or hepatic disease.

(5) Lidocaine has a low level of cardiotoxicity; the most common adverse effects are neurologic. In contrast to quinidine and procainamide, lidocaine has little effect on the autonomic nervous system (ANS).

b. Mexiletine (Mexitil)

(1) Mexiletine is an agent similar in action to lidocaine, but can be administered orally.

(2) Mexiletine is used primarily for long-term treatment of ventricular arrhythmias associated with previous MI.

4. ***Class IC***

a. Flecainide (Tambocor) and encainide (Enkaid)

(1) Flecainide is orally active; it is used for ventricular tachyarrhythmias and maintenance of sinus rhythm in patients with paroxysmal atrial fibrillation and/or atrial flutter.

(2) Encainide has been removed from the U.S. market but is available for use in patients already treated with the drug (compassionate use).

(3) Use of these drugs is limited by their propensity to cause proarrhythmic actions; cautious use is recommended in patients with sinus node dysfunction, post MI, and CHF.

b. Propafenone (Rythmol)
   (1) Propafenone has a spectrum of action similar to that of quinidine.
   (2) Propafenone possesses β-adrenoceptor antagonist activity.
   (3) This drug is approved for the treatment of supraventricular arrhythmias and suppression of life-threatening ventricular arrhythmias.
   (4) Propafenone may cause bradycardia, CHF, or new arrhythmias.

D. Treatment of tachyarrhythmias: Class II drugs

1. ***Mechanism.*** Class II drugs are **β-adrenoceptor antagonists,** including **propranolol,** which act by reducing sympathetic stimulation. They inhibit phase 4 depolarization, depress automaticity, prolong AV conduction, and decrease heart rate (except for agents that have sympathomimetic activity) and contractility.
2. ***Major drugs*** (see Table 4-2)
   a. **Propranolol** (Inderal, generic), a nonselective β-adrenoceptor antagonist, and the more selective β_1-adrenoceptor antagonists acebutolol (Sectral) and esmolol (Brevibloc) are used to treat ventricular arrhythmias. Esmolol is ultrashort acting, is administered by infusion, and is used to titrate block during surgery.
   b. **Propranolol, metoprolol** (Lopressor), **nadolol** (Corgard), and **timolol** (Blocadren) are frequently used to prevent recurrent MI.
3. ***Therapeutic uses***
   a. Class II drugs are used to treat **tachyarrhythmias** caused by increased sympathetic activity. They also are used for a variety of other arrhythmias, including atrial flutter and atrial fibrillation.
   b. These drugs **prevent reflex tachycardia** produced by vasodilating agents. They are sometimes used for digitalis toxicity.
4. ***Adverse effects.*** The adverse effects of class II drugs include **arteriolar vasoconstriction** and **bronchospasm.** Bradycardia, heart block, and myocardial depression may occur. **Atropine** or **isoproterenol** may be used to alleviate bradycardia.

E. Treatment of tachyarrhythmias: Class III drugs.

Class III drugs prolong action potential duration and effective refractory period. These drugs act by interfering with outward K^+ currents or slow inward Na^+ currents.

1. ***Amiodarone (Cordarone)***
   a. Amiodarone is structurally related to thyroxine. It **increases refractoriness,** and it also depresses sinus node automaticity and slows conduction.
   b. The **long half-life** of amiodarone (14–100 days) increases the risk of toxicity.
   c. The plasma concentration of amiodarone is not well correlated with its effects. Although electrophysiologic effects may be seen within hours after parenteral administration, effects on abnormal rhythms may not be seen for several days. The antiarrhythmic effects may last for weeks or months after the drug is discontinued.
   d. Amiodarone is used for treatment of refractory life-threatening ventricular arrhythmias in preference to lidocaine; additional uses include the treatment of atrial and/or ventricular arrhythmias including conversion of atrial fibrillation and the suppression of arrhythmias in patients with implanted defibrillators; it also possesses antianginal and vasodilatory effects. Amiodarone is a first-line agent for patients unresponsive to CPR.
   e. Amiodarone produces dose-related and cumulative **adverse effects** (especially **GI-related** effects) in about 70% of patients. Serious noncardiac adverse effects include pulmonary fibrosis and interstitial pneumonitis. Other adverse effects include photosensitivity, "gray man syndrome," corneal microdeposits, and thyroid disorders (due to iodine in the drug preparation).
2. ***Ibutilide (Corvert)***
   a. Ibutilide is a class III antiarrhythmic agent indicated for rapid conversion of atrial fibrillation or atrial flutter to normal sinus rhythm.
   b. Ibutilide must be administered by IV infusion.
   c. Ibutilide blocks slow inward Na^+ currents and prolongs the action potential duration, thereby causing a slowing of the sinus rate and AV conduction velocity.

3. ***Sotalol (Betapace, Sorine)***
   a. Solatol prolongs the cardiac action potential, increases the duration of the refractory period, and has nonselective β-adrenoceptor antagonist activity.
   b. Uses include treatment of atrial arrhythmias or life-threatening ventricular arrhythmias, and treatment of sustained ventricular tachycardia.
   c. Its adverse effects include significant proarrhythmic actions, dyspnea, and dizziness.
4. ***Dofetilide (Tikosyn)***
   a. Dofetilide is approved for the conversion and maintenance of normal sinus rhythm in atrial fibrillation or atrial flutter.
   b. Dofetilide is a potent inhibitor of K^+-channels and has no effect on conduction velocity.
   c. Adverse effects include serious arrhythmias and conduction abnormalities.
5. ***Bretylium (Bretylol)***
   a. Bretylium is a useful class III antiarrhythmic that is no longer commercially available because of manufacturing difficulties.
   b. Bretylium **inhibits** the **neuronal release of catecholamines,** and it also has some direct antiarrhythmic action. It has properties of class II drugs.
   c. Bretylium **prolongs ventricular action potential** but not atrial action potential.
   d. This drug is used intravenously for **severe refractory ventricular tachyarrhythmias** and also for prophylaxis and treatment of **ventricular fibrillation.**

F. Treatment of tachyarrhythmias: Class IV drugs

1. ***Mechanism***
   a. Class IV drugs selectively block L-type calcium channels.
   b. These drugs prolong nodal conduction and effective refractory period and have predominate actions in nodal tissues.
2. ***Verapamil (Calan, Isoptin)***
   a. Verapamil is a phenylalkylamine that blocks both **activated and inactivated slow calcium channels.** Tissues that depend on L-type calcium channels are most affected, and it has equipotent activity on the AV and SA nodes and in cardiac and vascular muscle tissues.
   b. Although verapamil is excreted primarily by the kidney, dose reduction is necessary in the presence of hepatic disease and in the elderly. Bioavailability following oral administration is about 20%; much lower doses are required when administered intravenously.
   c. Verapamil is useful in reentrant **supraventricular tachycardia,** and it can also reduce ventricular rate in **atrial flutter** and **fibrillation.**
   d. Verapamil has **negative inotropic action** that limits its use in damaged hearts; it can lead to AV block when given in large doses or in patients with partial blockage. Verapamil can precipitate sinus arrest in diseased patients, and it causes peripheral vasodilation.
   e. The **adverse cardiac effects** of verapamil, including sinus bradycardia, transient asystole, and other arrthythmias, may be exacerbated in individuals taking **β-adrenoceptor antagonists;** this can be reversed by atropine, β-adrenoceptor agonists, or calcium. Verapamil should not be used in patients with abnormal conduction circuits as in Wolff-Parkinson-White syndrome.

G. Treatment of tachyarrhythmias: Class V drugs

1. ***Adenosine (Adeno-jec, Adenocard)***
   a. Adenosine acts through specific **purinergic (P_1)** receptors.
   b. Adenosine causes an increase in potassium efflux and decreases calcium influx. This hyperpolarizes cardiac cells and decreases the calcium-dependent portion of the action potential.
   c. Adenosine is the drug of choice for the treatment of **paroxysmal supraventricular tachycardia,** including those associated with Wolff-Parkinson-White syndrome.
   d. Adverse effects are relatively minor, including flushing, dizziness, and headache.
2. ***Digoxin*** can control ventricular response in atrial flutter or fibrillation.

H. Treatment of bradyarrhythmias

1. ***Atropine***
   a. Atropine **blocks the effects of acetylcholine.** It elevates sinus rate and AV nodal and SA conduction velocity, and it decreases refractory period.

b. Atropine is used to treat **bradyarrhythmias** that accompany MI.

c. Atropine produces adverse effects that include dry mouth, mydriasis, and cycloplegia; it may induce arrhythmias.

2. *Isoproterenol (Isuprel)*

a. Isoproterenol **stimulates β-adrenoceptors** and increases heart rate and contractility.

b. Isoproterenol is used to **maintain adequate heart rate** and cardiac output in patients with AV block.

c. Isoproterenol may cause tachycardia, anginal attacks, headaches, dizziness, flushing, and tremors.

III. ANTIANGINAL AGENTS

A. Goal of therapy. The goal of therapy with antianginal agents is to restore the balance between oxygen supply and demand in the ischemic region of the myocardium.

B. Types of angina

1. *Classic angina (angina of exercise).* Classic angina occurs when oxygen demand exceeds oxygen supply, usually because of diminished coronary flow.

2. *Vasospastic (Prinzmetal's, or variant) angina.* Vasospastic angina results from reversible coronary vasospasm that decreases oxygen supply and occurs at rest. Some individuals have **mixed angina,** in which both exercise-induced and resting attacks may occur.

C. Nitrates and nitrites

1. *Structure and mechanism*

a. Nitrates and nitrites are polyol esters of nitric acid and nitrous acid, respectively, and relax vascular smooth muscle.

b. Nitrates and nitrites activate guanylate cyclase and increase cyclic guanine nucleotides. This activates cGMP-dependent kinases, ultimately leading to dephosphorylation of myosin light chain and relaxation of the contractile apparatus.

c. These drugs dilate all vessels. Peripheral venodilation decreases cardiac preload and myocardial wall tension; arterial dilation reduces afterload. Both of these actions lower oxygen demand by decreasing the work of the heart. Redistribution of coronary blood flow to ischemic regions is increased in nitrate-treated patients.

d. Nitrates and nitrites ameliorate the symptoms of classic angina predominantly through the improvement of hemodynamics. Variant angina is relieved through effects on coronary circulation.

e. Nitrates and nitrites form nitrosothiol in smooth muscle by reaction with glutathione. Tolerance occurs upon glutathione depletion.

2. *Bioavailability and selected drugs.* These drugs have a large first-pass effect due to the presence of high-capacity organic nitrate reductase in the liver, which inactivates drugs. Nitrates have a $t_{1/2}$ of less than 10 minutes.

a. Nitroglycerin (Cellegesic, Nitrek, others)

(1) Nitroglycerin is preferably administered sublingually for rapid delivery and short duration.

(2) Sustained-delivery systems (Transderm-Nitro, Nitrodisc) are available and are used to maintain blood levels. Aerosol, topical, intravenous, and oral preparations are also available.

b. Amyl nitrite is a **volatile liquid** that is **inhaled.** An unpleasant odor and extensive cutaneous vasodilation render it **less desirable** than **nitroglycerin.**

c. Isosorbide dinitrate (Isordil, Sorbitrate, others)

(1) Isosorbide dinitrate has active initial metabolites.

(2) This drug is administered orally or sublingually; it has better oral bioavailability and a longer half-life (up to 1 h) than nitroglycerin. Timed-release oral preparations are available with durations of action up to 12 hours.

(3) Isosorbide mononitrate (Imdur, Monoker) has comparable actions with a longer plasma half-life.

3. ***Therapeutic uses***
   a. Sublingual **nitroglycerin** is most often used for severe, recurrent **Prinzmetal's angina.**
   b. Continuous infusion or slowly absorbed preparations of nitroglycerin (including the transdermal patch) or derivatives with longer half-lives have been used for **unstable angina** and for **CHF in the presence of MI.**
4. ***Adverse effects***
   a. Nitrates and nitrites produce **vasodilation,** which can lead to orthostatic hypotension, reflex tachycardia, throbbing headache (may be dose limiting), blushing, and a burning sensation. Continuous exposure may lead to tolerance.
   b. Large doses produce **methemoglobinemia** and cyanosis.

D. β-Adrenoceptor antagonists

1. β-Adrenoceptor antagonists decrease heart rate, blood pressure, and contractility, resulting in **decreased myocardial oxygen requirements.** Combined therapy with nitrates is often preferred in the treatment of angina pectoris because of the decreased adverse effects of both agents.
2. β-Adrenoceptor antagonists are contraindicated in the presence of bradycardia, AV block, and asthma.

E. Calcium channel-blocking agents

1. ***Mechanism.*** Calcium channel-blocking agents produce a blockade of L-type (slow) calcium channels, which decreases contractile force and oxygen requirements. Agents cause **coronary vasodilation** and **relief of spasm;** they also dilate peripheral vasculature and decrease cardiac afterload.
2. ***Pharmacologic properties***
   a. Calcium channel-blocking agents can be administered orally. When administered intravenously, they are effective within minutes.
   b. These drugs are useful for **both variant and chronic stable angina** and are also used in instances where nitrates are ineffective or when β-adrenoceptor antagonists are contraindicated.
   c. Serum lipids are not increased.
   d. These drugs produce **hypotension,** and **edema** is a common adverse effect.
3. ***Selected drugs***
   a. Verapamil (Calan, Isoptin)
      (1) Verapamil produces slowed conduction through the AV node (predominant effect); this may be an unwanted effect in some situations (especially in the treatment of hypertension).
      (2) Verapamil may produce AV block when used in combination with β-adrenoceptor antagonists. The toxic effects of verapamil include myocardial depression, heart failure, and edema.
      (3) Verapamil also has peripheral vasodilating effects that can reduce afterload and blood pressure.
      (4) The peripheral effects of verapamil can produce headache, reflex tachycardia, and fluid retention.
   b. Nifedipine (Adalat, Procardia), isradipine (DynaCirc), nisoldipine (Sular), and nicardipine (Cardene)
      (1) These dihydropyridine calcium-channel blockers have predominant actions in the peripheral vasculature; they decrease afterload and to a lesser extent preload, and lower blood pressure.
      (2) These drugs have **significantly less direct effect on the heart** than verapamil.
   c. Diltiazem (Cardizem)
      (1) Diltiazem, a benzothiazepine, is intermediate in properties between verapamil and the dihydropyridines.
      (2) Diltiazem is used to treat variant (Prinzmetal's) angina, either naturally occurring or drug-induced and stable angina.

F. Dipyridamole (Persantine)

1. Dipyridamole is a nonnitrate coronary vasodilator that interferes with uptake of the vasodilator **adenosine.** It potentiates the effect of **PGI_2** (prostacyclin, epoprostenol) and dilates resistance vessels and inhibits platelet aggregation.
2. Dipyridamole may be used for **prophylaxis of angina pectoris,** but the efficacy of this drug is not proved.
3. Dipyridamole produces adverse effects that include the worsening of angina, dizziness, and headache.

IV. ANTIHYPERTENSIVE DRUGS

A. Principles of blood pressure regulation

1. **Blood pressure** is regulated by the following:
   a. Cardiac output
   b. Peripheral vascular resistance
   c. Volume of intravascular fluid (controlled at the kidney)
2. **Baroreflexes adjust moment-to-moment blood pressure.** Carotid baroreceptors respond to stretch, and their activation inhibits sympathetic discharge.
3. The **renin–angiotensin system** provides tonic, longer-term regulation of blood pressure. Reduction in renal perfusion pressure results in increased reabsorption of salt and water. Decreased renal pressure stimulates **renin production** and leads to enhanced levels of **angiotensin II.** This agent in turn causes resistance vessels to constrict and stimulates aldosterone synthesis, which ultimately increases the absorption of sodium by the kidney.

B. Goal of therapy

1. The goal of therapy is to **reduce elevated blood pressure,** which would ultimately lead to **end-organ damage, increased risk of stroke, and MI.**
2. This goal is achieved through the use of various drug classes, and treatment often involves a **combination of agents** (Table 4-3).

C. Diuretics increase sodium excretion and lower blood volume.

1. ***Thiazide diuretics***
   a. Thiazide diuretics are effective in lowering blood pressure 10–15 mm Hg.
   b. When administered alone, thiazide diuretics can provide relief for **mild or moderate hypertension.**
   c. Thiazide diuretics are used in combination with sympatholytic agents or vasodilators in **severe hypertension.**
2. ***Loop diuretics*** are used in combination with sympatholytic agents and vasodilators for hypertension refractory to thiazide treatment.
3. ***Potassium-sparing diuretics*** are used to avoid potassium depletion, especially when administered with cardiac glycosides.

D. Adrenoceptor antagonists

1. ***β-Adrenoceptor antagonists*** (see Table 2-1)
   a. Propranolol (Inderal)
      (1) Propranolol antagonizes catecholamine action at both β_1- and β_2-receptors. It produces sustained reduction in peripheral vascular resistance.
      (2) Blockade of cardiac β_1-adrenoceptors reduces heart rate and contractility. β_2-Adrenoceptor blockade increases airway resistance and decreases catecholamine-induced glycogenolysis and peripheral vasodilation.
      (3) Blockade of β-adrenoceptors in the CNS decreases sympathetic activity.
      (4) Propranolol also decreases renin release.
      (5) Propranolol is used in mild-to-moderate hypertension.

table 4-3 Some Antihypertensive Drugs

Class	Drug	Adverse Effects	Therapeutic Use
Diuretics			
Thiazide and thiazide-related agents	Chlorothiazide, hydrochlorothiazide, chlorthalidone, metolazone, indapamide	Hypokalemia, hyperuricemia, hypersensitivity reactions, hyperglycemia	Alone to treat moderate hypertension; in combination with other classes of drugs to treat severe hypertension
Loop	Furosemide, bumetanide, ethacrynic acid	Hypokalemia, hypotension, volume depletion, hypomagnesemia, hyperuricemia, hyperglycemia, hypocalcemia	In the presence of azotemia
Potassium-sparing agents	Triamterene, spironolactone, amiloride	Hyperkalemia	Used in combination with a thiazide or loop diuretic
Peripheral sympatholytics			
β-Adrenergic antagonists	Nonselective (β_1 and β_2): propranolol, timolol, nadolol, pindolol, penbutolol, carteolol; β_1-selective; acebutolol, atenolol, metoprolol	Most adverse effects are mild, rarely requiring withdrawal of drug: fatigue, depression, reduced exercise tolerance, bradycardia, CHF, bronchoconstriction in presence of asthma, gastrointestinal disturbances, masked hypoglycemia, increased triglycerides, decreased low-density lipoprotein cholesterol	All grades of hypertension; may be combined with a diuretic for additive effects, or with a diuretic plus an α-adrenoceptor antagonist for resistant hypertension; also diminish cardiac oxygen demand
α_1- and β-Adrenoceptor antagonists	Carvedilol, labetalol	Similar to propranolol; more likely to cause orthostatic hypotension and sexual dysfunction	
α_1-Adrenoceptor antagonists	Prazosin, terazosin, doxazosin	First-dose syncope, orthostatic hypotension, palpitations, anticholinergic effects	As single agents in mild-to-moderate hypertension; may be useful with a diuretic and a β-adrenoceptor antagonist
Inhibitors of renin–angiotensin			
Angiotensin-converting enzyme (ACE) inhibitors	Captopril, enalapril, lisinopril, ramipril, quinapril	Hyperkalemia, rash, dysgeusia, cough; individuals with high plasma renin activity may experience excessive hypotension	Mild-to-severe hypertension
Angiotensin II receptor antagonists	Losartan potassium	Hyperkalemia	Similar to ACE inhibitors

Renin inhibitor	Aliskiren	Dizziness	Similar to ARBs
Calcium-channel blockers	Verapamil, diltiazem, nicardipine, nifedipine, isradipine, felodipine	Negative inotropic effects, peripheral edema	Broad range of hypertensive patients; cautious use in presence of heart failure
Central sympatholytics	Methyldopa, clonidine, guanabenz	Dry mouth, sedation, lethargy, depression	Chronic hypertension
Adrenergic neuronal blocking drugs	Guanadrel	Orthostatic hypotension; severe hypotension in presence of pheochromocytoma	Severe refractory hypertension
	Reserpine	GI disturbances, mental depression	Mild-to-moderate hypertension
Vasodilators			
Arteriolar vasodilators	Hydralazine, minoxidil	Lupuslike syndrome may occur with hydralazine; minoxidil may cause severe volume retention	Sometimes for hypertension refractory to β-blocker/thiazide diuretic combination; in combination with a diuretic and often a β-blocker
Arteriolar and venule vasodilator	Sodium nitroprusside	Excessive decrease in blood pressure may occur	Emergency situations where rapid reduction in blood pressure is desired

b. Nadolol (Corgard), timolol (Blocadren), carteolol (Cartrol), pindolol (Visken), penbutolol (Levatol)
   (1) These drugs are similar in action to propranolol and block both β_1- and β_2-adrenoceptors.
   (2) Nadolol has an extended duration of action.
   (3) Pindolol, carteolol, and penbutolol have partial agonist activity (sympathomimetic).
c. Metoprolol (Lopressor), atenolol (Tenormin), acebutolol (Sectral), bisprolol (Zebeta)
   (1) These drugs are relatively selective for β_1-adrenoceptors.
   (2) Acebutolol has partial agonist activity.
d. Abrupt discontinuation of β-adrenoceptor blockers can worsen angina and increase risk of MI. Dose should be gradually reduced over a period of several weeks.

2. ***α-Adrenoceptor antagonists***
   a. α-Adrenoceptor antagonists **lower total peripheral resistance** by preventing stimulation (and consequent vasoconstriction) of α-receptors, which are located predominantly in resistance vessels of the skin, mucosa, intestine, and kidney. These drugs **reduce pressure** by dilating resistance and conductance vessels.
   b. The effectiveness of these drugs diminishes in some patients because of tolerance.
      (1) Prazosin (Minipress), terazosin (Hytrin), and doxazosin (Cardura)
         (a) These drugs are α_1-selective antagonists.
         (b) These drugs are used in treating **hypertension,** especially in the presence of CHF but use has diminished because no evidence of reduced cardiovascular events with doxazosin was found in a large clinical trial.
         (c) Prazosin, terazosin, and doxazosin are often administered with a diuretic and a β-adrenoceptor antagonist.
         (d) These drugs may produce initial orthostatic hypotension. Other adverse effects are minimal.
      (2) Phentolamine (Regitine) and phenoxybenzamine (Dibenzyline)
         (a) Phentolamine and phenoxybenzamine antagonize α_1- and α_2-adrenoceptors.
         (b) These drugs are used primarily in treating **hypertension** in the presence of **pheochromocytoma.** Phentolamine is administered parenterally; phenoxybenzamine is administered orally.

3. ***Labetalol (Normodyne, Trandate) and carvedilol (Coreg)***
   a. Labetalol is an α- and β-adrenoceptor antagonist.
   b. Labetalol reduces heart rate and contractility, slows AV conduction, and decreases peripheral resistance.
   c. Labetalol is available for both oral and IV administration.
   d. Labetalol is useful for treating hypertensive emergencies and in the treatment of **hypertension of pheochromocytoma.**
   e. Labetalol does not cause reflex tachycardia.
   f. Carvedilol has a significantly greater ratio of β to α antagonist activity than labetalol.

E. Agents that affect the renin–angiotensin system

1. ***Angiotensin converting enzyme (ACE) inhibitors*** (see section B above)
   a. ACE inhibitors reduce vascular resistance and blood volume; they lower blood pressure by decreasing total peripheral resistance.
   b. ACE inhibitors include **captopril** (Capoten), **enalapril** (Vasotec), **lisinopril** (Prinivil, Zestril), **ramipril** (Altace), **fosinopril** (Monopril), **benazepril** (Lotensin), **moexipril** (Univasc), **quinapril** (Accupril), perindopril (Aceon), and trandolapril (Mavik).
   c. These drugs are useful in treating **mild-to-severe hypertension.** Recent studies have established beneficial effect in patients with angina, CHF, cardiac ischemia, and post-MI.
   d. ACE inhibitors may be less effective in African Americans than in Caucasians.
2. ***Angiotensin II receptor antagonists, losartan potassium (Cozaar)*** (see Table 4-1)
   a. These drugs block angiotensin II type-1 (AT-1) receptors.
   b. The effects of these drugs are similar to those seen with ACE inhibitors.
   c. These drugs are effective as monotherapy for hypertension.

3. ***Inhibitors of renin activity, aliskiren (Tekturna)***
   a. Aliskiren inhibits renin and thereby reduces the production of all angiotensins.
   b. Initial clinical trials have combined aliskiren with a diuretic or an ARB and its effectiveness seems comparable to ARBs.
   c. Adverse effects are fewer compared to ACE inhibitors but include diarrhea, headache, and dizziness.

F. Calcium channel-blocking agents

1. Calcium channel-blocking (CCB) agents inhibit the entry of calcium into cardiac and smooth muscle cells by blocking the L-type Ca^{2+}-channel; they lower blood pressure by reducing peripheral resistance.
2. CCBs used for treatment of hypertension include verapamil, nifedipine, nicardipine, nisoldipine (Sular), isradipine (DynaCirc), amlodipine (Norvasc), felodipine (Plendil), and diltiazem.
3. CCBs are effective in the treatment of **mild-to-moderate hypertension.**
4. When combined with a β-adrenoceptor antagonist, these agents may lower blood pressure to a greater extent than when either class of drug is administered separately.
5. Short-acting preparations of the dihydropyridines such as nifedipine have been associated with an increase in cardiovascular mortality and events, including MI and increased anginal attacks.

G. Other drugs

1. ***Centrally acting sympathomimetic agents*** reduce peripheral resistance, inhibit cardiac function, and increase pooling in capacitance venules.
   a. Methyldopa (Aldomet)
      (1) Methyldopa has an active metabolite, α-methylnorepinephrine, a potent false neurotransmitter.
      (2) Methyldopa activates presynaptic inhibitory α-adrenoceptors and postsynaptic α_2-receptors in the CNS and reduces sympathetic outflow. It decreases total peripheral resistance.
      (3) Methyldopa reduces pressure in standing and supine positions.
      (4) Methyldopa is used to treat mild-to-moderate hypertension; it can be added to the regimen when a diuretic alone is not successful.
      (5) Methyldopa produces adverse effects that include drowsiness, dry mouth, and GI upset. Sexual dysfunction may occur and reduce compliance.
   b. Clonidine (Catapres)
      (1) Clonidine stimulates postsynaptic α_2-adrenoceptors in the central nervous system (CNS) and causes reduction in total peripheral resistance.
      (2) Clonidine is frequently combined with a diuretic.
      (3) Clonidine commonly produces drowsiness and lethargy, dry mouth, and constipation.
      (4) This drug is available as a transdermal patch (Catapres-TTS) that allows weekly dosing.
   c. Guanabenz acetate (Wytensin)
      (1) Guanabenz acetate activates central α_2-adrenoceptors and inhibits sympathetic outflow from the brain, which results in reduced blood pressure.
      (2) This drug is used in mild-to-moderate hypertension, most commonly in combination with a diuretic.
      (3) Guanabenz acetate most commonly produces sedation and dry mouth as adverse effects but with reduced frequency compared to clonidine.
2. ***Adrenergic neuronal blocking drugs***
   a. Reserpine
      (1) Reserpine eliminates norepinephrine release in response to nerve impulse by preventing vesicular uptake. It depletes norepinephrine from sympathetic nerve terminals in the periphery and in the adrenal medulla.
      (2) Reserpine is used in mild-to-moderate hypertension.
      (3) Reserpine most commonly produces GI disturbances. Mental depression, sometimes severe, may result, especially with high doses; use of reserpine is contraindicated in patients with a history of depression.

3. ***Vasodilators***
   a. Vasodilators relax smooth muscle and lower total peripheral resistance, thereby lowering blood pressure.
   b. The use of vasodilators is declining as a result of newer modalities, such as ACE inhibitors and calcium channel-blocking agents, which are more effective with fewer adverse effects.
      (1) Hydralazine (Apresoline)
         (a) Hydralazine reduces blood pressure directly by **relaxing arteriolar muscle.** This effect is probably mediated by increasing K^+ efflux and decreasing Ca^{2+} influx, and increasing the production of nitric oxide.
         (b) Hydralazine elicits the baroreceptor reflex, necessitating **coadministration** with a **diuretic** to counteract sodium and water retention and a β-blocker to prevent tachycardia.
         (c) This drug is used to treat **chronic hypertension** and in **hypertensive crises** accompanying acute glomerular nephritis or eclampsia.
         (d) Hydralazine may cause a lupuslike syndrome.
      (2) Minoxidil (Loniten)
         (a) Minoxidil has effects similar to hydralazine. Minoxidil acts to increase K^+ efflux, which hyperpolarizes cells and reduces the activity of L-type (voltage-sensitive) calcium channels. Minoxidil vasodilates predominantly arteriolar vessels.
         (b) Minoxidil also elicits the **baroreceptor reflex,** necessitating use of a **β-adrenoceptor antagonist** and a **diuretic.**
         (c) Minoxidil is useful for long-term therapy of **refractory hypertension.**
         (d) Minoxidil produces **hirsutism,** an advantage in formulations that are now used to reduce hair loss in both males and females.
      (3) Sodium nitroprusside (Nipride, Nitropress)
         (a) Sodium nitroprusside dilates both resistance and capacitance vessels; it increases heart rate but not output.
         (b) This drug is frequently used in **hypertensive emergencies** because of its rapid action. Continuous infusion is necessary to maintain effects.
         (c) Sodium nitroprusside is usually administered with **furosemide.**
         (d) On initial infusion, sodium nitroprusside may cause excessive vasodilation and hypotension.
         (e) Sodium nitroprusside can be converted to cyanide and thiocyanate. The accumulation of cyanide and **risk of toxicity** are minimized by concomitant administration of **sodium thiosulfate** or hydroxocobalamin.
      (4) Diazoxide (Hyperstat)
         (a) Diazoxide is used intravenously to reduce blood pressure rapidly, usually in an emergency situation.
         (b) Diazoxide is administered with **furosemide** to prevent fluid overload.
         (c) This drug is **declining in use** because of its unpredictable action and adverse effects.
4. ***Fenoldopam (Corlopam)*** is a selective **agonist at dopamine DA_1 receptors** that increases renal blood flow while reducing blood pressure. Administered by infusion, it is a useful drug in the control of emergency hypertension.
5. ***Specialized vasodilators***
   a. Drugs used to treat pulmonary hypertension
      (1) **Ambrisentan (Letaris) is a selective endothelin A receptor antagonist used to treat pulmory hypertension.** Plasma endothelin-1 is elevated in patients with pulmonary hypertension. Ambrisentan is administered orally. Peripheral edema is a common adverse effect of endothelin receptor antagonists.
      (2) **Bosentan** antagonizes both endothelin A and B receptors and reduces pulmonary hypertension. Headache and edema are common side effects.
      (3) Use of both ambrisentan and bosentan is controlled by access programs.
   b. Drugs used to treat erectile dysfunction
      (1) Drugs in this class include **sildenafil** citrate (Viagra, Revatio), **tadalafil** (Cialis), and **vardenafil** hydrochloride (Levitra).

(2) Viagra was originally developed as an antianginal and antihypertensive agent but proved very effective in treating erectile dysfunction.

(3) These agents specifically **inhibit phosphodiesterase type V,** the class of enzymes that are responsible for the breakdown of cGMP. The type V isoform is expressed in reproductive tissues and the lung. Inhibition of the breakdown of cGMP enhances the vasodilatory action of NO in the corpus callosum and in the pulmonary vasculature.

(4) These agents are useful in the treatment of erectile dysfunction, and sildenafil citrate is approved for treatment of pulmonary hypertension.

(5) The most common adverse effects of the phosphodiesterase type V inhibitors are headache, flushing, ocular disturbances, and abdominal pain. The most serious adverse effects are cardiovascular: arrhythmias, heart block, cardiac arrest, stroke, and hypotension.

(6) These drugs are contraindicated in patients taking nitrates, because of exacerbation of the effects of these drugs, or in patients taking α_1-adrenoceptor antagonists such as doxazosin.

V. DRUGS THAT LOWER PLASMA LIPIDS

A. Overview

1. Dietary or pharmacologic reduction of elevated plasma cholesterol levels can reduce the risk of atherosclerosis and subsequent cardiovascular disease. The exact factors linking elevated cholesterol levels to heart disease are not yet known.

2. The association between cardiovascular disease and elevated plasma triglycerides is less dramatic, but it is becoming more recognized. In addition, **elevated triglycerides** can produce life-threatening pancreatitis.

3. ***Hyperlipoproteinemias***

a. **Cholesterol** is a nonpolar, poorly water-soluble substance, transported in the plasma in particles that have a hydrophobic core of cholesteryl esters and triglycerides surrounded by a coat of phospholipids, free cholesterol (nonesterified), and one or more apoproteins. These lipoprotein particles vary in the ratio of triglyceride to cholesteryl ester as well as in the type of apoprotein; they are identified as **low-density lipoprotein (LDL)** particles, **very-low-density lipoprotein (VLDL)** particles, **intermediate-density lipoprotein (IDL)** particles, and **high-density lipoprotein (HDL)** particles.

b. Diseases of plasma lipids can be manifest as an elevation in triglycerides or as an elevation in cholesterol. In several of the complex or combined hyperlipoproteinemias, both **triglycerides and cholesterol can be elevated.**

B. Drugs useful in treating hyperlipidemias

1. ***Inhibitors of cholesterol biosynthesis (statins)***

a. These drugs include **lovastatin** (mevinolin) (Mevacor), **simvastatin** (Zocor), **pravastatin** (Pravachol), and **fluvastatin** (Lescol), **atorvastatin** (Lipitor), and **rosuvastatin** (Crestor).

b. Drugs that inhibit cholesterol biosynthesis are quite effective at lowering LDL cholesterol and total cholesterol.

(1) Mechanism

(a) These drugs function as competitive inhibitors of 3-hydroxy-3-methylglutaryl-coenzyme A reductase (HMG-CoA reductase), the rate-limiting enzyme in cholesterol biosynthesis. Reduced cholesterol synthesis results in a compensatory increase in the hepatic uptake of plasma cholesterol mediated by an increase in the number of LDL receptors.

(b) These drugs **reduce total cholesterol** by as much as 30%–50%; LDL cholesterol can be reduced by as much as 60% (rosuvastatin).

(2) Therapeutic uses. Inhibitors of cholesterol biosynthesis are effective in reducing cholesterol levels in familial and nonfamilial hypercholesterolemias.

(3) Recent clinical trials have established that statins interfere with osteoclast-mediated bone resorption and may reduce osteoporosis. These drugs may also interfere with intracellular localization of certain oncogenes and thereby reduce the incidence of some cancers. They also have weak anti-inflammatory activity.

(4) The adverse effects of these drugs include **myositis,** rhabdomyolysis, anxiety, irritability, **hepatotoxicity,** and **elevations in aminotransferases.**

2. ***Nicotinic acid (niacin) (Nicobid, Nicolar)***

a. Mechanism

(1) Nicotinic acid can exert cholesterol- and triglyceride-lowering effects at high concentrations (nicotinamide cannot do this). This is distinct from the role of this molecule as a vitamin, in which nicotinic acid is converted to nicotinamide and is used for biosynthesis of the cofactors NAD and NADP.

(2) Nicotinic acid reduces plasma VLDL by inhibiting the synthesis and esterification of fatty acids in the liver and reducing lipolysis in adipose tissue; it markedly decreases plasma triglyceride levels. As the substrate VLDL concentration is reduced, the concentrations of IDL and LDL also decrease, thereby reducing plasma cholesterol levels. HDL levels increase significantly.

(3) In much smaller doses, nicotinic acid can also be used as a vitamin supplement in the treatment of pellagra.

b. Adverse effects

(1) Nicotinic acid commonly produces flushing and an itching or burning feeling in the skin, which may reduce compliance. This is mediated by prostaglandin and histamine release and can be diminished by taking aspirin 30 minutes before taking nicotinic acid.

(2) Nicotinic acid produces hepatic effects, including increased transaminase activities; hyperglycemia; GI disturbances and peptic ulcer; renal effects that include elevated plasma uric acid; and macular edema.

3. ***Fibric acid analogues***

a. Fenofibrate (Antara, Triglide, Lofibra)

(1) Mechanism

(a) Fibrates stimulate the activity of peroxisome proliferating activating receptors (PPARα), a class of nuclear receptor. Activation of these receptors alters the transcription of a number of genes involved in triglyceride metabolism including lipoprotein lipase and apolipoprotein CIII. This **increases** the **peripheral catabolism of VLDL** and **chylomicrons,** resulting in a reduction in the plasma concentration of VLDL, most notably in triglycerides.

(b) Fibrates **reduce hepatic synthesis of cholesterol,** which further reduces plasma triglycerides.

(2) Therapeutic uses

(a) Fenofibrate can be used to treat **hyperlipidemia** of several etiologies, especially hypertriglyceridemia due to dysbetalipoproteinemia, a defect in apolipoprotein E that impairs clearance of chylomicron remnants and VLDL.

(b) Fenofibrate is ineffective in primary chylomicronemia (caused by a deficiency in lipoprotein lipase) and has little effect on reducing plasma cholesterol levels.

(c) Fenofibrate has antidiuretic action in individuals with mild or moderate **diabetes insipidus.**

(3) Adverse effects and contraindications

(a) Fenofibrate produces cholelithiasis and cholecystitis, GI intolerance, nausea, mild diarrhea, and myalgia.

(b) This drug frequently causes dermatologic reactions and drowsiness, as well as decreased libido in a small percentage of men.

(c) Fenofibrate can **displace** other albumin-bound drugs, most notably the **sulfonylureas** and **warfarin.**

(d) Fenofibrate must be used cautiously in individuals with impaired renal or hepatic function.

b. Gemfibrozil (Lopid)

(1) Gemfibrozil is a fibrate that is more effective than fenofibrate in some circumstances and has some unique biologic activities.

(2) The therapeutic uses of gemfibrozil are identical to those of fenofibrate; it may be more active in reducing triglycerides than fenofibrate.

4. ***Ezetimibe (Zetia)***

a. Ezetimibe acts within the intestine to reduce cholesterol absorption. Cholesterol is absorbed from the small intestine by a process that includes specific transporters that have not been completely characterized. Ezetimibe appears to block one or more of these cholesterol transporters, reducing cholesterol absorption.

b. Ezetimibe used alone produces a reduction in plasma cholesterol of about 18% and about a 10% decline in triglyceride levels. When combined with a statin, reductions in plasma cholesterol as high as 72% have been reported in clinical trials.

c. Ezetimibe appears to be well tolerated, with the most common adverse effects being fatigue, abdominal pain, and diarrhea.

5. ***Bile acid sequestrants.*** These agents include **cholestyramine** (Questran), **colestipol** (Colestid), and **colesevelam** (WelChol)

a. Structure and mechanism

(1) Bile acid sequestrants are large copolymers (resins) of hydrocarbons that can bind bile salts. Cholestyramine and colestipol exchange a chloride anion for a bile acid.

(2) These resins are hydrophilic, but they are not absorbed across the intestine.

(3) In the intestine, the resins bind bile salts and prevent enterohepatic reutilization of bile acids. In addition, they impair the absorption of dietary cholesterol.

b. Therapeutic uses. Bile acid sequestrants are effective in **reducing plasma cholesterol** (10%–20%) in patients with some normal LDL receptors. This excludes patients who completely lack functional LDL receptors because of a genetic defect (homozygous familial hypercholesterolemia).

c. Adverse effects

(1) These agents are generally quite safe, because they are not absorbed in the intestine.

(2) Bile acid sequestrants produce GI disturbances (constipation, nausea, and discomfort), which may reduce compliance. Colesevelam has fewer GI side effects than the other resins.

(3) These drugs interfere with the absorption of anionic drugs (e.g., digitalis, warfarin).

DRUG SUMMARY TABLE

ACE Inhibitors
Captopril (Capoten, generic)
Enalapril (Vasotec, generic)
Fosinopril (Monopril, generic)
Lisinopril (Prinivil, Zestril, generic)
Quinapril (Accupril)
Benazepril (Lotensin, generic)
Moexipril (Univasc, generic)
Perindopril (Aceon)
Ramipril (Altace)
Trandolapril (Mavik)

Angiotensin-Receptor Blockers
Losartan (Cozaar)
Valsartan (Diovan)
Irbesartan (Avapro)
Candesartan (Atacand)
Telmisartan (Micardis)
Eprosartan (Teveten)
Olmesartan (Benicar)

Renin Inhibitor
Aliskiren (Tekturna)

Drugs Used in CHF
Digoxin (Lanoxin)
Dobutamine
Dopamine
Nesiritide (Natrecor)

Antiarrhythmics
Inamrinone
Milrinone
Quinidine (Quinidex)
Procainamide (Pronestyl)
Disopyramide (Norpace)
Lidocaine (Xylocaine)
Mexiletine (Mexitil)
Flecainide (Tambocor)
Encainide (Enkaid)
Propafenone (Rythmol)
Propranolol (Inderal)
Acebutolol (Sectral)
Esmolol (Brevibloc)
Metoprolol (Lopressor)
Nadolol (Corgard)
Timolol (Blocadren)
Amiodarone (Cordarone)
Ibutilide (Corvert)

Antihypertensive Agents
Hydralazine (Apresoline)
Minoxidil (Loniten)
Sodium nitroprusside (Nipride)
Diazoxide (Hyperstat)

Specialized Vasodilators
Ambrisentan (Letaris)
Bosentan (Tracler)
Sildenafil citrate (Viagra, Revatio)
Tadalafil (Cialis)
Vardenafil hydrochloride (Levitra)
Solatol (Betapace)
Dofetilide (Tikosyn)
Bretylium (Bretylol)
Verapamil (Calan)
Adenosine (Adeno-jec)
Atropine (generic)
Isoproterenol (Isuprel)

Antianginal Agents
Nitroglycerin (Cellegesic)
Amyl nitrite (generic)
Isosorbide dinitrate (Isordil)
Nifedipine (Adalat)
Isradipine (DynaCirc)
Nisoldipine (Sular)
Nicardipine (Cardene)
Diltiazem (Cardizem)
Dipyridamole (Persantine)

Antihypertensive Agents
Hydrochlorothiazide
Furosemide
Spironolactone
Eplerenone (Inspra)
Nadolol (Corgard)
Timolol (Blocadren)
Carteolol (Cartrol)
Pindolol (Visken)
Penbutolol (Levatol)
Metoprolol (Lopressor)
Atenolol (Tenormin)
Acebutolol (Sectral)
Bisprolol (Zebeta)
Labetalol (Normodyne)
Carvedilol (Coreg)
Terazosin (Hytrin)
Prazosin (Minipress)
Doxazosin (Cardura)
Phentolamine (Regitine)
Phenoxybenzamine (Dibenzyline)
Methyldopa (Aldomet)
Clonidine (Catapres)
Guanabenz acetate (Wytensin)
Reserpine

Lipid Lowering Drugs
Lovastatin (Mevacor)
Simvastatin (Zocor)
Pravastatin (Pravachol)
Fluvastatin (Lescol)
Atorvastatin (Lipitor)
Rosuvastatin (Crestor)
Nicotinic acid (Nicobid)
Fenofibrate (Antara)
Gemfibrozil (Lopid)
Ezetimibe (Zetia)
Cholestyramine (Questran)
Colestipol (Colestid)
Colesevelam (WelChol)

Review Test for Chapter 4

Directions: Each of the numbered items or incomplete statements in this section is followed by answers or by completions of the statement. Select the ONE lettered answer or completion that is BEST in each case.

1. A patient with a long history of cardiovascular disease develops worsening ventricular arrhythmias. Which of the following drugs is most likely to be the cause of the arrhythmia?

(A) Quinidine
(B) Propanolol
(C) Dobutamine
(D) Methyldopa

2. A patient is admitted into the emergency room and manifests ventricular tachycardia following an acute myocardial infarction (MI). This arrhythmia is life threatening and must be controlled immediately. Which of the following drugs would be best to quickly control the condition?

(A) Dobutamine
(B) Digitalis
(C) Quinidine
(D) Lidocaine
(E) Atropine

3. A woman who is undergoing a endocrine work-up to diagnose the cause of a large multinodular goiter develops atrial fibrillation. Which of the following would be best to treat this arrhythmia?

(A) Verapamil
(B) Propranolol
(C) Digitalis
(D) Bretylium
(E) Tocainide

4. A 57-year-old man with atrial flutter is initially treated with quinidine to control the arrhythmia. He is released from the hospital, and while his condition improves, sporadic arrhythmias continue. Which of the following drugs might be used as an adjunct to quinidine in the treatment of the atrial flutter?

(A) Digitalis
(B) Lidocaine
(C) Procainamide
(D) Nifedipine
(E) Propranolol

5. A 16-year-old boy is brought to the hospital by ambulance following a car accident causing serious head injuries. His blood pressure is 220/170 mm Hg. Funduscopy reveals retinal damage, and you administer nitroprusside via infusion. Control of the hypertension requires 72 hours and you notice the patient becoming increasingly fatigued and nauseous. The mostly likely cause of these symptoms is

(A) Production of thiocyanate from nitroprusside
(B) Negative inotropic activity of nitroprusside
(C) Renal precipitation of nitroprusside
(D) Accumulation of nitroprusside because of its long half-life
(E) Production of hydroxocobalamin.

6. A 66-year-old man presents to your office with a 5-month history of dry cough. He denies any other symptoms. His past medical history includes a recent myocardial infarction (MI), after which he was placed on several medications. He does not smoke, nor has he had a history of asthma. You decide that a medication side effect is the most likely cause of this patient's symptoms. Which medication might this be?

(A) Lisinopril
(B) Nitroglycerin
(C) Lovastatin
(D) Digoxin
(E) Quinidine

7. Since the side effects of the medication you prescribed preclude the patient in the above scenario from taking it, you switch him to therapy with an agent that is said to produce similar mortality benefits, while working via a slightly different mechanism of action. What agent is it?

(A) Furosemide
(B) Captopril

(C) Losartan
(D) Esmolol
(E) Ezetimibe

8. A 54-year-old woman is diagnosed with congestive heart failure (CHF). You prescribe captopril, a medication proven to reduce her mortality. This agent delivers several benefits to patients with CHF. Which of the following effects is caused by this drug?

(A) It has a high affinity for angiotensin II receptors
(B) It promotes increased peripheral vascular resistance
(C) It decreases cardiac output and increases afterload
(D) It causes venodilation and induces natriuresis
(E) It increases preload

9. A 76-year-old man has suffered from atrial fibrillation for many years. This condition has been under good control with amiodarone and diltiazem until recently, when he started experiencing palpitations and came back to see you. You decide to start the patient on digoxin therapy. How does this medication work?

(A) It decreases intracellular sodium and increases intracellular potassium
(B) It lowers intracellular calcium
(C) It decreases stroke volume and cardiac output
(D) It diminishes elimination of sodium and water
(E) It increases vagal activity and decreases sympathetic tone

10. A 47-year-old woman is admitted for treatment of acute myocardial ischemia. Her prior medication included digoxin for atrial fibrillation. She also suffers from hypertension, for which she is currently not taking anything. Before you discharge her home, you decide to add a medication that works well for hypertension. While she is still on the floor she develops a dangerous arrhythmia, which you are fortunately able to treat promptly. Which medication you added likely increased the effects of digoxin that this patient was already taking?

(A) Valsartan
(B) Hydrochlorothiazide
(C) Hydralazine
(D) Tadalafil
(E) Lovastatin

11. A 55-year-old woman is admitted to the surgical intensive care unit after having a coronary artery bypass grafting of four of her coronary vessels. Overnight she develops hypotension, and her cardiac output, as measured by the Swan-Ganz catheter, is significantly lower than it had been post-surgery. You decide to give her a dose of milrinone. This results in an increase in her cardiac output. How does this medication work?

(A) It is a cholinergic agonist
(B) It reduces left ventricular filling pressure
(C) It potentiates cardiac phosphodiesterase type 3
(D) It decreases cyclic AMP (cAMP)
(E) It decreases intracellular calcium

12. You are taking care of a 64-year-old man who had just undergone a right hemicolectomy for colon cancer. His blood pressure has been low, and you want to find out whether the shock that this patient is experiencing is related to a possible intraabdominal infection as a consequence of his surgery or is due to his preexisting congestive heart failure (CHF). After analyzing the Swan-Ganz catheter measurements, you deduce that the picture is most compatible with cardiogenic shock. You recall from your pharmacology class that dobutamine can be used successfully for such patients. Which of the following is true regarding dobutamine?

(A) It acts on dopamine receptors
(B) It activates α-receptors
(C) It activates cyclic AMP (cAMP)-related pathways
(D) It increases peripheral resistance
(E) It produces bradycardia

13. A 75-year-old woman, who is admitted for management of her recent stroke, develops increased blood pressure, up to 195/105, with a heart rate of 95. Her physician is worried about the possibility of cerebral hemorrhage into the preexisting infarct and decides to administer a fast-acting vasodilating agent, which is also commonly used for severe decompensated congestive heart failure (CHF). Which medication did the doctor use?

(A) Nitroprusside
(B) Furosemide
(C) Dobutamine
(D) Losartan
(E) Digoxin

14. While doing your medicine clerkship, you hear an announcement that a CPR team should immediately report to the room of one of the patients. Being an inquisitive student, you decide to observe how the code team manages this unfortunate patient's CPR. The rhythm monitor displays ventricular fibrillation that is quickly converted to atrial fibrillation with rapid ventricular response. The senior resident orders amiodarone to be administered to this patient. Since you forgot how this agent works, you ask one of the residents to explain how this medication works. The resident replies that he is busy, but tells you it is a class III antiarrhythmic agent. What is the mechanism of action of this agent?

(A) It is a β-receptor antagonist
(B) It blocks fast sodium channels
(C) It decreases refractoriness
(D) It interferes with outward potassium current
(E) It has a relatively short half-life

15. Although the rhythm is now under control in the patient described in the question 14, his rate is still rather high, into the 140s–150s. The rhythm strip is consistent with supraventricular tachycardia. The resident that was testing you before is now less busy and asks you what medication he should use next, given that he has in mind an agent that can also be used as an antimalarial. Which agent is it?

(A) Digoxin
(B) Propranolol
(C) Flecainide
(D) Verapamil
(E) Quinidine

Answers and Explanations

1. **The answer is A.** Quinidine is associated with QT interval prolongation and torsade de point arrhythmias. Propranolol can cause heart block. Dobutamine rarely causes ventricular arrhythmias.

2. **The answer is D.** Lidocaine is the best agent for management of ventricular tachycardia associated with acute myocardial infarction (MI). Dobutamine, digitalis, quinidine, and atropine can all induce tachyarrhythmias. Lidocaine does not slow conduction and has little effect on atrial function.

3. **The answer is B.** Hyperthyroidism apparently increases β-adrenoceptors. β-Adrenoceptor antagonists such as propranolol can actually decrease symptoms of hyperthyroidism.

4. **The answer is A.** Quinidine acts to prolong refractoriness and slow conduction rather than as a negative inotropic agent. The ability of digitalis to decrease conduction through the atrioventricular (AV) node makes its effects compatible with quinidine to reduce atrial flutter. Lidocaine must be administered parenterally. The effects of procainamide are synergistic with quinidine, increasing the risk of toxicity; nifedipine has little antiarrhythmic effect.

5. **The answer is A.** The toxicity of nitroprusside is caused by the release of cyanide and the accumulation of thiocyanate. Hydroxocobalamin is used to reduce the toxicity of nitroprusside through the formation of the less toxic cyanocobalamin.

6. **The answer is A.** Angiotensin-converting enzyme (ACE) inhibitors commonly cause dry nonproductive cough. Nitroglycerin can cause headaches. Lovastatin commonly causes liver dysfunction. Digoxin can cause arrhythmias, and quinidine is known to cause muscle weakness.

7. **The answer is C.** Losartan is an angiotensin receptor blocker (ARB) that produces effects similar to those of angiotensin converting enzyme (ACE) inhibitors while causing less cough and angioedema. Furosemide is a loop diuretic that is used in congestive heart failure. Captopril is an example of another ACE inhibitor. Esmolol is an antiarrhythmic agent. Ezetimibe is a lipid-lowering drug.

8. **The answer is D.** Angiotensin converting enzyme (ACE) inhibitors cause venodilation and induce natriuresis, thereby reducing preload. A high affinity for angiotensin II receptors represents the mechanism of action of angiotensin-receptor blockers. ACE inhibitors counteract increased peripheral resistance, increase cardiac output, and decrease afterload.

9. **The answer is E.** Digoxin, a cardiac glycoside, increases vagal activity, resulting in inhibition of the sinoatrial (SA) node and delayed conduction through the atrioventricular (AV) node. It also decreases sympathetic tone. Cardiac glycosides increase intracellular sodium while decreasing intracellular potassium; increase intracellular calcium; and increase stroke volume and therefore cardiac output. Cardiac glycosides enhance elimination of sodium and water.

10. **The answer is B.** Hydrochlorothiazide, a diuretic, is known to cause hypokalemia, a state in which the actions of digoxin can be potentiated to a dangerous level. Valsartan is generally not used as a sole agent for hypertension. Hydralazine lowers blood pressure, but it does not generally cause marked electrolyte disturbances. Tadalafil is an agent used for erectile dysfunction. Lovastatin is an HMG-CoA inhibitor, used for hypercholesterolemia.

11. **The answer is B.** Milrinone reduces left ventricular filling pressure and thus enhances cardiac output. It is related to the anticholinergic agent biperiden. Milrinone inhibits cardiac phosphodiesterase type 3. It increases cyclic AMP (cAMP), and therefore intracellular calcium.

12. **The answer is C.** Dobutamine increases cyclic AMP (cAMP)-mediated phosphorylation and the activity of calcium channels. It does not act on dopamine receptors or α-receptors; it only acts

on β_1-receptors. Dobutamine does not substantially affect peripheral resistance. This agent produces mild tachycardia.

13. **The answer is A.** Nitroprusside is a vasodilating agent that can be used in hypertensive emergencies. Furosemide is used for long-term treatment of congestive heart failure (CHF). Dobutamine does not significantly affect the vessels to produce vasodilation. Losartan is an angiotensin converting enzyme (ACE) inhibitor that is used in long-term care of CHF. Digoxin is another long-term agent used in CHF and certain arrhythmias.

14. **The answer is D.** Amiodarone is a class III antiarrhythmic agent that interferes with outward potassium current. β-Receptor antagonists are considered class II antiarrhythmics. Class I antiarrhythmics block fast sodium channels. Amiodarone prolongs the effective refractory period. It has a rather long half-life, up to 100 days.

15. **The answer is E.** Quinidine is used for supraventricular tachycardia and is used to maintain sinus rhythm after conversion of atrial fibrillation. It also has antimalarial properties. Digoxin can be used in long-term management of atrial fibrillation. Propranolol is a class II antiarrhythmic agent. Flecainide is a class IC agent that can be used for ventricular tachyarrhythmias. Verapamil is a class IV antiarrhythmic agent.

chapter 5

Drugs Acting on the Central Nervous System

I. SEDATIVE–HYPNOTIC DRUGS

A. Definitions

1. ***Sedation*** is characterized by decreased anxiety, motor activity, and cognitive acuity.
2. ***Hypnosis*** is characterized by drowsiness and an increased tendency to sleep.

B. Benzodiazepines (Table 5-1)

1. ***General properties***
   a. Benzodiazepines have a **great margin of safety** over previously available sedative–hypnotic agents (Fig. 5-1). With the notable exception of several relatively new nonbenzodiazepine agents (**zolpidem, zaleplon, eszopiclone, buspirone**), previously available sedative–hypnotic agents (e.g., barbiturates, chloral hydrate, ethanol) produce a dose-dependent continuum of central nervous system (CNS) depression, leading ultimately to coma and death.
   b. Benzodiazepines have qualitatively similar therapeutic actions. However, because of quantitative differences in their relative lipid solubility, biotransformation, and elimination half-life, some benzodiazepines are marketed for specific therapeutic purposes.
2. ***Mechanism of action*** (Fig. 5-2)
   a. Benzodiazepines facilitate γ-aminobutyric acid (GABA)-mediated inhibition of neuronal activity in the CNS.
   b. They bind to a benzodiazepine receptor (there are at least two subtypes, BZ1 and BZ2) that is part of, but distinct from, the pentameric $GABA_A$-receptor–chloride channel complex that consists of at least four distinct subunits (α, β, γ, δ) and their multiple isoforms in different proportions. A major form of the complex in the brain consists of 2α subunits, 2β subunits, and 1γ subunit.
   c. Benzodiazepines **allosterically increase GABA affinity and the frequency of GABA-stimulated chloride channel opening,** chloride conductance, and neuronal hyperpolarization; they also inhibit depolarization by excitatory neurotransmitters. These drugs have no action in the absence of GABA.
3. ***Pharmacologic properties***
   a. Generally, benzodiazepines are administered orally to treat anxiety and sleep disorders. Some can be given parenterally (e.g., **chlordiazepoxide, diazepam, lorazepam, and midazolam**).
   b. The onset of benzodiazepine action is related to the relative degree of lipid solubility, which can vary 50-fold or more. Benzodiazepines that are highly lipid soluble (e.g., **midazolam, flurazepam, triazolam, and diazepam**) have a more rapid onset of action than benzodiazepines that are relatively less lipid soluble.
   c. Redistribution from the brain to peripheral tissues is considered an important factor in terminating the actions of single, or intermittent, nonaccumulating doses of the most highly lipid-soluble benzodiazepines.
   d. Hepatic metabolism accounts for the clearance of all benzodiazepines. However, there is sometimes little correlation between the plasma half-life ($t_{1/2}$) of the parent drug and the

table 5-1 Benzodiazepine Indications

Drug (Half-Life)	Primary Indications
Short acting ($t_{1/2}$ <5 h)	
Midazolam	Preanesthetic
Triazolam	Insomnia, preanesthetic
Intermediate acting ($t_{1/2}$ 5–24 h)	
Alprazolam[a]	Anxiety, antidepressant
Clonazepam	Seizures
Estazolam	Insomnia
Lorazepam	Anxiety, insomnia, seizures, preanesthetic
Oxazepam	Anxiety
Temazepam	Insomnia
Long-lasting ($t_{1/2}$ >24 h)	
Chlordiazepoxide[b,d]	Anxiety, preanesthetic, withdrawal states
Clorazepate[b,c]	Anxiety, seizures
Diazepam[b,d]	Anxiety, preanesthetic, seizures, withdrawal states
Flurazepam	Insomnia
Prazepam[b,c]	Anxiety
Quazepam	Insomnia

[a] For panic disorders.
[b] Converted to the long-acting, active metabolite.
[c] Prodrug.
[d] For withdrawal from ethanol and other sedative-hypnotics

duration of its action. Active metabolites, particularly **desmethyldiazepam,** result from acid hydrolysis in the stomach (as with the prodrug clorazepate) or phase I hepatic microsomal oxidation (*N*-dealkylation, aliphatic hydroxylation) and extend the plasma half-life of some benzodiazepines (e.g., chlordiazepoxide, diazepam, prazepam) to as long as 60 hours or more.

e. Biotransformation (ring hydroxylation and glucuronidation) to inactive metabolites is the most important factor for terminating the actions of less lipid-soluble benzodiazepines (**estazolam, lorazepam, oxazepam**). These are excreted by the kidney.

f. With long-term multiple-dose therapy, the rate and extent of accumulation of benzodiazepines and active metabolites or their disappearance after discontinuing administration is directly related to their elimination half-life and clearance.

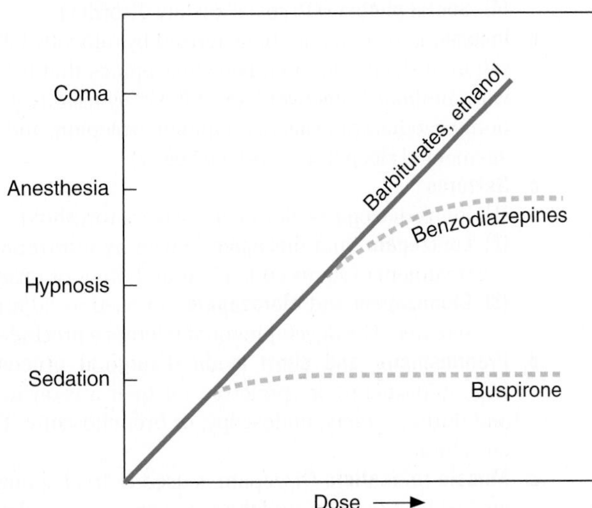

FIGURE 5-1. Theoretical dose–response relationships for sedative–hypnotic drugs and buspirone.

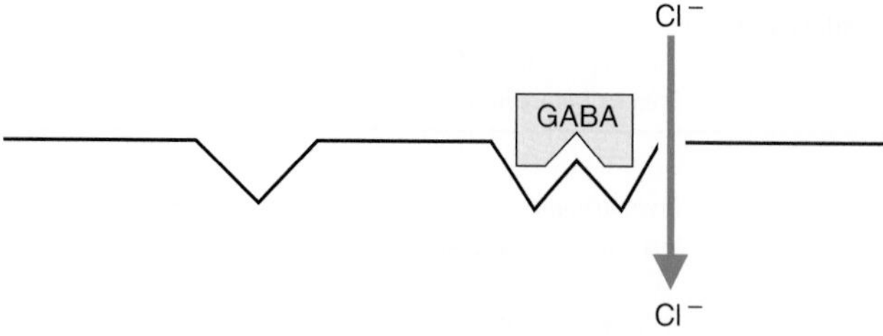

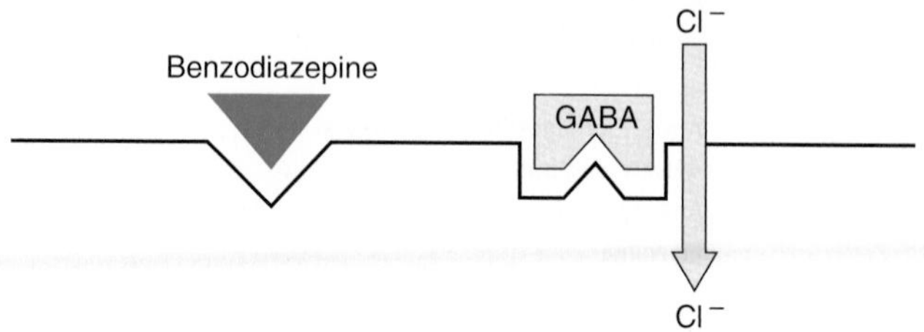

FIGURE 5-2. Representation of GABA-receptor–chloride channel receptor complex. Binding of GABA to its receptor causes the closed chloride channel to open. Binding of benzodiazepine to its receptor allosterically enhances binding of GABA. This causes increased chloride conductance and further hyperpolarization of the cell, making it less excitable.

g. Clearance of benzodiazepines is decreased in the elderly and in patients with liver disease. In these patients, doses should be reduced.

4. ***Therapeutic uses*** (see Table 5-1)

a. Benzodiazepines are effective and safe for the **short-term treatment of anxiety disorders.** Selective serotonin-reuptake inhibitors (SSRIs; see III E below) are preferred for long-term treatment of the following anxiety disorders as well as first-line therapy for obsessive–compulsive disorder (OCD) and posttraumatic stress disorder (PTSD), in which benzodiazepines may worsen symptoms.

(1) **Generalized anxiety disorders** (GADs; characterized by feelings of severe apprehension, tension, and uneasiness that disrupt normal function)

(2) **Situational anxiety disorders** (SADs; e.g., frightening medical or dental procedures)

(3) **Panic disorders** (PDs; irrational, intense apprehension that may include symptoms of a heart attack) with or without agoraphobia. Because of its apparent greater specificity, alprazolam is widely used for urgent care.

(4) **Social phobia** (SP; social anxiety disorder)

b. **Insomnia.** Insomnia is characterized by difficulty falling or staying asleep or inadequate duration of sleep. Although benzodiazepines that have a rapid onset and sufficient duration with minimal "hangover" are still widely used (e.g., triazolam, triazepam, flurazepam), the nonbenzodiazepine agents zolpidem, zaleplon, and eszopiclone are now preferred for management of sleep disorders (see below).

c. **Seizures**

(1) Benzodiazepines elevate the seizure threshold.

(2) **Lorazepam** (and **diazepam**), given by intravenous (IV) infusion, is preferred for initial treatment of status epilepticus and drug- or toxin-induced seizures.

(3) **Clonazepam** and **clorazepate** are used as adjuncts for absence, myoclonic, and atonic seizures. The development of tolerance precludes their long-term use.

d. **Preanesthetic and short medical/surgical procedures.** Shorter-acting benzodiazepines (e.g., midazolam) are preferred for their anxiolytic, sedative, and amnestic actions before and during surgery, endoscopy, or bronchoscopy. These drugs do not produce full surgical anesthesia.

e. **Muscle relaxation.** Diazepam is used to treat spontaneous muscle spasms, spasms associated with endoscopy, and the spasticity of cerebral palsy.

f. **Acute mania** of bipolar disorder for the initial management of agitation

g. **Physical dependence.** Long-acting benzodiazepines, such as diazepam and chlordiazepoxide, are used to reduce the withdrawal symptoms of physical dependence associated with the long-term use of shorter-acting benzodiazepines and other sedative-hypnotic drugs, including alcohol and the barbiturates.

5. ***Adverse effects, contraindications, and drug interactions***
   a. Benzodiazepines commonly produce **daytime drowsiness, sedation, and ataxia** that may impair judgment and interfere with motor skills, particularly in the elderly. In the treatment of insomnia, these adverse effects are more likely to occur with longer-acting benzodiazepines.
   b. These drugs may cause **rebound insomnia** on discontinuation.
   c. **In the elderly,** benzodiazepines infrequently cause **reversible confusion and amnesia** as well as blurred vision, hypotension, tremor, and constipation.
   d. These drugs may **depress respiration** at higher than hypnotic doses, an effect that can be exaggerated in patients with chronic obstructive pulmonary disease (COPD) or obstructive sleep apnea (OSA).
   e. Benzodiazepines, particularly when given intravenously, may decrease blood pressure and decrease heart rate in patients with impaired cardiovascular function.
   f. These drugs cause rare paradoxical excitement.
   g. Benzodiazepines **enhance CNS depression when taken in combination with other drugs that depress the CNS,** most notably alcohol.
   h. Drugs and grapefruit juice that inhibit CYP3A4 can extend the duration of benzodiazepine action.
6. ***Tolerance, abuse, and dependence***
   a. With long-term administration, tolerance develops to the sedative-hypnotic and anticonvulsant actions of benzodiazepines but not to their anxiolytic action. Patients exhibit **cross-tolerance** with other sedative-hypnotic agents, including **alcohol** and **barbiturates.**
   b. The abuse potential of benzodiazepines is low compared with that of other classes of sedative-hypnotic drugs except when there is already a history of substance abuse.
   c. Signs of withdrawal after long-term benzodiazepine use (3–4 months) may include anxiety and insomnia, and also GI disturbances, headache, and tremor. Perceptual distortions, delusions, and seizures have also been reported. Withdrawal occurs sooner and is more severe after abrupt discontinuation of shorter-acting benzodiazepines; the effects associated with withdrawal can be minimized by tapering the dose reduction or substituting longer-acting benzodiazepines such as diazepam.

C. Flumazenil

1. Flumazenil is a **competitive antagonist** at benzodiazepine receptors.
2. Flumazenil is used to prevent or reverse the CNS effects from benzodiazepine overdose or to speed recovery from the effects of benzodiazepines used in anesthetic and diagnostic procedures; it may precipitate withdrawal. Its short duration of action often necessitates multiple dosing.

D. Zolpidem, zaleplon, and eszopiclone

1. Zolpidem, zaleplon, and eszoplicone are widely used for short-term treatment of **insomnia**; Zolpidem has some minimal anxiolytic activity as well.
2. These drugs, which act on a specific subtype of the benzodiazepine receptor BZ1 (omega1) to reduce chloride conductance, have a similar mechanism of action but are structurally unrelated to the benzodiazepines.
3. Dosage of these drugs should be reduced in the elderly and in patients with hepatic impairment.
4. These drugs have only **weak muscle-relaxing or anticonvulsant activity,** with **reduced potential compared to the benzodiazepines for tolerance, abuse, physical dependence, or rebound insomnia.**
5. Their actions are blocked or reversed by flumazenil.
6. Adverse effects include modest daytime sedation, headache, and GI upset. Eszopiclone is reported to also produce dry mouth, some sedation, and an unpleasant taste.

E. Buspirone

1. Buspirone is a **nonbenzodiazepine** that selectively relieves anxiety without the sedation, hypnosis, general CNS depression, or drug abuse liability of the benzodiazepines (see Fig. 5-1). It has no other benzodiazepine-like activities.

2. Buspirone is used primarily to treat generalized anxiety disorder, particularly in the elderly, who are more susceptible to the CNS depressant action of the benzodiazepines.
3. Buspirone is a **partial agonist** at serotonin (5-HT_{1A})-receptors.
4. A week or more of administration may be required to achieve the therapeutic effects of buspirone.
5. Buspirone may cause **nervousness, restlessness, dysphoria, tachycardia, or GI distress** more often than benzodiazepines. It causes **pupillary constriction.**

F. Ramelteon

1. Ramelteon is a selective agonist at **melatonin MT1- and MT2-receptors** that is prescribed for patients who have difficulty falling asleep.
2. Ramelteon is rapidly absorbed and metabolized to an active longer-acting metabolite.
3. This drug has no direct effect on GABA receptors.
4. This drug is metabolized by CYP1A2 and thus should be used cautiously in patients with liver disease or who use drugs that inhibit this enzyme.
5. Adverse effects include dizziness, fatigue, and certain endocrine alterations.

G. Other sedative–hypnotics. Barbiturates, chloral hydrate (rapidly metabolized in the liver to its active form, trichloroethanol), and meprobamate have been largely supplanted by benzodiazepines, the newer nonbenzodiazepine sedative–hypnotic agents, and the SSRIs for treatment of anxiety and sleep disorders.

1. ***Barbiturates (amobarbital, pentobarbital, secobarbital; see also phenobarbital)*** (Table 5-2; see also VII C 1 and X C 3)
   a. Barbiturates are weak organic acids (substituted barbituric acid).
   b. Barbiturates are classified according to the rate of onset and duration of the therapeutic action. **Redistribution** from highly vascular (e.g., brain) to less-vascular tissues (e.g., muscle, fat) is **responsible for the short duration of highly lipid-soluble barbiturates** (e.g., **thiopental**). Metabolism (oxidation and conjugation in the liver) and excretion are more important determinants for less lipid-soluble barbiturates. About 25% of a dose of **phenobarbital** is excreted unchanged. Alkalinization of the urine enhances excretion and shortens its duration of action.
   c. Barbiturates **interact with a binding site on the GABA-receptor–chloride channel complex** that is separate from the benzodiazepine receptor. At low doses, barbiturates allosterically **prolong the GABA-induced opening of chloride channels** and enhance GABA-inhibitory neurotransmission; at higher doses, these drugs have GABA-mimetic activity (they open chloride channels independently of GABA).
   d. With long-term use, these drugs, particularly **phenobarbital,** may **induce the synthesis of hepatic microsomal enzymes** and increase their own metabolism or the metabolism of numerous other drugs.

table 5-2 Classification and Indications of Barbiturates

Drug and Classification	Indications
Ultra-short acting Thiopental (Pentothal) Methohexital (Brevital) Thiamylal (Surital)	Intravenous general anesthesia
Intermediate acting Amobarbital (Amytal) Pentobarbital (Nembutal) Secobarbital (Seconal)	Preanesthetic medication and regional anesthesia; sedation and hypnosis (largely supplanted by benzodiazepines)
Long acting Phenobarbital (Luminal) Mephobarbital (Mebaral)	Seizure disorders; withdrawal syndrome from sedative– hypnotics

e. Barbiturates **increase porphyrin synthesis** by the induction of hepatic δ-aminolevulinic acid synthase, and they can precipitate acute intermittent porphyria.

f. The use of these drugs as sedative–hypnotic agents is almost obsolete, supplanted by benzodiazepines and other nonbenzodiazepine sedative–hypnotic agents. (**Pentobarbital** is used to some extent; **phenobarbital** is still widely used as an anticonvulsant; **thiopental** [and other ultra-short-acting barbiturates] is used as an IV general anesthetic.) The barbiturates are limited by their strong sedation effects, rapid tolerance, drug interactions, abuse potential, and lethality in overdose.

g. Barbiturates produce **dose-related respiratory depression** with cerebral hypoxia, possibly leading to coma or death; this effect results from abuse or suicide attempt. Treatment includes ventilation, gastric lavage, hemodialysis, osmotic diuretics, and (for **phenobarbital**) alkalinization of urine.

h. Barbiturates depress the medullary vasomotor center, with circulatory collapse.

i. Use of barbiturates is contraindicated in patients with pulmonary insufficiency.

j. Hepatic and renal disease may prolong barbiturate action.

k. **Phenobarbital** and **pentobarbital** are occasionally used to treat the physical dependence associated with long-term use of sedative–hypnotic drugs.

l. **Amobarbital, pentobarbital,** and **secobarbital** are drugs of abuse (see X C 3).

II. ANTIPSYCHOTIC (NEUROLEPTIC) DRUGS

A. Classification

1. Antipsychotic drugs may be classified as either **conventional** or **atypical.**
2. ***Conventional antipsychotic drugs*** are often subclassified according to their oral milligram potency (high potency or low potency).
   - **a.** **High-potency** drugs (**piperazine phenothiazines, e.g., fluphenazine;** and **haloperidol**) are more likely to produce extrapyramidal reactions.
   - **b.** **Low-potency** drugs (**aliphatic phenothiazines, e.g., triflupromazine; piperidine phenothiazines, e.g., thioridazine**) are less likely to produce acute extrapyramidal reactions and more likely to produce sedation and postural hypotension.
3. ***Atypical antipsychotic agents*** **(e.g., risperidone, olanzapine)** have generally replaced the conventional drugs for initial treatment of first-episode patients. **Clozapine** is reserved for treatment-resistant patients.
4. Other **conventional heterocyclic antipsychotic drugs** such as **loxapine** and **molindone,** with intermediate potency, have no clear advantage over other conventional drugs.

B. Mechanism of therapeutic action

1. The therapeutic action of the conventional antipsychotic drugs is correlated best with **antagonist activity** at **postjunctional dopamine D_2-receptors,** where dopamine normally inhibits adenylyl cyclase activity.
2. The therapeutic action of the atypical antipsychotic drugs is correlated with antagonist activity at both 5-HT_2-receptors and dopamine D_2- or D_4-receptors. Aripiprazole is a partial agonist at dopamine D_2-receptors and, like ziprasidone, also stimulates serotonin 5-HT_{1A}-receptors.
3. The therapeutic action is best correlated with the actions of these drugs in the mesolimbic and mesocortical areas of the CNS.

C. Pharmacologic properties

1. Most of these drugs show little correlation between plasma levels and therapeutic action. Plasma levels are monitored primarily for compliance and toxicity.
2. Most antipsychotic drugs are highly lipophilic and have **long half-lives** (10–20 h). They are metabolized by liver microsomal oxidation and conjugation. Thioridazine is metabolized to mesoridazine, which accounts for most of the parent compound's effects.
3. Esterification of fluphenazine and haloperidol (fluphenazine decanoate, haloperidol decanoate) results in long-acting depot forms (2- to 3-week duration of action) that can be used to

manage compliance issues. **Plasma esterases** convert the parent compound to the active drug when the ester diffuses into the bloodstream.

D. Therapeutic uses

1. *Schizophrenia*

a. Antipsychotic drugs produce an **immediate quieting action.** However, their antipsychotic effects, including decreased symptoms of thought disorders, paranoid features, delusions, hostility, hallucinations (the positive symptoms of schizophrenia) and, to a lesser degree, decreased withdrawal, apathy, and blunted affect (the negative symptoms of schizophrenia), typically take longer to occur (a week or more). Atypical antipsychotic drugs, particularly **clozapine,** have a seemingly greater effect on negative symptoms than the conventional agents.

b. These drugs **curb acute psychotic attacks** and delay subsequent relapses.

2. *Other selected therapeutic uses*

a. **Acute mania in bipolar disorder**

b. **Atypical psychotic disorders** (e.g., following surgery or myocardial infarction)

c. **Depression with psychotic manifestations**

d. **Tourette syndrome (haloperidol or pimozide** [Orap]), to suppress severe tics and vocalization

e. Severe nausea or vomiting associated with a variety of diseases, radiation treatment, and cancer chemotherapy, as well as postoperative nausea and vomiting. Conventional antipsychotic agents, with the exception of thioridazine, have strong antiemetic activity due to dopamine D_2-receptor blockade in the chemoreceptor trigger zone of the medulla. The most commonly used are the phenothiazine **prochlorperazine,** which is marketed only as an antiemetic, and **promethazine,** which has no antipsychotic activity.

E. Adverse effects and contraindications. Selection of a specific antipsychotic agent for therapeutic use is often based on its associated adverse effects rather than therapeutic efficacy. The adverse effects of antipsychotic agents are due to their antagonist actions at dopamine D_2- and histamine H_1-receptors (and possibly serotonin receptors) in the CNS and to their antagonist actions at muscarinic cholinoceptors and α-adrenoceptors in the periphery.

1. *Central nervous system*

a. **Extrapyramidal syndromes** (see Tables 5-3 and 5-4)

(1) These adverse effects are related to a **dopamine-receptor blockade** in the basal ganglia (and elsewhere in the CNS) that leads to an imbalance in dopamine and acetylcholine actions in the nigrostriatal pathway.

(2) These effects are a major cause of **noncompliance.**

(3) Extrapyramidal effects are **most likely to occur with high-potency conventional antipsychotic drugs** that have a high affinity for postjunctional dopamine D_2-receptors in the basal ganglia. They are less likely to occur with low-potency conventional antipsychotic drugs such as **thioridazine,** which have lower affinity for dopamine D_2-receptors than high-potency drugs. With the exception of **risperidone,** they are also unlikely to occur with atypical antipsychotic drugs such as **clozapine** and **olanzapine.** Extrapyramidal effects are also less likely to occur with those conventional agents that also have substantial antagonist activity at cholinoceptors in the basal ganglia.

(4) These effects can sometimes spontaneously remit.

(5) Extrapyramidal syndromes include the following:

(a) **Acute dystonia**

(i) Acute dystonia is characterized by spastic retrocollis or torticollis. Respiration may be compromised.

(ii) This condition is often elicited during the first week of therapy.

(iii) Acute dystonia can be controlled with more-centrally acting antimuscarinic drugs such as **benztropine** and **biperiden,** with the antihistamine **diphenhydramine (Benadryl)** (which has central anticholinergic activity), and by reducing the antipsychotic drug dose, which may lead to an increase in psychotic symptoms.

table 5-3 Potency and Selected Adverse Effects of Representative Conventional Antipsychotic Drugs

Drugs	Oral Dose (mg)	Extrapyramidal Effects[a]	Autonomic Effects	Sedation
Conventional drugs				
Aliphatic phenothiazines				
Chlorpromazine	100	++	+++	+++
Triflupromazine	50	++	+++	+++
Piperidine phenothiazines				
Thioridazine[b,c]	100	+	+++	+++
Mesoridazine[c]	50	+	+++	+++
Piperazine phenothiazines				
Trifluoperazine	10	+++	++	++
Fluphenazine[d]	5	+++	++	++
Butyrophenones				
Haloperidol	2	+++	+	+
Other related drugs				
Molindone[c]	20–200	+++	++	++
Loxapine	20–250	+++	++	++

[a] Excluding tardive dyskinesia.
[b] Cardiotoxicity.
[c] No antiemetic activity.
[d] Esterification (enanthate or decanoate) results in depot form.

(b) Akathisia is the irresistible compulsion to be in motion.

(i) This condition can develop as early as the first 2 weeks of treatment or as late as 60 days into therapy.

(ii) Akathisia, like acute dystonia, can be controlled by drugs with antimuscarinic activity and by the β-receptor antagonist **propranolol.**

(c) Parkinsonian-like syndrome

(i) Parkinsonian-like syndrome is characterized by tremors, bradykinesia, rigidity, and other signs of parkinsonism.

(ii) This syndrome can develop from 5 days to weeks into treatment.

(iii) Parkinsonian-like syndrome can be controlled with antimuscarinic drugs (e.g., **benztropine, biperiden**) or by reducing the antipsychotic drug dose.

b. Tardive dyskinesia

(1) Tardive dyskinesia is much more likely with conventional antipsychotic agents than atypical agents. It does not occur with **clozapine.**

table 5-4 Selected Adverse Effects of Atypical Antipsychotic Drugs

Atypical Drugs	Extrapyramidal Effects[a]	Hypotensive Activity	Sedation	Weight Gain	Increased Prolactin
Aripiprazole	+/–	+	+/–	+/–	+/–
Clozapine[b]	+/–	++	+	+++	+/–
Olanzapine	+/–	+	++	+++	+/–
Quetiapine	+/–	++	++	++	+/–
Risperidone[c]	++	+	+	+	++
Ziprasidone[d]	+/–	+/–	+	+/–	+/–

[a] Excluding tardive dyskinesia.
[b] Agranulocytosis.
[c] Little extrapyramidal effects at low doses.
[d] QTc prolongation.

(2) Tardive dyskinesia is primarily characterized by disfiguring orofaciolingual movements (tics), but it occasionally includes dystonic movements of the trunk.

(3) These effects may be the result of a developing supersensitivity of the postjunctional dopamine receptors in the CNS, perhaps in the basal ganglia.

(4) Tardive dyskinesia generally occurs after months to years of drug exposure; it may be exacerbated or precipitated by the discontinuation of therapy.

(5) Tardive dyskinesia is **often irreversible.**

(6) Tardive dyskinesia has an estimated incidence of 10%–20%; it is more likely to occur in the elderly or in institutionalized patients who receive long-term, high-dose therapy.

(7) The only effective treatment for antipsychotic drug-induced tardive dyskinesia is the discontinuation of drug therapy.

c. **Neuroleptic malignant syndrome**

(1) Neuroleptic malignant syndrome is most likely in patients sensitive to the extrapyramidal effects of the conventional high-potency antipsychotic agents.

(2) This syndrome is characterized by autonomic instability, muscle rigidity, diaphoresis, profound hyperthermia, and myoglobinemia.

(3) This condition occurs, often explosively, in 1% of patients; it is **associated with a 20% mortality rate.**

(4) This condition is treated by discontinuing drug therapy and initiating supportive measures, including the use of **bromocriptine** to overcome the dopamine receptor blockade and the use of muscle relaxants such as **diazepam** and perhaps **dantrolene** to reduce muscle rigidity.

d. **Sedation** (see Tables 5-3 and 5-4)

(1) The sedation effects, **more likely with low-potency antipsychotic agents** and with the atypical agents, are due to a central histamine H_1-receptor blockade.

(2) These effects may be mild to severe. The elderly are particularly at risk.

(3) **The effects** may be temporary.

e. **Confusional state with memory impairment.** This effect is likely with antipsychotic agents with pronounced antimuscarinic activity.

f. **Seizures**

(1) Seizures are especially more common with **chlorpromazine, clozapine, and olanzapine.**

(2) This effect is due to a lowering of the seizure threshold; antipsychotic drugs may precipitate or unmask epilepsy.

2. ***Autonomic nervous system*** (see Tables 5-3 and 5-4)

a. **α-Adrenoceptor blockade**

(1) Blockade of α-adrenoceptors, **more likely to occur with conventional low-potency and atypical antipsychotic agents,** causes **orthostatic hypotension** and possibly syncope, as a result of peripheral vasodilation; central depression of the vasomotor center may also contribute. This effect may be severe and may result in reflex tachycardia. Elderly patients and those with heart disease are more at risk. The effect may be temporary.

(2) This blockade also causes impotence and inhibition of ejaculation.

b. **Muscarinic cholinoceptor blockade**

(1) Blockade of muscarinic cholinoceptors, more common with conventional low-potency antipsychotic agents and with the atypical agent clozapine, produces an atropine-like effect, resulting in dry mouth and blurred vision.

(2) This blockade may also produce constipation, tachycardia, and difficulty in urination leading to urine retention. The effect may be temporary.

(3) Muscarinic cholinoceptor blockade more rarely causes paralytic ileus and severe bladder infections.

(4) Elderly patients are more at risk

3. ***Endocrine and metabolic disturbances,*** likely with most conventional antipsychotic agents and the atypical agent **risperidone,** are due to dopamine (D_2)-receptor antagonist activity in the pituitary, resulting in **hyperprolactinemia** (see Table 5-4).

a. In **women,** these disturbances include spontaneous or induced **galactorrhea, loss of libido,** and delayed ovulation and menstruation or amenorrhea.

b. In **men,** these disturbances include **gynecomastia** and **impotence.**

c. **Weight gain,** which is likely with most conventional antipsychotic agents and the atypical antipsychotic agents, **clozapine** and **olanzapine,** may be due in part to histamine H_1-receptor antagonist activity (see Table 5-4).

4. ***Other adverse effects***

a. **Withdrawal-like syndrome**

(1) This syndrome is characterized by **nausea, vomiting, insomnia,** and **headache** in 30% of patients, especially those receiving low-potency antipsychotic drugs.

(2) These symptoms may persist for up to 2 weeks.

(3) The symptoms can be minimized with a tapered reduction of drug dosage.

b. **Cardiac arrhythmias**

(1) Cardiac arrhythmias result from a quinidine-like effect in which there is local anesthetic activity with an increased likelihood of heart block.

(2) Cardiac arrhythmias are more likely with **thioridazine** and **ziprasidone,** which can prolong the Q-T interval and lead to conduction block and sudden death.

c. **Blood dyscrasias** are rare, except in the case of **clozapine,** which may induce agranulocytosis in up to 3% of patients and, therefore, is used only when other drug groups prove ineffective.

d. **Cholestatic jaundice,** which is caused primarily by **chlorpromazine**

e. **Photosensitivity**

(1) The effect is specific to **chlorpromazine;** it includes dermatitis (5%), rash, sunburn, and pigmentation, and it may be irreversible.

(2) Chlorpromazine and high-dose **thioridazine** also produce retinitis pigmentosa.

F. **Overdose.** Overdose with antipsychotics is rarely fatal, except when caused by thioridazine or mesoridazine (and possibly ziprasidone), which may result in drowsiness, agitation, coma, ventricular arrhythmias, heart block, or sudden death.

G. **Drug interactions**

1. Antipsychotics have potentiated sedative effects in the presence of **CNS depressants** (e.g., sedative–hypnotics, opioids, antihistamines).
2. Certain antipsychotic drugs produce additive anticholinergic effects with tricyclic antidepressants, antiparkinsonian drugs, and other drugs with anticholinergic activity.

III. ANTIDEPRESSANT DRUGS

A. **Classification** (Table 5-5). Antidepressant drugs are classified into four groups: 1) **tricyclic antidepressants (TCAs);** 2) **SSRIs;** 3) **atypical (heterocyclic second- and third-generation) antidepressants;** and 4) **monoamine oxidase inhibitors (MAOIs).**

B. **Mechanism of action** (see Table 5-5)

1. ***TCAs and atypical antidepressant drugs***

a. TCAs and atypical antidepressant drugs **potentiate** the actions of **norepinephrine, serotonin,** or **both by blocking their uptake by transporters into prejunctional nerve endings,** the major route for their physiologic inactivation.

b. Exceptions include

(1) **Amoxapine,** which also blocks dopamine receptors

(2) **Trazodone** and **nefazodone,** which are antagonists at postjunctional 5-HT_2-receptors and also block prejunctional serotonin 5-HT_1-autoreceptors

(3) **Mirtazapine,** which has serotonin 5-HT_2-receptor antagonist activity and also blocks α_2-adrenoceptors

(4) **Bupropion,** the mechanism of action of which is unclear.

2. ***SSRIs.*** SSRIs are selective inhibitors of serotonin uptake.

table 5-5 Relative Activity of Selected Antidepressant Drugs on Norepinephrine and Serotonin Prejunctional Neuronal Uptake

Drug and Classification	Inhibition of Norepinephrine Uptake	Inhibition of Serotonin Uptake
Tricyclic antidepressants		
Tertiary amines		
Amitriptyline	++	+++
Imipramine	++	+++
Trimipramine	+	0
Doxepin	+	++
Clomipramine	+++	+++
Secondary amines		
Desipramine	+++	0
Nortriptyline	++	+++
Protriptyline	+++	0
Dibenzoxazepine		
Amoxapine[a]	++	+
Selective serotonin reuptake inhibitors		
Fluoxetine	0/+	+++
Paroxetine	0	+++
Sertraline	0	+++
Citalopram	0	+++
Escitalopram	0	+++
Fluvoxamine	0	+++
Atypical antidepressants		
Trazodone[b]	0	++
Maprotiline	+++	0
Bupropion	0/+	0/+
Venlafaxine	++	+++
Nefazodone[b]	0	0/+
Mirtazapine[c]	0	0
Duloxetine	+++	+++

[a] Has dopamine-receptor antagonist activity.
[b] Has serotonin 5-HT_1–receptor antagonist activity at prejunctional receptors.
[c] Has serotonin 5-HT_2-receptor and α_2-adrenoceptor antagonist activity.

3. ***MAOIs (Phenelzine, Tranylcypromine)***
   a. MAOIs rapidly, nonselectively, and essentially irreversibly **inhibit the activity of enzymes MAO-A and MAO-B.** Inhibition of MAO-A, which preferentially degrades norepinephrine and serotonin, is responsible for the therapeutic efficacy of MAOIs as antidepressants (MAO-B degrades dopamine preferentially).
   b. MAOIs act as "suicide" enzyme inhibitors, with inhibition continuing for up to 2–3 weeks after their elimination from the body.
4. ***Therapeutic efficacy***
   a. All antidepressant drugs have similar therapeutic efficacy, although individual patients may respond better to one drug than another. Selection is often based on associated adverse effects.
   b. Therapeutic efficacy of these drugs **occurs after several weeks of antidepressant administration** and is closely associated with adaptive changes over the same time period, including **decreased cyclic AMP (cAMP) accumulation and a reduction (down-regulation) of postjunctional β-adrenoceptors,** as well as an increase in responsiveness of postjunctional serotonin 5-HT_{1A}-receptors. **Adaptive desensitization** of prejunctional norepinephrine and serotonin autoreceptors may also be factors.
   c. Adaptive changes in neurotropic factors have also been implicated.

C. Therapeutic uses

1. ***Major depressive disorder***
   a. Antidepressant drugs elevate mood, increase physical activity and mental alertness, increase appetite and sexual drive, improve sleep patterns, and reduce preoccupation with morbid thoughts.
   b. These drugs are effective in 70% of patients.
   c. SSRIs are preferred over TCAs because of their more limited toxicity.
   d. MAOIs are used rarely, usually only when TCAs have proved ineffective or for "atypical" depression.
2. ***Bipolar affective disorder.*** The depressed phase of bipolar affective disorder is often treated with antidepressants given in combination with lithium or other drugs used to control mania.
3. ***Anxiety disorders*** (SSRIs, although unlike benzodiazepines, their full efficacy may not be seen for weeks).
   a. **Generalized anxiety disorder (GAD)** and **panic disorder (PD)**
   b. **Obsessive–compulsive disorder (OCD),** which is also treated with **clomipramine**.
   c. **Social phobia (SP), situational anxiety disorder (SAD)**, and **post-traumatic stress disorder (PTSD)**.
4. ***Enuresis***
   a. **Although not the preferred strategy,** tricyclic antidepressants like **imipramine** are used to suppress enuresis in children (over age 6) and adults.
   b. The exact mechanism of action is uncertain.
5. ***Attention-deficit/hyperactivity disorder (ADHD).*** TCAs (e.g., **imipramine**, **desipramine**) are useful in patients unresponsive or intolerant to stimulants; however, there is some concern regarding reports of toxicity in preadolescents. **Atomoxetine**, a selective inhibitor of norepinephrine reuptake that has some structural similarities to TCA, is also approved for the treatment of ADHD.
6. ***Chronic pain***
   a. TCAs and **venlafaxine** are often used for chronic pain of unknown origin. SSRIs are ineffective. **Duloxetine** is approved for treatment of neuropathic pain associated with diabetes.
   b. These drugs may work directly on pain pathways, but the exact mechanism of action is unknown.
7. Other indications
   a. **Bulemia**
   b. **Premenstrual dysphoric disorder**

D. Tricyclic antidepressants (TCAs)

1. ***Pharmacologic properties***
   a. TCAs are generally highly lipid-soluble and have relatively long half-lives.
   b. TCAs are metabolized by ring hydroxylation and glucuronide conjugation or by demethylation; monodemethylation of the tertiary amines **imipramine** and **amitriptyline** results in the active secondary amine metabolites **desipramine** and **nortriptyline,** respectively.
   c. Plasma levels are used primarily to monitor compliance and toxicity.
2. ***Adverse effects*** (Table 5-6). The adverse effects of TCAs are often accounted for by their antagonist activity at α-adrenoceptors, muscarinic cholinoceptors, histamine H_1-receptors, and others.
   a. **CNS**
      (1) **Sedation** is common and probably due to antagonist activity at CNS histamine H_1 receptors.
      (2) **Confusion and memory dysfunction** are central anticholinergic effects and are more common in the elderly.
      (3) **Mania** occasionally occurs in patients with an underlying bipolar affective disorder ("switch" reaction).
      (4) **Agitation** and **psychosis** may worsen in psychotic patients.
      (5) **Tremor** occurs in 10% of patients and is managed with **propranolol.**
      (6) **Seizures** occur occasionally because of lowered seizure threshold; they are more common with tertiary amines.

table 5-6 Relationship Between Blockade of Neurotransmitter Receptors and Antidepressant-Induced Adverse Effects

Receptor Subtype	Adverse Effects
Histamine H_1-receptors	Sedation Weight gain Hypotension Potentiation of CNS depressants
Muscarinic receptors	Dry mouth Blurred vision Urinary retention Constipation Memory dysfunction Tachycardia
α_1-Adrenoceptors	Postural hypotension Reflex tachycardia
α_2-Adrenoceptors	Blockade of antihypertensive effects of clonidine, α-methyldopa
Serotonin 5-HT_2-receptors	Ejaculatory dysfunction

Reprinted and adapted with permission from Charney DS, et al. Treatment of depression. In: Schatzberg AF, Nemeroff CB, eds. Textbook of Psychopharmacology. Washington, DC: American Psychiatric Press, 1995:578. (Adapted from Richelson, EJ: Side effects of old and new generation antidepressants: a pharmacologic framework. Clin Psychiatry 1991;9:13–19.)

(7) **Movement disorders** are occasionally produced by **amoxapine;** these effects are due to dopamine-receptor antagonist activity.

b. **Cardiovascular system**

(1) **Postural hypotension,** which may be severe and may be temporary, is probably due to peripheral α_1-adrenoceptor blockade; it may result in reflex tachycardia.

(2) Tachycardia, conduction defects, and arrhythmias

(a) These effects are particularly common with overdose, particularly with **imipramine.**

(b) Patients with preexisting heart block or compensated cardiac output are at risk.

c. **Autonomic nervous system**

(1) Autonomic nervous system effects reflect the **muscarinic cholinoceptor antagonist activity** of TCAs. The effects may be temporary.

(2) TCA use commonly produces dry mouth, blurred vision, difficulty in urination, and constipation.

(3) TCAs more rarely may precipitate narrow-angle glaucoma or paralytic ileus or cause urine retention.

(4) These effects are more common in the elderly.

d. Rebound/discontinuation effects

(1) Common effects include dizziness, nausea, headache, and fatigue.

(2) The effects may persist for up to 2 months.

(3) Tapered withdrawal minimizes effects.

e. **Other adverse effects**

(1) TCAs often produce **weight gain** that can be extensive.

(2) TCAs can cause **sexual dysfunction.**

(3) **TCAs** may increase **suicidal ideation** for children, adolescents, and young adults; **"blackbox" warning.**

(4) These drugs produce rare but serious hematologic changes, including hemolytic anemia and agranulocytosis.

(5) TCAs infrequently cause allergic reactions and obstructive jaundice.

(6) **Atomoxetine** may increase suicidal thoughts in children and adolescents.

3. ***Overdose and toxicity.*** Overdose of TCAs produces severe anticholinergic and antiadrenergic signs, respiratory depression, arrhythmias, shock, seizures, coma, and death. Treatment is supportive and includes sodium bicarbonate for cardiac toxicity, benzodiazepines for seizures, and IV fluids and norepinephrine for hypotension.

4. ***Drug interactions***
   a. TCAs potentiate the CNS depressant effects of **alcohol** and other drugs with similar activity.
   b. TCAs potentiate the pressor activity of **norepinephrine.**
   c. TCAs have additive anticholinergic effects with **antiparkinsonian drugs, antipsychotic drugs,** and other drugs with anticholinergic activity.
   d. TCAs block α-adrenoceptors and thus reduce the antihypertensive action of **clonidine** and **α-methyldopa.**
   e. Interaction with **MAOIs** can cause excitement, hyperpyrexia, and a hypertensive episode. This "serotonin syndrome" (see III E 3 c) also may occur with TCAs that more selectively block serotonin reuptake.

E. Selective serotonin reuptake inhibitors (SSRIs)

1. ***Adverse effects*** (see Table 5-6). Overall, SSRIs produce fewer serious adverse effects than TCAs, including little sedation, postural hypotension, anticholinergic activity, and cardiovascular toxicity.
   a. **Headache** that is generally temporary
   b. **Sexual dysfunction** in up to 40% of all patients, which is a leading cause of noncompliance
   c. **Gastric irritation** that is generally transient and includes nausea and heartburn
   d. **Weight loss** initially followed in some patients by weight gain
   e. **Stimulation** that is mild and often transient, may be experienced as dysphoria, and is marked by agitation, anxiety, increased motor activity, insomnia, tremor, and excitement
   f. **Apathy** (flattened affect) occurs in some patients.
   g. **Rebound/discontinuation** effects like those for TCAs are most likely to occur with **paroxetine.**
2. ***Overdose and toxicity.*** With only a few reported seizures in overdose, SSRIs are remarkably safe in comparison to other antidepressants. This accounts for their relative popularity. However, SSRIs may increase **suicidal ideation** for children, adolescents, and young adults; **"blackbox" warning.**
3. ***Drug interactions***
   a. **Fluoxetine** and **paroxetine** inhibit liver microsomal enzymes (CYP2D6) and thus can rarely potentiate the actions of other drugs metabolized by the same enzymes.
   b. SSRIs have a rare and potentially fatal interaction with MAOIs called "**serotonin syndrome**" that includes tremor, hyperthermia, muscle rigidity, and cardiovascular collapse.

F. Atypical antidepressant agents (selected).

The pharmacologic properties of atypical antidepressant agents are similar to those of TCAs.

1. ***Trazodone, nefazodone, mirtazapine***
   a. These drugs are **highly sedating;** they cause drowsiness and dizziness.
   b. These drugs cause insomnia and nausea.
   c. **Trazodone** may cause **postural hypotension** in the elderly and a rare **priapism** in men.
   d. **Trazodone** has no significant anticholinergic activity; it has fewer autonomic and cardiovascular effects than TCAs and is safer than TCAs in overdose.
   e. **Mirtazepine** causes marked **weight gain.**
2. ***Bupropion***
   a. Bupropion has no significant anticholinergic activity or hypotensive activity; it causes little sexual dysfunction.
   b. Bupropion is more likely than TCAs to cause **seizures,** particularly at high therapeutic doses.
   c. Like SSRIs, bupropion causes stimulation, insomnia, and weight loss.
   d. Bupropion is also marketed as Zyban, a sustained-release aid for smoking cessation.
3. ***Maprotiline*** is highly sedating. The seizure risk with maprotiline may be 4% at high therapeutic doses. Also, cardiotoxicity is much higher in overdose.
4. ***Amoxapine***
   a. **Movement disorders** similar to those caused by antipsychotic agents, including tardive dyskinesia, are occasionally produced by amoxapine; these effects are due to dopamine-receptor antagonist activity.
   b. Overdose of amoxapine causes seizures.

5. ***Venlafaxine*** causes nausea, dizziness, sexual disturbances, anxiety, and insomnia.
6. ***Duloxetine*** causes GI disturbances (nausea, constipation, diarrhea, and vomiting), sexual disturbances, insomnia, and sedation.

G. Monoamine oxidase inhibitors (MAOIs)

1. ***Pharmacologic properties***
   a. **Tranylcypromine** and **phenelzine** are used infrequently because of their potential for serious drug interactions.
   b. **Phencyclidine** is inactivated by acetylation; genetically slow acetylators may show exaggerated effects.
2. ***Adverse effects*** include postural hypotension, headache, dry mouth, sexual dysfunction (phenelzine), weight gain, and sleep disturbances.
3. ***Overdose and toxicity.*** Uncommon results of overdose of MAOIs include agitation, hyperthermia, seizures, hypotension, or hypertension.
4. ***Drug interactions***
   a. MAOIs may result in headache, nausea, cardiac arrhythmias, hypertensive crisis, and, rarely, **subarachnoid bleeding and stroke** in the presence of indirectly acting sympathomimetics (e.g., **tyramine from certain foods**). These effects are due to the release of increased stores of catecholamines resulting from inhibition of monoamine oxidase.
   b. These can potentiate the pressor effect of high doses of directly acting sympathetic amines.
   c. MAOIs may cause a "serotonin syndrome" in the presence of SSRIs, certain TCAs, and opioids such as meperidine.
   d. MAOIs result in additive sedation and CNS depression in the presence of barbiturates, alcohol, and opioids.

IV. LITHIUM

A. Mechanism of action (see Fig. 1-1D)

1. The mechanism of action for lithium is unclear, although it may be directly related to the **inhibition of phospholipid turnover** (lithium inhibits inositol monophosphatase) and, consequently, decreased activity of the second messengers diacylglycerol (DAG) and inositol 1,4,5-trisphosphate (IP_3).
2. Lithium also has reported effects on nerve conduction; on the release, synthesis, and action of biogenic amines; and on calcium metabolism.

B. Pharmacologic properties

1. This drug is eliminated almost entirely by the kidney; 80% is reabsorbed in the proximal renal tubule.
2. Lithium has a low therapeutic index; plasma levels must be monitored continuously.

C. Therapeutic uses

1. ***Acute mania or bipolar affective disorder***
   a. Lithium normalizes mood in 70% of patients. The onset of the therapeutic effect takes 2–3 weeks; antipsychotic agents and benzodiazepines can be used in the initial stages of the disease to control acute agitation.
   b. The anticonvulsants **carbamazepine, valproic acid,** and **lamotrigene** have been used successfully either alone or as adjuncts to lithium therapy; the dose is similar to that used to treat epilepsy. The mechanism of action for these drugs is unknown (see VII).
2. ***Prophylaxis of bipolar affective disorder,*** for which lithium is often administered with a TCA (may precipitate mania)

D. Adverse effects

1. Adverse effects are common at therapeutic doses of 0.5–1.4 mmol/L or slightly higher.
2. These effects include **nausea, vomiting, diarrhea, fine tremor, polydipsia, edema,** and **weight gain.**

3. Lithium administration produces **polyuria,** which occurs as the kidney collecting tubule becomes unresponsive to antidiuretic hormone (reversible). More rarely, decreased renal function occurs with long-term treatment, similar to nephrogenic diabetes insipidus.
4. Adverse effects of lithium also include **benign, reversible thyroid enlargement** caused by reducing tyrosine iodination and the synthesis of thyroxine. Lithium more rarely causes hypothyroidism.
5. Lithium is generally **contraindicated** during the first trimester of pregnancy because of the possible risk of fetal congenital abnormalities. Renal clearance of lithium increases during pregnancy. Breast-feeding is not recommended because lithium is secreted in breast milk with possible neonate dysfunction.

E. Drug interactions

1. Sodium depletion is increased by **low-salt diets, thiazide diuretics, furosemide, ethacrynic acid,** or severe vomiting or diarrhea. This depletion results in increased renal reabsorption of lithium and an **increased chance for toxicity.**
2. Renal clearance of lithium is decreased and the chance of toxicity is enhanced by some nonsteroidal anti-inflammatory drugs (e.g., **indomethacin and phenylbutazone**).

F. Toxicity

1. At a toxicity level **above 2 mmol/L,** confusion (important first sign of toxicity), drowsiness, vomiting, ataxia, dizziness, and severe tremors develop.
2. At a toxicity level **above 2.5 mmol/L,** clonic movements of the limbs, seizures, circulatory collapse, and coma occur.
3. Treatment includes discontinuing lithium administration, hemodialysis, and the use of anticonvulsants.

V. OPIOID ANALGESICS AND ANTAGONISTS

A. Definitions

1. ***Opioids*** are drugs with morphine-like activity that produce analgesia (i.e., reduce pain) without the loss of consciousness and can induce tolerance and physical dependence. Opioids are also referred to as narcotic analgesics.
2. ***Opiates*** are drugs derived from opium (e.g., morphine, heroin), a powdered, dried exudate of the fruit capsule (poppy) of the plant *Papaver somniferum.* Opium alkaloids (e.g., **thebaine**) are used to make semisynthetic opioids. Other opioids are prepared **synthetically** (e.g., **methadone**).
3. ***Opiopeptins*** (endogenous opioid peptides) are natural substances of the body that have opioid-like activity.
   a. Opiopeptins are localized in discrete areas of the CNS and in a number of peripheral tissues including the GI tract, kidney, and biliary tract.
   b. Opiopeptins are derived from distinct polypeptide precursors.
      (1) Preproopiomelanocortin contains β-endorphin (also adrenocorticotropic hormone [ACTH] and melanocyte-stimulating hormone).
      (2) Preproenkephalin contains the pentapeptides *met*-enkephalin and *leu*-enkephalin.
      (3) Preprodynorphin contains dynorphins A and B and neoendorphins α and β.

B. Mechanism of action

1. Opioids such as morphine are believed to mimic the effects of opiopeptins by interaction with one or more several **distinct receptors** (μ, κ, δ). Each opioid receptor has **distinct subtypes** (e.g., μ_1, μ_2). Opioids with mixed agonist–antagonist properties may act as agonists at one opioid receptor and antagonists at another (e.g., **pentazocine**) or as partial agonists (e.g., **buprenorphine**).
   a. Interaction with **μ-receptors** contributes to supraspinal and spinal analgesia, respiratory depression, sedation, euphoria, decreased GI transit, and physical dependence.

b. Interaction with κ-**receptors** contributes to supraspinal and spinal analgesia, sedation, and miosis.
c. The significance of interaction with δ-**receptors** is unclear, but it may contribute to analgesia.
d. β-Endorphins, the enkephalins, and dynorphins have their highest affinity for, respectively, μ-, δ-, and κ- receptors.

2. Opioids produce **analgesia** and their other actions by mechanisms that are not completely understood.
   a. All opioids activate inhibitory guanine nucleotide binding proteins (G_i; see Fig. 1-1C).
   b. Opioids **inhibit adenylyl cyclase activity,** resulting in a reduction in intracellular cAMP and decreased protein phosphorylation.
   c. Opioids **promote the opening of potassium channels** to increase potassium conductance, which hyperpolarizes and inhibits the activity of postjunctional cells.
   d. Opioids **close voltage-dependent calcium channels** on prejunctional nerve terminals to inhibit release of neurotransmitters (e.g., the release of glutamate and the release of substance P in the spinal cord).
   e. Opioids **raise the threshold to pain** by interrupting pain transmission through ascending pathways (substantia gelatinosa in the dorsal horn of the spinal cord, ventral caudal thalamus) and activating the descending modulatory pathways (periaqueductal gray area in the midbrain, rostral ventral medulla) in the CNS.
   f. Opioids also raise the threshold to pain by action on peripheral sensory neurons.
   g. Opioids **decrease emotional reactivity to pain** through actions in the limbic areas of the CNS.

C. Psychologic dependence and compulsive drug use

1. The euphoria and other pleasurable activities produced by opioid analgesics, particularly when self-administered intravenously, can result in the development of psychologic dependence with compulsive drug use. This development may be reinforced by the development of physical dependence (see below).
2. Although physical dependence is not uncommon when opioids are used for therapeutic purposes, psychologic dependence and compulsive drug use are not.

D. Tolerance and physical dependence

1. ***Tolerance***
   a. Tolerance occurs gradually with repeated administration; a larger opioid dose is necessary to produce the same initial effect.
   b. Tolerance is due to a direct neuronal effect of opioids in the CNS (i.e., cellular tolerance).
   c. Tolerance varies in degree (Table 5-7).
   d. Tolerance can be conferred from one opioid agonist to others (cross-tolerance).
2. ***Physical dependence*** occurs with the development of tolerance to opioids.
   a. **Abstinent withdrawal**
      (1) Abstinent withdrawal is a syndrome revealed with discontinuation of opioid administration.
      (2) Abstinent withdrawal is characterized by drug-seeking behavior and physical signs of autonomic hyperexcitability that may include "goose bumps" ("going cold turkey"),

table 5-7 Relative Development of Tolerance to Opioid Actions

Substantial	Minimal
Analgesia	Constipation
Respiratory depression	Seizures
Euphoria and dysphoria	Miosis
Sedation	Antagonist action
Nausea and vomiting	
Cough suppression	

muscle spasms ("kicking the habit"), hyperalgesia, lacrimation, rhinorrhea, yawning, sweating, restlessness, dilated pupils, anorexia, irritability, tremor, diarrhea, and flushing.

(3) Abstinent withdrawal peaks at 48–72 hours.

(4) This type of withdrawal is generally not life threatening, except in dependent neonates and the severely debilitated.

(5) Abstinent withdrawal can be reversed by readministration of opioid.

b. Precipitated withdrawal

(1) Precipitated withdrawal is induced by administration of an opioid antagonist such as naloxone.

(2) Precipitated withdrawal peaks sooner and more explosively than abstinent withdrawal and is more severe.

(3) Precipitated withdrawal is more difficult to reverse with opioid agonists than abstinent withdrawal.

E. Morphine: prototype

1. *Pharmacologic properties*

a. Morphine is usually given parenterally, but it can be given orally or rectally.

b. Morphine undergoes extensive first-pass metabolism with glucuronide conjugation (morphine-6-glucuronide may possess analgesic activity). Dosage adjustment of morphine is necessary in patients with hepatic insufficiency.

c. Morphine has a plasma half-life ($t_{1/2}$) of 2–3 hours; its duration of action is 3–6 hours.

2. *Therapeutic uses of morphine and other opioids* (Table 5-8)

a. Analgesia

(1) Morphine is used for analgesia in severe preoperative and postoperative pain, as well as for the pain of terminal illness; it is used to treat the visceral pain of trauma, burns, cancer, acute myocardial infarction (MI), and renal or biliary colic. Higher doses are necessary for intermittent sharp pain.

(2) Morphine produces analgesia by increasing the threshold for the sensation of pain and by dissociating the perception of pain from the sensation. There is significant interpatient variability in this latter effect.

(3) In addition to analgesia, decreased anxiety, sedation that is marked by drowsiness, inability or decreased ability to concentrate, loss of recent memory, and occasional euphoria are useful additional properties of morphine in frightening disorders, such as MI and terminal illness.

b. Diarrhea

(1) The antidiarrheal effect of morphine is a pharmacologic extension of its constipating effect (see below). For this reason, morphine is often used after an ileostomy or colostomy.

table 5-8 Indications for Morphine and Other Opioids

Indication	Opioid Used
Analgesia	Morphine, hydromorphone
Dyspnea	Morphine
Diarrhea	Diphenoxylate, loperamide
Cough	Codeine when not controlled by nonnarcotic cough suppressants
Preanesthesia	Fentanyl often used for its short duration of action (1–2 h)
Regional anesthesia	Morphine, fentanyl
Cardiovascular surgery	High-dose fentanyl as primary anesthetic because it produces minimal cardiac depression
Withdrawal or maintenance therapy	Methadone substitution for treatment of opioid dependence; clonidine, an α-adrenoceptor agonist, is also used for withdrawal because it suppresses autonomic components

(2) **Morphine** is an effective treatment for diarrhea at a less-than-analgesic dose.

(3) **Codeine** is popular because of its reduced abuse liability. **Diphenoxylate** (with atropine to reduce the likelihood of parenteral use) and **loperamide** are used widely, because at therapeutic doses, their actions are confined primarily to the GI tract and because their insolubility precludes IV use.

(4) No significant development of tolerance occurs to the antidiarrheal action of **morphine.**

c. **Acute pulmonary edema**

(1) Morphine relieves the dyspnea (feeling of shortness of breath and the struggle to breathe) associated with acute pulmonary edema secondary to left ventricular failure.

(2) This effect may be due to 1) decreased peripheral resistance with a decreased afterload and decreased venous tone with a decreased preload; 2) decreased anxiety of the patient; and/or 3) depression of the respiratory center and the CNS response to hypoxic drive.

d. **Myocardial infarction.** Vasodilation and the subsequent decreased cardiac preload are of additional therapeutic benefit when morphine is used for the pain of MI. **Pentazocine** and **butorphanol** increase preload and are contraindicated for the treatment of MI.

e. **Cough**

(1) Opioids are used to produce a direct depression of the cough center in the medulla when the cough is not controlled by nonopioids. **Codeine,** at a subanalgesic dose, is widely used for severe cough.

(2) The receptors are unique in that the cough reflex is depressed by both L-isomers and D-isomers of opioids (D-isomers are without analgesic action).

f. **Anesthesia applications**

(1) **Preanesthetic medication** or supplement to anesthetic agents during surgery

(a) Opioids are used for analgesic and sedative or anxiolytic effects.

(b) **Fentanyl** is often used for its short duration of action relative to morphine.

(2) **Regional analgesia** (epidural or intrathecal administration)

(a) **Morphine** and **fentanyl** are used to achieve long-lasting analgesia that is mediated through action on the spinal cord.

(b) There is a reduced incidence of adverse effects, but delayed respiratory depression, nausea, vomiting, and pruritus often occur.

(3) High-dose **fentanyl** or congeners (or **morphine**) are used as primary anesthetic in cardiovascular surgery because of their minimal cardiac depression.

g. **Physical dependence.** Opioids (**methadone, buprenorphine**) are used to mitigate the withdrawal symptoms of physical dependence caused by other opioids, including heroin.

3. ***Adverse effects and contraindications of morphine and other opioids***

a. **Respiratory depression**

(1) Respiratory depression is generally not a serious clinical problem except in several special circumstances.

(2) Respiratory depression with opioid use is due to the direct inhibition of the respiratory center in the brainstem and to decreased sensitivity of the respiratory center to CO_2 with decreased hypoxic drive; it leads to decreased respiratory rate, minute volume, and tidal exchange.

(3) Opioids are contraindicated if there is a preexisting decrease in respiratory reserve (e.g., emphysema) or excessive respiratory secretions (e.g., obstructive lung disease).

(4) These drugs are contraindicated in patients with head injury. Cerebral vasodilation results from the increased pCO_2 caused by respiratory depression and may result in increased cerebral vascular pressure, which may lead to exaggerated respiratory depression and altered brain function.

(5) Opioids should be used cautiously during pregnancy because they may prolong labor and cause fetal dependence.

(6) Clinical or accidental opioid overdose with respiratory depression may be treated with artificial ventilation; this may be sufficient for the treatment of respiratory depression or coma. Opioid antagonists can be used to reverse respiratory depression.

b. **Constipation**

(1) Constipation results from increased tone with decreased coordinated GI motility, increased anal sphincter tone, and inattention to the defecation reflex.

(2) This effect is mediated through actions on the GI tract, **to inhibit release of acetylcholine,** and on the CNS.
(3) There is no clinically significant tolerance to this effect.

c. **Hypotension**
(1) Opioids inhibit the vasomotor center in the brainstem, causing peripheral vasodilation; they also inhibit compensatory baroreceptor reflexes and increase histamine release.
(2) Opioids should be used cautiously in patients in shock or with reduced blood volume. The elderly are particularly susceptible.

d. **Nausea and vomiting**
(1) This common effect of opioids is caused by the direct stimulation of the chemoreceptor trigger zone (CTZ) in the area postrema of the medulla, which leads to activation of the vomiting center; there is also a direct vestibular component.
(2) This effect is blocked by dopamine-receptor antagonists.
(3) This effect is self-limiting because of the subsequent direct inhibition by morphine of the vomiting center.

e. **Pneumonia** is a potential result of a reduced cough reflex when opioids are used for analgesia, particularly when respiration is compromised.

f. **Sedative activity with drowsiness** places ambulatory patients at risk for accidents. A paradoxical dysphoria occasionally develops.

g. **Pain from biliary or urinary tract spasm**
(1) This pain is due to the increased muscle tone of smooth muscle in the biliary tract, the sphincter of Oddi, and the ureters and bladder.
(2) These spasms may result in a paradoxical increase in pain when opioids are used to alleviate the pain associated with the passing of urinary or biliary stones if the dose is insufficient to induce centrally mediated analgesia.

h. **Urine retention**
(1) This effect, more common in the elderly, is due primarily to decreased renal plasma flow. Other contributing factors include increased tone with decreased coordinated contractility of the ureters and bladder, increased urethral sphincter tone, and inattention to the urinary reflex.
(2) Catheterization is necessary in some instances.
(3) Opioids should be used cautiously in patients with prostatic hypertrophy or urethral stricture.

i. **Psychologic or physical dependence.** The risk for the development of psychologic dependence or physical dependence is not a valid excuse to withhold opioids and thereby provide inadequate relief from pain, particularly in the terminally ill.

j. **Miosis**
(1) Opioid stimulation of the Edinger-Westphal nucleus of the oculomotor nerve results in "pinpoint" pupils even in the dark. This effect is mediated by acetylcholine and blocked by atropine.
(2) No tolerance develops to this effect.
(3) During severe respiratory depression and asphyxia, miosis may revert to mydriasis.

4. ***Drug interactions***
a. **Drugs that depress the CNS** add to or potentiate the respiratory depression caused by opioids (e.g., sedative–hypnotic agents).
b. **Antipsychotic and antidepressant agents** with sedative activity potentiate the sedation produced by opioids.
c. In the presence of opioids, particularly meperidine, **MAOIs** produce severe hyperthermia, seizures, and coma.

F. Other strong opioid agonists

1. ***Hydromorphone, oxymorphone, levorphanol, and heroin***
a. These drugs have actions similar to those of morphine.
b. **Oxymorphone** has little antitussive activity.
c. Heroin (not approved for clinical use) is more lipid soluble and faster acting than morphine, producing greater euphoria, which accounts for its popularity as a drug of abuse.

2. ***Fentanyl, sufentanil, alfentanil, remifentanil***
   a. Fentanyl and other subtypes are administered parenterally. They have a shorter duration of action than morphine. **Remifentanil** is rapidly metabolized by blood and tissue esterases.
   b. Fentanyl is available as a transdermal patch and lozenge on a stick for breakthrough cancer pain.
   c. Fentanyl is administered as a preanesthetic and intraoperative medication for its analgesic, anxiolytic, and sedative properties.
   d. Fentanyl (or **morphine**) is used in high doses as a **primary anesthetic** for **cardiovascular surgery** because it produces minimal cardiac depression.
   e. Fentanyl is used to supplement the analgesia and sedative-hypnotic effects of nitrous oxide and halothane in a "balanced anesthesia" approach. Morphine also is used for this indication.
   f. Fentanyl is infrequently used in the combination product **fentanyl/droperidol** (Innovar) to induce neuroleptanalgesia. This combination permits a wakeful state when patient cooperation is needed (intubations, minor surgical procedures, changing burn dressings).
   g. These drugs may cause severe truncal rigidity when administered by rapid IV at a high dose.
3. ***Methadone (also levomethadyl acetate)***
   a. Methadone, like morphine, has good analgesic activity. It is administered orally and has a longer duration of action than morphine.
   b. Methadone is associated with a less severe withdrawal syndrome than morphine; it is often substituted for other opioids as a treatment for physical dependence because it allows a smoother withdrawal with tapered dose reduction. It is also used for maintenance therapy of the heroin-dependent addict.
4. ***Meperidine***
   a. Meperidine has a shorter duration of action than morphine.
   b. Meperidine appears to produce less neonatal respiratory depression than morphine and may be preferred in obstetrics.
   c. High doses may cause CNS excitation (tremors, delirium, hyperreflexia) and seizures due to formation of a metabolite, normeperidine.
   d. Meperidine causes severe restlessness, excitement, and fever when administered with MAOIs.
   e. Meperidine use may result in mydriasis and tachycardia due to weak anticholinergic activity.
   f. Meperidine has no effect on the cough reflex.

G. Weak agonists

1. ***Codeine, oxycodone, and hydrocodone*** are partial opioid receptor agonists used for moderate pain.
   a. They are orally effective and undergo less first-pass metabolism than morphine.
   b. These drugs are usually used in combination with other analgesics such as acetaminophen, aspirin, or ibuprofen (e.g., **codeine**/acetaminophen = Tylenol with codeine; **hydrocodone**/acetaminophen = Vicodin, Lortab; **oxycodone**/aspirin = Percodan; and **oxycodone**/acetaminophen = Percocet).
   c. These drugs are associated with less respiratory depression than morphine and have less dependence liability. Overdose with codeine produces seizures.
2. ***Propoxyphene***
   a. Propoxyphene is used as an analgesic; however, it has lower efficacy than codeine. It is usually used in combination with aspirin or acetaminophen.
   b. Propoxyphene has low abuse liability but can produce respiratory depression and dependence.
   c. Propoxyphene may cause seizures at high doses.

H. Mixed agonist–antagonists/Partial agonists

1. ***Buprenorphine, pentazocine, nalbuphine, and butorphanol***
   a. **Buprenorphine** is a partial agonist at opioid μ-receptors.
   b. **Pentazocine, nalbuphine, and butorphanol** are opioid κ-receptor agonists with partial agonist or antagonist activity at opioid μ-receptors.

2. These drugs are used for **moderate pain.**
3. **Buprenorphine**, like methadone, is used for heroin detoxification.
4. Severe respiratory depression, although uncommon, is resistant to naloxone reversal.
5. These drugs have less dependence liability than morphine.
6. These drugs, except **nalbuphine**, can increase cardiac preload and should not be used to treat the pain of MI.
7. These drugs can precipitate withdrawal if administered to patients already receiving strong opioid agonists.
8. **Pentazocine** occasionally causes dysphoria, hallucinations, and depersonalization and is not commonly used in clinical practice.

I. Tramadol

1. In addition to weak opioid μ-receptor agonist activity, tramadol also weakly blocks reuptake of serotonin and norepinephrine—effects that appear to account for its analgesic action.
2. It may have special use for neuropathic pain.
3. Tramadol is associated with an increased risk of seizures and is contraindicated in patients with epilepsy.
4. Its actions are only partially reversed by naloxone.
5. Tramadol should not be administered to patients taking MAOIs.

J. Opioid antagonists

1. ***Naloxone and naltrexone (also nalmefene)*** are competitive inhibitors of the actions of opioids.
2. These drugs will **precipitate opioid withdrawal.**
3. Naloxone has a relative short duration of action of 1–2 hours. It is used to diagnose opioid dependence and to treat acute opioid overdose. Because of its short duration of action, multiple doses may need to be administered.
4. Naltrexone has a duration of action of up to 48 hours. It is approved for use to help decrease craving for alcohol.

K. Antidiarrheal agents (see also Chapter 8 VII B)

1. ***Diphenoxylate/atropine, difenoxin, and loperamide*** are taken orally for the symptomatic treatment of diarrhea.
2. Diphenoxylate is only available combined with atropine to minimize parenteral misuse.
3. Insolubility of diphenoxylate limits its absorption across the GI tract. Loperamide does not penetrate the brain.
4. These drugs have minimal dependence liability or other centrally mediated opioid-like effects at therapeutic doses.

L. Antitussive agents

1. ***Dextromethorphan,*** an opioid isomer, is an over-the-counter cough medication that, like codeine, is used for its antitussive activity. However, it has little or no analgesic or addictive properties at therapeutic doses. Some constipation and sedation have been noted.

VI. ANTIPARKINSONIAN DRUGS AND DRUGS USED TO TREAT ALZHEIMER DISEASE

A. Idiopathic parkinsonian disease

1. Idiopathic parkinsonian disease is characterized by resting tremor, rigidity, bradykinesia, loss of postural reflexes, and, occasionally, behavioral manifestations.
2. Idiopathic parkinsonian disease is a result of the **progressive degeneration of dopamine (DA)-producing neurons** in the substantia nigra pars compacta that is thought to cause an imbalance in DA and acetylcholine (ACh) action on neurons of the corpus striatum, which 1) controls

motor activity by pathways leading to the thalamus and cerebral cortex and 2) modulates DA output by a feedback loop to the substantia nigra.

3. The net effect of the reduced output of DA (and relative increase in ACh activity) is a net loss of inhibitory regulation of the neuronal release of GABA in the corpus striatum, which leads to the characteristic movement disorders associated with parkinsonian disease.
4. A parkinsonian-like syndrome also may be induced by antipsychotic drugs, e.g., **haloperidol**.

B. Therapeutic goal. Because it is not yet possible to reverse the degenerative process, drugs are used to **increase DA** activity or to **reduce** excitatory interneuron **ACh** activity, in order to **restore** their **balance** in the corpus striatum.

C. Levodopa (L-dopa), carbidopa, and levodopa/carbidopa

1. ***Mechanism of action*** (see Fig. 1-1C). Levodopa is a levorotatory isomer of dopa that is prejunctionally decarboxylated in the CNS to restore DA activity in the corpus striatum, where it interacts with postjunctional dopamine D_2- and D_3-receptors to activate inhibitory G proteins, inhibit adenylyl cyclase, decrease cAMP levels, and open potassium channels.
2. ***Pharmacologic properties***
   a. Levodopa is **absorbed rapidly** and enters the CNS where it is decarboxylated to dopamine. Absorption is delayed by food and influenced by the rate of gastric emptying and, through competition for absorption sites, by dietary amino acids.
   b. Levodopa is usually administered with **carbidopa** in a fixed combination (as Sinemet). A controlled-release preparation is available.
      (1) Carbidopa (α-methyldopa hydrazine) is an L-amino acid decarboxylase inhibitor that acts peripherally, does not cross the blood–brain barrier, and has little effect of its own.
      (2) In the presence of carbidopa, less levodopa is decarboxylated by dopa decarboxylase to dopamine in the periphery; therefore, the therapeutic dose of levodopa can be reduced by up to 80%, substantially minimizing nausea and vomiting and adverse cardiovascular effects.
3. ***Therapeutic effects***
   a. Clinical improvement, including major improvement in functional capacity and quality of life, occurs in 70% of patients after several weeks of treatment.
   b. Tremor is more resistant to therapy, and there is little improvement of dementia.
   c. The **therapeutic effects** of L-dopa last for about **2–5 years.** It is believed that neuronal regeneration progresses to the extent that the remaining functional neurons are unable to process and store (as dopamine) enough exogenously administered L-dopa to compensate for the decreased endogenous dopamine levels.
4. ***Adverse effects and contraindications***
   a. **Dyskinesias**
      (1) Dyskinesias are the major limiting factor in therapy.
      (2) Dyskinesias occur in 80% of patients and are characterized by a variety of repetitive involuntary abnormal movements (e.g., dystonia, tics, ballismus, tremor, myoclonus) affecting the face, trunk, and limbs.
      (3) Dyskinesias may be relieved by **decreasing** the dose of **levodopa,** but the parkinsonian symptoms may then increase.
   b. **Akinesias** are characterized by decreased voluntary movement that lasts for a few minutes or several hours and occur with increasing frequency with continued levodopa treatment.
      (1) **End-of-dose akinesia**
         (a) Each dose of L-dopa improves mobility for a period of time but is followed by the rapid return of muscle rigidity and akinesia before the end of the dosing interval.
         (b) Increasing the dose and frequency of L-dopa administration may relieve these symptoms but may also induce dyskinesias.
      (2) **"On–off" akinesia**
         (a) "On–off" akinesia is a rapid fluctuation between showing no beneficial effects of L-dopa and showing beneficial effects with dyskinesias. "On–off" akinesia may be a sign of the latter stage of dopamine neuron degeneration.

(b) Clinical improvement can be obtained with continuous IV infusion and, in some instances, with sustained release formulations of **levodopa/carbidopa.**

(3) **Akinesia paradoxica**

(a) Akinesia paradoxica is a sudden freezing of movement.

(b) Akinesia paradoxica often follows an episode of dyskinesia and is often precipitated by stress.

c. **Behavioral effects**

(1) Behavioral effects may include anxiety, insomnia, and early-onset psychosis due to exacerbation of a preexisting psychotic problem.

(2) There are also occasional late-onset (2 years) dream alterations (vivid dreams, nightmares), visual hallucinations, and drug-induced psychoses characterized by paranoia and confusional states.

d. **Nausea and vomiting**

(1) Nausea and vomiting occur in 80% of patients; this effect is attenuated if levodopa is taken with carbidopa, with food, in divided doses, or with nonphenothiazine antiemetics.

(2) This effect is due to the direct effects of dopamine on the GI tract and on the chemoreceptor trigger zone (CTZ) in the CNS. Tolerance to the emetic effect may develop.

e. **Cardiovascular effects**

(1) The uncommon cardiovascular effects of levodopa include postural hypotension (activation of vascular dopamine receptors), occasional hypertension, and (rarely), tachycardia, arrhythmias (dopamine action at α- and β-adrenergic receptors), and atrial fibrillation due to increased circulating catecholamines.

(2) The incidence of the hypotensive effect of levodopa is reduced with carbidopa.

f. **Mydriasis.** Mydriasis and precipitation of an attack of acute glaucoma can develop.

5. ***Drug interactions and contraindications***

a. The therapeutic action of levodopa is reduced by **antiemetic or antipsychotic drugs** that block dopamine receptors.

b. **Natural aromatic amino acids** (tryptophan, histidine, phenylalanine, tyrosine) decrease the absorption of levodopa.

c. Levodopa should not be used with **MAO_A inhibitors.** This combination can cause a severe hypertensive crisis.

d. In the absence of carbidopa, peripheral levels of levodopa are decreased by **pyridoxine** (vitamin B_6), which increases the activity of dopa decarboxylase and increases conversion of levodopa to dopamine in the periphery.

e. The use of levodopa is **contraindicated in patients with psychosis, narrow-angle glaucoma, and peptic ulcer disease.**

D. Other Antiparkinsonian Agents

1. ***Pramipexole, ropinirole, and bromocriptine***

a. Characteristics

(1) **Pramipexole** is a relatively selective dopamine D_3-receptor agonist; **ropinirole** is a relatively selective dopamine D_2-receptor agonist; **bromocriptine** is a dopamine D_2- (and D_1-) receptor agonist.

(2) These drugs are often given in combination with levodopa for optimal treatment or are alternative first-line drugs when levodopa is not tolerated. **Bromocriptine** is also used to treat hyperprolactinemia.

(3) **Pramipexole** is excreted unchanged; dosage adjustments may be necessary in patients with renal insufficiency. **Ropinirole,** which is also approved to treat **restless leg syndrome,** is metabolized by CYP1A2; dosage adjustments may be necessary in the presence of other drugs that are metabolized by the same enzymes.

b. **Adverse effects**

(1) These drugs have the same adverse effects, cautions, and contraindications as levodopa, although the severity of their effects may differ.

(2) These drugs may induce profound hypotension after an initial dose. Nausea, vomiting, and constipation may be problematic.

(3) Behavioral manifestations are more common and severe than with levodopa.

(4) Rarely, uncontrolled sleep occurs with **pramipexole** and **ropinirole.**

2. ***Amantadine***

a. **Characteristics**

(1) Amantadine is an antiviral drug that **increases the release of dopamine** in the CNS by an unknown mechanism.

(2) Amantadine is useful in the early stages of parkinsonism or as an adjunct to levodopa therapy. The therapeutic effect of this drug may diminish in a few weeks.

b. **Adverse effects**

(1) Amantadine is associated with a reversible occasional headache, insomnia, confusion, hallucinations, and peripheral edema.

(2) Long-term use of amantadine may lead to reversible discoloration of the skin (livedo reticularis) or, more rarely, congestive heart failure.

(3) Overdose may cause a toxic psychosis and seizures.

3. ***Selegiline, Rasagilene***

a. **Characteristics**

(1) Selegilene and rasagilene are **selective MAO-B inhibitors** that decrease dopamine metabolism in the CNS and prolong its action.

(2) These drugs are used as initial therapy or as adjuncts to levodopa therapy for Parkinson disease.

b. **Adverse effects.** These drugs are well tolerated. Selegiline causes an occasional mild amphetamine-like stimulating action (amphetamine is one of the metabolites).

c. These drugs should be avoided by patients taking SSRIs, TCAs, and **meperidine,** because of the possibility of precipitating a "serotonin syndrome."

4. ***Entacapone and tolcapone***

a. These drugs **inhibit catechol-o-methyltransferase (COMT),** thereby reducing the peripheral metabolism of levodopa. The decreased clearance of L-dopa increases its CNS bioavailability.

b. **Entacapone, acts only in the periphery.** It decreases metabolism of levodopa to make more available to the brain; **Tolcapone** acts in the periphery and the brain. In the brain, it inhibits the degradation of dopamine.

c. **Entacapone**, in a combined product (Stalevo), is used to augment the effect of **carbidopa/levodopa.**

d. **Adverse effects** of these drugs include GI disturbances, postural hypotension, sleep disturbances, and an orange discoloration of the urine. **Entacapone** is preferred because tolcapone has been associated (rarely) with acute, fatal hepatic failure.

e. These drugs can exacerbate dysphoria, nausea, and other adverse effects of levodopa; downward dose adjustment of levodopa is necessary.

5. ***Benztropine, biperidin, orphenadrine, procyclidine, and trihexyphenidyl***

a. **Characteristics**

(1) These drugs **block muscarinic receptors** and suppress overactivity of cholinergic interneurons in the striatum; they have a somewhat greater ratio of CNS to peripheral activity.

(2) These drugs are often used in the initial stages of mild parkinsonism, often in combination with levodopa. They have a significant effect on tremor and rigidity but little effect on bradykinesia and postural reflexes. These drugs are effective in 25% of patients, many of whom become refractory.

b. **Adverse effects, contraindications, and drug interactions**

(1) These drugs are associated with occasional restlessness, sedation, confusion, mood changes, dry mouth, mydriasis, constipation, tachycardia, and arrhythmias.

(2) These drugs are contraindicated in patients with prostatic hypertrophy, obstructive GI disease (e.g., paralytic ileus) and narrow-angle glaucoma.

(3) To avoid precipitating these conditions, these drugs should not be administered to patients taking other drugs with anticholinergic activity (e.g., tricyclic antidepressants, antihistamines).

E. Alzheimer disease

1. ***Donepezil, rivastigmine, galantamine, and tacrine*** are **acetylcholinesterase inhibitors** (see also Chapter 2 II B) used to treat Alzheimer disease, a disease characterized functionally by a loss of memory and biochemically and cellularly by accumulation of β-amyloid plaques, formation of neurofibrillary tangles, and loss of cortical neurons.
2. ***Memantine,*** a noncompetitive **inhibitor of *N*-methyl-d-aspartate (NMDA) receptors** that has few side effects, is also used to treat Alzheimer disease.
3. These drugs have only a short-term, modest effect and do nothing to halt the progression of neurodegeneration.
4. ***Adverse effects*** of the acetylcholinesterase inhibitors include GI dysfunction and muscle cramps. **Tacrine** is associated with liver toxicity.

VII. ANTIEPILEPTIC DRUGS

A. Drug treatment of seizures

1. **Epilepsy,** a chronic disease, occurs in approximately 1% of the population. Antiepileptic drugs (AEDs) are effective, at least to some degree, for about 80% of these patients. Life-long treatment may be necessary.
2. It may take weeks to establish adequate drug plasma levels and to determine the adequacy of therapeutic improvement. **Lack of compliance** is responsible for many treatment failures.
3. AEDs are **most effective** and have the **least adverse effects** when they are used as **monotherapy.** Addition of a second drug to the therapeutic regimen should be gradual, as should discontinuance of the initial drug before the substitution of an alternative drug, because seizures may occur on withdrawal.
4. Some AEDs have **teratogenic potential.** This may call for the reduction or termination of therapy during pregnancy or before planned pregnancy. However, maternal seizures also present a significant risk to the fetus.
5. AEDs may also be used to treat seizures that result from various neurologic disorders, as well as from metabolic disturbances, trauma, and exposure to certain toxins.
6. AEDs may increase the risk of suicidal ideation.

B. Classification of epilepsies and drug selection.

Epilepsies are characterized by either focal or generalized abnormal neuronal discharges. Drug selection, based on seizure classification, is listed below in the order of general choice.

1. ***Partial seizures***
   a. **Simple:** Localized discharge; consciousness unaltered
   b. **Complex:** Localized discharge that becomes widespread; accompanied by loss of consciousness
      (1) **Phenytoin, carbamazepine, lamotrigine**
      (2) Valproic acid, phenobarbital
2. ***Generalized seizures***
   a. **Tonic-clonic** (grand mal): Dramatic bilateral movements with either clonic jerking of the extremities or tonic rigidity of the entire body; accompanied by loss of consciousness
      (1) **Phenytoin, carbamazepine**
      (2) Topiramate, other newer AEDs
   b. **Absence** (petit mal): Sudden onset of altered consciousness that lasts 10–45 seconds, with up to hundreds of seizures per day; begins in childhood or adolescence
      (1) **Ethosuximide**
      (2) Valproic acid (when absence seizures coexist with tonic-clonic seizures)
      (3) clonazepam, lamotrigine, topiramate
   c. **Myoclonic** syndromes: Lightninglike jerks of one or more extremities occurring singly or in bursts of up to a hundred; accompanied by alteration of consciousness
      (1) **Valproic acid, lamotrigine**
      (2) Other newer AEDs

3. ***Status epilepticus:*** Prolonged seizure (>20 min) of any of the types previously described; the most common is life-threatening generalized tonic-clonic status epilepticus. Treatment is **IV diazepam** or **lorazepam** followed by **IV fosphenytoin** (or phenytoin) or **phenobarbital.**

C. Mechanism of action

1. ***Phenytoin, carbamazepine, valproic acid, and lamotrigine*** block sodium channels and inhibit the generation of action potentials. Their effect is "use dependent," that is, related to their selective binding and prolongation of the inactivated state of the sodium channel (see IX below). They also decrease neurotransmission by actions on prejunctional neurons.
   a. **Valproic acid at higher concentrations reduces low-threshold T-type Ca^{2+} current.**
   b. **Lamotrigine probably has additional therapeutically relevant actions.**
2. ***Ethosuximide*** reduces the low-threshold T-type Ca^{2+} current that provides the pacemaker activity in the thalamus.
3. ***Barbiturates*** (e.g., phenobarbital) and **benzodiazepines** (e.g., diazepam, lorazepam, clonazepam) facilitate GABA-mediated inhibition of neuronal activity.

D. Phenytoin, fosphenytoin

1. ***Pharmacologic properties***
   a. **Phenytoin** is absorbed well after oral administration, but its rate and extent of absorption can be altered considerably by its formulation.
   b. **Phenytoin** is metabolized by microsomal enzymes and excreted primarily as glucuronide. Its plasma half-life is approximately 24 hours at therapeutic doses. In some patients, metabolic enzymes become saturated at low doses, and half-life increases as the dose and plasma concentration increase, resulting in a steady-state mean **plasma concentration that varies disproportionately with dose** (Fig. 5-3).
   c. A steep dose response and **low therapeutic index** require that **phenytoin** plasma levels be carefully monitored.
   d. **Fosphenytoin** is available for parenteral administration as a replacement for phenytoin. Compared with phenytoin, fosphenytoin allows more rapid loading, intramuscular (IM) administration (phenytoin precipitates by the IM route), and IV administration, with minimal vascular erosion.
2. ***Adverse effects and toxicity***
   a. **Common:** Nystagmus (occurs early), diplopia and ataxia (most common), slurred speech, blurred vision, mental confusion, hirsutism (an issue particularly for females), gingival hyperplasia (can be minimized with good dental hygiene)
   b. **Rare:** With long-term use, coarsening of facial features, with mild peripheral neuropathy, and osteomalacia; idiosyncratic reactions requiring drug discontinuance (e.g., exfoliative dermatitis; blood dyscrasias, including agranulocytosis)
   c. **Fetal malformation** ("fetal hydantoin syndrome") includes growth retardation, microencephaly, and craniofacial abnormalities (e.g., cleft palate) and is possibly due to an epoxide metabolite of phenytoin.
3. ***Drug interactions***
   a. Phenytoin stimulates hepatic metabolism by microsomal enzyme induction and thereby reduces plasma concentrations of numerous drugs, including AEDs such as **carbamazepine** and **valproic acid,** and some **antibiotics, oral anticoagulants,** and **oral contraceptives.**
   b. The plasma concentration of phenytoin is increased by drugs that inhibit its hepatic metabolism (e.g., **cimetidine, isoniazid**).
   c. The plasma concentration of phenytoin is decreased by drugs that stimulate hepatic metabolism (e.g., **carbamazepine**).

E. Carbamazepine, Oxcarbazepine

1. ***Pharmacologic properties***
   a. **Carbamazepine** has good oral absorption although there is significant interpatient variability in its rate of absorption. An extended-release preparation is available. Its 10,11-epoxide metabolite may have some intrinsic toxicity.

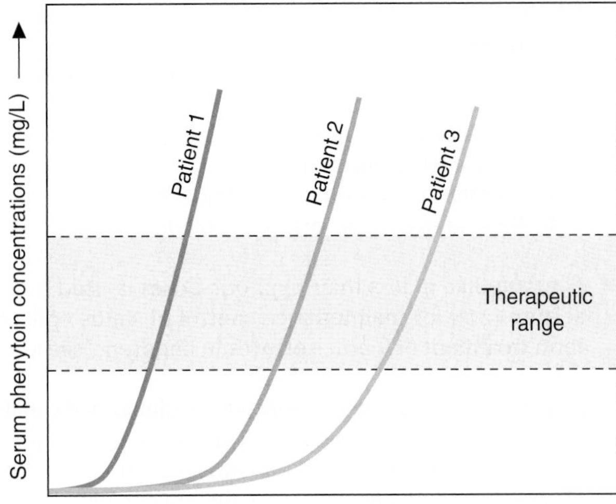

FIGURE 5-3. Nonlinear accumulation and variable serum levels of phenytoin dosage among different patients. (Modified with permission from Jusko WJ. Bioavailability and disposition kinetics of phenytoin in man. In: Kellaway P, Peterson I. Quantitative Analytic Studies in Epilepsy. New York: Raven Press, 1976:128.)

b. **Carbamazepine** induces microsomal enzymes and increases its own hepatic clearance (autometabolism), thus reducing its half-life from more than 30 hours to less than 20 hours. Gradual dosage adjustment is required early in therapy.
c. **Carbamazepine** is the drug of choice to treat trigeminal neuralgia and other pain syndromes (phenytoin is occasionally used); it is also used to treat bipolar affective disorder.
d. **Oxcarbazepine** is a prodrug whose actions are similar to those of carbamazepine; it has a short half-life of 1–2 hours. Its activity is due to a 10-hydroxy metabolite with a half-life of 10 hours. It may have a better adverse effect profile and be a less potent inducer of hepatic microsomal enzymes than carbamazepine.

2. ***Adverse effects and toxicity***
   a. **Common:** Diplopia and ataxia (most common), GI disturbances; sedation at high doses
   b. **Occasional:** Retention of water and hyponatremia; rash, agitation in children
   c. **Rare:** Idiosyncratic blood dyscrasias and severe rashes
3. ***Drug interactions***
   a. Carbamazepine induces microsomal enzymes and increases the hepatic clearance of numerous drugs including phenytoin and valproic acid.
   b. Plasma concentration of carbamazepine is increased by numerous drugs that inhibit hepatic metabolism.

F. Valproic acid

1. ***Pharmacologic properties***
   a. Valproic acid is also used to treat bipolar affective disorder and is used for migraine prophylaxis.
   b. **Valproic acid** inhibits the metabolism of other drugs including **phenytoin** and **carbamazepine.**
   c. **Divalproex sodium** (Depakote) is a 1:1 enteric formulation of valproic acid and valproate sodium that is absorbed more slowly than valproic acid and is often preferred by patients.
2. ***Adverse effects and toxicity***
   a. **Common:** GI disturbances and hair loss
   b. **Uncommon:** Weight gain, sedation, ataxia, and tremor at high doses
   c. **Rare:** Idiosyncratic hepatotoxicity; may be fatal in infants and in patients using multiple anticonvulsants.
   d. **Fetal malformations:** Spina bifida; orofacial and cardiovascular anomalies have been reported.

G. Ethosuximide

1. ***Pharmacologic properties***
   a. Although it is effective in fewer patients with absence seizures than valproic acid, ethosuximide is often the drug of choice because of its greater safety.
   b. **Phensuximide** and **methsuximide** are congeners with limited utility.
2. ***Adverse effects and toxicity***
   a. **Common:** GI disturbances, **fatigue, dizziness**
   b. **Rare:** Idiosyncratic rashes and blood dyscrasias

H. Phenobarbital at less than hypnotic doses is used most often as a first-line drug for neonatal seizures and for maintenance control of status epilepticus. On occasion it is used for short-term treatment of febrile seizures in children. (see also I F).

I. Benzodiazepines: Diazepam, lorazepam, clonazepam, and clorazepate (see also I B)

1. Diazepam and lorazepam are highly effective in short-term treatment of status epilepticus.
2. Clonazepam is effective for treatment of absence seizures. Clorazepate is used to treat complex partial seizures. Sedation is the their major adverse effect.

J. Other anticonvulsant agents (for partial and generalized tonic-clonic seizures)

1. ***Lamotrigine*** acts like phenytoin and carbamazepine. Its half-life is reduced by drugs that induce microsomal enzymes (e.g., phenytoin and carbamazepine) and is increased by valproic acid. Adverse effects include headache, ataxia, dizziness, and (rarely) a rash that may be life-threatening, particularly in children.
2. ***Gabapentin,*** among other activities, alters GABA metabolism to increase GABA levels in the brain. It is also used to treat neuropathic pain and postherpetic neuralgia. Its adverse effects include dizziness, ataxia, and tremor.
3. ***Topiramate*** acts like phenytoin and carbamazepine and may also act to facilitate the inhibitory action of GABA through an undetermined interaction with the GABA receptor. FDA approved for migraine headache prophylaxis. It suppresses weight loss and has been used to treat patients with eating disorders. Adverse effects include fatigue, nervousness, and memory dysfunction. Acute myopia and glaucoma may limit its use. Nephrolithiasis has been reported.
4. ***Tiagabine*** inhibits GABA uptake by interaction with its transporter. Dizziness is the most common adverse effect. Confusion and ataxia may limit its use.
5. ***Levetiracetam*** acts by an unknown mechanism. Its adverse actions include dizziness.
6. ***Felbamate*** may act at therapeutic levels at the glycine binding site to block the *N*-methyl-d-aspartate (NMDA) glutamate receptor. It alters the metabolism of other AEDs. Its use is limited by development of aplastic anemia (1:3,000) and severe hepatitis with liver failure (1:10,000).
7. ***Zonisamide*** acts at the sodium channel and possibly the voltage-dependent calcium channel. Adverse effects include drowsiness, confusion, and rashes.
8. ***Pregabalin,*** an analogue of gabapentin, is used to treat partial seizures. It binds to voltage-gated calcium channels and reduces release of excitatory neurotransmitters. It is also approved for use in treating postherpetic neuralgia and diabetic peripheral neuropathy. Its major adverse effects are dizziness, dry mouth, blurred vision, and weight gain. It is a schedule V controlled substance because of reports that it causes euphoria.

VIII. GENERAL ANESTHETICS

A. Overview of general anesthetics

1. ***General anesthesia*** is characterized by a loss of consciousness, analgesia, amnesia, skeletal muscle relaxation, and inhibition of autonomic and sensory reflexes.
2. ***Balanced anesthesia***
   a. Balanced anesthesia refers to a combination of drugs used to take advantage of individual drug properties while attempting to minimize their adverse actions.

b. In addition to inhalation anesthetics and neuromuscular junction (NMJ)-blocking drugs, other drugs, such as barbiturates, opioids, and benzodiazepines, are administered preoperatively, intraoperatively, and postoperatively to ensure smooth induction, analgesia, sedation, and smooth recovery.

3. ***Stages and planes of anesthesia.*** The stages and planes of anesthesia identify the progression of physical signs that indicate the depth of anesthesia. Newer, more potent agents progress through these stages rapidly, and therefore, the stages are often obscured. Mechanical ventilation and the use of adjunct drugs also obscure the signs indicating the depth of anesthesia.
   a. Stage I: Analgesia, amnesia
   b. Stage II: Loss of consciousness (may be excitement)
   c. Stage III: Surgical anesthesia
      (1) Four planes have been described relating to increased depth of anesthesia. Plane IV includes maximal pupil dilation, apnea, and circulatory depression.
      (2) The loss of the eyelash reflex and a pattern of respiration that is regular in rate and depth are the most reliable signs of stage III anesthesia.
   d. Stage IV: Respiratory and cardiovascular failure

B. Inhalation anesthetics

1. ***Nitrous oxide, isoflurane, desflurane, sevoflurane, halothane, and enflurane***
   a. **Nitrous oxide, isoflurane, desflurane,** and **sevoflurane** are the most commonly used inhalation anesthetics. The more blood-soluble agents, **halothane** and **enflurane,** are used less often. All except nitrous oxide are halogenated volatile liquids.
   b. These agents are nonflammable and nonexplosive. They decrease cerebral vascular resistance with increased perfusion of the brain.
   c. These anesthetics are all respiratory depressants; consequently, assisted or controlled ventilation is usually necessary during surgical anesthesia.
   d. Concentrations of halogenated inhalation anesthetics that produce good skeletal muscle relaxation generally produce unacceptable dose-related cardiovascular depression; consequently, NMJ-blocking drugs are commonly used for surgical muscle relaxation. Also, they are generally administered with nitrous oxide, which decreases the extent of cardiovascular and respiratory depression at equivalent anesthetic depths.

2. ***Mechanism of anesthetic action.*** Inhalation and intravenous anesthetic agent interaction with **discrete protein binding sites in nerve endings to activate ligand-gated ion channels** best explains their mechanism of action. These channels include the following (see also Fig. 1-1A):
   a. **$GABA_A$-receptor chloride channels,** where these anesthetic agents directly and indirectly facilitate a GABA-mediated increase in chloride (Cl^-) conductance to hyperpolarize and inhibit neuronal membrane activity
   b. **Ligand-gated potassium (K^+) channels,** where these anesthetic agents increase potassium conductance to hyperpolarize and inhibit neuronal membrane activity

3. ***Potency*** (Table 5-9)
   a. **Minimum alveolar concentration (MAC)** is a relative term defined as the minimum alveolar concentration at steady state (measured in volume/volume percent) that results in immobility in 50% of patients when exposed to a noxious stimulus, such as a surgical incision. Inhalant anesthetics have a steep dose–response relationship.
   b. The lower the MAC value, the more potent the agent; for example, **nitrous oxide** has a MAC of more than 100, indicating that immobility can generally only be achieved under hyperbaric conditions, whereas **isoflurane** has a MAC of 1.2, indicating immobility can be achieved at a relatively low concentration.
   c. MAC is an additive function for inhaled anesthetic agents.
   d. MAC will decrease with increasing age, pregnancy, hypothermia, and hypotension; MAC decreases in the presence of adjuvant drugs such as other general anesthetics, opioids, sedative–hypnotics, or other CNS depressants. It is independent of gender and weight.

4. ***Solubility*** (see Table 5-9)
   a. The rate at which the partial pressure of an inhalation anesthetic reaches equilibrium between various tissues, notably the CNS, and inspired air depends primarily on the solubility of the drug in blood.

table 5-9 Properties of Inhalation Anesthetics

Anesthetic	Blood–Gas Partition Coefficient (λ)	Oil–Gas Partition Coefficient	Minimum Alveolar Concentration (%) (MAC)
Nitrous Oxide	0.47	1.4	>100
Halothane	2.3	224	0.75
Enflurane	1.8	95	1.7
Isoflurane	1.5	98	1.4
Desflurane	0.42	??	2.0

b. The relative solubility of an inhalation anesthetic in blood relative to air is defined by its blood–gas partition coefficient, lambda (λ), which is directly related to the pharmacokinetics of an anesthetic (see Table 5-9):

$$\lambda = [\text{anesthetic}]\text{ in blood} / [\text{anesthetic}]\text{ in gas}$$

Relatively few molecules of an anesthetic with low solubility in blood are necessary to increase its partial pressure in blood. This results in its rapid equilibrium in the CNS and a rapid onset of action (e.g., **nitrous oxide, desflurane, sevoflurane**).

(1) Increasing the anesthetic concentration in inspired air will increase the rate of induction (Fick's law). For anesthetic agents of moderate solubility (e.g., **halothane**), a higher concentration can be used initially to more rapidly achieve adequate anesthesia.

(2) Increased rate and depth of ventilation, such as that produced by mechanical hyperventilation or CO_2 stimulation, will increase the partial pressure more rapidly for anesthetics with intermediate or high blood solubility.

(3) Changes in the rate of pulmonary blood flow to and from the lungs will change the rate of rise of arterial tension, particularly for anesthetic agents with intermediate-to-low solubility. Increased pulmonary flow from, for example, increased cardiac output decreases the rate of rise in partial pressure by presenting a larger volume of blood into which the anesthetic can dissolve. Conversely, decreased pulmonary flow, such as occurs during shock, increases the rate of induction of anesthesia.

(4) The less soluble an anesthetic (low blood:gas partition coefficient), the more rapid its elimination and the more rapid the patient's recovery from anesthesia (e.g., **nitrous oxide, desflurane, sevoflurane**). For soluble anesthetics, the longer the exposure, the longer the time to recovery, because of accumulation of anesthetic in various tissues. Other factors that affect recovery include pulmonary ventilation and pulmonary blood flow.

5. ***Pharmacology of commonly used inhalation anesthetics***

a. Nitrous oxide (N_2O)

(1) Advantages

(a) Nitrous oxide is an anesthetic gas that has **good analgesic and sedative properties** but no skeletal muscle relaxant properties.

(b) Nitrous oxide is often **used in combination with other inhalation anesthetics** to increase their rate of uptake and to add to their analgesic activity while reducing their adverse effects. When given in large volumes, it increases the volume of uptake of a second blood-soluble gas such as **halothane (second-gas effect),** which then speeds the induction of anesthesia.

(c) This anesthetic is often supplemented in balanced anesthesia with other sedative–hypnotics, analgesics, and skeletal muscle relaxants.

(2) Disadvantages

(a) Nitrous oxide **lacks sufficient potency to produce surgical anesthesia.**

(b) Nitrous oxide is commonly associated with **postoperative nausea and vomiting.**

(c) Nitrous oxide **inactivates methionine synthase** with long-term exposure (e.g., recreational use). This may cause inhibition of DNA and protein synthesis and result in anemia or leukopenia.

b. Isoflurane

(1) Advantages

(a) Isoflurane produces more **rapid induction and emergence** than halothane.

(b) Isoflurane undergoes minimal metabolism.

(c) Isoflurane has **good analgesic** and **sedative–hypnotic** effects.

(2) Disadvantages

(a) Isoflurane **sensitizes the heart to catecholamines (less likely than halothane).**

(b) Isoflurane **decreases vascular resistance** and dilates the coronary vasculature, which, depending on a number of factors that influence cardiac function, could be beneficial in patients with ischemic heart disease. However, paradoxically, isoflurane may precipitate cardiac ischemia in patients with underlying coronary heart disease.

c. Desflurane

(1) Advantages

(a) Desflurane produces more **rapid induction and rapid emergence** than isoflurane and, therefore, is often preferred for outpatient surgical procedures.

(b) Enflurane undergoes minimal metabolism and, therefore, rarely produces organ toxicity.

(2) Disadvantages

(a) Desflurane is especially **irritating to the airway** and may cause coughing, laryngospasm, and increased secretions with breath holding.

(b) Special dispensing equipment for desflurane is necessary because of its low boiling point (23.5°C).

(c) Desflurane, like isoflurane, decreases vascular resistance.

(d) Desflurane increases heart rate and causes sympathetic stimulation at high concentrations.

d. Sevoflurane

(1) Advantages

(a) Sevoflurane produces a very **rapid and smooth induction and rapid recovery** with no respiratory irritation. It is widely used for pediatric anesthesia.

(b) Sevoflurane causes **bronchodilation,** an effect that is useful for patients with respiratory difficulties.

(2) Disadvantage. Sevoflurane produces fluoride ions during its liver metabolism that potentially could be **nephrotoxic.**

e. Halothane

(1) Advantages

(a) Halothane has a **pleasant odor** and produces a **smooth and relatively rapid induction.** It is usually administered with nitrous oxide.

(b) This anesthetic has fair **analgesic** and **skeletal muscle and uterine relaxant** properties; it has excellent **hypnotic properties.**

(2) Disadvantages

(a) Halothane **decreases cardiac output.** The result may be a fall in blood pressure.

(b) Halothane **sensitizes the heart to endogenous and exogenous catecholamines,** producing extrasystoles and transient arrhythmias.

(c) Halothane may result in an **unpredictable hepatotoxicity,** possibly due to a reactive free radical toxic metabolite, trifluoroacetic acid (on average >40% is metabolized during most anesthetic procedures). However, incidence of this hepatotoxicity is extremely rare (1 in 10,000–30,000).

f. Enflurane

(1) Advantages

(a) Enflurane produces a **rapid induction and recovery** with little excitation.

(b) Enflurane produces good **analgesia, muscle relaxation,** and **hypnosis.** It is less likely than halothane to sensitize the heart to catecholamines or cause arrhythmias.

(2) Disadvantages

(a) It is **pungent,** which may result in breath holding or coughing; thus, this anesthetic is less well accepted by children.

(b) At high concentrations, enflurane produces **CNS stimulation** with mild twitching or tonic-clonic movements; hypocapnia exaggerates these effects. It should be avoided in patients with epilepsy or other seizure disorders.

(c) Enflurane **reduces cardiac output** and may cause a decrease in blood pressure.

(d) Enflurane is contraindicated in patients with renal failure because some is **metabolized to fluoride ion** that is excreted by the kidney.

6. ***Additional effects of inhalation anesthetics***
   a. Inhalation anesthetics are bronchodilators, particularly **halothane** and **sevoflurane,** which allows use in patients with underlying respiratory problems.
   b. **Methoxyflurane** is now rarely used in humans. It is highly metabolized, resulting in dose-related fluoride-induced renal toxicity.
   c. Inhalation anesthetics, except **nitrous oxide,** relax uterine muscle, an advantage during certain obstetrical procedures.
   d. Inhalation anesthetics increase cerebral blood flow, which may indirectly result in increased intracranial pressure. Patients with brain tumor or head injury are at risk.
   e. Genetically susceptible patients may (rarely) develop potentially lethal **malignant hyperthermia**, which includes tachycardia, hypertension, acid–base and electrolyte abnormalities, muscle rigidity, and hyperthermia. These effects stem from increased free calcium levels in skeletal muscle cells. Treatment is supportive with **dantrolene,** a muscle relaxant that blocks calcium channels.
   f. Inhalation anesthetics cause vasodilation and hypothermia by lowering the metabolic rate and lowering the set point for thermoregulatory vasoconstriction.

C. Intravenous anesthetics and preanesthetic drugs

1. ***Barbiturates: thiopental (also methohexital)*** (see also I F 1 and X C 3)
   a. Thiopental, which is highly lipid soluble, is administered IV to induce anesthesia and results in a smooth, pleasant, and rapid induction and minimal postoperative nausea and vomiting, although there may be a "hangover."
   b. Thiopental has a rapid onset (~20 seconds) and has a short duration of action (5–10 min) due to redistribution from highly vascular tissue, particularly brain tissue, to less vascular tissue such as muscle and adipose tissue.
   c. The action of thiopental in the CNS is similar to that of inhalation anesthetics; it can produce profound respiratory and cardiovascular depression. Thiopental has no analgesic or muscle relaxant properties.
   d. Use of thiopental is an absolute contraindication for patients with acute intermediate porphyria or variegate porphyria.
2. ***Benzodiazepines*** (see also I B)
   a. **Diazepam, lorazepam, and midazolam** may be administered orally or IV and are used preoperatively for sedation and to reduce anxiety. They can be used intraoperatively with other drugs as part of balanced anesthesia. These drugs are used as sole agents for surgical and diagnostic procedures that do not require analgesia (endoscopy, cardiac catheterization, changing burn dressings).
   b. Benzodiazepines, particularly **midazolam,** produce a clinically useful anterograde amnesia.
   c. **Midazolam** has a more rapid onset and shorter elimination time than **diazepam** and **lorazepam** and produces less cardiovascular depression.
3. ***Opioids: fentanyl, sufentanil, and remifentanil*** (see also V)
   a. Opioids are administered preoperatively as adjuncts to inhalation and IV anesthetic to reduce pain.
   b. **Remifentanil** have a rapid onset of action; **remifentanil** has a short duration of action due to metabolism by nonspecific esterases in the blood and certain tissues.
   c. At high doses, these drugs (and **morphine**) are used to achieve general anesthesia during cardiac surgery when circulatory stability is important (may be combined with muscle relaxants and **nitrous oxide** or very small doses of inhalation anesthetic).
   d. **Fentanyl** and **droperidol,** a butyrophenone similar to haloperidol that has antiemetic and sedating properties, are used in fixed combination (Innovar) with **nitrous oxide** or, more

rationally, as individual agents to achieve motor inactivity, reduced anxiety, and amnesia (i.e., neuroleptanalgesia) for minor diagnostic and surgical procedures in which patients can still be responsive to commands.

e. Opioids increase the risk of preoperative and postoperative nausea and vomiting.

4. *Etomidate*

a. Etomidate is a nonbarbiturate anesthetic used like thiopental for rapid-onset, short-duration anesthesia. Unlike thiopental, it causes minimal cardiorespiratory depression, which is useful for treatment of at-risk patients.

b. Etomidate has no analgesic effect.

c. Etomidate produces the following adverse effects: pain at injection site, unpredictable and often severe myoclonus during induction of hypnosis, suppression of adrenocortical function (with continued use), and postoperative nausea and vomiting.

5. *Propofol*

a. Propofol, which has replaced thiopental as the **agent of choice for rapid sedation and rapid-onset and short-duration anesthesia,** is administered IV. It is rapidly metabolized in the liver.

b. Propofol is widely used for outpatient surgical procedures, in intensive care settings, and in balanced anesthesia.

c. Propofol produces no analgesia; it produces minimal postoperative nausea and vomiting.

d. Propofol produces the following adverse effects: pain at injection site and systemic hypotension from decreased systemic vascular resistance.

6. *Ketamine*

a. Ketamine produces a **dissociative anesthesia,** an effect in which patients feel dissociated from their surroundings; analgesia; and amnesia, with or without loss of consciousness.

b. This drug is thought to **block the effects of glutamic acid at NMDA-receptors.**

c. Ketamine has an analgesic effect on superficial pain but not visceral pain. It also has an amnestic action.

d. Ketamine is a potent cardiovascular stimulant; it is useful for patients in cardiogenic or septic shock.

e. At low doses it is used in infants and children (trauma, minor surgical and diagnostic procedures, changing dressings).

f. Ketamine's adverse effects include frequent distortions of reality, terrifying dreams, and delirium, particularly in adults.

IX. LOCAL ANESTHETICS

A. Overview of local anesthetics

1. Local anesthetics produce a transient and reversible loss of sensation in a circumscribed region of the body **without loss of consciousness.** Smaller nonmyelinated dorsal root type C nerve fibers and lightly myelinated delta type A nerve fibers, which carry pain and temperature sensations (and also sympathetic type C unmyelinated postganglionic nerve fibers), are blocked before larger, heavily myelinated type A fibers, which transmit sensory proprioception and motor functions.
2. Local anesthetics are generally classified as either **esters** or **amides** and are usually linked to a lipophilic aromatic group and to a hydrophilic, ionizable tertiary (sometimes secondary) amine. Most are weak bases with pK_a values between 8 and 9, and at physiologic pH they are primarily in the charged, cationic form.
3. The potency of local anesthetics is positively correlated with their lipid solubility, which may vary 16-fold, and negatively correlated with their molecular size.
4. These anesthetics are selected for use on the basis of the duration of drug action (short, 20 min; intermediate, 1–1.5 h; long, 2–4 h), effectiveness at the administration site, and potential for toxicity.

B. Mechanism of action. Local anesthetics act by blocking sodium channels and the conduction of action potentials along sensory nerves. Blockade is voltage dependent and time dependent.

1. At rest, the voltage-dependent sodium (Na^+) channels of sensory nerves are in the resting (closed) state. Following the action potential the Na^+ channel becomes active (open) and then converts to an inactive (closed) state that is insensitive to depolarization. Following repolarization of the plasma membrane there is a slow reversion of channels from the inactive to the resting state, which can again be activated by depolarization. During excitation the cationic charged form of local anesthetics interacts preferentially with the inactivated state of the Na^+ channels on the inner aspect of the sodium channel to **block sodium current** and **increase the threshold for excitation.**
2. This results in a dose-dependent decrease in impulse conduction and in the rate of rise and amplitude of the action potential. This is more pronounced in rapidly firing axons, suggesting that local anesthetics gain access to the inner axonal membrane by traversing sodium channels while they are more often in an open configuration. Access to the inner axonal membrane may also occur by passage of the more lipophilic anesthetic molecules directly through the plasma membrane.

C. Pharmacologic properties

1. ***Administration and absorption***
   a. Local anesthetics, except cocaine, are poorly absorbed from the GI tract. They are administered topically, by infiltration into tissues to bathe local nerves, by injection directly around nerves and their branches, and by injection into epidural or subarachnoid spaces.
   b. The rate and extent of absorption to and from nerves are important in determining the rate of onset of action and termination of action and also the potential for systemic adverse effects. Their **absorption rate is correlated with the relative lipid solubility of the uncharged form** and is influenced by the dose and the drug's physicochemical properties, as well as by tissue blood flow and drug binding.
      (1) **Reduced pH,** as in inflamed tissues, increases the prevalence of the cationic form, which reduces diffusion into nerves and thereby reduces local anesthetic effectiveness.
      (2) **"Carbonation"** of local anesthetic solutions (saturation with carbon dioxide) can decrease intracellular pH, which increases the prevalence and activity of the cationic active form inside the nerve.
   c. All local anesthetics, except **cocaine,** are vasodilators at therapeutic doses. Coadministration of a vasoconstrictor (e.g., **epinephrine**) with a local anesthetic (generally of short or intermediate duration of action) reduces local blood flow. This reduces systemic absorption of the local anesthetic from the site of application, prolongs its action, and reduces its potential for toxicity. **Epinephrine** should not be coadministered for nerve block in areas such as fingers and toes that are supplied with end-arteries because it may cause **ischemia or necrosis,** and it should be used cautiously in patients in labor and in patients with thyrotoxicosis or cardiovascular disease.
2. ***Metabolism***
   a. **Ester-type** local anesthetics are metabolized by **plasma butyrylcholinesterase** and thus have very short plasma half-lives. The metabolic rate of these anesthetics is decreased in patients with decreased or genetically atypical cholinesterase.
   b. **Amide-type** local anesthetics are metabolized at varying rates and to varying extents by **hepatic microsomal enzymes** (dealkylation and conjugation). They are excreted in metabolized and uncharged form by the kidney. The rate of metabolism of these anesthetics is decreased in patients with liver disease or decreased hepatic blood flow, or by drugs that interfere with cytochrome P-450 enzymes (e.g., **cimetidine, alfentanil, midazolam**).

D. Specific drugs and their therapeutic uses

1. ***Amides***
   a. **Lidocaine**
      (1) **Lidocaine** is the prototype amide; it has an intermediate duration of action.
      (2) **Lidocaine** is generally preferred for infiltration blocks and for epidural anesthesia.
   b. **Mepivacaine**
      (1) Mepivacaine has an intermediate duration of action that is longer than that of lidocaine.

(2) Mepivacaine has actions similar to those of lidocaine, but it causes less drowsiness and sedation.
(3) Mepivacaine is not used topically.

c. **Prilocaine**
(1) Prilocaine has an intermediate duration of action that is longer than that of lidocaine.
(2) Prilocaine has actions similar to those of lidocaine, but it is less toxic.
(3) This anesthetic is not used topically or for subarachnoid anesthesia.
(4) Prilocaine should not be used in patients with cardiac or respiratory disease or in those with idiopathic or congenital methemoglobinemia because toluidine metabolites may produce methemoglobin. Methemoglobinemia can be reversed by administration of methylene blue.

d. **Bupivacaine, Ropivacaine, Etidocaine**
(1) These drugs have a long duration of action.
(2) **Bupivacaine** has greater cardiotoxicity than other amide local anesthetics.
(3) **Ropivacaine** may have less cardiotoxicity than bupivacaine.
(4) **Etidocaine** has a rapid onset of action.

2. ***Esters***

a. **Procaine**
(1) Procaine has a slow onset and is short acting.
(2) Procaine is ineffective topically.

b. **Chloroprocaine**
(1) Chloroprocaine has a rapid onset and short duration of action. It is very rapidly metabolized by plasma cholinesterase.
(2) Chloroprocaine has less reported toxicity than procaine.

c. **Cocaine** (also see X D)
(1) Cocaine is a short-acting, naturally occurring alkaloid that is used medically only for the topical anesthesia of mucous membranes.
(2) Systemically, cocaine will block the uptake of catecholamines into nerve terminals and may induce intense vasoconstriction.
(3) Adverse effects of cocaine include euphoria, CNS stimulation, tachycardia, restlessness, tremors, seizures, and arrhythmias.
(4) Cocaine should be used cautiously in patients with hypertension, cardiovascular disease, or thyrotoxicosis, and with other drugs that potentiate catecholamine activity.
(5) Cocaine is a schedule II controlled substance that is subject to abuse.

d. **Tetracaine**
(1) Tetracaine is long acting but has a slow onset of action (>10 min).
(2) Tetracaine is often preferred for spinal anesthesia and for ophthalmologic use.
(3) Tetracaine is not generally used for peripheral nerve blocks, infiltration blocks, or lumbar epidural nerve blocks.

e. **Dibucaine**
(1) Dibucaine is long acting but has a slow onset of action (15 min).
(2) Dibucaine is used only for topical anesthesia.

f. **Benzocaine** and **butamben picrate.** These anesthetics are used topically only to treat sunburn, minor burns, and pruritus.

g. **Proparacaine** is used topically for ophthalmology when rapid onset and short duration are desirable.

3. ***Other local anesthetics***

a. **Dyclonine** has a rapid onset of action and is used topically.
b. **Pramoxine** is used topically but is too irritating for the eye or nose.

E. **Adverse effects and toxicity.** Adverse effects are generally an extension of therapeutic action to block the membrane sodium channel. They are usually the result of overdose or inadvertent injection into the vascular system. Systemic effects are most likely to occur with administration of the amide class.

1. ***CNS***

a. Adverse CNS effects include light-headedness, dizziness, restlessness, tinnitus, tremor, and visual disturbances. Lidocaine and procaine may cause sedation and sleep.

b. At high blood concentrations, local anesthetics produce nystagmus, shivering, tonic-clonic seizures, respiratory depression, coma, and death.
c. Adverse CNS effects are treated by maintenance of airway and assisted ventilation, IV diazepam for seizures (or prophylactically), and succinylcholine to suppress muscular reactions.

2. ***Cardiovascular system***
   a. Adverse cardiovascular system effects develop at relatively higher plasma levels than do adverse CNS effects.
   b. Bradycardia develops as a result of the block of cardiac sodium channels and the depression of pacemaker activity.
   c. Hypotension develops from arteriolar dilation and decreased cardiac contractility.
   d. These adverse effects are treated with IV fluids and vasopressor agents.
3. ***Allergic reactions***
   a. Allergic reactions include rare rash, edema, and anaphylaxis.
   b. These reactions are usually associated with ester-type drugs such as **procaine** that are metabolized to derivatives of *para*-aminobenzoic acid.

X. DRUGS OF ABUSE

A. Overview

1. Drugs of abuse generally act on the CNS to modify the user's mental state, although some are used for enhancing physical performance.
2. Long-term use may lead to the development of tolerance and to the development of psychologic or physical dependence, or both.
3. Complications related to parenteral drug administration under unsterile conditions or to the coadministration of adulterants are extremely common (e.g., thrombophlebitis, local and systemic abscesses, viral hepatitis, HIV infection).

B. Definitions

1. Drug abuse is the nonmedical, self-administered use of a drug that is harmful to the user. Commonly abused drugs include opioid (narcotic) analgesics (e.g., heroin), general CNS depressants (e.g., ethanol, barbiturates such as pentobarbital), inhalants (e.g., toluene, nitrous oxide, amyl nitrate), sedative–hypnotics (e.g., alprazolam, diazepam), CNS stimulants (e.g., cocaine, amphetamines, nicotine), hallucinogens (e.g., LSD, mescaline, phencyclidine), and marijuana (cannabis).
2. Drug addiction is a nonmedical term that refers to the drug abuser's overwhelming preoccupation with the procurement and use of a drug.
3. Tolerance is the decreased intensity of a response to a drug following its continued administration. A larger dose often can produce the same initial effect.
   a. **Metabolic tolerance** (pharmacokinetic tolerance): The rate of drug elimination increases with long-term use because of stimulation of its own metabolism (autometabolism).
   b. **Cellular tolerance** (pharmacodynamic tolerance): Biochemical adaptation or homeostatic adjustment of cells to the continued presence of a drug. The development of cellular tolerance may be due to a compensatory change in the activity of specific neurotransmitters in the CNS caused by a change in their levels, storage, or release or to changes in the number or activity of their receptors.
   c. **Cross-tolerance.** Tolerance to one drug confers at least partial tolerance to other drugs in the same drug class (e.g., between **heroin** and **methadone;** between **ethanol** and **diazepam**).
   d. Tolerance is often, but not always, associated with the development of physical dependence.
   e. The degree of tolerance varies considerably among different classes of drugs of abuse (e.g., **cocaine**$\gg$**marijuana**).
4. Dependence refers to the biologic need to continue to take a drug.
   a. **Psychologic dependence:** Overwhelming compulsive need to take a drug (drug-seeking behavior) to maintain a sense of well-being. Psychologic dependence may be related to

increased dopamine activity in the "brain reward system" (includes the mesolimbic dopaminergic pathway from the ventral midbrain to the nucleus accumbens and other limbic structures including the prefrontal cortex and limbic and motor systems). Development of psychologic dependence generally precedes development of physical dependence but does not necessarily lead to it.

b. **Physical dependence:** A latent hyperexcitability that is revealed when administration of a drug of abuse is discontinued after its long-term use ("abstinent withdrawal"). Continued drug use is necessary to avoid the abstinent withdrawal syndrome.

(1) The **abstinent withdrawal syndrome** is characterized by effects that are often opposite to the short-term effects of the abused drug and that often include activation of the sympathetic nervous system. The severity of the withdrawal syndrome is directly related to the dose of the drug, how long it is used, and its rate of elimination.

(2) **"Precipitated withdrawal"** that follows administration of an antagonist (e.g., **naloxone, flumazenil**) has a more explosive onset and shorter duration than abstinent withdrawal.

(3) The development of physical dependence, the mechanism of which is not understood, is always associated with the development of tolerance.

(4) The degree of physical dependence varies considerably among different drugs of abuse (**heroin**$\gg$**marijuana**).

c. **Cross-dependence:** Ability of one drug to substitute for another drug in the same drug class to maintain a dependent state or to prevent withdrawal (e.g., **diazepam** for ethanol; **methadone** for heroin).

C. General CNS depressants

1. *Ethanol*

a. **Mechanism of action**

(1) The precise mechanism of action for ethanol on the CNS is unknown. It may be related to changes in membrane fluidity with changes in membrane protein functions, particularly signaling pathways.

(2) Among many other actions, ethanol has a direct effect on $GABA_A$-receptors to acutely enhance the inhibitory action of GABA in the CNS. It also has an inhibitory effect on glutamate activation of NMDA-glutamate receptors in the CNS.

b. **Acute pharmacologic effects**

(1) General CNS depression

(a) At **low-to-moderate levels** in nontolerant individuals (50–100 mg/dL), inhibition of inhibitory CNS pathways (disinhibition) occurs, resulting in decreased anxiety and disinhibited behavior with slurred speech, ataxia, and impaired judgment (drunkenness).

(b) At **moderate-to-toxic levels** (100–300 mg/dL), a dose-dependent general inhibition of the CNS occurs with increasing sedation and respiratory depression and decreasing mental acuity and motor function.

(c) At **toxic levels** (>300 mg/dL), CNS depression can result in coma, profound respiratory depression, and death. **Acute toxicity with respiratory depression** is a serious medical emergency. Respiratory support and avoidance of aspiration of vomitus may be sufficient, but the patient may also require restoration of fluid and electrolyte balance, thiamine to prevent Wernicke-Korsakoff syndrome, and treatment of hypoglycemia.

(2) **Depressed myocardial contractility** possibly caused by the ethanol metabolite acetaldehyde

(3) Cutaneous vasodilation

(a) Cutaneous vasodilation is due to probable inhibitory effects on the vasomotor and thermoregulatory centers.

(b) Hypothermia may be significant in cases of severe overdose or in cold environments.

(4) **Diuresis** develops due to an increase in plasma fluid volume and inhibition of antidiuretic hormone release from the posterior pituitary.

(5) **GI effects** include increased salivation, decreased GI motility, GI irritation, and occasional nausea and vomiting.

c. Long-term pharmacologic effects

(1) Liver disease

(a) Liver disease, manifested by a progression from reversible fatty liver to alcohol hepatitis, and to irreversible cirrhosis and liver failure, is the most common adverse effect of long-term ethanol consumption.

(b) Other contributing factors to liver disease may include reduced glutathione as a free radical scavenger, damage to mitochondria, and a background of malnutrition.

(2) Peripheral neuropathy with paresthesias of the hands and feet

(3) Wernicke's encephalopathy with ataxia, confusion, abnormal eye movements and **Korsakoff's psychosis** with impairment of memory that is often irreversible (**Wernicke-Korsakoff syndrome**). This effect is associated with **thiamine deficiency** secondary to malnutrition.

(4) Pancreatitis and gastritis. Direct erosion by ethanol of pancreatic acinar cells may lead to pancreatitis. Likewise, the direct action of ethanol may erode the GI epithelium and decrease GI mucosal defense barriers, resulting in GI bleeding, gastritis, esophagitis, and pancreatitis.

(5) Heart disease

(a) Cardiomyopathy may develop due to ethanol-induced membrane disruption with decreased mitochondrial activity, among other effects.

(b) Arrhythmias (and seizures) may develop during "binge" drinking or during the ethanol withdrawal syndrome.

(c) Hypertension, which may be reversible

(d) Moderate, long-term consumption of ethanol may decrease the risk of coronary heart disease possibly due to an ethanol-induced increase in high-density lipoproteins (HDL) or to its antioxidant or anti-inflammatory effects.

(6) Fetal alcohol spectrum disorder

(a) Fetal alcohol spectrum disorder results from maternal abuse of ethanol.

(b) Fetal alcohol syndrome is characterized by retarded growth, microencephaly, poorly developed coordination, mental retardation, and congenital heart abnormalities.

(c) Severe behavioral abnormalities can occur in the absence of dysmorphology. There is also an increased rate of spontaneous abortions.

(7) Other long-term effects include mild anemia, hypoglycemia, gynecomastia, testicular atrophy, and cancer of the GI tract.

d. Pharmacologic properties

(1) Ethanol is rapidly absorbed from the stomach and small intestine and is rapidly distributed in total body water. Absorption is delayed by food.

(2) Ethanol is oxidized at low plasma concentrations to acetaldehyde by the liver cytosolic enzyme **alcohol dehydrogenase** (ADH), with the generation of reduced nicotinamide adenine dinucleotide (NADH). ADH is also found in the stomach and brain. At higher blood concentrations (>100 mg/dL) ethanol is also oxidized to acetaldehyde by liver microsomal enzymes. Acetaldehyde is further oxidized by mitochondrial **aldehyde dehydrogenase** to acetate, which is further metabolized to CO_2 and H_2O.

(a) Plasma ethanol levels achieved with even one or two alcoholic beverages results in hepatic metabolism that shows **zero-order kinetics** (due to a functional saturation of alcohol dehydrogenase) so that the rate of ethanol elimination is independent of plasma concentration, with the attendant increased risk of accumulation (in the adult, approximately 6–8 g or 7.5–10 mL of alcohol is metabolized per hour).

(b) Women demonstrate less activity of a stomach alcohol dehydrogenase than men, with resulting higher blood alcohol levels after oral administration of a similar dose. The generally higher fat and blood ratio in women also contributes to the increased effect of ethanol.

(c) Certain **Asian populations** have a genetic alteration in aldehyde dehydrogenase that increases their sensitivity to ethanol because of the relatively greater accumulation of acetaldehyde.

e. Therapeutic uses. Ethanol is used as an antiseptic, as a solvent for other drugs, and as a treatment to prevent methanol-induced toxicity.

f. Drug interactions/contraindications

(1) Ethanol has an additive or potentiative CNS depression and possible respiratory arrest activity with other drugs that also have CNS depressant effects (the **benzodiazepines, antihistamines, antipsychotics, antidepressants**).

(2) Short-term ethanol use decreases the metabolism and augments the effects of many drugs (e.g., **phenytoin, warfarin**) because of its inhibitory effects on liver microsomal enzymes.

(3) Long-term ethanol use increases the metabolism and thereby decreases the effect of numerous drugs by induction of liver cytochrome P-450 enzymes (e.g., **phenytoin, warfarin, barbiturates;** also, inhibition of the usual metabolic pathway results in increased production of a toxic metabolite by an alternative metabolic pathway).

(4) Ethanol use is contraindicated during pregnancy, and in patients with ulcers, liver disease, and seizure disorders.

g. Tolerance and dependence

(1) Tolerance to the intoxicating and euphoric effects of ethanol develops with long-term use. Tolerance to ethanol is related to neuronal adaptation and also to some increased autometabolism. A lesser degree of tolerance develops to the potentially lethal action of ethanol. There is cross-tolerance to other CNS depressants, including the benzodiazepines and barbiturates, but not the opioids.

(2) Psychologic dependence (see above)

(3) Physical dependence and withdrawal syndrome

(a) Symptoms occurring over 1–2 days include anxiety, apprehension, irritability, insomnia, and tremor. More severe cases progress to signs of anorexia, nausea, vomiting, autonomic hyperactivity, hypertension, diaphoresis, and hyperthermia. The most severe cases progress to delirium (agitation, disorientation, modified consciousness, visual and auditory hallucinations, and severe autonomic hyperexcitability also referred to as **"delirium tremens")** and seizures.

(b) The **acute withdrawal syndrome** usually subsides within 3–7 days. This withdrawal syndrome can be life threatening in debilitated individuals.

(4) Management of ethanol abuse

(a) In addition to maintenance and nutritional (e.g., thiamine replacement) and electrolyte therapy and long-term psychologic support, treatment may include prevention or reversal of seizures with a benzodiazepine or **phenytoin,** and administration of a long-acting benzodiazepine (e.g., **diazepam**) as a substitute for ethanol, followed by tapered dose reduction over several weeks.

(b) Disulfiram is used as an adjunct in the supervised treatment of alcoholism, although compliance is low.

(i) Disulfiram **inhibits aldehyde dehydrogenase,** resulting in the accumulation of toxic levels of acetaldehyde, with nausea, vomiting, flushing, headache, sweating, hypotension, and confusion lasting up to 3 hours.

(ii) Disulfiram can be toxic in the presence of small amounts of alcohol (e.g., the amount in some over-the-counter [OTC] preparations). Other drugs with disulfiram-like activity include **metronidazole, sulfonylureas,** and some **cephalosporins**).

(iii) Disulfiram is absorbed rapidly; its peak effect takes 12 hours. The elimination of disulfiram is slow, so its action may persist for several days.

(c) Naltrexone, an orally effective opioid-receptor antagonist, **reduces craving for ethanol** and reduces the rate of relapse of alcoholism.

(d) Acamprosate reduces the incidence of relapse and prolongs abstinence from ethanol. It acts as a competitive inhibitor at the NMDA glutamate receptor.

2. *Methanol (wood alcohol)*

a. Methanol is metabolized by alcohol dehydrogenase to formaldehyde, which is then oxidized to formic acid, which is toxic.

b. Methanol produces blurred vision and other visual disturbances ("snowstorm") when poisoning has occurred. In severe poisoning, bradycardia, acidosis, coma, and seizures are common.

c. Treatment of methanol toxicity includes the administration of ethanol to slow the conversion of methanol to formaldehyde (ethanol has a higher affinity for alcohol dehydrogenase). In addition to other supportive measures, dialysis is used to remove methanol, and bicarbonate is administered to correct acidosis.

d. **Fomepizole,** an inhibitor of alcohol dehydrogenase that reduces the rate of accumulation of formaldehyde, is also used to treat methanol (and ethylene glycol) toxicity.

3. ***Barbiturates (secobarbital, pentobarbital, g-hydroxybutyric acid) and benzodiazepines*** (see also I F 1 and VIII C 1)

a. Adverse effects, drug interactions, and contraindications

(1) Barbiturates produce drowsiness at hypnotic doses; they can interfere with motor and mental performance.

(2) Barbiturates potentiate the depressant effects of other CNS depressants or drugs with CNS depressant activity such as antidepressants.

(3) Barbiturates produce dose-related respiratory depression with cerebral hypoxia, possibly leading to coma or death. Treatment includes ventilation, gastric lavage, hemodialysis, osmotic diuretics, and (for phenobarbital) alkalinization of urine.

(4) **γ-Hydroxybutyric acid** (GHB) has been used as a "date rape" drug.

b. **Tolerance and dependence.** Abuse and psychologic dependence are more likely with the shorter-acting, more rapidly eliminated drugs (**pentobarbital, amobarbital, secobarbital**). The abuse potential of the barbiturates exceeds that of the benzodiazepines.

(1) **Tolerance**

(a) Neuronal adaptation (cellular tolerance) and increased metabolism due to induction of hepatic microsomal enzymes (metabolic tolerance) both contribute to the development of tolerance.

(b) **Cross-tolerance** occurs with other CNS depressants, including the benzodiazepines and **ethanol.**

(c) Tolerance develops less readily to the potentially lethal respiratory depression.

(2) **Physical dependence**

(a) **Withdrawal symptoms** include restlessness, anxiety, and insomnia. More severe symptoms of withdrawal include tremor, autonomic hyperactivity, delirium, and potentially life-threatening tonic-clonic seizures.

(b) For a smoother withdrawal, **chlordiazepoxide** or **phenobarbital** is substituted for shorter-acting barbiturates.

D. CNS stimulants

1. ***Cocaine and amphetamine/methamphetamine (Desoxyn)*** (and dextroamphetamine [Dexedrine]; also methylene-dioxymethamphetamine [MDMA, "Ecstasy"], 2,5-dimethoxy-4-methylamphetamine [DOM, "STP"], and methylenedioxyamphetamine [MDA], which in addition to their amphetamine-like activity also heighten responses to sensory stimulation)

a. **Mechanism of action**

(1) **Cocaine blocks the dopamine transporter** (also norepinephrine and serotonin transporters at higher doses) in the CNS to inhibit uptake of dopamine into nerve terminals in the mesolimbic pathway that includes the "brain reward" center.

(2) **Amphetamine** also blocks the uptake of biogenic amines, but its major effect is to **increase the release of prejunctional neuronal catecholamines,** including dopamine and norepinephrine. Amphetamine also exhibits some direct sympathomimetic action and weakly inhibits MAO.

b. **Pharmacologic properties**

(1) **Cocaine** is inhaled (snorted) or smoked (free-base form, "**crack cocaine**"); **amphetamine,** usually in the form of **methamphetamine,** is taken orally, IV, or smoked in a form referred to as "**ice.**"

(2) Short-term, repeated IV administration or smoking (referred to as a "**spree" or "run"**) results in intense euphoria **("rush")** as well as increased wakefulness, alertness, self-confidence, and ability to concentrate. Use also increases motor activity and sexual urge and decreases appetite.

(3) **Cocaine** has a much shorter duration of action (~1 hour) than amphetamine.

(4) **Cocaine** is metabolized by plasma and liver cholinesterase; genetically slow metabolizers are more likely to show severe adverse effects. A nonenzymatic metabolite, **benzoylecgonine,** is measurable for 5 days or more after a spree and is used to detect cocaine use.

c. **Therapeutic uses**

(1) **Cocaine** is used as a **local anesthetic** for ear, nose, and throat surgery. It is the only one with inherent vasoconstrictor activity (see also IX D 2 c).

(2) **Methylphenidate** (Ritalin), an amphetamine congener

(a) **Attention-deficit/hyperactivity disorder** (ADHD); also **amphetamine.** This drug decreases behavioral problems, aggression, noncompliance, and negativity associated with ADHD.

(b) **Narcolepsy (methylphenidate).** This drug causes an increase in wakefulness and sleep latency.

d. **Short-term and adverse effects**

(1) Short-term, repeated IV administration or smoking results in intense **euphoria** as well as increased wakefulness, alertness, self-confidence, and ability to concentrate. Use also increases motor activity and sexual urge and decreases appetite. Adverse effects may occur during this same time or from overdose and are due to excessive sympathomimetic activity. These adverse effects include the following:

(2) **Anxiety, inability to sleep, hyperactivity, sexual dysfunction,** and stereotypic and sometimes **dangerous behavior,** often followed by exhaustion ("crash") with increased appetite and increased sleep with disturbed sleep patterns (the withdrawal pattern)

(3) **Toxic psychosis**

(a) Toxic psychosis is marked by paranoia and tactile and auditory hallucinations.

(b) This condition is usually reversible, but it may be permanent.

(4) **Necrotizing arteritis**

(a) Necrotizing arteritis is produced by **amphetamine.**

(b) This effect sometimes results in brain hemorrhage and renal failure.

(5) **Perforation of the nasal septum** from the vasoconstrictor effects of "snorting" **cocaine**

(6) **Cardiac toxicity** caused by **cocaethylene** that forms when cocaine and ethanol are taken together

(7) **Fetal abnormalities** and early childhood learning disabilities from the maternal use of **cocaine** ("cocaine babies")

(8) **Overdose**

(a) Overdose results in tachycardia, hypertension, hyperthermia, and tremor.

(b) Overdose, particularly with **cocaine,** may cause hypertensive crisis with **cerebrovascular hemorrhage and MI.**

(c) Overdose occasionally produces seizures, coronary vasospasm, cardiac arrhythmias, shock, and death.

(d) Overdose is more likely with "crack" and "ice."

e. **Tolerance and dependence**

(1) Extremely strong psychologic dependence to these drugs develops.

(2) Tolerance, which may reach extraordinary levels, can develop.

(3) The withdrawal-like syndrome includes long periods of sleep, increased appetite, anergia, depression, and drug craving.

2. ***Nicotine*** is a constituent of tobacco, along with various gases (e.g., carbon monoxide, nitrosamines, hydrogen cyanide) and particulate matter.

a. **Mechanism of action:** Nicotine mimics the action of ACh at cholinergic nicotinic receptors of ganglia, in skeletal muscle, and in the CNS.

b. **Pharmacologic properties**

(1) Nicotine is a volatile liquid alkaloid that is well absorbed from the lung after smoking and is rapidly distributed.

(2) Nicotine is rapidly metabolized in the liver: it has a plasma half-life ($t_{1/2}$) of approximately 1 hour.

(3) Nicotine may cause nausea and vomiting in the early stages of smoking. It increases psychomotor activity and cognitive function, increases release of adrenal catecholamines and antidiuretic hormone (ADH), increases blood pressure and heart rate, and increases tone and secretions of the GI tract.

c. **Adverse effects.** Nicotine use contributes to cancer of the lungs, oral cavity, bladder, and pancreas; obstructive lung disease; coronary artery disease; and peripheral vascular disease.

d. **Tolerance and dependence**

(1) Tolerance

(a) Tolerance to the subjective effects of nicotine develops rapidly.

(b) Tolerance is primarily cellular; there is some metabolic tolerance.

(2) Dependence

(a) Nicotine produces strong psychologic dependence; it activates the "brain reward system" (increased activity of dopamine in the nucleus accumbens).

(b) The withdrawal-like syndrome indicative of physical dependence occurs within 24 hours and persists for weeks or months. Dizziness, tremor, increased blood pressure, drug craving, irritability, anxiety, restlessness, difficulty in concentration, drowsiness, headache, sleep disturbances, increased appetite, GI complaints, nausea, and vomiting may occur.

e. **Medications and replacement therapies**

(1) **Nicotine polacrilex** is a **nicotine resin** contained in a chewing gum that, when used as a nicotine replacement, has therapeutic value for diminishing withdrawal symptoms while the patient undergoes behavioral modification to overcome psychologic dependence. It has an objectionable taste and may cause stomach discomfort, mouth sores, and dyspepsia.

(2) A nicotine **transdermal patch** containing nicotine is also available. Local skin irritation is a common problem. A nicotine nasal spray is also available (which may cause nasal irritation) as is a nicotine inhaler, which may cause local irritation of the mouth and throat. Because of potential nicotine overdose, the gum or nicotine patch should be used with caution in patients who continue to use cigarettes.

(3) **Other available pharmacologic therapies** that have been used with some reported success include **varenicline** (nicotine), **clonidine** (α_2-adrenoceptor agonist), **nortriptyline** and **bupropion** (antidepressant agents), and **selegiline** (MAOI).

E. Hallucinogens (psychotomimetics)

1. *LSD (d-lysergic acid diethylamide); also mescaline, psilocybin*

a. LSD is an extremely potent synthetic drug that, when taken orally, causes altered consciousness, euphoria, increased sensory awareness ("mind expansion"), perceptual distortions, and increased introspection.

b. Its mechanism of action is unknown but may be related to its action as an **agonist at neuronal postjunctional serotonin receptors** (5-HT_{1A}- and 5-HT_{1C}).

c. The sympathomimetic activity of LSD includes pupillary dilation, increased blood pressure, and tachycardia.

d. **Adverse effects** of LSD include alteration of perception and thoughts with misjudgment, changes in sense of time, visual hallucinations, dysphoria, panic reactions, suicide (bad trips), "flashbacks," and psychosis; treatment includes benzodiazepines for sedation.

e. A high degree of tolerance to the behavioral effects of LSD develops rapidly.

f. Cross-tolerance develops with mescaline and psilocybin, hallucinogens that are less potent than LSD.

g. Dependence and withdrawal do not occur with these hallucinogens.

2. *Phencyclidine (PCP, "angel dust")*

a. PCP is a veterinary anesthetic used initially in humans as a dissociative anesthetic (replaced by ketamine, a drug that also has some hallucinatory activity).

b. PCP is taken orally and IV; it is also "snorted" and smoked.

c. The behavioral actions related to PCP are thought to be related to its **antagonist activity at NMDA receptors** for the excitatory amino acid glutamate.

d. Low doses of PCP produce a state resembling ethanol intoxication. High doses cause euphoria, hallucinations, changed body image, and an increased sense of isolation and loneliness; it also impairs judgment and increases aggressiveness.
e. Overdose with PCP may result in seizures, respiratory depression, cardiac arrest, and coma. Treatment of PCP overdose includes maintenance of respiration, control of seizures, reduction of sensory input, and therapy directed at behavioral manifestations, possibly including benzodiazepine or antipsychotic drug therapy.

F. Marijuana (cannabis), dronabinol (Marinol)

1. The active ingredient in marijuana is **Δ-9 tetrahydrocannabinol;** it acts as an agonist to inhibit adenylyl cyclase through G-protein–linked cannabinoid receptors, whose normal CNS function is unknown.
   a. **Cannabinol CB1-receptors,** which account for most CNS effects, are localized to cognitive and motor areas of the brain. Cannabinol **CB2-receptors** are found in the immune system among other peripheral organs.
   b. **Anandamide and 2-arachidonylglycerol,** naturally occurring ligands that are derived from arachidonic acid, are agonists at **CB1-receptors;** their normal physiologic function is unclear.
2. Marijuana is mostly smoked, but can be taken orally. It is very lipid soluble. The effects of smoking are immediate and last up to 2–3 hours.
3. The **initial phase** of marijuana use (the "high") consists of euphoria, uncontrolled laughter, loss of sense of time, and increased introspection. The **second phase** includes relaxation, a dreamlike state, sleepiness, and difficulty in concentration. At extremely high doses, acute psychosis with depersonalization has been observed.
4. The physiologic effects of marijuana include increased pulse rate and a characteristic reddening of the conjunctiva.
5. Marijuana, and its analogue dronabinol, is used therapeutically to decrease intraocular pressure for the treatment of glaucoma, as an antiemetic in cancer chemotherapy, and to stimulate appetite in patients with AIDS.
6. Tolerance, although documented in animals, is difficult to demonstrate in man except among long-term high-dose users, for whom a mild form of psychologic and physical dependence has been noted.
7. Adverse effects of marijuana, some of which are controversial, include the following:
   a. Long-term effects similar to those of cigarette smoking, including periodontal disease.
   b. Exacerbation of preexisting paranoia or psychosis
   c. "Amotivational syndrome," may be more related to user's personality type
   d. Impairment of short-term memory and disturbances of the immune, reproductive, and thermoregulatory systems

DRUG SUMMARY TABLE

Sedative–Hypnotic Drugs
Benzodiazepines
Alprazolam (Xanax, generic)
Clonazepam (Klonopin)
Clorazepate (Tranxene, generic)
Chlordiazepoxide (Librium)
Diazepam (Valium, generic)
Estazolam (ProSom, generic)
Flurazepam (Dalmane, generic)
Halazepam (Paxipam)
Lorazepam (Ativan, generic)
Midazolam (Versed)
Oxazepam (Serax, generic)
Prazepam (Centrax)
Quazepam (Doral)
Temazepam (Restoril, generic)
Triazolam (Halcion, generic)

Nonbenzodiazepines
Buspirone (BuSpar)
Eszopiclone (Lunesta)
Zaleplon (Sonata)
Zolpidem (Ambien)

Melatonin receptor agonists
Ramelteon (Rozerem)

Barbiturates
Amobarbital (Amytal)
Pentobarbital (Nembutal, generic)
Secobarbital (Seconal, generic)

Benzodiazepine receptor antagonists
Flumazenil (Romazicon)

Antipsychotic (Neuroleptic) Drugs
Conventional
Chlorpromazine (Thorazine, generic)
Triflupromazine (Vesprin)
Thioridazine (Mellaril, generic)
Loxapine (Loxitane)
Mesoridazine (Serentil)
Molindone (Moban)
Trifluoperazine (Stelazine, generic)
Fluphenazine (Prolixin, Permitil)
Perphenazine (Trilafon)
Thiothixene (Navane, generic)
Haloperidol (Haldol, generic)
Atypical
Aripiprazole (Abilify)
Clozapine (Clozaril)
Olanzapine (Zyprexa)

Quetiapine (Seroquel)
Risperidone (Risperdal)
Ziprasidone (Geodon)
Other
Pimozide (Orap)
Prochlorperazine (Compazine)

Antidepressant Drugs
Tricyclic Antidepressants
Amitriptyline (Elavil, others, generic)
Imipramine (Tofranil, others, generic)
Trimipramine (Surmontil)
Doxepin (Sinequan, others, generic)
Clomipramine (Anafranil, generic)
Desipramine (Norpramin, Pertofrane, generic)
Nortriptyline (Aventyl, Pamelor, generic)
Protriptyline (Vivactil, generic)
Amoxapine (Asendin, generic)
Selective Serotonin Reuptake Inhibitors
Citalopram (Celexa)
Escitalopram (Lexapro)
Fluoxetine (Prozac, generic)
Fluvoxamine (Luvox)
Paroxetine (Paxil)
Sertraline (Zoloft)
Atypical Antidepressants
Bupropion (Wellbutrin)
Duloxetine (Cymbalta)
Maprotiline (Ludiomil)
Mirtazapine (Remeron)
Nefazodone (Serzone)
Trazodone (Desyrel, generic)
Venlafaxine (Effexor)
Monoamine Oxidase Inhibitors
Phenelzine (Nardil)
Tranylcypromine (Parnate)

Opioid Analgesics, Antagonists, and Antitussives
Opioid Analgesics
Alfentanil (Alfenta)
Buprenorphine (Buprenex, others)
Butorphanol (Stadol, generic)
Codeine (generic)
Fentanyl (Sublimaze, generic)
Hydrocodone (Used only in analgesic combinations)
Hydromorphone (Dilaudid, generic)
Levomethadyl acetate (ORLAAM)
Levorphanol (Levo-Dromoran, generic)
Meperidine (Demerol, generic)
Methadone (Dolophine, generic)
Morphine (generic)
Nalbuphine (Nubain, generic)
Oxycodone (generic)
Oxymorphone (Numorphan)
Pentazocine (Talwin)
Propoxyphene (Darvon, generic)
Remifentanil (Ultiva)
Sufentanil (Sufenta, generic)
Tramadol (Ultram)
Opioid Antagonists
Nalmefene (Revex)
Naloxone (Narcan)
Naltrexone (ReVia, Depade)

Antidiarrheal Agents
Difenoxin (Motofen)
Diphenoxylate/atropine (Lomotil)
Loperamide (Imodium)

Antitussive Agents
Dextromethorphan (Benylin DM, others, generic)

Antiparkinsonian Drugs
Amantadine (Symmetrel, others)
Benztropine (Cogentin, others)
Biperidin (Akineton)
Bromocriptine (Parlodel)
Carbidopa (Lodosyn)
Entacapone (Comtan)
Levodopa (Dopar, Larodopa)
Levodopa 1 Carbidopa (Sinemet)
Orphenadrine (various)
Pramipexole (Mirapex)
Procyclidine (Kemadrin)
Rasagiline (Azilect)
Ropinirole (Requip)
Selegiline (deprenyl) (Eldepryl, generic)
Tolcapone (Tasmar)
Trihexyphenidyl (Artane, others)

Drugs Used to Treat Alzheimer Disease
Donepezil (Aricept)
Galantamine (Reminyl)
Memantine (Axura)
Rivastigmine (Exelon)
Tacrine (Cognex)

Antiepileptic Drugs
Carbamazepine (Tegretol)
Clonazepam (Klonopin)
Clorazepate (Tranxene)
Diazepam (Valium)
Ethosuximide (Zarontin)
Felbamate (Felbatol)
Fosphenytoin (Cerebyx)
Gabapentin (Neurontin)
Lamotrigine (Lamictal)
Levetiracetam (Keppra)
Lorazepam (Ativan)
Methsuximide (Celontin)
Oxcarbazepine (Trileptal)
Phenobarbital (Luminal)
Phensuximide (Milontin)
Phenytoin (Dilantin)
Pregabalin (Lyrica)
Primidone (Mysoline)
Tiagabine (Gabitril)
Topiramate (Topamax)
Valproic acid (Depakene)
Zonisamide (Zonegran)

Anesthetic Agents
Desflurane (Suprane)
Diazepam (Valium, generic)
Droperidol (Inapsine, generic)
Droperidol + Fentanyl (Innovar)
Enflurane (Enflurane, Ethrane)
Etomidate (Amidate)
Halothane (Fluothane, generic)
Isoflurane (Isoflurane, Forane)
Ketamine (Ketalar, generic)
Lorazepam (Ativan, generic)
Methohexital (Brevital Sodium)
Methoxyflurane (Penthrane)
Midazolam (Versed, generic)
Nitrous oxide
Propofol (Diprivan, generic)
Sevoflurane (Ultane)
Thiopental (Pentothal, generic)

Local Anesthetics
Benzocaine (generic)
Bupivacaine (Marcaine, Sensorcaine, generic)
Butamben picrate
Chloroprocaine (Nesacaine, generic)
Cocaine (Generic)
Dibucaine (Nupercainal, generic)
Dyclonine (Dyclone)
Etidocaine (Duranest)
Lidocaine (Xylocaine, others, generic)
Mepivacaine (Carbocaine, others, generic)
Pramoxine (Tronothane, others)
Prilocaine (Citanest)
Procaine (Novocain, generic)
Proparacaine (Alcaine, others, generic)
Ropivacaine (Naropin)
Tetracaine (Pontocaine)

Medications (selected) for Drug Abuse
Opioids
Clonidine (Catapres, generic)
L-Acetylmethadol (ORLAAM)
Methadone (Dolophine, generic)
Ethanol
Acamprosate (Campral)
Diazepam (Valium, generic)
Disulfiram (Antabuse, generic)
Lorazepam (Ativan, Alzapam, generic)
Naltrexone (ReVia)
Oxazepam (Serax, generic)
Thiamine (generic)
Methanol
Ethanol
Fomepizole (Antizol)
Nicotine
Bupropion (Zyban)
Nicotine replacements (Nicorette, Nicoderm, generic)
Nortriptyline (Aventyl, Pamelor, generic)
Selegiline (Eldepryl, generic)
Varenicline (Chantix)

Review Test for Chapter 5

Directions: Each of the numbered items or incomplete statements in this section is followed by answers or by completions of the statement. Select the ONE lettered answer or completion that is BEST in each case.

1. A 42-year-old businessman visits a psychiatrist for what he describes as a very "embarrassing problem." The patient has found it difficult to make it to work on time because he keeps driving back to his house to make sure that the garage door is shut. He has begun waking up 2 hours early to facilitate these obsessions and compulsions. He is otherwise without additional complaints. The psychiatrist is concerned that the patient has developed obsessive–compulsive disorder (OCD) and has him try which of the following?

(A) Imipramine
(B) Clomipramine
(C) Atomoxetine
(D) Propranolol
(E) Desipramine

2. A 56-year-old truck driver is on disability for a back injury he sustained while making a delivery 3 months ago. He has been on several opioid drugs but continues to complain of "nagging back pain." The pain specialist he sees decides to try treating him with an antidepressant approved for the management of chronic pain. Which of the following would he chose?

(A) Fluoxetine
(B) Promethazine
(C) Trazodone
(D) Prochlorperazine
(E) Venlafaxine

3. A 56-year-old man recently suffered a myocardial infarction (MI). He is on numerous medications, many of which are metabolized by the cytochrome P-450 system. He now presents to the psychiatrist with difficulty sleeping and decreased appetite and reports "no longer enjoying golf like I used to." Recognizing that depression is common in patients who have recently had an MI, the psychiatrist decides to start the patient on selective serotonin reuptake inhibitor (SSRI) therapy. Given his multiple medications, which SSRI should be avoided?

(A) Fluoxetine
(B) Tranylcypromine
(C) Sertraline
(D) Escitalopram
(E) Phenylzine

4. The above patient returns for follow-up 6 months later. He has joined a health club and has lost several pounds and notes "feeling better mentally." However, upon questioning he still has not returned to the activities he once enjoyed and is still not sleeping or eating well. The psychiatrist recommends increasing the dose of his selective serotonin reuptake inhibitor (SSRI). The patient reluctantly admits that he has not been taking his medication because of some of the side effects. Which one is likely to be the most bothersome?

(A) Weight gain
(B) Tachycardia
(C) Headache
(D) Sexual dysfunction
(E) Tremor

5. A 36-year-old man has been smoking two packs of cigarettes a day for the last 20 years. He is concerned that his health has deteriorated, and he has a persistent hacking cough. He also states that he doesn't want to "get lung cancer and die, like my father did." He has tried nicotine patches with no success and wants to know if there is any "pill" he could try. What medication could the physician recommend?

(A) Mirtazapine
(B) Citalopram
(C) Phenelzine
(D) Buspirone
(E) Bupropion

6. A 23-year-old man is brought to the emergency room after he was found walking the streets naked while proclaiming himself "the son of God." His urine toxicology screen comes back negative for illicit drugs or alcohol. During the interview with the on-call psychiatrist, the patient displays flight of ideas as he jumps from topic to topic. The physician recommends starting the patient on lithium therapy for acute mania. Which of the following is associated with lithium use?

(A) Urinary retention
(B) Weight loss
(C) Fine tremor
(D) A wide therapeutic margin
(E) Hyperthyroidism

7. A first-year surgery intern has rotated on numerous surgical services during the first year, including general surgery, cardiothoracic surgery, urology, surgical oncology, trauma surgery, and colorectal surgery. He has gotten quite used to liberally ordering morphine for pain control. However, which of the following is an absolute contraindication to opioid use?

(A) Closed head injury
(B) Myocardial infarction
(C) Acute pulmonary edema
(D) Renal colic
(E) Biliary colic

8. A 5-year-old child is admitted to the hospital with a low-grade fever and a persistent cough that has resulted in vomiting episodes following prolonged coughing spells. His throat culture is negative, his fever has resolved, and all that is left is a slight cough. He is discharged from the hospital by the pediatrician who recommends an over-the-counter opioid antitussive. Which of the following does he recommend?

(A) Tramadol
(B) Propoxyphene
(C) Loperamide
(D) Dextromethorphan
(E) Naloxone

9. An anesthesia resident is on his first case alone. The surgeons are preparing the patient's abdomen for their eventual incision when the attending physician enters the operating room and asks the anesthesia resident if the patient is anesthetized. Which of the following is the most reliable sign that surgical anesthesia has been reached?

(A) Analgesia
(B) Amnesia
(C) Loss of consciousness
(D) Maximum papillary dilation
(E) Loss of eyelash reflex

10. A 16-year-old patient visits his dentist for a routine checkup. He finds that his wisdom teeth are severely impacted and need to be removed. The oral surgeon to whom he is referred plans on using an agent that has good analgesic and sedative properties but does not cause skeletal muscle relaxation. Which agent has these ideal properties?

(A) Enflurane
(B) Nitrous oxide
(C) Thiopental
(D) Halothane
(E) Isoflurane

11. A 6-year-old child was badly burned when his house caught on fire. He sustained full-thickness burns on approximately 40% of his body. He has spent many months enduring multiple skin-grafting procedures. To aid in reducing the pain associated with dressing changes, he is given ketamine IV. This drug has been associated with which of the following adverse reactions?

(A) Irritation to the respiratory airways
(B) Sensitization of the heart to catecholamines
(C) Reduction of cardiac output
(D) Malignant hyperthermia
(E) Distortion of reality and terrifying dreams

12. A patient sees an otolaryngologist with complaints of recurrent sinusitis. The surgeon decides to perform sinus surgery to debride the scarred sinus tissue. During the procedure the surgeon elects to use an agent that has good local anesthesia as well as vasoconstrictive properties. What agent might he use?

(A) Cocaine
(B) Procaine
(C) Tetracaine
(D) Lidocaine
(E) Mepivacaine

13. A 28-year-old alcoholic woman learns that she is pregnant after missing her last two menstrual periods. She received poor prenatal care, missing many of her appointments. The neonatologist that cared for her child at birth learned that the mother did not refrain from her normal heavy alcohol binges throughout her pregnancy. Which of the following is the most likely consequence of such abuse to the child during pregnancy?

(A) Abruptio placentae and learning difficulties as the child ages

(B) Spina bifida and orofacial defects
(C) Fetal hemorrhage and defects in fetal bone formation
(D) Microcephaly, retarded growth, and congenital heart defects
(E) Growth retardation, microcephaly, and craniofacial abnormalities

14. A 16-year-old boy is brought to the emergency room at 4 am by his friends, who report that the patient was at an all-night rave party and was agitated, hyperactive, and hypersexual. The physician learns that the boy took several pills, which his friends thought were "ecstasy" (methylenedioxymethamphetamine). Which of the following describes the mechanism of this "party" drug?

(A) Antagonistic activity at the *N*-methyl-d-aspartate (NMDA) receptor for glutamic acid
(B) Binding to the cannabinol CB1 receptor
(C) Increased release of dopamine and norepinephrine
(D) Mimics the action of acetylcholine
(E) Agonist at postjunctional serotonin receptors

15. A 31-year-old lawyer is transferred to the emergency room after collapsing at a party. He complained of chest pain, and an electrocardiogram demonstrated ventricular fibrillation, for which he received cardioversion. A primary survey of the patient showed little trauma, with the exception of a perforated nasal septum. A close friend accompanied the patient and confides in you that the patient was "doing" an illicit substance at the party. Which of the following is the most likely?

(A) Phencyclidine (PCP)
(B) γ-Hydroxybutyric acid (GHB)
(C) Lysergic acid diethylamide (LSD)
(D) Cocaine
(E) Marijuana

Answers and Explanations

1. **The answer is B.** Clomipramine, a tricyclic antidepressant (TCA) that inhibits serotonin uptake as well as the selective serotonin- reuptake inhibitors (SSRIs), is used for the treatment of obsessive–compulsive disorder (OCD). Imipramine is a tricyclic agent that is used specifically to suppress enuresis in children and is metabolized to yet another TCA, desipramine. Atomoxetine is a newer tricyclic drug that is used in the management of attention-deficit/hyperactivity disorder (ADHD). Propranolol is a β-blocker used to treat the tremor some patients experience while taking a TCA.

2. **The answer is E.** Venlafaxine and some tricyclic antidepressants are used in the management of chronic pain. Promethazine and prochlorperazine are two dopamine receptor blockers, without antipsychotic activity, used to treat nausea and vomiting. Trazodone is an atypical antidepressant that is highly sedating and has been associated with orthostatic hypotension and priapism. Fluoxetine is a selective serotonin reuptake inhibitor (SSRI). SSRIs are not effective therapy for chronic pain.

3. **The answer is A.** Both fluoxetine and paroxetine inhibit cytochrome P-450 and thus need to be used with caution as they can potentiate the action of other drugs metabolized by this system. Tranylcypromine and phenelzine are monoamine oxidase inhibitors (MAOIs) that, when used with selective serotonin reuptake inhibitors (SSRIs), can cause a potentially fatal "serotonin syndrome." Sertraline and escitalopram are two SSRIs that are not metabolized by the P-450 system and might be good choices for this individual.

4. **The answer is D.** Sexual dysfunction is a common complaint with selective serotonin reuptake inhibitors (SSRIs), occurring in up to 40% of all patients, and a leading cause of noncompliance. Weight loss is usually experienced initially with SSRIs, and some persons may eventually gain weight. Headache is associated with SSRIs, although it is often transient. Tremor and tachycardia are side effects that are more typical with tricyclic antidepressants (TCAs).

5. **The answer is E.** Bupropion is an atypical antidepressant that is useful as an aid in smoking cessation. Mirtazapine is another atypical agent used in the treatment of depression that blocks both serotonin and α-adrenergic receptors. Phenelzine is an MAOI, sometimes used for depression. Citalopram is a selective serotonin reuptake inhibitor (SSRI), which are typically not used for smoking cessation. Buspirone is an antianxiety drug useful in situations where nonsedating agents are favored.

6. **The answer is C.** Lithium use is associated with a fine tremor that can often be successfully managed with β-blockers. Lithium is associated with polydipsia and polyuria, not urinary retention. Likewise, the other choices are opposite what might be expected with lithium use, as patients experience weight gain and hypothyroidism. Lithium has a narrow therapeutic margin, with therapeutic doses not too much lower than toxic doses.

7. **The answer is A.** Opioids are contraindicated in cases of head trauma, as they increase cerebral vascular pressure and may cause hemorrhage and/or herniation. Morphine is used during myocardial infarction, as it decreases cardiac preload and chest pain. Morphine is also used to reduce dyspnea associated with acute pulmonary edema. Renal colic, pain due to a kidney stone passing through the ureter, or biliary colic, which is a similar pain associated with gallstones passing through biliary ducts, are both well managed with morphine.

8. **The answer is D.** Dextromethorphan is an opioid isomer available in over-the-counter cough remedies. It has no analgesic properties and limited abuse potential. Tramadol is a weak μ-opioid-receptor agonist, which also blocks serotonin and norepinephrine uptake and is used for neuropathic pain. Propoxyphene is a weak opioid agonist usually used in combination with aspirin or acetaminophen. Loperamide is an opioid that does not cross the blood–brain barrier

and is used for the treatment of diarrhea. Naloxone is an opioid antagonist used to reverse opioid overdose.

9. **The answer is E.** Loss of eyelash reflex and a pattern of respiration that is regular and deep are the most reliable indications of stage III, or surgical, anesthesia. Analgesia and amnesia are characteristics of stage I anesthesia, whereas loss of consciousness is associated with stage II anesthesia. Maximum papillary dilation also occurs during stage III anesthesia, but closer to the progression to stage IV anesthesia, an undesirable stage associated with respiratory and cardiovascular failure.

10. **The answer is B.** Nitrous oxide is an anesthetic gas that has good analgesic and sedative properties without the skeletal muscle–relaxing effects. It is often used in the vignette setting but can be used along with other inhaled agents, decreasing their concentrations and thus their side effects. Enflurane produces anesthesia, hypnosis, and muscle relaxation, as do the others, and is very pungent. Thiopental is a barbiturate that is too short acting for this application. Halothane has a pleasant odor but can result in an unpredictable hepatotoxicity. Isoflurane is associated with more rapid induction and recovery than halothane and may have some benefits in patients with ischemic heart disease.

11. **The answer is E.** Ketamine is a dissociative anesthetic related to phencyclidine (PCP) and is thought to block glutamic acid *N*-methyl-d-aspartate (NMDA) receptors. Its use is associated with distortions of reality, terrifying dreams, and delirium, more commonly in adults. Malignant hyperthermia may be associated with any of the inhaled anesthetics, such as halothane, in genetically prone individuals. Halothane and isoflurane sensitize the heart to catecholamines. Desfluramine is especially irritating to airways, and enflurane can reduce cardiac output.

12. **The answer is A.** Cocaine is ideal for such surgery because of its topical activity; it does not require the addition of epinephrine, as it has intrinsic vasoconstrictive activity that aids in hemostasis. Like cocaine, procaine and tetracaine are both ester-type compounds; however, procaine is not topically active and tetracaine is used primarily for spinal anesthesia and ophthalmologic procedures. Lidocaine is an amide anesthetic preferred for infiltrative blocks and epidural anesthesia. Mepivacaine is another amide local anesthetic, although not topically active, which, like all such agents, acts by blocking sodium channels.

13. **The answer is D.** Fetal alcohol syndrome is a leading cause of congenital abnormalities, especially microcephaly, growth retardation, and congenital heart defects. Abruptio placentae and learning difficulties are more typical with maternal use of cocaine during pregnancy. Spina bifida and orofacial defects are associated with valproic acid use during pregnancy, and the anticonvulsant phenytoin is associated with fetal growth retardation, microcephaly, and craniofacial abnormalities. Fetal hemorrhage and bone malformation are a consequence of warfarin use during pregnancy.

14. **The answer is C.** Like other amphetamines, ecstasy increases the release of dopamine and norepinephrine. Its use is becoming more common in more affluent areas and is often associated with parties. Phencyclidine (PCP) is an antagonist at the *N*-methyl-d-aspartate (NMDA) receptor for glutamic acid, causing euphoria and hallucinations. Marijuana causes euphoria, uncontrollable laughter, loss of time perception, and increased introspection. It binds to the cannabinol CB-1 receptor. Nicotine is a powerful stimulant in tobacco products and works by mimicking the effects of acetylcholine. Lysergic acid diethylamide (LSD) is an agonist of the postjunctional serotonin receptors.

15. **The answer is D.** Cocaine is cardiotoxic and can cause arrhythmias that can be life threatening. These effects are even more likely when alcohol is also consumed. Cocaine causes vasoconstriction, and snorting the drug causes necrosis and eventual perforation of the nasal septum. γ-Hydroxybutyric acid (GHB) is a barbiturate that is used as a "date rape" drug. Lysergic acid diethylamide (LSD) causes increased sensory awareness, perceptual distortions, and altered consciousness. Phencyclidine (PCP) can cause euphoria, hallucinations, an increased sense of isolation and loneliness, and increased aggression. Marijuana causes euphoria, laughter, a loss of time perception, and increased introspection.

chapter 6

Autocoids, Ergots, Anti-inflammatory Agents, and Immunosuppressive Agents

I. HISTAMINE AND ANTIHISTAMINES

A. Histamine (Fig. 6-1). Histamine is a small molecule produced by decarboxylation of the amino acid histidine; it is catalyzed by the enzyme L-histidine decarboxylase in a reaction that requires pyridoxal phosphate.

1. *Synthesis*

a. Histamine is found in many tissues, including the brain; it is stored and found in the highest amounts in mast cells and basophils. Mast cells, which are especially abundant in the respiratory tract, skin (especially hands and feet), gastrointestinal (GI) tract, and blood vessels, store histamine in a granule bound in a complex with heparin, adenosine triphosphate (ATP), and an acidic protein.

b. Release of histamine can occur by two processes:

(1) Energy- and Ca^{2+}-dependent degranulation reaction. The release of histamine from mast cells is induced by immunoglobulin E (IgE) fixation to mast cells (sensitization) and subsequent exposure to a specific antigen; complement activation (mediated by immunoglobulin G or immunoglobulin M) may also induce degranulation.

(2) Energy- and Ca^{2+}-independent release (displacement). Displacement is induced by drugs such as morphine, tubocurarine, guanethidine, and amine antibiotics. In addition, mast cell damage, which is caused by noxious agents such as venom or by mechanical trauma, can release histamine.

2. *Mechanism of action*

a. Histamine (H_1)-receptors

(1) H_1-receptors are found in the brain, heart, bronchi, GI tract, vascular smooth muscles, and leukocytes.

(2) H_1-receptors are membrane bound and coupled to G-proteins, specifically $G_{q/11}$, and their activation causes an increase in phospholipase A_2 and D activity, increases in diacylglycerol and intracellular Ca^{2+}, and increased cyclic guanosine 5′-monophosphate (cGMP).

(3) Activation of H_1-receptors in the brain increases wakefulness.

(4) Activation of H_1-receptors in vessels causes vasodilation and an increase in permeability.

(5) Activation of H_1-receptors typically stimulates nonvascular smooth muscle.

b. Histamine (H_2)-receptors

(1) H_2-receptors are membrane bound; they are found in the brain, heart, vascular smooth muscles, leukocytes, and parietal cells.

(2) The response of H_2-receptors is coupled via $G\alpha_s$ to increased cyclic AMP (cAMP) production.

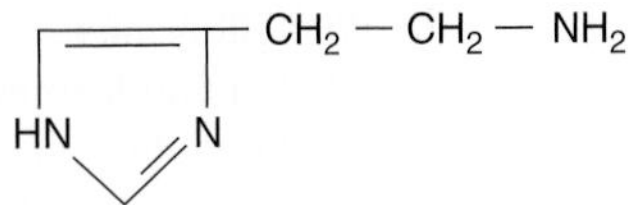

FIGURE 6-1. Structure of histamine.

(3) Activation of H_2-receptors increases gastric acid production, causes vasodilation, and generally relaxes smooth muscles.

c. Histamine (H_3)-receptors

(1) H_3-receptors are found in the central nervous system (CNS) and peripheral nervous system (PNS) at presynaptic nerve terminals.

(2) H_3-receptors are membrane bound and coupled to $G_{i/o}$; their activation increases intracellular Ca^{2+} and decreases cAMP.

(3) Stimulation of H_3-receptors on nerve cells causes a decrease in histamine release; in the CNS, stimulation of H_3 modulates the release of dopamine, acetylcholine, serotonin, and norepinephrine. Activation of H_3-receptors on the vagus nerve decreases acetylcholine (ACh) release. H_3 receptors may participate in cognitive function and eating behavior.

d. Histamine (H_4)-receptors

(1) H_4-receptors are found on hematopoietic cells and in the spleen, thymus, and colon.

(2) Stimulation of H_4 receptors increases chemotaxis of mast cells and leukocytes cells toward sites of inflammation.

(3) H_4 receptors are coupled to G_i/G_o and thereby inhibit the production of cAMP and increase intracellular Ca^{2+}.

B. Histamine agonists

1. ***Prototypes.*** These agents include **histamine, betahistin**, and **impromidine.**
   - a. **Betazole** has approximately tenfold greater activity at H_2-receptors than at H_1-receptors.
   - b. **Impromidine** is an investigational agent; its ratio of H_2 to H_1 activity is about 10,000.
   - c. Methimepip is an H_3-specific agonist.
2. ***Uses.*** The uses of histamine agonists are primarily diagnostic. These agents are used in **allergy testing** to assess histamine sensitivity and in the **test of gastric secretory function** (they have been largely supplanted for this use by **pentagastrin** [Peptavlon], a synthetic peptide analogue of gastrin with fewer adverse effects).
3. ***Adverse effects.*** The adverse effects of these agents can be quite severe; they include flushing, a burning sensation, hypotension, tachycardia, and bronchoconstriction.

C. Histamine (H_1)-receptor antagonists are competitive inhibitors at the H_1-receptor (see Table 6-1).

1. ***Classification***

a. First-generation agents

(1) Alkylamines

- **(a)** Alkylamines include **chlorpheniramine** and **brompheniramine.**
- **(b)** These agents produce slight sedation.
- **(c)** Alkylamines are the antihistamines used most frequently in the United States.

(2) Ethanolamines

- **(a)** Ethanolamines include **diphenhydramine, doxylamine,** and **clemastine; dimenhydrinate** is an equimolar combination of diphenhydramine and 8-chlorotheophylline.
- **(b)** Ethanolamines produce marked **sedation; doxylamine** is marketed only as a sleeping aid.
- **(c)** Ethanolamines also act as **antiemetics.**

(3) Ethylenediamines

- **(a)** Ethylenediamines include **pyrilamine** and **antazoline.**
- **(b)** Ethylenediamines produce moderate **sedation** and can cause **GI upset.**

(4) Piperazines

- **(a)** Piperazines include **meclizine** and **cyclizine.**
- **(b)** Piperazines produce marked **adverse GI effects** and **moderate sedation.**
- **(c)** These agents have **antiemetic and antivertigo activities.**

(5) Phenothiazines

(a) Phenothiazines include **promethazine** and **cyproheptadine.**

(b) Phenothazines produce marked **sedation.**

(c) These agents have **antiemetic activity.**

(d) Phenothiazines are also weak α-adrenoceptor antagonists.

(6) Methylpiperidines

(a) Methylpiperidines include **cyproheptadine.**

(b) Methylpiperidines have antihistamine, anticholinergic, and antiserotonin activities.

b. Second-generation agents

(1) Piperidines

(a) Loratadine (Claritin), desloratadine (Clarinex). Poor CNS penetration. Little or no anticholinergic activity and greatly reduced sedation compared with earlier agents. Desloratadine is the active metabolite of loratadine and has about 15-fold greater affinity for the H_1 receptor than the parent compound.

(b) Fexophenadine is structurally different than the other piperidine antihistamines; sedative activity is low but dose dependent.

(2) Clemastine is a second-generation ethanolamine with a much longer duration of action than dimenhydramine; it has some antiemetic activity.

(3) Alkylamines: acrivastine (Semprex-D). Acrivastine is not associated with cardiac effects.

(4) Cetirizine (Zyrtec)

(a) Cetirizine is not associated with cardiac abnormalities.

(b) Cetirizine has poor penetration into the CNS.

(c) Cetirizine is less sedating; it is ineffective for motion sickness or antiemesis.

(5) Levocirizine (Xyzal) is an active (L) isomer of citirizine.

2. *Pharmacologic properties* (Table 6-1)

a. Histamine (H_1)-receptor antagonists are well absorbed after oral administration. The effects of these agents are usually seen in 30 minutes (with maximal effects at 1–2 h); the duration of action is 3–8 hours for first-generation compounds and 3–24 hours for second-generation compounds.

b. H_1-receptor antagonists are lipid soluble; most first-generation agents cross the blood–brain barrier, a property reduced but not eliminated with second-generation agents.

table 6-1 Major Pharmacologic Properties of H_1-Receptor Antagonists

Drug Class	Prototype	Duration of Action	Antihistamine Potency	Anticholinergic Potency	Antiemetic Potency	Sedative Effect
First-generation agents						
Alkylamines	Chlorpheniramine	4–25 h	+++	++	Marginal	+
Ethanolamines	Diphenhydramine	4–6 h	++	+++	+++	+++
	Dimenhydrinate	4–8 h	++	++	+	+++
	Clemastine	10–24 h	++	++	+	+
Ethylenediamines	Pyrilamine	4–6 h	+	++	Marginal	+
Piperazines	Cyclizine	4–24 h	++	++	+++	+
Phenothiazines	Promethazine	4–24 h	+/+++	+++	++++	+++
Methylpiperidines	Cyproheptadine	6–8 h	++	++	++	++
Second-generation agents						
Alkylamines	Acrivastine	6–8 h	++++	Marginal	None	Marginal
Piperazines	Cetirizine	12–24 h	++++	+	Marginal	+ 14%
	Levocitirizine	12–24 h	++++	+	Marginal	6%
Piperidines	Loratadine	24 h	++	None	None	8%
	Desloratadine	24 h	++++	None	None	2.1%
	Fexofenadine	12 h	++++	None	None	1.3%

c. H_1-receptor antagonists are metabolized in the liver; many induce microsomal enzymes and alter their own metabolism and that of other drugs.

3. ***Pharmacologic actions***
   a. Many H_1-receptor antagonists, especially the **ethanolamines, phenothiazines,** and **ethylenediamines,** have muscarinic–cholinergic antagonist activity.
   b. Most of these agents are effective local anesthetics, probably because of a blockade of sodium channels in excitable tissues. **Dimenhydrinate** and **promethazine** are potent local anesthetics.
   c. H_1-receptor antagonists relax histamine-induced contraction of bronchial smooth muscle and have some use in allergic bronchospasm.
   d. These agents block the vasodilator action of histamine.
   e. H_1-receptor antagonists inhibit histamine-induced increases in capillary permeability.
   f. These agents block mucus secretion and sensory nerve stimulation.
   g. H_1-receptor antagonists, especially the first-generation agents, frequently cause CNS depression (marked by sedation, decreased alertness, and decreased appetite). In children and some adults, these agents stimulate the CNS.
4. ***Therapeutic uses***
   a. **Treatment of allergic rhinitis and conjunctivitis.** Clemastine is approved for the treatment of rhinorrhea. Many antihistamines are used to treat the common cold, based on their anticholinergic properties, but they are only marginally effective for this use. Diphenhydramine also has an antitussive effect not mediated by H_1-receptor antagonism.
   b. **Treatment of urticaria** and **atopic dermatitis,** including hives
   c. **Sedatives.** Several **(doxylamine, diphenhydramine)** are marketed as over-the-counter (OTC) sleep aids.
   d. Prevention of **motion sickness**
   e. Appetite suppressants
5. ***Adverse effects*** (significantly reduced with second-generation agents)
   a. H_1-receptor antagonists produce sedation (synergistic with alcohol and other depressants), dizziness, and loss of appetite.
   b. These agents can cause GI upset, nausea, and constipation or diarrhea.
   c. H_1-receptor antagonists produce anticholinergic effects (dry mouth, blurred vision, and urine retention).
   d. Two second-generation H_1 antagonists, astemizole and terfenadine (a prodrug of fexofenadine) were discontinued or removed from the market because they were associated with Q-T prolongation and ventricular tachycardias.

D. Histamine (H_2)-receptor antagonists (see also Chapter 8 III C 1)

1. Histamine (H_2)-receptor antagonists include **cimetidine** (Tagamet), **ranitidine** (Zantac), **famotidine** (Pepcid AC), and **nizatidine** (Axid).
2. These agents are competitive antagonists at the H_2-receptor, which predominates in the gastric parietal cell.
3. H_2-receptor antagonists are used in the treatment of GI disorders, including heartburn and acid-induced indigestion.
4. These agents promote the healing of **gastric and duodenal ulcers** and are used to treat hypersecretory states such as **Zollinger-Ellison syndrome.**

E. The chromones: cromolyn (Intal), nedocromil sodium (Tilade)

1. These are poorly absorbed salts; they must be administered by **inhalation.**
2. They inhibit the release of histamine and other autocoids from the mast cell.
3. Each is used prophylactically in the treatment of **asthma;** they do not reverse bronchospasm.
4. These agents produce adverse effects that are usually confined to the site of application; these effects include **sore throat** and **dry mouth.**
5. Nedocromil sodium appears to be more effective in reducing **bronchospasm** caused by exercise or cold air.

II. SEROTONIN AND SEROTONIN ANTAGONISTS

A. Serotonin (5-hydroxytryptamine, 5-HT)

1. *Biosynthesis and distribution*

a. Serotonin is synthesized from the amino acid L-tryptophan by hydroxylation and decarboxylation.

b. Approximately 90% of serotonin is found in the enterochromaffin cells of the GI tract. Much of the remaining 10% is found in the platelets; small amounts are found in other tissues, including the brain. Platelets acquire serotonin from the circulation during passage through the intestine by a specific and highly active uptake mechanism.

c. Serotonin is stored in granules as a complex with ATP.

d. The major breakdown product of serotonin is **5-hydroxyindoleacetic acid (5-HIAA).**

2. *Mechanism of action.*

Serotonin acts on several classes of 5-HT receptors, which are located on cell membranes of many tissues:

a. **5-HT$_1$** (subtypes 5-HT$_{1A}$ through 5-HT$_{1F}$). 5-HT$_1$ receptors are coupled to an inhibition in cAMP; stimulation contracts arterial smooth muscle, especially in carotid and cranial circulation. At presynaptic sites, neuronal serotonin release is inhibited.

b. **5-HT$_2$** (subtypes 5-HT$_{2A}$ through 5-HT$_{2C}$). 5-HT$_2$ receptors are coupled to an increase in phospholipase C activity; stimulation causes contraction of vascular and intestinal smooth muscle and increases microcirculation and vascular permeability. Stimulation of this receptor on platelet membranes causes platelet aggregation; in the CNS, this receptor mediates hallucinogenic effects.

c. **5-HT$_3$** receptors are coupled to a ligand-gated ion channel. Stimulation of this receptor in the area postrema causes nausea and vomiting; stimulation on peripheral sensory neurons causes pain.

d. **5-HT$_4$** receptors increase cAMP; in the GI tract, these receptors mediate an increase in secretion and peristalsis.

e. **5-HT$_{5a,b}$** are expressed in the brain and are coupled to a decrease in cAMP.

f. **5-HT$_6$** and **5-HT$_7$** have been cloned and appear to be coupled to an increase in cAMP biosynthesis. 5-HT$_6$ receptors appear to be involved in anxiety and cognitive function. 5-HT$_7$ receptors are involved in thermoregulation, learning memory, and mood.

B. Serotonin agonists (see Table 6-2)

1. *Buspirone (BuSpar)*

a. Buspirone is a relatively specific 5-HT$_{1A}$-receptor agonist.

b. Buspirone is useful for the management of **anxiety disorders.**

c. Therapeutic actions can take as long as 2 weeks to appear.

2. *Triptans:* sumatriptan, rizatriptan, eletriptan, zolmitriptan, almotriptan, frovatriptan, naratriptan

a. The "triptans" as a class are 5-HT$_{1D}$- and 5-HT$_{1B}$-receptor agonists and have 5-HT$_{1F}$ agonist activity. Activation of 5-HT$_{1D}$ receptors inhibits vasodilation and inflammation of the meninges and pain transmission and the release of vasodilator substances such as calcitonin gene-related peptide (CGRP) in trigeminal neurons. 5-HT$_{1B}$ agonist activity results in vasoconstriction of dilated cerebral vessels.

b. The major use of the triptans is the treatment of **acute migraine;** about 50%–80% of patients report relief from pain within 2 hours. Triptans may be useful to treat cluster headaches.

c. Sumatriptan has 5-HT$_{1B}$ activity in coronaries, and chest pain is an adverse effect of this agent. Adverse effects of this class include flushing, hypertension, nausea, and vomiting.

d. Due to the serotonin-agonist activities, triptans are under clinical investigation for irritable bowel syndrome.

e. All are available as oral agents. Sumatriptan and zolmitriptan are also available as nasal sprays, and sumatriptan is also available for subcutaneous injection.

3. *Trazodone (Desyrel)*

a. The parent drug is metabolized to *m*-chlorophenylpiperazine, an activator of 5-HT$_{1B}$ and 5-HT$_2$ receptors. It also blocks the reuptake of serotonin.

b. Trazodone is used to treat **depression.**

table 6-2 Drugs that Interact with Serotonin Receptors

Drug	Receptor	Action
Buspirone	5-HT_{1a} agonist	Anxiolytic
Sumatriptan	5-$HT_{1D,\ 1B,\ 1F}$ agonist	Acute migraine
Almotriptan	5-$HT_{1D,\ 1B,\ 1F}$ agonist	Acute migraine
Dolasetron (Anzemet)	5-HT_3 antagonist	Antiemetic
Granisetron (Kytril)	5-HT_3 antagonist	Antiemetic
Ondansetron (Zofran)	5-HT_3 antagonist	Antiemetic
Alosetron	5-HT_3 antagonist	Severe irritable bowel
Risperidone	5-$HT_{2A,\ 2C}$ antagonist (and D_2 antagonist)	Atypical antipsychotic

4. ***Tegaserod (Zelnorm), Alosetron (Lotronox)***
   a. Tegaserod is a specific 5-HT_4 agonist used to treat irritable bowel syndrome and constipation.
   b. Tegaserod speeds gastric emptying and reduces GI sensitivity.
   c. Alosetron is a 5-HT3 antagonist and can have severe side effects; its use is restricted to women.

C. **Serotonin antagonists**
1. ***Cyproheptadine***
   a. Cyproheptadine is a potent H_1-receptor antagonist of the phenothiazine class; it also blocks both 5-HT_1 and 5-HT_2 receptors.
   b. Cyproheptadine is used most frequently to limit diarrhea and intestinal spasms produced by **serotonin-secreting carcinoid tumors** and postgastrectomy **dumping syndrome.**
   c. Cyproheptadine produces sedation and anticholinergic actions.
2. ***Ondansetron, granisetron, dolasetron, palonosetron***
   a. These drugs are 5-HT_3-receptor antagonists.
   b. The 5-HT_3-receptor antagonists are highly effective in treating the nausea and vomiting associated with chemotherapy and radiation therapy and have become the primary agents used with these therapies.
   c. Administered intravenously (IV) or orally; IV administration 30 minutes before anticancer treatment is the most effective.
3. ***Clozapine***
   a. While clozapine mainly blocks D_1 and D_4 receptors, it also blocks 5-HT_{2A} and 5-HT_{2C} receptors and has mixed acetylcholine muscarinic antagonist/agonist activities.
   b. Clozapine is an atypical **antipsychotic** with reduced extrapyramidal effects.
4. ***Risperidone (Risperdal)***
   a. Risperidone is an antagonist at 5-HT_{2A}, 5-HT_{2C}, and dopamine (D_2) receptors.
   b. Risperidone is an **atypical antischizophrenic agent** with reduced extrapyramidal activity.

D. **Other serotonergic agents.** ***Fluoxetine (Prozac)*** and other SSRIs (see also Chapter 5, Table 5-5). The actions of this class of antidepressants are presumed to be due to decreased serotonin uptake into neurons.

III. ERGOTS

A. **Structure.** Ergots include a wide variety of compounds sharing the tetracyclic ergoline nucleus that are produced by the fungus *Claviceps purpurea.* These agents have a strong structural similarity to the neurotransmitters norepinephrine, dopamine, and serotonin.
1. ***Amine ergot alkaloids*** include **methysergide, lysergic acid** and **LSD,** and **methylergonovine.**
2. ***Peptide ergot alkaloids*** include **ergotamine (Ergomar), dihydroergotamine (Migranol), ergocristine, ergonovine, bromocriptine (Parlodel), cabergoline, and pergolide (Permax).**

table 6-3 Pharmacologic Properties of Ergots

Drug	Receptor	Target Tissue and Response	Therapeutic Uses	Toxicity
Methylergonovine	α-Adrenoceptor agonist	Uterine smooth muscle contraction	Postpartum hemorrhage	Hypertension, nausea
Ergotamine	α-Adrenoceptor agonist, 5-HT receptor agonist	Vascular smooth muscle; vasoconstriction	Acute migraine attacks	Nausea, diarrhea
Methysergide	5-HT receptor antagonist	Vascular smooth muscle; prevent initial vasoconstriction	Migraine prophylaxis	Fibroblastic changes
Bromocriptine, pergolide	Dopamine agonists	Breast, uterus, pituitary; suppress lactation and decrease growth hormone levels	Hyperprolactinemia, amenorrhea, acromegaly	Dose-related effects, ranging from nausea to parkinsonian-like symptoms

B. Mechanism of action

1. Ergots display varying degrees of agonist or antagonist activity in three receptor types: α-adrenoceptors, dopamine receptors, and serotonin receptors.
2. The pharmacologic application of ergots is determined by the relative affinity and efficacy of the individual agents for these receptor systems. Many agents exhibit partial agonist activities and thus can cause either stimulatory or inhibitory effects.

C. Pharmacologic properties (Table 6-3)

1. Ergots may be administered parenterally, rectally, sublingually, as inhalants, or orally, and vary widely in their absorption. Amine alkaloids are slowly and relatively poorly absorbed; the peptide alkaloids are completely absorbed.
2. Ergots are extensively metabolized to compounds of varying activity and half-life.

D. Therapeutic uses

1. ***Postpartum hemorrhage***
   a. **Methylergonovine** (Methergine) is the most uterine-selective agent; causes prolonged and forceful **contraction of uterine smooth muscle.**
   b. Ergots should not be used to induce labor.
   c. Uterine sensitivity varies with hormonal status; the uterus at term is most sensitive.
2. ***Migraine***
   a. **Ergotamine** (Ergomar, Ergostat) is widely used for relief of an acute migraine attack.
      (1) The major effect of ergotamine is **cerebral vasoconstriction;** it reverses the rebound vasodilation that is the probable cause of pain.
      (2) Ergotamine acts as a central 5-HT receptor and α-adrenoceptor agonist.
      (3) Ergotamine is most effective if administered in the early (prodromal) stages of attack to reverse rebound vasodilation.
      (4) Ergotamine is frequently **combined with caffeine,** which probably increases absorption.
      (5) Ergotamine produces long-lasting and cumulative effects; weekly dosage must be strictly limited.
   b. **Methysergide** (Sansert) is used for **prophylaxis of migraine.**
      (1) Methysergide acts as a serotonin-receptor ($5\text{-HT}_{2A,C}$) antagonist, and it inhibits initial vasoconstriction in the early stages of a migraine.
      (2) Methysergide is effective in 60% of patients for the prophylaxis of migraine; it is ineffective after the onset of an attack.
      (3) The cumulative toxicity of methysergide requires drug-free periods of 3–4 weeks every 6 months.
   c. **Propranolol** and other **β-adrenergic antagonists** are also effective agents for the prophylaxis of migraine.

3. ***Hyperprolactinemia***
   a. **Bromocriptine mesylate** (Parlodel) and **pergolide** (Permax), **cabergoline,** dopaminergic agonists, cause specific **inhibition of prolactin secretion** (elevated prolactin secretion can induce infertility and amenorrhea in women and galactorrhea in men and women).
   b. These agents are used to treat prolactin-secreting tumors of the pituitary, to counteract central dopaminergic antagonists, and to suppress normal lactation.
   c. Bromocriptine mesylate and pergolide are used as adjuncts to agents such as **levodopa** in the management of **Parkinson disease** (not a prolactin-lowering effect).
   d. These agents reduce growth hormone secretion.

E. Adverse effects

1. The most serious adverse effect is **prolonged vasospasm;** this can lead to gangrene and is most frequently caused by **ergotamine** and **ergonovine.**
2. The most common side effect is **GI disturbance.**
3. **Methysergide toxicity** includes retroperitoneal fibroplasia and coronary and endocardial fibrosis, as well as CNS stimulation and hallucinations.

IV. EICOSANOIDS

A. Overview

1. Eicosanoids are a large group of autocoids with potent effects on virtually every tissue in the body; these agents are derived from metabolism of 20-carbon, unsaturated fatty acids **(eicosanoic acids).**
2. The eicosanoids include the prostaglandins, thromboxanes, leukotrienes, hydroperoxyeicosatetraenoic acids **(HPETEs),** and hydroxyeicosatetraenoic acids **(HETEs).**

B. Biosynthesis (Fig. 6-2)

1. **Arachidonic acid,** the most common precursor of the eicosanoids, is formed by two pathways:

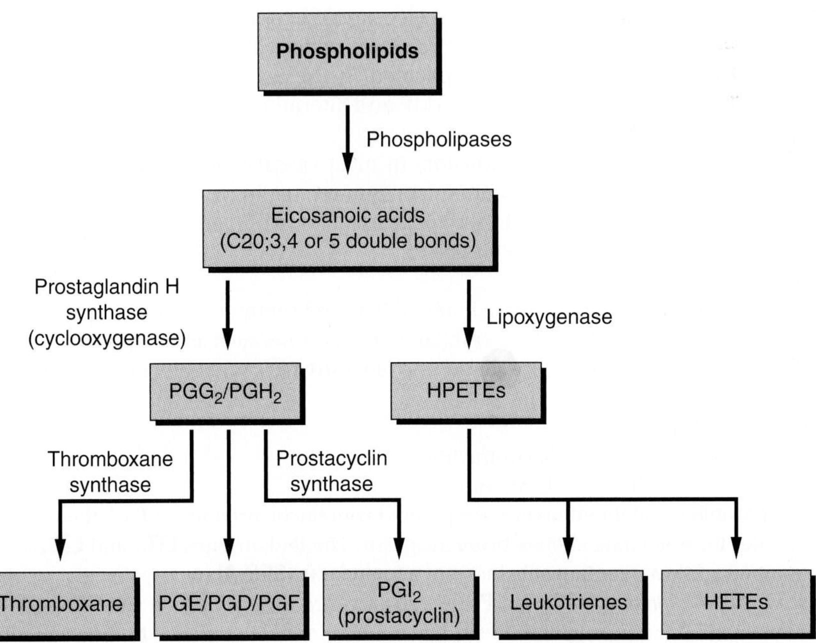

FIGURE 6-2. Biosynthesis of eicosanoids.

a. **Phospholipase A_2**-mediated production from membrane phospholipids; this pathway is inhibited by glucocorticoids.
b. **Phospholipase C** in concert with diglyceride lipase can also produce free arachidonate.
2. **Eicosanoids** are **synthesized** by two pathways:
   a. The **prostaglandin H synthase (COX, cyclooxygenase) pathway** produces **thromboxane,** the primary prostaglandins (**prostaglandin E,** or PGE; **prostaglandin F,** or PGF; and **prostaglandin D,** or PGD), and **prostacyclin (PGI_2).**
      (1) There are **two forms** of **COX: COX-1** is located in endothelial cells, platelets, kidney, GI tract, and many other locations; **COX-2** is found in great abundance in connective tissues.
      (2) The **COX-1** enzyme is expressed at fairly constant levels and may provide protective action on gastric mucosa, on endothelium, and in the kidney.
      (3) The **COX-2** enzyme is highly inducible by numerous factors associated with inflammation. Current theories suggest that the COX-2 isoform is predominantly associated with **eicosanoid production** in inflammation.
   b. The **lipoxygenase pathway** produces the HPETEs, HETEs, and the leukotrienes.
      (1) 5-Lipoxygenase produces 5-HPETEs, which are subsequently converted to 5-HETEs and then to leukotrienes.
      (2) 12-Lipoxygenase produces 12-HPETEs, which are converted to 12-HETEs.
   c. Additional metabolites of the HPETEs, hepoxilins and lipoxins have been identified, but their biologic role is unclear.
3. The eicosanoids all have short plasma half-lives (typically 0.5–5 min). Most catabolism occurs in the lung.
   a. Prostaglandins are metabolized by prostaglandin 15-OH dehydrogenase (PDGH) to 15-keto metabolites, which are excreted in the urine.
   b. **Thromboxane A_2 (TXA_2)** is rapidly hydrated to the less active TXB_2.
   c. **PGI_2** is hydrolyzed to 6-keto-$PGF_{1\alpha}$.
4. Various eicosanoids are synthesized throughout the body; synthesis can be very tissue specific:
   a. **PGI_2** is synthesized in endothelial and vascular smooth muscle cells.
   b. **Thromboxane** synthesis occurs primarily in platelets.
   c. **HPETEs, HETEs,** and the **leukotrienes** are synthesized predominantly in mast cells, white blood cells, airway epithelium, and platelets.

C. Actions. There is no universal mediator of eicosanoid action. A separate cell-surface receptor appears to mediate the activities of each class of metabolite. Virtually all of the known second-messenger systems have been implicated in the action of the eicosanoids, including stimulation or inhibition of cAMP and cGMP and alterations in Ca^{2+} flux.

1. ***Vascular smooth muscle***
   a. **PGE_2** and **PGI_2** are potent vasodilators in most vascular beds. **PGE_2** also antagonizes the effects of vasoconstrictor substances such as norepinephrine.
   b. **$PGF_{2\alpha}$** causes arteriolar vasodilation and constriction of superficial veins.
   c. **Thromboxane** is a potent vasoconstrictor.
2. ***Inflammation***
   a. **PGE_2** and **PGI_2** cause an increase in blood flow and promote, but do not cause, edema. PGE also potentiates the effect of other inflammatory agents such as bradykinin.
   b. **HETEs** (5-HETE, 12-HETE, 15-HETE) and **leukotrienes** cause chemotaxis of neutrophils and eosinophils.
3. ***Bronchial smooth muscle***
   a. **PGFs** cause smooth muscle contraction.
   b. **PGEs** cause smooth muscle relaxation.
   c. **Leukotrienes** and **thromboxane** are potent bronchoconstrictors and are the most likely candidates for mediating allergic bronchospasm. The leukotrienes **LTC_4** and **LTD_4** are the components of **slow-reacting substance of anaphylaxis (SRS-A).**
4. ***Uterine smooth muscle.*** **PGE_2** and **$PGF_{2\alpha}$** cause contraction of uterine smooth muscle in pregnant women. The nonpregnant uterus has a more variable response to prostaglandins; **$PGF_{2\alpha}$** causes contraction, and **PGE_2** causes relaxation.

5. ***GI tract***
   a. **PGE_2** and **$PGF_{2\alpha}$** increase the rate of longitudinal contraction in the gut and decrease transit time.
   b. The **leukotrienes** are potent stimulators of GI smooth muscle.
   c. **PGE_2** and **PGI_2** inhibit acid and pepsinogen secretion in the stomach. In addition, prostaglandins increase mucus, water, and electrolyte secretion in the stomach and the intestine.
6. ***Blood***
   a. **TXA_2** is a potent inducer of platelet aggregation.
   b. **PGI_2** and **PGE_2** inhibit platelet aggregation.
   c. **PGEs** induce erythropoiesis by stimulating the renal release of erythropoietin.
   d. **5-HPETE** stimulates release of histamine; **PGI_2** and **PGD** inhibit histamine release.

D. Therapeutic uses

1. ***Induction of labor at term.*** Induction of labor is produced by infusion of **$PGF_{2\alpha}$** (carboprost tromethamine) (Hemabate) or **PGE_2** (dinoprostone) (Prostin E).
2. ***Therapeutic abortion.*** Infusion of **carboprost tromethamine** or administration of vaginal suppositories containing **dinoprostone** is effective in inducing abortion in the second trimester. Currently, these prostaglandins are combined with **mifepristone (RU486)** to induce first-trimester abortion.
3. ***Maintenance of ductus arteriosus*** is produced by **PGE_1** (Prostin VR) infusion; PGE_1 will maintain patency of the ductus arteriosus, which may be desirable before surgery.
4. ***Treatment of peptic ulcer.*** **Misoprostol** (Cytotec), a methylated derivative of PGE_1, is approved for use in patients taking high doses of nonsteroidal anti-inflammatory drugs (NSAIDs) to reduce gastric ulceration.
5. ***Erectile dysfunction.*** Alprostadil (PGE_1) can be injected directly into the corpus cavernosum or administered as a transurethral suppository to cause vasodilation and enhance tumescence.

E. Adverse effects of eicosanoids include local pain and irritation, bronchospasm, and GI disturbances, including nausea, vomiting, cramping, and diarrhea.

F. Pharmacologic inhibition of eicosanoid synthesis

1. **Phospholipase A2-mediated** release of eicosanoic precursors, such as arachidonic acid, is inhibited by glucocorticoids, in part by the action of annexin-1 (lipocortin).
2. **Aspirin** and most **NSAIDs** inhibit synthesis of prostaglandin G (PGG) and prostaglandin H (PGH) by their actions on the **cyclooxygenase pathways.** Aspirin can increase the synthesis of eicosanoids through the lipoxygenase pathway, perhaps by increasing substrate concentration.
3. **Eicosatetraenoic acid** is an arachidonic acid analogue that inhibits both cyclooxygenase and lipoxygenase activity.
4. Imidazole derivatives such as **dazoxiben** appear to inhibit thromboxane synthase preferentially.

V. NONSTEROIDAL ANTI-INFLAMMATORY DRUGS (NSAIDS) (TABLE 6-4)

A. Overview

1. The inflammatory response is complex, involving the immune system and the influence of various endogenous agents, including prostaglandins, bradykinin, histamine, chemotactic factors, and superoxide free radicals formed by the action of lysosomal enzymes.
2. Aspirin, other salicylates, and newer drugs with diverse structures are referred to as **NSAIDs** to distinguish them from the anti-inflammatory glucocorticoids. NSAIDs are used to **suppress the symptoms of inflammation associated with rheumatic disease.** Some are also used to relieve **pain** (analgesic action) and **fever** (antipyretic action).

table 6-4 Nonsteroidal and Analgesic Compounds and Their Therapeutic Effectiveness

Chemical Class	Prototype	Analgesia	Antipyresis	Anti-inflammatory
Salicylates	Aspirin	+++	+++	+++
Para-aminophenols	Acetaminophen	+++	+++	Marginal
Indoles	Indomethacin	+++	++++	++++
Pyrrol acetic acids	Tolmentin, mefenamic acid	+++	+++	+++
Propionic acids	Ibuprofen, naproxen	++++	+++	++++
Enolic acids	Phenylbutazone, piroxicam	+++	+++	++++
Alkanones	Nabumetone	++	++	+++
Sulfonamide	Celecoxib	++++	+++	++++

B. Mechanism of action

1. *Anti-inflammatory effect*

a. The anti-inflammatory effect of NSAIDs is due to the inhibition of the enzymes that produce prostaglandin H synthase (cyclooxygenase, or COX), which converts arachidonic acid to **prostaglandins,** and to **TXA_2** and **prostacyclin.**

b. Aspirin irreversibly inactivates COX-1 and COX-2 by acetylation of a specific serine residue. This distinguishes it from other NSAIDs, which reversibly inhibit COX-1 and COX-2.

c. NSAIDs have no effect on lipoxygenase and therefore do not inhibit the production of leukotrienes.

d. Additional anti-inflammatory mechanisms may include interference with the potentiative action of other mediators of inflammation (bradykinin, histamine, serotonin), modulation of T-cell function, stabilization of lysosomal membranes, and inhibition of chemotaxis.

2. *Analgesic effect*

a. PGE_2 and PGI_2 are the most important prostaglandins involved in pain. Inhibition of their synthesis is a primary mechanism of NSAID-mediated analgesia.

(1) Prostaglandins sensitize pain receptors and processing; peripheral input via C and Aδ fibers and TRPV-1 Ca^{2+} channels

- NSAID primary hyperalgesia

(2) Afferent input processed in dorsal horn (prostaglandins inhibit GABA and glycine inhibitory interneurons)

- NSAID secondary hyperalgesia

(3) Prostaglandins produce changes in central pain processing that leads to **allodynia:** painful sensation cause by normally innocuous stimuli.

b. NSAIDs prevent the potentiating action of prostaglandins on endogenous mediators of peripheral nerve stimulation (e.g., bradykinin).

3. *Antipyretic effect.*

The antipyretic effect of NSAIDs is believed to be related to inhibition of production of prostaglandins induced by interleukin-1 (IL-1) and interleukin-6 (IL-6) in the hypothalamus and the "resetting" of the thermoregulatory system, leading to vasodilatation and increased heat loss.

C. Therapeutic uses

1. *Inflammation*

a. NSAIDs are first-line drugs used to arrest inflammation and the accompanying pain of rheumatic and nonrheumatic diseases, including **rheumatoid arthritis, juvenile arthritis, osteoarthritis, psoriatic arthritis, ankylosing spondylitis, Reiter syndrome,** and **dysmenorrhea.** Pain and inflammation of bursitis and tendonitis also respond to NSAIDs.

b. NSAIDs do not significantly reverse the progress of rheumatic disease; rather, they slow destruction of cartilage and bone and allow patients increased mobility and use of their joints.

c. Treatment of chronic inflammation requires use of these agents at doses well above those used for analgesia and antipyresis; consequently, the incidence of adverse drug effects is increased. Drug selection is generally dictated by the patient's ability to tolerate the adverse effects, and the cost of the drugs.

d. Anti-inflammatory effects may develop only after several weeks of treatment.

2. *Analgesia.* NSAIDs **alleviate mild-to-moderate pain** by decreasing PGE- and PGF I_2 ie PGI_2-mediated increases in pain receptor sensitivity. They are less effective than opioids, and they are more effective against pain associated with integumental structures (pain of muscular and vascular origin, arthritis, and bursitis) than with pain associated with the viscera.

3. *Antipyresis.* NSAIDs **reduce elevated body temperature** with little effect on normal body temperature.

4. *Miscellaneous uses.* Aspirin **reduces** the **formation of thrombi** and is used prophylactically to reduce recurrent transient ischemia, unstable angina, and the incidence of thrombosis after coronary artery bypass grafts.

D. Aspirin (acetylsalicylic acid) and nonacetylated salicylates include sodium salicylate, magnesium salicylate, choline salicylate, sodium thiosalicylate, sulfasalazine (Azulfidine), mesalamine (Asacol), and salsalate.

1. *Pharmacologic properties*

a. Salicylates are weak organic acids; **aspirin** has a pK_a of 3.5.

b. These agents are rapidly absorbed from the intestine as well as from the stomach, where the low pH favors absorption. The rate of absorption is increased with rapidly dissolving (buffered) or predissolved (effervescent) dosage forms.

c. Salicylates are hydrolyzed rapidly by plasma and tissue esterases to acetic acid and the active metabolite **salicylic acid.** Salicylic acid is more slowly oxidized to gentisic acid and conjugated with glycine to **salicyluric acid** and to ether and ester glucuronides.

d. Salicylates have a $t_{1/2}$ of 3–6 hours after short-term administration. Long-term administration of high doses (to treat arthritis) or toxic overdose increases the $t_{1/2}$ to 15–30 hours because the enzymes for glycine and glucuronide conjugation become saturated.

e. Unmetabolized salicylates are excreted by the kidney. If the urine pH increases to above 8, clearance is increased approximately fourfold as a result of decreased reabsorption of the ionized salicylate from the tubules.

2. *Therapeutic uses*

a. Salicylates are used to treat **rheumatoid arthritis, juvenile arthritis,** and **osteoarthritis,** as well as other inflammatory disorders. 5-Amino salicylates (mesalamine, sulfasalazine) can be used to treat **Crohn disease.**

b. Salicylic acid is used **topically** to treat **plantar warts, fungal infections,** and **corns;** use is based on the destruction of keratinocytes and dermal epithelia by the free acid.

c. Aspirin has significantly greater antithrombotic activity than other NSAIDs and is useful in preventing or reducing the risk of myocardial infarction in patients with a history of myocardial infarction, angina, cardiac surgery, and cerebral or peripheral vascular disease.

3. *Adverse effects*

a. GI effects

(1) GI effects are the most common adverse effects of high-dose **aspirin** use (70% of patients); these effects may include nausea, vomiting, diarrhea, constipation, dyspepsia, epigastric pain, bleeding, and ulceration (primarily gastric).

(2) These GI effects are thought to be due to a direct chemical effect on gastric cells and a decrease in the production and cytoprotective activity of prostaglandins, which leads to gastric tissue susceptibility to damage by hydrochloric acid.

(3) The GI effects may contraindicate **aspirin** use in patients with an active ulcer. Aspirin may be taken with prostaglandins to reduce gastric damage.

(4) Substitution of enteric-coated or timed-release preparations, or the use of **nonacetylated salicylates,** may decrease gastric irritation. Gastric irritation is not prevented by using buffered tablets.

b. Hypersensitivity (intolerance)

(1) Hypersensitivity is relatively **uncommon with the use of aspirin** (0.3% of patients); hypersensitivity results in rash, bronchospasm, rhinitis, edema, or an anaphylactic reaction with shock, which may be life threatening. The incidence of intolerance is highest in patients with asthma, nasal polyps, recurrent rhinitis, or urticaria. Aspirin should be avoided in such patients.

(2) **Cross-hypersensitivity** may exist to other **NSAIDs** and to the yellow dye tartrazine, which is used in many pharmaceutical preparations.

(3) Hypersensitivity is not associated with **sodium salicylate** or **magnesium salicylate.**

(4) The use of **aspirin** and other **salicylates** to control fever during viral infections (influenza and chickenpox) in children and adolescents is associated with an increased incidence of **Reye syndrome,** an illness characterized by vomiting, hepatic disturbances, and encephalopathy that has a 35% mortality rate. **Acetaminophen** is recommended as a substitute for children with **fever of unknown etiology.**

c. **Miscellaneous adverse effects and contraindications**

(1) Salicylates occasionally **decrease** the **glomerular filtration rate,** particularly in patients with renal insufficiency.

(2) Salicylates occasionally produce **mild hepatitis,** usually asymptomatic, particularly in patients with systemic lupus erythematosus, juvenile or adult rheumatoid arthritis, or rheumatic fever.

(3) These agents **prolong bleeding time. Aspirin** irreversibly inhibits platelet COX-1 and COX-2 and, thereby, **TXA_2** production, suppressing platelet adhesion and aggregation. The use of salicylates is contraindicated in patients with bleeding disorders, such as hypothrombinemia, hemophilia, hepatic disease, and vitamin K deficiency, and use should be avoided in patients receiving anticoagulants such as coumarin and **heparin.**

(4) Salicylates are not recommended during pregnancy; they may induce **postpartum hemorrhage** and lead to **premature closure** of the **fetal ductus arteriosus.**

4. ***Drug interactions***

a. The **action of anticoagulants** may be enhanced by their displacement by aspirin from binding sites on serum albumin. Aspirin also displaces **tolbutamide, phenytoin,** and other drugs from their plasma protein-binding sites.

b. The hypoglycemic action of **sulfonylureas** may be enhanced by displacement from their binding sites on serum albumin or by inhibition of their renal tubular secretion by aspirin.

c. Usual analgesic doses of **aspirin** (<2 g/day) decrease renal excretion of **sodium urate** and antagonize the uricosuric effect of **sulfinpyrazone** and **probenecid; aspirin** is contraindicated in patients with gout who are taking uricosuric agents.

d. **Antacids** may alter the absorption of **aspirin.**

e. **Aspirin** competes for tubular secretion with **penicillin G** and prolongs its half-life.

f. **Corticosteroids** increase renal clearance of **salicylates.**

g. **Alcohol** may increase GI bleeding when taken with aspirin.

5. ***Toxicity***

a. In adults, **salicylism** (tinnitus, hearing loss, vertigo) occurs as initial sign of toxicity after **aspirin** or **salicylate overdose** or poisoning.

b. In children, the common signs of toxicity include **hyperventilation** and **acidosis,** with accompanying lethargy and hyperpnea.

c. Disturbance of acid–base balance results in **metabolic acidosis** in infants and young children and in **compensated respiratory alkalosis** in older children and adults. **Salicylate toxicity** initially increases the medullary response to carbon dioxide, with resulting hyperventilation and respiratory alkalosis. In infants and young children, increases in lactic acid and ketone body production result in metabolic acidosis. With increased severity of toxicity, respiratory depression occurs, with accompanying respiratory acidosis.

d. The uncoupling of oxidative phosphorylation by **aspirin** results in **hyperthermia** and **hypoglycemia,** particularly in infants and young children. Nausea, vomiting, tachycardia, hyperpnea, dehydration, and coma may develop.

e. **Treatment** includes correction of acid–base disturbances, replacement of electrolytes and fluids, cooling, alkalinization of urine with bicarbonate to reduce salicylate reabsorption, forced diuresis, and gastric lavage or emesis.

E. Other nonsteroidal anti-inflammatory drugs

1. ***Overview***

a. Like aspirin, these agents are used for the treatment of **inflammation** associated with rheumatic and nonrheumatic diseases.

b. NSAIDs are absorbed rapidly after oral administration. These agents are extensively bound to plasma proteins, especially albumin. They cause drug interactions due to the displacement of other agents, particularly anticoagulants, from serum albumin; these interactions are similar to those seen with **aspirin.**

c. NSAIDs are metabolized in the liver and excreted by the kidney; the half-lives of these agents vary greatly (from 1 to 45 h, with most between 10 and 20 h). The required frequency of administration may influence drug choice because of possible problems with compliance.

d. These agents commonly produce **GI disturbances;** they demonstrate **cross-sensitivity with aspirin** and with each other. Other adverse effects, such as hypersensitivity, are generally the same as for aspirin; the cautions and contraindications are also similar to those for aspirin.

e. NSAIDs are associated with non–dose-related instances of acute renal failure and nephrotic syndrome, and they may lead to renal toxicity in combination with angiotensin-converting enzyme (ACE) inhibitors. **Indomethacin, meclofenamate, tolmetin,** and **phenylbutazone** are generally more toxic than other NSAIDs.

2. ***Ibuprofen, naproxen (Naprosyn, Aleve), fenoprofen (Nalfon), and ketoprofen (Orudis)***

a. These agents are propionic acid derivatives.

b. There is no reported interaction of **ibuprofen** or **ketoprofen** with anticoagulants. **Fenoprofen** has been reported to induce **nephrotoxic syndrome.**

c. Long-term use of ibuprofen is associated with an increased incidence of hypertension in women.

3. ***Sulindac (Clinoril), tolmetin (Tolectin), and ketorolac (Toradol)***

a. Sulindac and tolmetin are pyrrole acetic acid derivatives. **Sulindac** is a prodrug that is oxidized to a sulfone and then to the active sulfide, which has a relatively long $t_{1/2}$ (16 h) because of enterohepatic cycling.

b. **Tolmetin** has minimal effect on platelet aggregation; it is associated with a higher incidence of anaphylaxis than other NSAIDs. Tolmetin has a relatively short $t_{1/2}$ (1 h).

c. **Ketorolac** is a potent analgesic with moderate anti-inflammatory activity that can be administered IV or topically in an ophthalmic solution.

4. ***Indomethacin (Indocin)***

a. Indomethacin is the drug of choice for treatment of **ankylosing spondylitis** and **Reiter syndrome;** it is also used for acute gouty arthritis.

b. Indomethacin is also used to speed the closure of **patent ductus arteriosus** in premature infants (otherwise, it is not used in children); it inhibits the production of prostaglandins that prevent closure of the ductus.

c. Indomethacin is not recommended as a simple analgesic or antipyretic because of the potential for severe adverse effects.

d. Bleeding, ulceration, and other adverse effects are more likely with **indomethacin** than with most other NSAIDs. Headache is a common adverse effect; tinnitus, dizziness, or confusion also occasionally occurs.

5. ***Piroxicam (Feldene)***

a. Piroxicam is an oxicam derivative of enolic acid.

b. Piroxicam has $t_{1/2}$ of 45 hours.

c. Like **aspirin** and **indomethacin, bleeding** and **ulceration** are more likely with piroxicam than with other NSAIDs.

6. ***Meclofenamate (Meclomen) and mefenamic acid (Ponstel)***

a. Meclofenamate and mefenamic acid have $t_{1/2}$ of 2 hours.

b. A relatively high incidence of GI disturbances is associated with these agents.

7. ***Nabumetone (Relafen)***

a. Nabumetone is another chemical class of **NSAIDs,** but it has **similar effects.**

b. Compared with NSAIDs, nabumetone is associated with **reduced inhibition of platelet function** and **reduced incidence of GI bleeding.**

c. Nabumetone inhibits COX-2 more than COX-1.

8. ***Other NSAIDs*** include flurbiprofen (Ansaid), diclofenac (Voltaren), and etodolac (Lodine). Flurbiprofen is also available for topical ophthalmic use.
9. ***COX-2 selective agents***
   a. Several agents, celecoxib (Celebrex), rofecoxib (Vioxx), valdecoxib (Bextra), that inhibit COX-2 more than COX-1 have been developed and approved for use. The relative COX-2/COX-1 specificity of these agents is about 10, 35, and 30, respectively.
   b. The rationale behind development of these drugs was that inhibition of COX-2 would reduce the inflammatory response and pain but not inhibit the cytoprotective action of prostaglandins in the stomach, which is largely mediated by COX-1.
   c. Concern has arisen due to a doubling in the incidence of heart attack and stroke in patients taking rofecoxib and valdecoxib. This appears to be classwide adverse effect, but only rofecoxib and valdecoxib have been removed from the market. Valdecoxib has also been associated with serious adverse skin reactions. One possible explanation, as illustrated in Figure 6-3, is that inhibition of COX-2-mediated production of the vasodilator PGI_2 by endothelial cells, while not affecting the prothrombotic actions of COX-1 in platelets, increases the chance of blood clots.
   d. While the incidence of GI adverse effects is reduced with COX-2 selective inhibitors (especially the frequency of endoscopically detected microerosions), there have still been occurrences of serious GI adverse effects with these agents.
   e. Celecoxib remains on the market and is approved for osteoarthritis and rheumatoid arthritis; pain including bone pain, dental pain, and headache; and ankylosing spondylitis.

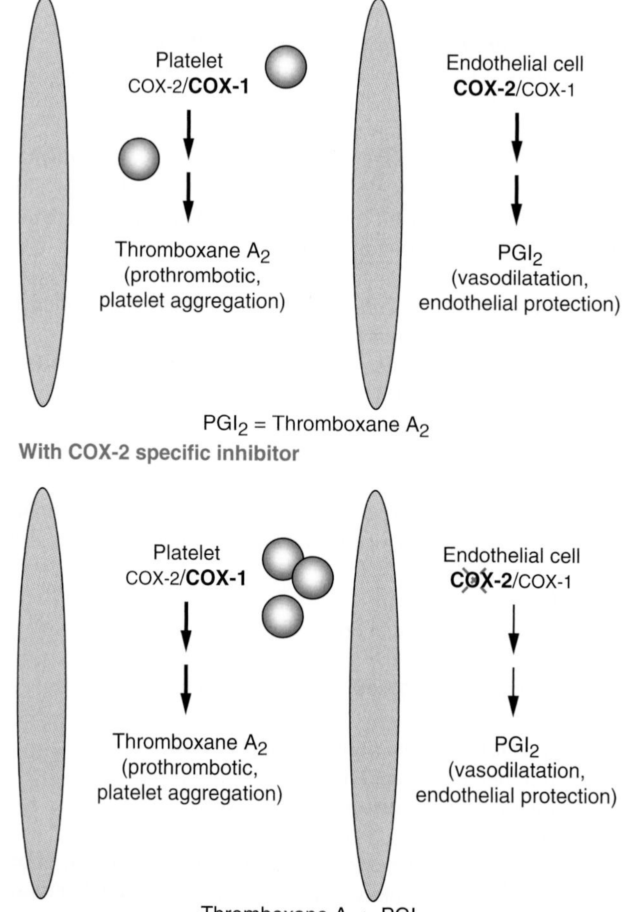

FIGURE 6-3. COX-2 inhibition and increased risk of cardiovascular accident.

F. Other anti-inflammatory drugs are used in the more advanced stages of some rheumatoid diseases.

1. ***Aurothioglucose (Solganal), gold sodium thiomalate (Myochrysine), and auranofin (Ridaura)***
   a. Aurothioglucose, gold sodium thiomalate, and auranofin are gold compounds that may **retard** the **destruction of bone and joints** by an unknown mechanism.
   b. These agents have long latency.
   c. **Aurothioglucose** and **gold sodium thiomalate** are administered intramuscularly (IM). **Auranofin** is administered orally and is 95% bound to plasma proteins.
   d. These agents can produce **serious GI disturbances, dermatitis,** and **mucous membrane lesions.** Less common effects include hematologic disorders such as aplastic anemia and proteinuria, with occasional nephrotic syndrome.
2. ***Penicillamine (Cuprimine, Depen)***
   a. Penicillamine is a chelating drug (will chelate gold) that is a metabolite of **penicillin.**
   b. Penicillamine has **immunosuppressant activity,** but its mechanism of action is unknown.
   c. This agent has long latency.
   d. The incidence of severe adverse effects is high; these effects are similar to those of the gold compounds.
3. ***Methotrexate***
   a. Methotrexate is an antineoplastic drug used for **rheumatoid arthritis** in patients who do not respond well to NSAIDs or glucocorticoids.
   b. Methotrexate commonly produces **hepatotoxicity.**
4. ***Chloroquine and hydrochloroquine (Plaquenil)***
   a. Chloroquine and hydrochloroquine are **antimalarial drugs.**
   b. These agents have immunosuppressant activity, but their mechanism of action is unknown.
   c. Used to treat joint pain associated with lupus and arthritis
5. ***Adrenocorticosteroids***

G. Nonopioid analgesics and antipyretics

1. ***Overview***
   a. **Aspirin, NSAIDs,** and **acetaminophen** are useful for the treatment of mild-to-moderate pain associated with integumental structures, including **pain of muscles and joints, postpartum pain,** and **headache.**
   b. These agents have **antipyretic activity** and, **except for acetaminophen,** have anti-inflammatory activity at higher doses.
   c. These agents act by an unknown mechanism to reduce pain and temperature. Their peripherally mediated analgesic activity and centrally mediated antipyretic activity are correlated with the inhibition of prostaglandin synthesis.
2. ***Acetaminophen***
   a. Unlike aspirin and other NSAIDs, acetaminophen does not displace other drugs from plasma proteins; it causes minimal gastric irritation, has little effect on platelet adhesion and aggregation, and does not block the effect of uricosuric drugs on uric acid secretion.
   b. Acetaminophen has no significant anti-inflammatory or antiuricosuric activity.
   c. Acetaminophen is administered orally and is rapidly absorbed. It is metabolized by hepatic microsomal enzymes to sulfate and glucuronide.
   d. Acetaminophen is a **substitute for aspirin** to treat mild-to-moderate pain for selected patients who are intolerant to aspirin, have a history of peptic ulcer or hemophilia, are using anticoagulants or a uricosuric drug to manage gout, or are at risk for Reye syndrome. Acetaminophen can be administered in pregnancy with greater safety than aspirin.
   e. Overdose with acetaminophen results in accumulation of a minor metabolite, *N*-acetyl-*p*-benzoquinone, which is responsible for hepatotoxicity. When the enzymes for glucuronide and sulfate conjugation of acetaminophen and the reactive metabolite become saturated, an alternative glutathione conjugation pathway (cytochrome P-450 dependent) becomes more important. If hepatic glutathione is depleted, the reactive metabolite accumulates and may cause hepatic damage by interaction with cellular macromolecules, such as DNA and RNA. Overdose is treated by emesis or gastric lavage and oral administration of ***N*-acetylcysteine** within 1 day to neutralize the metabolite.

table 6-5 Selected Disease-Modifying Antiarthritic Drugs

Drug	Characteristic	Molecular Target	Use
Adalimumab	Anti-TNF-α antibody	Plasma & tissue TNF-α	Rheumatoid arthritis
Infiximab	Anti-TNF-α antibody	Plasma & tissue TNF-α	Rheumatoid arthritis, Crohn disease, uveitis, psoriasis
Etanercept	TNF-receptor fusion protein	Plasma & tissue TNF-α	Rheumatoid arthritis, psoriasis
Anakinra	Recombinant IL-1a	Interleukin-1	Rheumatoid arthritis
Abatacept	Anti CD80/CD86 antibody	T cells	Rheumatoid arthritis

f. Long-term use of acetaminophen has been associated with a three-fold increase in kidney disease; and women taking more than 500 mg/day had a doubling in the incidence of hypertension.

H. Disease-modifying antiarthritic drugs (DMAARDs)

1. ***Tumor necrosis factor (TNF)*** plays an important causative role in rheumatoid arthritis, and this has led to development of drugs that specifically target this ligand or its receptor to treat the disease. TNF-α is responsible for inducing IL-1 and IL-6 and other cytokines that further the disease.
2. ***Anti-TNF-a drugs*** (Table 6-5)
   - **a. Infiximab** (Remicade) is a recombinant antibody with human constant and murine variable regions that specifically binds TNF-α, thereby blocking its action.
     - **(1)** Approved for use for rheumatoid arthritis, Crohn disease, psoriasis, and other autoimmune diseases
     - **(2)** Administered by IV infusion at 2-week intervals initially and repeated at 6 and 8 weeks
   - **b. Adalimumab** (Humira) is approved for the treatment of rheumatoid arthritis. It is a humanized (no murine components) anti-TNF-α antibody administered subcutaneously every other week.
   - **c. Etanercept** (Enbrel) is a fusion protein composed of the ligand-binding pocket of a TNF-α receptor fused to an IgG1 Fc fragment. The fusion protein has two TNF-binding sites per IgG molecule and is administered subcutaneously weekly.
   - **d.** The most serious adverse effect is **infection** including tuberculosis, immunogenicity, and lymphoma. Injection site infections are common.
3. ***Anti IL-1 drugs.*** **Anakinra** (Kineret) is a recombinant protein essentially identical to IL-1a, a soluble antagonist of IL-1 that binds to the IL-1 receptor but does not trigger a biologic response. Anakinra is a competitive antagonist of the IL-1 receptor. It is approved for use for the treatment of rheumatoid arthritis. It has a relatively short half-life and must be administered subcutaneously daily.

I. Other Immunosuppressive Biologicals

1. **Alefacept (Amevive)**
   - **a.** Alefacept is a recombinant fusion protein composed of the extracellular domain of LFA-3 and a portion of human IgG heavy chain. This protein acts as an antagonist of the LFA-3/CD2 interaction and causes a marked decrease in the number of CD2 T cells.
   - **b.** Alefacept is administered IV or IM.
   - **c.** Treatment with alefacept has demonstrated a rapid improvement and lessening of the severity of **psoriasis**, a disease with an autoimmune component.
2. **Rituximab (Rituxan)**
   - **a.** Rituximab is an engineered monoclonal antibody to **CD20**, a B-lymphocyte differentiation antigen on pre-B and mature B-lymphocytes. Rituximab binding to the surface of B-cells results in their destruction.
   - **b.** Rituximab, in combination with methotrexate, is approved for use in rheumatoid arthritis unresponsive to other therapies. It is also approved for treating refractory or large B-cell non-Hodgkin lymphoma.

3. **Abatacept** (Orencia)
   a. T-cell activation requires co-stimulation by an antigen presenting cell. **Abatacept blocks the co-stimulatory signal.** It is a fusion protein consisting of a portion of human CTLA4 and a fragment of the Fc domain of human IgG1. Abatacept mimics endogenous CTLA4 and competes with CD28 for CD80 and CD86 binding. This prevents complete T-cell activation, reduces T-cell proliferation, and reduces plasma cytokine levels.
   b. **Abatacept** is approved for use in rheumatoid arthritis.
   c. The most common side effect with its use is **infection.**
4. **Efalizumab** (Raptiva)
   a. **Efalizumab** is a monoclonal antibody that binds to CD11a of T cells. A component of T-cell activation is an interaction of CD-11a with ICAM-1. Efalizumab binding to T cells prevents their activation without their destruction.
   b. Efalizumab has proven effective in treating psoriasis. Its most adverse effects are nausea, headache, chills, and fever.

VI. DRUGS USED FOR GOUT

A. Gout
1. Gout is a familial disease characterized by recurrent hyperuricemia and arthritis with severe pain; it is caused by **deposits of uric acid** (the end-product of purine metabolism) in joints, cartilage, and the kidney.
2. Acute gout is treated with nonsalicylate NSAIDs, particularly **indomethacin,** or with **colchicine.**
3. Chronic gout is treated with the uricosuric agent **probenecid** or **sulfinpyrazone,** which increases the elimination of uric acid, or **allopurinol,** which inhibits uric acid production.

B. Colchicine
1. Colchicine is an alkaloid with anti-inflammatory properties; it is used for relief of inflammation and pain in **acute gouty arthritis.** Reduction of inflammation and relief from pain occur 12–24 hours after oral administration.
2. The mechanism of action in acute gout is unclear. Colchicine prevents polymerization of tubulin into microtubules and inhibits leukocyte migration and phagocytosis. Colchicine also inhibits cell mitosis.
3. The adverse effects after oral administration, which occur in 80% of patients at a dose near that necessary to relieve gout, include **nausea, vomiting, abdominal pain,** and particularly **diarrhea.** IV administration reduces the risk of GI disturbances and provides faster relief (6–12 h) but increases the risk of sloughing skin and subcutaneous tissue. Higher doses may (rarely) result in liver damage and blood dyscrasias.

C. NSAIDs
1. Historically, **indomethacin** has been the NSAID most often used to treat **acute gout** attacks; however, because they have fewer adverse effects, the use of **naproxen** and **sulindac** is increasing.
2. NSAIDs are preferred to the more disease-specific colchicine because of the diarrhea associated with the use of colchicine.

D. Probenecid
1. Probenecid is an organic acid that reduces urate levels by acting at the anionic transport site in the renal tubule to prevent reabsorption of uric acid.
2. These agents are used for **chronic gout,** often in combination with **colchicine.**
3. Probenecid and sulfinpyrazone undergo rapid oral absorption.
4. These agents inhibit the excretion of other drugs that are actively secreted by renal tubules, including **penicillin,** NSAIDs, cephalosporins, and **methotrexate.** Dose reduction of these drugs may be warranted.

5. Increased urinary concentration of uric acid may result in the formation of urate stones (**urolithiasis**). This risk is decreased with the ingestion of large volumes of fluid or alkalinization of urine with potassium citrate.
6. Low doses of uricosuric agents and salicylates inhibit uric acid secretion. Aspirin is contraindicated in gout.
7. Common adverse effects include **GI disturbances** and **dermatitis;** rarely, these agents cause blood dyscrasias.

E. Allopurinol (Lopurin, Zyloprim)

1. Allopurinol is used to treat **chronic, tophaceous gout** because it reduces the size of the established tophi; **colchicine** is administered concomitantly during the first week of therapy to prevent gouty arthritis.
2. Allopurinol inhibits the synthesis of uric acid by inhibiting **xanthine oxidase,** an enzyme that converts hypoxanthine to xanthine and xanthine to uric acid. Allopurinol is metabolized by xanthine oxidase to alloxanthine, which also inhibits xanthine oxidase. Allopurinol also inhibits de novo purine synthesis.
3. Allopurinol commonly produces **GI disturbances** and **dermatitis.** This agent more rarely causes hypersensitivity, including fever, hepatic dysfunction, and blood dyscrasias. Allopurinol should be used with caution in patients with liver disease or bone marrow depression.

VII. IMMUNOSUPPRESSIVE AGENTS

A. Inhibition of immune response

1. ***Nonspecific inhibition.*** **Azathioprine, cyclophosphamide,** and **methotrexate** suppress immune function by their cytotoxic action achieved through a variety of mechanisms, particularly by inhibition of DNA synthesis. Generally, immunosuppressive activity is achieved at nearly toxic doses.
2. ***Specific inhibition*** (Fig. 6-4). **Glucocorticoids, cyclosporine, tacrolimus** (Prograf), and sirolimus (rapamycin) (Rapamune) inhibit the activation or actions of specific cells of the immune system and are generally less toxic than the nonspecific agents.
3. ***Suppression*** of the immune system increases the risk of opportunistic viral, bacterial, and fungal infections.
4. ***Development of tolerance.*** To overcome an allergic reaction, small quantities of antigen are administered gradually to develop tolerance, most probably as a result of the induction of IgG antibodies to neutralize a subsequent IgE reaction with the allergen.

B. Use of immunosuppressive agents

1. Immunosuppressive agents are used to treat syndromes or diseases that reflect **imbalances in the immune system,** including rheumatoid arthritis, systemic lupus erythematosus, inflammatory bowel disease, chronic active hepatitis, lipoid nephrosis, Goodpasture syndrome, and autoimmune hemolytic anemia.
2. Immunosuppressive agents are also used to **prevent allograft rejection,** which results when cytotoxic T lymphocytes develop in response to incompatible transplanted organs.

C. Individual agents

1. ***Glucocorticoids***
   a. Glucocorticoids are thought to interfere with the cell cycle of activated lymphoid cells and stimulate apoptosis in some lymphoid lineages.
   b. Glucocorticoids are used for a wide variety of immunologically mediated diseases.
   c. Glucocorticoids are important agents in suppressing allograft rejection; they are often used in **combination** with either **cyclosporine** or a cytotoxic agent.
2. ***Cyclosporine (Sandimmune, Neoral)***
   a. Cyclosporine is a potent immunosuppressive cyclic polypeptide that binds to cyclophilin and inhibits T-helper cell activation, mostly by inhibiting transport to the nucleus of the

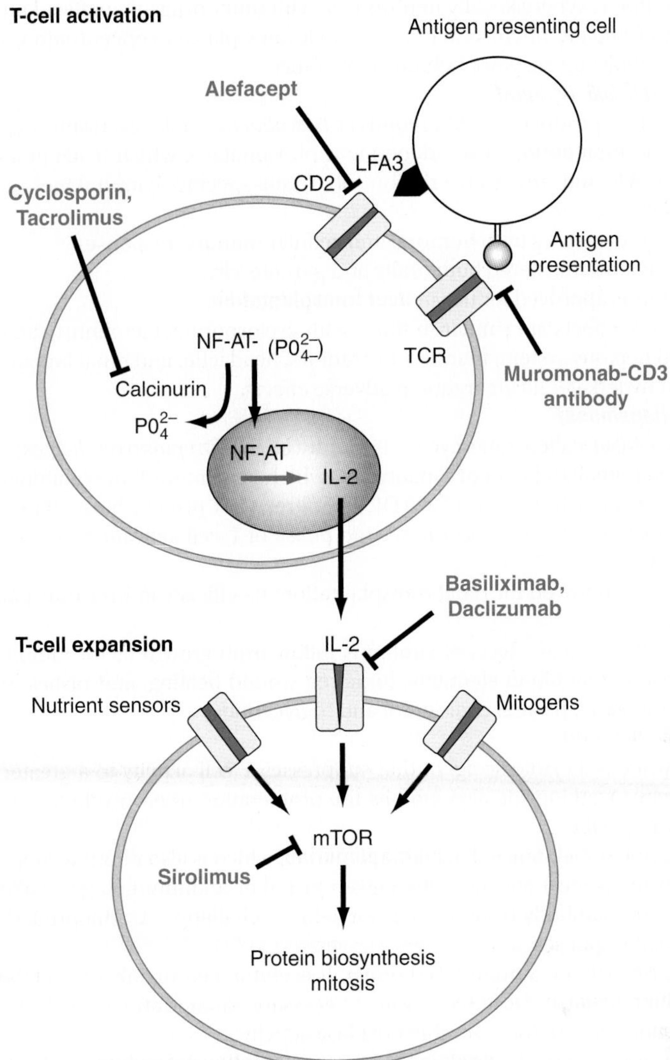

FIGURE 6-4. Sites of action of immunomodulators.

transcription factor NF-AT and subsequently the production of interleukin-2 and the first phase of T-cell activation.

b. Cyclosporine has variable absorption from the GI tract (20%–50%). Doses must be established by monitoring the blood levels. Cyclosporine has a biphasic $t_{1/2}$, with a terminal phase of 10–25 hours; it is metabolized in the liver and eliminated primarily in bile.

c. Cyclosporine is most often administered IV; a microemulsion (Neoral) permits oral dosing but still requires careful blood monitoring.

d. The main use of cyclosporine is in **short- and long-term suppression of organ rejection in transplants** of the kidney, liver, and heart. It is generally used in combination with glucocorticoids.

e. **Cyclosporine as an ophthalmic emulsion** (Restasis) is used to increase tear production in patients with ocular inflammation associated with keratoconjunctivitis sicca.

f. Cyclosporine causes **nephrotoxicity** in 25%–75% of patients, with a reduction in glomerular filtration and renal plasma flow; **hypertension** in 30% of patients; **neurotoxicity** (tremor and seizures) in 5%–50% of patients; and **hirsutism** and **gingival hyperplasia** in 10%–30% of patients.

g. Cyclosporine is synergistically nephrotoxic with other drugs that affect kidney function. Inhibition of hepatic microsomal enzymes elevates plasma concentration; the induction of drug-metabolizing enzymes enhances clearance.

3. *Tacrolimus (FK-506) (Prograf)*

a. Tacrolimus is produced by *Streptomyces tsukubaensis.* Like cyclosporine, it decreases the activity of **calcineurin,** a Ca^{2+}-dependent phosphatase, which leads to a decrease in nuclear NF-AT and the transcription of T-cell–specific lymphokines and early T-cell activation.

b. Tacrolimus decreases both humoral and cellular immune responses.

c. This agent is administered both orally and parenterally.

d. Tacrolimus is approved for use in **liver transplantation.**

e. The adverse effects are similar to those with cyclosporine; tacrolimus can damage the kidneys and nervous system, manifest by tremors, headache, and renal impairment. Hypertension and hyperkalemia are frequent adverse effects.

4. *Sirolimus (Rapamune)*

a. Sirolimus (also called rapamycin) is produced by *Streptomyces hygroscopius.* It inhibits mTOR (mammalian target of rapamycin), which is an important component of several signaling pathways. Inhibition of mTOR interferes with protein biosynthesis and delays the G1-S transition, which blocks the second phase of T-cell activation; B-cell differentiation is also inhibited.

b. Sirolimus is approved for renal transplantation; its efficacy in liver transplant has not been determined.

c. Many of the adverse effects of sirolimus follow from growth factor inhibition and include suppression of all blood elements, impaired wound healing, and rashes; metabolic effects include increased plasma cholesterol and triglycerides.

5. *Azathioprine (Imuran)*

a. Azathioprine is a cytotoxic agent that suppresses T-cell activity to a greater degree than B-cell activity. Azathioprine also inhibits the proliferation of promyelocytes in the marrow. It is S-phase specific.

b. Azathioprine is metabolized to **mercaptopurine,** which is also immunosuppressive.

c. Azathioprine is most effective when given just after an immunologic challenge. This agent may enhance antibody response if given before a challenge. Azathioprine is not effective on established responses.

d. Azathioprine can be administered orally. It is eliminated mainly by metabolic degradation by **xanthine oxidase.** Dose reduction is necessary when azathioprine is administered with **allopurinol,** which reduces xanthine oxidase activity.

e. Azathioprine is used with **prednisone** in **transplantation procedures** and in some diseases of the immune system, including **systemic lupus erythematosus** and **rheumatoid arthritis.**

f. The major adverse effect associated with this agent is bone marrow suppression. At higher doses, occasional nausea and vomiting, GI disturbances, and hepatic dysfunction occur.

6. *Cyclophosphamide (Cytoxan, Neosar)*

a. Cyclophosphamide is an alkylating agent developed as an anticancer drug.

b. Cyclophosphamide suppresses B lymphocytes to a greater degree than T cells.

c. This agent is the drug of choice in the treatment of **Wegener granulomatosis;** it is also used in severe cases of **rheumatoid arthritis** and other autoimmune disorders.

d. Cyclophosphamide causes adverse effects that include cystitis and cardiomyopathy.

7. *Methotrexate (Folex, Mexate)*

a. Methotrexate is an anticancer agent that has immunosuppressive action.

b. Methotrexate inhibits replication and function of T cells and possibly B cells.

c. Methotrexate has been used for **graft rejection** and for autoimmune and inflammatory diseases.

d. This agent has also proved beneficial in the treatment of **severe psoriasis** that is refractory to other agents.

e. **Hepatotoxicity** is the major adverse effect.

8. *Immunosuppressive antibody reagents*

a. Antithymocyte globulin (Atgam)

(1) Polygonal antibodies raised against human thymic lymphocytes

(2) Following intravenous administration, T lymphocytes are removed from the circulation, resulting in decreased T-cell–mediated immune response.
(3) Used to treat allograft rejection and to prevent rejection
(4) Adverse effects include serum sickness and nephritis

b. ***Muromonab-cd3 antibody (Orthoclone OKT3)***
(1) Monoclonal antibodies that recognize the CD3 surface glycoprotein on T lymphocytes
(2) Attachment of antibodies to CD3 impairs antigen recognition by T cells.
(3) Following IV administration, T-cell levels fall rapidly and immune responses are impaired.
(4) Used to prevent acute allograft rejection
(5) Adverse effects include cytokine release syndrome, anaphylactoid reactions, and CNS toxicity.

c. ***Basiliximab (Simulect) and daclizumab (Zenopax)***
(1) Both are monoclonal antibodies against CD25, one of the subunits of the IL-2 receptor.
(2) Both reduce the incidence and the severity of renal transplant rejection, but they cannot be used to treat acute rejection.
(3) Side effects include shortness of breath, hypersensitivity reactions including itching and rash, and infections.

DRUG SUMMARY TABLE

Histamine H_1-receptor antagonists
Chlorpheniramine (generic)
Brompheniramine (generic)
Diphenhydramine (Benadryl, Compose, generic)
Doxylamine (Unisom, generic)
Clemastine (Tavist, Contact-D, others)
Dimenhydrinate (Dramamine, others)
Pyrilamine (generic)
Antazoline (Vasocon-A)
Meclizine (Antivert, others)
Cyclizine (Marezine)
Promethazine (Phenergan, others)
Cyproheptadine (Periactin)
Loratadine (Claritin)
Desloratadine (Clarinex)
Fexophenadine (Allegra)
Acrivastine (Semprex-D)
Cetirizine (Zyrtec)
Levocitirizine (Xyzal)

Chromones
Cromolyn (Intal)
Nedocromil sodium (Tilade)

Ergots
Methysergide (Sansert)
Methylergonovine (Methergine)
Ergotamine (Ergomar, Ergostat)
Dihydroergotamine (Migranol)
Bromocriptine (Parlodel)
Pergolide (Permax)

Eicosanoids
Carboprost tromethamine (Hemabate)
Dinoprostone (Prostin E)
Misoprostol (Cytotec)
Prostaglandin E_1 (Caverject)

Nonsteroidal Analgesics
Acetaminophen (generic)

Gold Salts
Aurothioglucose (Solganal)
Gold sodium thiomalate (Myochrysine)
Auranofin (Ridaura)

Other Anti-RA Drugs
Penicillamine (Cuprimine, Depen)
Methotrexate (Rheumatrex)
Chloroquine (Aralen)

DMAARDs
Infiximab (Remicade)
Adalimumab (Humira)
Etanercept (Enbrel)
Anakinra (Kineret)
Alefacept (Amevive)
Abatacept (Orencia)

Antigout Drugs
Probenecid (Benemid)
Allopurinol (Lopurin, Zyloprim)
Colchicine (generic)

Histamine H_2-receptor antagonists
Cimetidine (Tagamet)
Ranitidine (Zantac)
Famotidine (Pepcid AC)
Nizatidine (Axid)

Serotonin Receptor Agonists
Buspirone (BuSpar)
Sumatriptan (Imitrex)
Rizatriptan (Maxalt)
Eletriptan (Relpax)
Zolmitriptan (Zomig)
Almotriptan (Axert)
Frovatriptan (Frova)
Naratriptan (Amerge)
Trazodone (Desyrel)
Tegaserod (Zelnorm)

Serotonin-Receptor Antagonists
Cyproheptadine (Periactin)
Ondansetron (Zofran)
Granisetron (Kytril)
Dolasetron (Anzemet)
Palonosetron (Aloxi)
Clozapine (Clozaril)
Risperidone (Risperdal)

NSAIDs
Acetylsalicylic acid
Magnesium salicylate (Tricosal)
Sulfasalazine (Azulfidine)
Mesalamine (Asacol)
Salsalate (Amigesic, generic)
Ibuprofen (Advil, Motrin, generic)
Naproxen (Aleve, generic)
Fenoprofen (Nalfon)
Ketoprofen (Orudis)
Sulindac (Clinoril)
Tolmetin (Tolectin)
Ketoralac (Toradol)
Indomethacin (Indocin)
Piroxicam (Feldene)
Meclofenamate (Meclomen)
Mefenamic acid (Ponstel)
Nabumetone (Relafen)
Flurbiprofen (generic)
Diclofenac (Voltaren)
Etodolac (Lodine)
Celecoxib (Celebrex)

Immunosuppressive Drugs
Azathioprine (Imuran)
Cyclophosphamide (Cytoxan, Neosar)
Methotrexate (Folex, Mexate)
Cyclosporine (Sandimmune, Neoral)
Tacrolimus (FK-506) (Prograf)
Sirolimus (Rapamune)
Antithymocyte globulin (Atgam)
Muromonab-cd3 antibody (Orthoclone OKT3)
Basiliximab (Simulect)
Daclizumab (Zenopax)

Review Test for Chapter 6

Directions: Each of the numbered items or incomplete statements in this section is followed by answers or by completions of the statement. Select the ONE lettered answer or completion that is BEST in each case.

1. A long-haul truck driver comes into your asthma clinic complaining that he is sneezing constantly and has burning and watery eyes. He indicates that he seems to have a month or so of these symptoms every spring. Which of the following drugs would be most appropriate to treat this patient?

(A) Dimenhydrinate
(B) Scopolamine
(C) Fexofenadine
(D) Cetirizine

2. Following a prolonged first labor, an alert nurse notices persistent bleeding in the postpartum patient with no vaginal or cervical laceration, and her uterine fundus feels very soft. The patient's heart rate is mildly elevated, and her blood pressure is 105/55 mm Hg. Which of the following would be the best choice in this circumstance?

(A) Acetaminophen
(B) Buspirone
(C) Methylergonovine
(D) Methysergide

3. A 24-year old woman has a history of migraine headaches with accompanying aura. During her last attack, ergotamine was much less effective, and you decide to try an alternative to treat her current attack. Agonist activity at which of the following receptors would be the best target for your new treatment?

(A) Histamine H_1
(B) α-Adrenoreceptors
(C) Serotonin 5-HT_{1B}
(D) Prostaglandin FP

4. An elderly patient has a history of taking both prescription medications and over-the-counter (OTC) "pain killers" for her rheumatoid arthritis. She is not diabetic and has no history of kidney disease. She is admitted into your clinic in acute renal failure and comments that the pain in her hands has become much worse in the last week. Which of the following drugs is most likely responsible for the adverse renal effect?

(A) Ibuprofen
(B) Prednisone
(C) Colchicine
(D) Probenecid

5. A neonate is identified as having atrial septal defect of congenital origin that will require surgical repair. Adequate systemic perfusion requires that the patency of the ductus arteriosus be maintained. Which of the following agents would best accomplish this goal?

(A) Indomethacin
(B) PGE_1
(C) PGI_2
(D) celecoxib

6. A 24-year-old student has been taking over-the-counter (OTC) diphenhydramine for her allergy symptoms most of her life. Lately, however, she has had more frequent symptoms, so she increased the dose of the medication. She now asks her friend, who is a medical student, to explain to her how exactly this agent makes her more sleepy lately. What is the most likely answer regarding diphenhydramine?

(A) It blocks H_1-receptors in the brain
(B) It modulates the release of dopamine and serotonin
(C) It acts peripherally, since it does not cross the blood–brain barrier
(D) It exerts its effects via muscarinic–cholinergic agonist activity
(E) It contains tryptophan, which produces sedation

7. A 35-year-old man presents to his doctor with complaints of epigastric pain. He explains that he has been taking aspirin for many years for pain related to his low back injury. The doctor suspects gastritis and prescribes a trial of medication that might be helpful to this patient.

What medication did the physician most likely prescribe?

(A) Doxylamine
(B) Desloratadine
(C) Cetrizine
(D) Famotidine
(E) Buspirone

8. A 30-year-old woman has suffered from cyclical migraines for many years. She now presents to her physician asking for a medication designated specifically for migraines, not just a general pain reliever. Her physician decided to prescribe sumatriptan as a trial medication. The patient, who is a biochemist, would like to know how this medication works.

(A) It is a 5-HT_{1A} agonist
(B) It is a 5-HT_{1D} agonist
(C) It blocks reuptake of serotonin
(D) It is a 5-HT_3 antagonist
(E) It is a 5-HT_{2A} antagonist

9. A 35-year-old woman presents to her physician with a chief complaint of headaches. She states that her symptoms started several months ago and most recently have been associated with occasional vomiting. She also complains of milky discharge from her breasts and lack of menstruation in the last 3 months. Her physician orders a brain a magnetic resonance imaging (MRI) scan, and the patient is diagnosed with a large pituitary adenoma. Which medication would most likely benefit this patient if she is deemed not a good operative candidate?

(A) Methysergide
(B) Bromocriptine
(C) Ergotamine
(D) Aprotinin
(E) Allopurinol

10. A 24-year-old woman who is 42 weeks pregnant is admitted to the labor and delivery ward for induction of labor. A fetal heart monitor shows that the fetus is currently in no acute distress. Sterile examination shows the patient to be minimally dilated without significant effacement. She is given carboprost. Which eicosanoid does this medication represent?

(A) PGG
(B) TXA_2
(C) PGF_{2a}
(D) PGE_1
(E) PGH

11. A 70-year-old man suffers a myocardial infarction (MI). He is admitted to the cardiac intensive care unit and is given aspirin and a β-blocker. A catheterization procedure is scheduled. The patient's wife, who is a pharmacy technician, wants to know why the patient is being given aspirin and not another nonsteroidal anti-inflammatory drug (NSAID). What is the best answer to this question?

(A) Aspirin inhibits both COX-1 and COX-2
(B) Aspirin irreversibly binds to its binding site on the enzyme
(C) Aspirin is a weak acid
(D) Aspirin is excreted by the kidneys
(E) Aspirin has much greater antithrombotic activity

Answers and Explanations

1. **The answer is C.** Fexofenadine is a potent histamine H_1-receptor antagonist; its poor central nervous system (CNS) penetration reduces sedative effects. Cetirizine is a second-generation antihistamine, but it still has some sedating effects. Ranitidine is a histamine H_2-receptor antagonist.

2. **The answer is C.** Methylergonovine produces powerful contraction of uterine smooth muscle that can reduce postpartum bleeding. The other agents also interact with serotonin receptors but would not be effective in this case.

3. **The answer is C.** The "triptans" as a class are effective against acute migraine attacks and all act as agonists at serotonin 5-HT_{1B} and HT_{1D} receptors. Agonists at α-adrenergic receptors like epinephrine cause vasoconstriction but are not effective for migraine; antihistamines and agents that interfere with the prostaglandin FP receptor would not be effective either.

4. **The answer is A.** NSAIDs as a class are associated with renal toxicity. Prednisone is effective in alleviating the inflammation in rheumatoid arthritis but is not associated with adverse renal effects. Colchicine and probenecid are used to treat gout, not rheumatoid arthritis.

5. **The answer is B.** E-series prostaglandins are responsible for maintenance of the ductus. Inhibitors of prostaglandin biosynthesis, indomethacin and celecoxib, cause closure of the ductus.

6. **The answer is A.** Diphenhydramine blocks H_1-receptors in the brain, thereby producing sedation. The release of dopamine and serotonin is modulated via H_3-receptors. Diphenhydramine readily crosses the blood–brain barrier. This agent has muscarinic–cholinergic agonist properties. It is not known to contain tryptophan.

7. **The answer is D.** Famotidine is an H_2-blocker that is used for symptoms of gastritis. Doxylamine is an H_1-blocker that is used as a sleep aid. Desloratadine is an H_1-blocker that is used for allergy symptoms. Cetrizine is used for allergy symptoms as well. Buspirone is a serotonin agonist that is prescribed for anxiety.

8. **The answer is B.** Sumatriptan is a 5-HT_{1D} agonist. An example of an agent known as a 5-HT_{1A} agonist would be buspirone, an antianxiety agent. Fluoxetine is an example of a serotonin-reuptake inhibitor. Ondansetron, an antinausea medication, is a 5-HT_3 antagonist. The antipsychotic medication Risperdal is an example of a 5-HT_{2A} antagonist.

9. **The answer is B.** Bromocriptine is a dopaminergic agonist used to treat hyperprolactinemia, as with pituitary adenomas, or for suppression of normal lactation. It is also used for management of Parkinson disease. Methysergide is used for prophylaxis of migraine headaches. Ergotamine is used to treat acute migraine attacks. Aprotinin is used in cardiac surgery to reduce the amount of blood transfusions. Allopurinol is used to treat gout.

10. **The answer is C.** Carboprost tromethamine is used for induction of labor; it is a PGF_{2a} analog. PGG and PGH are prostaglandins that are inhibited by nonsteroidal anti-inflammatory drugs (NSAIDs). TXA_2 is a potent inducer of platelet aggregation. PGE_1 is used for maintenance of patency of ductus arteriosus.

11. **The answer is E.** Aspirin has a much greater antithrombotic activity than other nonsteroidal anti-inflammatory drugs (NSAIDs), which is why this agent is used for prevention of myocardial infarction (MI) in patients with a history of MI, angina, or cardiac surgery. Aspirin inhibits both COX-1 and COX-2; however, so do most other NSAIDs. Aspirin does not bind to COX but causes it to be covalently modified. Aspirin is a weak acid and is excreted by the kidneys; however, they are not the reason why aspirin is preferred over other NSAIDs in the setting of prevention of MI.

chapter 7

Drugs Used in Anemia and Disorders of Hemostasis

I. DRUGS USED IN THE TREATMENT OF ANEMIAS

A. Iron deficiency anemias

1. ***Iron***
   a. **Structure and storage of iron (Fig. 7-1)**
      (1) Iron is an integral component of heme. Approximately 70% of total body iron is found in hemoglobin. Heme iron is also an essential component of muscle myoglobin and of several enzymes, such as catalase, peroxidase, the cytochromes, and others.
      (2) Iron is stored in reticuloendothelial cells, hepatocytes, and intestinal cells as ferritin (a particle with a ferric hydroxide core and a surface layer of the protein apoferritin) and hemosiderin (aggregates of ferritin–apoferritin).
   b. **Absorption and transport**
      (1) Heme iron is much more readily absorbed across the intestine than inorganic iron.
      (2) Inorganic iron in the ferrous state (Fe^{2+}) is much more readily absorbed than that in the ferric state (Fe^{3+}); gastric acid and ascorbic acid promote the absorption of ferrous iron.
      (3) Iron is actively transported across the intestinal cell; it is then oxidized to ferric iron and stored as ferritin or transported to other tissues.
      (4) Iron is transported in the plasma bound to the glycoprotein transferrin; specific cell-surface receptors bind the transferrin–iron complex, and the iron is delivered to the recipient cell by endocytosis.
   c. **Regulation**
      (1) Except for menstruation and bleeding disorders, very little iron is lost from the body, and no mechanism exists for increasing excretion. Therefore, iron storage is regulated at the level of absorption.
      (2) When plasma iron concentrations are low, the number of transferrin receptors is increased, facilitating cellular absorption, and ferritin synthesis is decreased, reducing tissue iron storage.
      (3) When iron stores are high, intestinal absorption decreases; synthesis of transferrin receptors also decreases, inhibiting additional cellular uptake, and ferritin synthesis is increased.
2. ***Causes of iron deficiency anemia***
   a. **Bleeding** (approximately 30 mg of iron are lost in a normal menstrual cycle)
   b. Dietary deficiencies
   c. Malabsorption syndromes
   d. Increased iron demands such as pregnancy or lactation
3. ***Iron salt supplements***
   a. **Oral agents**
      (1) Several ferrous iron salts are available for oral use. All are essentially equivalent therapeutically if doses are adjusted according to iron content (gluconate, sulfate, and fumarate forms are 12%, 20%, and 33% iron by weight, respectively; a polysaccharide–iron complex is also available).

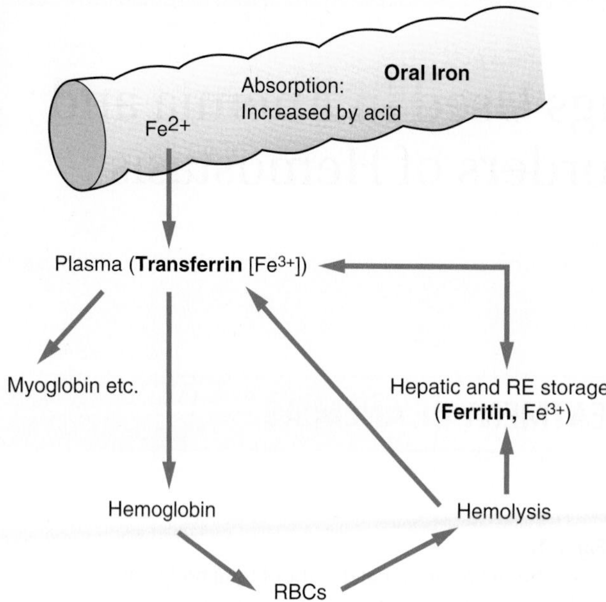

FIGURE 7-1. Absorption and circulation of iron within the body.

(2) Approximately 25% of orally administered iron is absorbed; a typical daily dose is 100–200 mg iron/day.

(3) Oral iron treatment may require 3–6 months to replenish body stores.

b. **Parenteral agents**

(1) A colloidal suspension of ferrous hydroxide and dextran can be administered by intravenous (IV) infusion or intramuscular injection.

(2) Parenteral agents may be useful in patients with iron absorption disorders caused by inflammatory bowel disease, small-bowel resection, gastrectomy, or hereditary absorption defects.

(3) Parenteral agents are indicated for patients with hypersensitivity reactions to oral iron salts.

(4) These agents are useful in severe anemic conditions in which rapid correction of iron deficiency is desired.

(5) Parenteral agents may be used to reduce toxic reactions on initiation of erythropoietin (epoetin alfa) therapy in patients with renal disease.

c. **Adverse and toxic effects**

(1) Iron salt supplements produce gastrointestinal (GI) upset (nausea, cramps, constipation, diarrhea).

(2) These supplements may cause hypersensitivity reactions (most common with parenteral administration), including bronchospasm, urticaria, and anaphylaxis.

(3) Fatal overdose (1–10 g) is possible; children are especially susceptible. Deferoxamine (Desferal), an iron-chelating agent, is used to treat iron toxicity. Administered systematically or by gastric lavage, deferoxamine binds iron and promotes excretion.

B. Red cell deficiency anemias

1. Red cell deficiency anemias are most commonly treated with erythropoesis-stimulating agents (ESAs).

2. ***Erythropoietin (EPO) (Epogen)***

a. **Properties**

(1) EPO is a glycoprotein produced mostly (90%) by the peritubular cells in the kidney; EPO is essential for normal reticulocyte production.

(2) Synthesis of EPO is stimulated by hypoxia.

(3) Erythropoietin is available as recombinant human EPO, **epoetin alfa, and darbepoetin. Darbepoeitin** is a second-generation ESA with a half-life about twice that of epoetin alfa. Administered parenterally (IV or subcutaneously).

b. **Mechanism of action**

(1) EPO increases the rate of proliferation and differentiation of erythroid precursor cells in the bone marrow.

(2) EPO induces the transformation of the most mature erythroid progenitor cell, erythroid colony-forming unit (CFU-E), to a proerythroblast.

(3) EPO increases the release of reticulocytes from marrow.

(4) EPO increases hemoglobin synthesis.

(5) The action of EPO requires adequate stores of iron.

c. **Therapeutic uses.** EPO is used to treat anemia in the following patients: acquired immune deficiency syndrome (**AIDS**) **patients** treated with zidovudine **(AZT)**, cancer patients undergoing **chemotherapy,** and patients in **renal failure;** all of these conditions and treatments produce anemia. EPO is also used in surgical patients to reduce the need for transfusions.

d. **Adverse and toxic effects** of EPO include hypertension, seizures, and headache probably caused by rapid expansion of blood volume. ESAs have been shown to increase the risk of death and serious cardiovascular events, both arterial and venous thromboembolic events including myocardial infarction (MI), stroke, congestive heart failure, and hemodialysis graft occlusion, when administered to target a hemoglobin concentration >12 g/dl.

C. Sideroblastic anemias

1. Sideroblastic anemias are characterized by decreased hemoglobin synthesis and intracellular accumulation of iron in erythroid precursor cells.
2. Sideroblastic anemias are often caused by agents that antagonize or deplete pyridoxal phosphate.
3. Sideroblastic anemias are sometimes seen in alcoholics, in patients undergoing antituberculin therapy with isoniazid and pyrazinamide, and in certain inflammatory and malignant disorders.
4. **Hereditary sideroblastic anemia** is an X-linked trait.
5. Sideroblastic anemia is treated with **pyridoxine** (vitamin B_6) administered orally (preferred route) or parenterally. Pyridoxine has variable efficacy with inherited forms of the disease.

D. Vitamin deficiency (megaloblastic) anemias

1. ***Vitamin B_{12}***

a. **Structure**

(1) Vitamin B_{12} is a complex, cobalt-containing molecule. Various groups are covalently linked to the cobalt atom, forming the cobalamins. The endogenous cobalamins in humans are methylcobalamin and 5-deoxyadenosylcobalamin.

(a) **Methylcobalamin** is a coenzyme essential for the production of methionine and *S*-adenosylmethionine from homocysteine and for the production of tetrahydrofolate from methyltetrahydrofolate.

(b) **Deoxyadenosylcobalamin** participates in the mitochondrial reaction that produces succinyl-CoA from methylmalonyl-CoA; vitamin B_{12} deficiency leads to the production of abnormal fatty acids.

(2) For pharmacologic use, vitamin B_{12} is supplied as the stable derivatives cyanocobalamin or hydroxocobalamin (AlphaRedisol).

b. **Transport and absorption**

(1) In the stomach, dietary vitamin B_{12} complexes with **intrinsic factor,** a peptide secreted by the parietal cells. The intrinsic factor–vitamin B_{12} complex is absorbed by active transport in the distal ileum.

(2) Vitamin B_{12} is transported in the plasma bound to the protein transcobalamin II and is taken up by and stored in hepatocytes.

c. **Actions and pharmacologic properties**

(1) Vitamin B_{12} is essential for normal DNA synthesis and fatty acid metabolism. A deficiency results in impaired DNA replication, which is most apparent in tissues that

are actively dividing, such as the GI tract and erythroid precursors. The appearance of large macrocytic (megaloblastic) red cells in the blood is characteristic of this deficiency. Vitamin B_{12} deficiency can also result in irreversible neurologic disorders.

(2) Vitamin B_{12}, along with vitamin B_6 and folic acid, participates in the metabolism of homocysteine to cysteine. Elevations in homocysteine are associated with accelerated atherosclerosis.

(3) Loss of vitamin B_{12} from the body is very slow (2 μg/day), and hepatic stores are sufficient for up to 5 years. Vitamin B_{12} is not synthesized by eukaryotic cells and is normally obtained from microbial synthesis.

(4) Parenteral administration of vitamin B_{12} is standard because the vast majority of situations requiring vitamin B_{12} replacement are due to malabsorption. Uncorrectable malabsorption requires life-long treatment.

(5) Improvement in hemoglobin concentration is apparent in 7 days and normalizes in 1–2 months.

d. Therapeutic uses

(1) Vitamin B_{12} is used to treat pernicious anemia (inadequate secretion of intrinsic factor with subsequent reduction in vitamin B_{12} absorption).

(2) Vitamin B_{12} is used after partial or total gastrectomy to mitigate the loss or reduction of intrinsic factor synthesis.

(3) Administration of vitamin B_{12} is used to replace vitamin B_{12} in deficiency caused by dysfunction of the distal ileum with defective or absent absorption of the intrinsic factor–vitamin B_{12} complex.

(4) Administration of vitamin B_{12} is necessary in patients with insufficient dietary intake of vitamin B_{12} (occasionally seen in strict vegetarians).

e. Adverse effects of vitamin B_{12} are uncommon, even at large doses. Hypokalemia and thrombocytosis can occur upon conversion of severe megaloblastic anemia to normal erythropoiesis with cyanocobalamin therapy.

2. *Folic acid (vitamin B_9) (Folacin, leucovorin)*

a. Folic acid is composed of three subunits: pteridine, *para*-aminobenzoic acid (PABA), and one to five glutamic acid residues.

(1) Folic acid typically occurs in the diet in a polyglutamate form that must be converted to the monoglutamyl form for absorption. Most folate is absorbed in the proximal portions of the small intestine and is transported to tissues bound to a plasma-binding protein. Folic acid requires reduction by dihydrofolate reductase to the active metabolite methyltetrahydrofolate.

(2) Leucovorin is a racemic mixture of the *d/l* stereoisomers of 5-formyltetrahydrofolic acid. It does not require metabolism by dihydrofolate reductase.

b. The cofactors of folic acid provide single carbon groups for transfer to various acceptors and are essential for the biosynthesis of purines and the pyrimidine **deoxythymidylate.** A deficiency in folic acid results in **impaired DNA synthesis;** mitotically active tissues such as erythroid tissues are markedly affected.

c. Catabolism and excretion of vitamin B_9 is more rapid than that of vitamin B_{12}; hepatic reserves are sufficient for only 1–3 months.

d. Folic acid and leucovorin are usually administered orally.

e. Folic acid is used to correct dietary insufficiency (commonly observed in the elderly), as a supplement during pregnancy to decrease the risk of neural tube defects, during lactation, and in cases of rapid cell turnover, such as hemolytic anemia. Leucovorin may be used to reverse the effects of the folate antagonists (see Chapter 12) methotrexate, pyrimethamine, and trimethoprim.

E. Sickle cell anemias

1. Hydroxyurea has been shown effective in reducing painful episodes by about 50%; the necessity of blood transfusions was also shown to be reduced. Hydroxyurea increases the production of **fetal hemoglobin,** which makes red cells resistant to sickling and reduces the expression of adhesion molecules such as L-selectin.

2. **Pentoxifylline** is a synthetic dimethylxanthine structurally similar to caffeine. The actions of pentoxifylline include increased erythrocyte flexibility and decreased blood viscosity. Pentoxifylline appears to inhibit erythrocyte phosphodiesterase, which causes an increase in erythrocyte cyclic adenosine 5′-monophosphate (cAMP) activity and an increase in membrane flexibility.

II. DRUGS ACTING ON MYELOID CELLS

A. **Myeloid growth factors** are glycoproteins produced by many cells including fibroblasts, endothelial cells, macrophages, and immune cells that act to stimulate proliferation and differentiation of one or more myeloid lineage.

1. ***Sargramostim (granulocyte–macrophage colony-stimulating factor, GM-CSF)***
   a. **Sargramostim** is a recombinant protein essentially identical to the native protein. Its principal action is to stimulate myelopoiesis in granulocyte–macrophage pathways as well as megakaryocytic and erythroid progenitor cells.
   b. **Clinical uses**
      (1) **Reduce the duration of neutropenia** and incidence of infection in patients receiving myelosuppressive chemotherapy or bone marrow transplantation
      (2) **Mobilize peripheral blood progenitor cells** prior to collection
      (3) **For bone marrow graft failure**
   c. Sargramostim is **administered IV,** and the most common adverse effects are **granulocytosis,** bone pain, fever, nausea, and rash.
2. ***Filgrastim, pegfilgrastin (granulocyte colony-stimulating factor, G-CSF)***
   a. Filgrastim is a recombinant protein that stimulates bone marrow production of neutrophils without increasing the number of basophils, eosinophils, or monocytes.
   b. Pegfilgrastin is filgrastin with a polypropylene glycol molecule added to the N-terminus.
   c. Its clinical uses are similar to those of sargramostim: reduction in the duration of neutropenia in patients on anticancer regimens and for patients with chronic severe neutropenia.
3. ***Oprelvekin (interleukin-11)***
   a. **Oprelvekin** is a genetically engineered form of **human interleukin-11.** IL-11 has a number of biologic activities in hematopoietic, lymphopoietic, hepatic, adipose, neuronal, and osteoclast cells.
   b. It is used clinically to prevent **severe chemotherapy-induced thrombocytopenia** and to reduce the need for platelet transfusions following myelosuppressive chemotherapy for nonmyeloid malignancies.

III. DRUGS USED IN HEMOSTATIC DISORDERS

A. **Anticoagulants (Fig. 7-2)**

1. ***Heparin***
   a. **Structure**
      (1) Heparin is a polymeric mixture of sulfated mucopolysaccharides. Commercial heparin contains 8–15 repeats of d-glycosamine-l-iduronic acid and d-glucosamine-d-glucuronic acid. It is highly negatively charged at physiologic pH.
      (2) Low-molecular-weight heparins are also available (dalteparin (Fragmin), enoxaparin (Lovenox)).
      (3) Heparin is synthesized as a normal product of many tissues, including the lung, intestine, and liver. Commercial preparations are derived from bovine lung or porcine intestinal extracts.
   b. **Actions**
      (1) Increases the activity of antithrombin by 1,000-fold
         (a) Antithrombin inhibits activated serine proteases in the clotting cascade, including IIa (thrombin), IXa, and Xa.

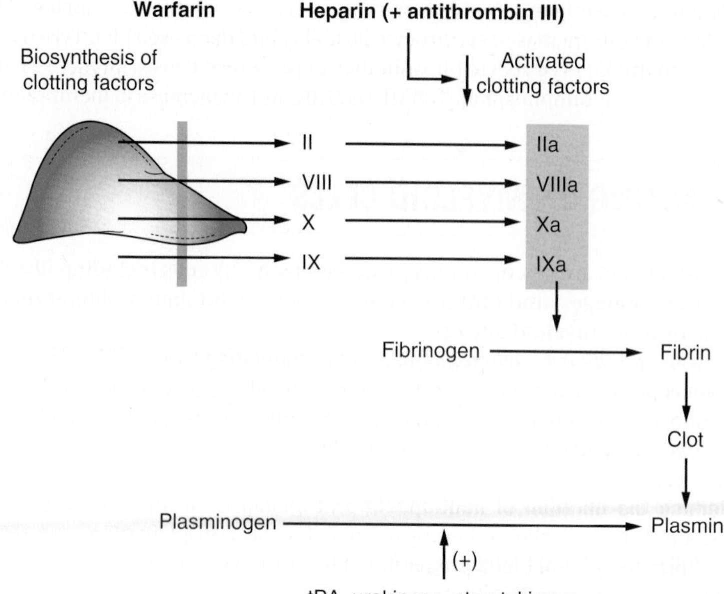

FIGURE 7-2. Sites of pharmacologic action of antithrombotic and fibrinolytic agents.

(b) **Heparin, antithrombin,** and the clotting factors form a ternary complex. The clotting factor is inactivated, and intact heparin is released and recycled in a catalytic manner. Some evidence suggests that additional anti-clotting factors, such as heparin cofactor II, may also be activated by heparin.

(c) The lower-molecular-weight heparins act mainly via antithrombin to inhibit factor Xa; they have little effect on inhibition of thrombin.

(2) Heparin has a direct anticoagulant activity (can inhibit clotting in vitro).

(3) Heparin releases lipoprotein lipase from vascular beds, which accelerates postprandial clearing of lipoproteins from the plasma.

c. Pharmacologic properties

(1) Heparin must be given parenterally (by slow infusion or deep subcutaneous injection); it is not injected intramuscularly because of the potential for hematoma formation.

(2) The half-life ($t_{1/2}$) of heparin is dose dependent. The principal advantage of the low-molecular-weight heparins is a greater pharmacokinetic predictability that allows once- or twice-a-day subcutaneous dosing without the need for monitoring.

(3) Heparin is metabolized in the liver by heparinase to smaller molecular weight compounds, which are excreted in the urine.

d. Therapeutic uses

(1) Heparin provides preoperative prophylaxis against deep vein thrombosis.

(2) Heparin is administered following acute MI (AMI) or pulmonary embolism.

(3) This agent reduces pulmonary embolism in patients with established thrombosis.

(4) Heparin prevents clotting in extracorporeal circulation devices.

e. Adverse effects

(1) Bleeding is a common adverse effect, especially in older women. An increased incidence of bleeding is also seen in patients with renal disease. Protamine sulfate, a highly positively charged mixture of peptides, can be administered IV if bleeding does not abate after the cessation of heparin therapy.

(2) Heparin causes thrombocytopenia in 25% of patients and severe platelet reductions in 5% of patients; heparin may induce antiplatelet antibodies and may also induce platelet aggregation and lysis.

(3) Heparin can cause hypersensitivity reactions, including chills, fever, urticaria, and anaphylaxis.
(4) Heparin may produce reversible alopecia.
(5) Osteoporosis and predisposition to fracture are seen with long-term use of heparin.

f. Contraindications and drug interactions

(1) Heparin is contraindicated in patients who are bleeding (internally or externally) and in patients with hemophilia, thrombocytopenia, hypertension, or purpura.
(2) Heparin is also contraindicated before and after brain, spinal cord, or eye surgery.
(3) Extreme caution is advised in the treatment of pregnant women; however, alternative agents (coumarin derivatives) are teratogenic.
(4) Heparin should not be administered with aspirin or other agents that interfere with platelet aggregation.
(5) Positively charged drugs, aminoglycosides, and some histamine-receptor antagonists can reduce the effectiveness of heparin therapy.

2. *Synthetic anticoagulants, fondaparinux*

a. Fondaparinux is a synthetic polysaccharide based on the antithrombin-binding region of heparin. Administered by subcutaneous injection, it behaves like the low-molecular-weight heparins in inactivating factor Xa.
b. Fondaparinux is approved for prophylaxis of thrombus formation in patients undergoing hip or knee surgery, treatment of pulmonary embolism, and deep vein thrombosis.

3. *Coumarin derivatives*

a. Structure

(1) Coumarin derivatives are derived from 4-hydroxycoumarin and include dicumarol, warfarin sodium, and phenprocoumon.
(2) Of these agents, warfarin has the best bioavailability and the least severe adverse effects.

b. Actions and pharmacologic properties

(1) Coumarin derivatives indirectly interfere with γ-carboxylation of glutamate residues in clotting factors II (prothrombin), VII, IX, and X, which is coupled to the oxidation of vitamin K. Continued production of functional clotting factors requires replenishment of reduced vitamin K from the oxidized form; this reduction is catalyzed by vitamin K epoxide reductase; which is directly inhibited by coumarin derivatives.
(2) Clotting factors are still synthesized, but at reduced levels, and are undercarboxylated and have greatly reduced biologic activity; clotting factors produced before coumarin therapy decline in concentration as a function of factor half-life. This causes a latency period of 36–48 hours before effects are seen. It does not affect established thrombi.
   (a) **Warfarin,** administered orally, has 100% bioavailability. Highly teratogenic and fetotoxic, with a $t_{1/2}$ of 2.5 days, warfarin is extensively (99%) bound to plasma albumin and can displace many other drugs from this site.
   (b) **Dicumarol** is much less well absorbed; a $t_{1/2}$ of approximately 2–10 days increases the potential for bleeding episodes.

c. Therapeutic uses

(1) The therapeutic uses of coumarin derivatives are similar to those of heparin; they also include treatment and prophylaxis of venous thrombosis and of pulmonary embolism. Coumarin derivatives are also indicated to reduce thromboembolism in patients with mechanical heart valves.
(2) Coumarin derivatives are also used to treat patients with atrial fibrillation, whose risk for a stroke is greatly increased.

d. Adverse effects

(1) Bleeding is a common adverse effect with oral anticoagulants; prothrombin times should be frequently monitored.
(2) Warfarin causes hemorrhagic infarction in the breast, intestine, and fatty tissues; it also readily crosses the placenta and can cause hemorrhage in the fetus. Warfarin causes defects in normal fetal bone formation; its teratogenic potential is high.

e. Drug interactions

(1) Amiodarone and sulfinpyrazone inhibit metabolism of the more active warfarin stereoisomer and increase drug activity.

(2) Aspirin and salicylates increase warfarin action by inhibiting platelet function and displacement of warfarin from plasma-binding sites.
(3) Antibiotics decrease microbial vitamin K production in the intestine.
(4) Barbiturates and rifampin decrease warfarin effectiveness by inducing microsomal enzymes.
(5) Oral contraceptives decrease warfarin effectiveness by increasing plasma clotting factors and decreasing antithrombin III.

4. ***Hirudin and analogues***
   a. **Hirudin,** a protein found in the saliva of the medicinal leech, directly binds to and **inhibits thrombin** in the circulation and within clots. It does not require antithrombin.
   b. Bivalirudin (Angiomax) is a synthetic 20-amino-acid peptide hirudin analogue; desirudin and lepirudin are recombinant hirudin analogues made in yeast. All are administered parenterally.
   c. These drugs are used in patients with unstable angina pectoris undergoing percutaneous transluminal coronary angioplasty (PTCA) and when combined with additional antiplatelet drugs (see below) in patients undergoing percutaneous coronary interventions. Lepirudin is approved for anticoagulation in patients with heparin-induced thrombocytopenia.
5. **Argatroban** and **lepirudin** are synthetic inhibitors of thrombin and are derived from arginine. They are useful in the management of patients at risk for heparin-induced thrombocytopenia

B. Hemostatic agents

1. ***Vitamin K_1 (phytonadione) and vitamin K_2 (menaquinone)***
   a. **Vitamin K_1** is found in foodstuffs and is available for oral or parenteral use. Adequate bile salts are required for oral absorption. **Vitamin K_2** is found in human tissues and is the form synthesized by intestinal bacteria. A pharmaceutical preparation of vitamin K_2 is not available.
   b. **Vitamin K** is required for posttranslational modification of clotting factors II, VII, IX, and X.
   c. Administration of vitamin K to newborns reduces the incidence of **hypothrombinemia of the newborn,** which is especially common in premature infants.
   d. IV administration is typical for patients with **dietary deficiencies** and for replenishment of normal levels reduced by **antimicrobial therapy or surgery.**
   e. IV **vitamin K_1** is effective in reversing **bleeding episodes induced by oral hypoglycemic agents.**
2. ***Plasma fractions***
   a. Plasma fractions must be administered IV.
   b. Plasma fractions are frequently prepared from blood or plasma pooled from multiple individuals; thus, they are associated with an increased risk of exposure to hepatitis and human immunodeficiency virus (HIV) (approximately 80% of hemophiliacs over age 30 are infected with HIV). Recombinant DNA techniques that permit in vitro synthesis of these products eliminate this danger.
      (1) Plasma protein preparations include the following:
         (a) **Lyophilized factor VIII concentrate** and **recombinant factor VIII**
         (b) **Cryoprecipitate** (plasma protein fraction obtained from whole blood)
         (c) **Concentrates of plasma** (contain variable amounts of factors II, IX, X, and VII)
         (d) **Lyophilized factor IX concentrates, recombinant factor IX**
         (e) **Recombinant factor VIIa**
         (f) **Recombinant thrombin**
         (g) **Antithrombin** (Thrombate III)
         (h) **Antiinhibitor coagulant complex (AICC)**
         - activated clotting factors
      (2) Therapeutic uses. Therapeutic uses include the treatment of various congenital defects of hemostasis, including the following:
         (a) **Hemophilia A** (classic hemophilia, due to a deficiency in factor VIII)
         (b) **Hemophilia B** (Christmas disease, due to a deficiency in factor IX)
         (c) **Hereditary antithrombin III deficiency**
3. ***Other agents that increase clotting capacity***
   a. **Desmopressin acetate** (DDAVP, Stimate) increases factor VIII activity and can be used before minor surgery in patients with **mild hemophilia A.**

b. **Danazol** is an impeded androgen that increases factor VIII synthesis. It is infrequently used in some anemias and refractory idiopathic thrombocytopenic purpura.

4. ***Inhibitors of fibrinolysis***
   a. **Aminocaproic acid**
      (1) Aminocaproic acid is a synthetic agent similar in structure to lysine.
      (2) Aminocaproic acid competitively inhibits plasminogen activation.
      (3) This agent is used as an adjunct in the treatment of hemophilia, for postsurgical bleeding, and in patients with hyperfibrinolysis.
   b. **Tranexamic acid (Cyklokapron).** Tranexamic acid is a more potent analogue of aminocaproic acid.

C. Antithrombotics

1. ***Aspirin***
   a. Aspirin and aspirin-like agents **decrease thromboxane A_2 production** in platelets by inhibiting cyclooxygenases type 1.
   b. At higher doses (>325 mg/day), aspirin may **reduce antithrombotic action** by decreasing endothelial cell synthesis of prostaglandin I_2 (PGI_2), which requires cyclooxygenase (type 2) activity. Low doses may impair prostaglandin synthesis in platelets to a greater extent than in endothelial cells and avoid this effect.
   c. Other NSAIDs (see Chapter 6) do not have comparable antithrombotic activity.
2. ***Dipyridamole (Persantine, Pyridamole)***
   a. Dipyridamole **inhibits the cellular uptake of adenosine,** which has vasodilating and antiaggregating activity.
   b. The use of dipyridamole as an antithrombotic agent is limited to prophylaxis (with warfarin) in patients with **prosthetic heart valves.**
3. ***Ticlopidine (Ticlid), clopidogrel (Plavix)***
   a. **Ticlopidine** irreversibly inhibits the platelet purinergic $P2Y_{12}$ receptor. This reduces the activation of glycoprotein IIb/IIIa and inhibits the binding of platelets to fibrinogen, thus **inhibiting platelet aggregation.**
   b. **Clopidogrel** is structurally similar and has the same mechanism of action.
   c. These agents are used for arterial thromboembolism prophylaxis in high-risk patients, stroke prophylaxis in patients with noncardioembolic TIA or stroke, and acute coronary syndrome.
   d. Adverse effects include bleeding, diarrhea, rash, and severe neutropenia. The incidence of adverse effects is lower with clopidogrel.
   e. Maximal effects are seen after several days of therapy; effects persist several days after treatment.
4. **Anagrelide (Agrylin)** is an antithrombopenic agent that inhibits megakaryocytes for treatment of patients with thrombocythemia.
5. **Cilostazol** inhibits platelet aggregation and has antithrombitic and vasodilatory actions, mediated in part by inhibition of phosphodisterase type III. It is approved for use in the treatment of claudication.
6. ***GPIIb/IIIa inhibitors***
   a. The abundant platelet glycoprotein GPIIa/IIIb plays a critical role in platelet aggregation (Fig. 7-3). GPIIa/IIIb is an integrin that, when activated, binds to fibrinogen. There are two GPIIa/IIIb binding sites on a fibrinogen molecule, thus permitting fibrinogen-mediated platelet aggregation.
   b. **Abciximab** is the Fab fragment of a chimeric monoclonal antibody that contains human and mouse IgG components. It binds to GPIIa/IIIb and blocks fibrinogen binding. It also binds to the vitronectin receptor.
   c. **Eptifibatide** is a small **synthetic peptide** that competes for fibrinogen binding **to GPIIa/IIIb.**
   d. **Tirofiban** (Aggrastat) is a peptide mimetic of low molecular weight (mol. wt. = 495) that binds to the GPIIa/IIIb receptor (and the vitronectin receptor).
   e. These drugs have been approved for use in patients undergoing percutaneous coronary intervention, for unstable angina, and for post-MI.
   f. All are administered by infusion.

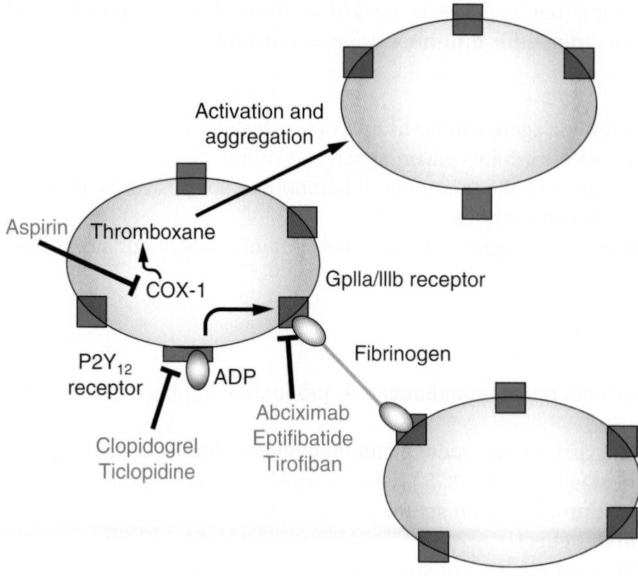

FIGURE 7-3. Sites of action of antiplatelet drugs.

g. The most common adverse effect is bleeding, especially if used in combination with heparin.

7. ***Dextran 40 and dextran 70, 75***
   a. These agents are plasma volume expanders that reduce erythrocyte aggregation and **impair fibrin polymerization and platelet function** in vivo by an unclear mechanism.
   b. Adverse effects include **respiratory distress, urticaria,** and (rarely) anaphylaxis.

D. **Thrombolytics** (Table 7-1). Fibrin clots are dissolved by the serine protease plasmin. Inactive plasminogen is converted to plasmin in vivo by peptides called **tissue plasminogen activators.**

1. ***Tissue plasminogen activator (tPA), alteplase (Activase), reteplase (Retavase), and tenecteplase (TNKase)***
   a. tPA is an endogenous protease that preferentially activates plasminogen bound to fibrin. **Alteplase** is a recombinant human protein produced in cultured cells.
   b. tPA is most specific to **fibrin-bound plasminogen;** local activation of plasmin reduces the incidence of systemic bleeding.

table 7-1 Properties and Uses of Thrombolytics

Drug	Composition	Properties	Uses
Alteplase	Recombinant natural human tPA	Activity more localized to fibrin clot	AMI; stroke
Reteplase	Recombinant fragment of human tPA	Smaller than native tPA; in theory, diffuses into fibrin clot more readily	AMI
Duteplase	Recombinant human tPA with a single amino acid change	Activity more localized to fibrin clot	AMI
Streptokinase	Bacterial glycoprotein; activates plasminogen	Not targeted specifically to fibrin in clots	AMI; deep vein thrombosis
Urokinase	Produced in the kidney; activates plasminogen	Not targeted specifically to fibrin in clots	Acute massive pulmonary emboli; AMI

AMI, acute myocardial infaction; tPA, tissue plasminogen activator.

c. Reteplase and tenecteplase are genetically engineered forms of human tPA and have a longer half-life, higher specificity for fibrin, and greater resistance to plasminogen activator inhibitor-1 (PAI-1) than native tPA. The increase in half-life permits administration as a bolus rather than by continuous infusion.

d. Antithrombotics are used in patients with **acute arterial thrombosis** including AMI and **stroke.** Use of thrombolytics has reduced morbidity and mortality associated with AMI and acute ischemic stroke. Outcomes following AMI and stroke are improved if administration occurs promptly after the event; recommendations are usually within 3–6 hours. tPA has also been used in the treatment of pulmonary embolism and for deep vein thrombosis.

e. The most common adverse effect of all thrombolytics is bleeding. Bleeding sites include both internal (intracranial, retroperitoneal, GI, genitourinary, respiratory) and superficial sites (venous cutdowns, arterial punctures, sites of recent surgical intervention).

2. ***Streptokinase***

a. Streptokinase is a nonenzyme protein that is isolated from streptococci; it binds to plasminogen to catalyze the conversion of plasminogen to active plasmin.

b. Streptokinase acts on both circulating plasminogen and fibrin-bound plasminogen.

c. Therapeutic uses of streptokinase include treatment of **AMI and stroke, acute pulmonary embolism, deep vein thrombosis,** and **reperfusion of occluded peripheral arteries.** It is also used, as are other thrombolytics, to **clear occluded venous catheters.**

d. The major adverse effect associated with streptokinase is **systemic bleeding.** Many individuals have antistreptococcal antibodies because of prior exposure to the bacteria; this can reduce effectiveness and complicate treatment.

e. Although streptokinase is commonly used in Europe, it is no longer marketed in the United States.

3. ***Urokinase***

a. Urokinase is a protease originally isolated from urine; the drug is now prepared in recombinant form from cultured kidney cells.

b. Urokinase activates circulating and fibrin-bound plasminogen.

c. Urokinase is approved for the treatment of pulmonary embolism. It is less antigenic than streptokinase and is indicated in patients sensitive to streptokinase.

DRUG SUMMARY TABLE

Drugs Used for Anemias
Iron salts (Fe-Max, Femiron, Feostat, many others)
Epoetin alfa (Epogen, Procrit)
Darbepoietin Alfa (Aranesp)
Pyridoxine (vitamin B_6) (Neuro-K)
Cyanocobalamin (vitamin B_{12}) (Betalin, Redisol)
Hydroxocobalamin (vitamin B_{12}) (AlphaRedisol)
Folic acid (vitamin B_9) (Folacin, Folicet)
Leucovorin (generic)
Hydroxyurea (Mylocel, Droxia)
Pentoxifylline (Pentopak)

Myeloid Growth Stimulators
Sargramostim (Leukine)
Filgrastim (Neupogen)
Pegfilgrastin (Neulasta)
Oprelvekin (Neumega)

Anticoagulants
Heparin (Calciparine, others)
Fondaparinex (Arixtra)
Warfarin (Coumadin)
Phenprocoumon (Liquamar)
Dicumarol (generic)
Bivalirudin (Angiomax)
Desirudin (Iprivask)
Lepirudin (Refludan)
Antithrombin (Thrombate III)
Argatroban (generic)

Hemostatic Agents
Phytonadione (vitamin K_1) (AquaMEPHYTON, Mephyton)
Factor VIII (Kogenate, Helixate)
Factor IX (AlphaNine, Profilnine)
Factor VIIa (NovoSeven)
Thrombin (Recothrom)
AICC (Feiba)
Desmopressin acetate (DDAVP, Stimate)
Danazol (Danacrine)

Antifibrinolytics
Aminocaproic acid (Amicar)
Tranexamic acid (Cyklokapron)

Antithrombotics
Aspirin
Dipyridamole (Persantine, Pyridamole)
Ticlopidine (Ticlid)
Clopidogrel (Plavix)
Anagrelide (Agrylin)
Cilostazol (generic)
Dextran (Dextran 40, others)

GPIIb/IIIa Inhibitors
Abciximab (ReoPro)
Eptifibatide (Integrilin)
Tirofiban (Aggrastat)

Thrombolytics
Alteplase (Activase)
Reteplase (Retavase)
Tenecteplase (TNKase)
Streptokinase (Kabikinase, Streptase)
Urokinase (Abbokinase)

Review Test for Chapter 7

Directions: Each of the numbered items or incomplete statements in this section is followed by answers or by completions of the statement. Select the ONE lettered answer or completion that is BEST in each case.

1. A patient is admitted to the hospital for gallbladder surgery, and although the surgery is successful, a case of ileus develops. This necessitates feeding the patient parenterally for 8 days. A nurse observes that the surgical wound and IV sites have begun to ooze small but constant amounts of blood. Which of the following would be the most appropriate treatment of this patient?

(A) Ticlopidine
(B) Factor VIII concentrate
(C) Urokinase
(D) Vitamin K
(E) Folic acid

2. A man undergoing chemotherapy for lung cancer complains of shortness of breath when climbing stairs and generalized fatigue. An electrocardiogram (ECG) appears normal, but his hematocrit level is 8.1. Which of the following would be most appropriate for this patient?

(A) Erythropoietin
(B) Digoxin
(C) Ticlopidine
(D) Vitamin B_6
(E) Enalapril

3. A 56-year old woman has a temporary loss of peripheral vision and dizziness that lasts for approximately 10 minutes. Her family history reveals that her mother had thromboembolemic disease, but her father was normal. Which of the following would be the best outpatient prophylactic regimen for this patient 2 days after these symptoms appeared?

(A) Anistreplase
(B) Clopidogrel
(C) Heparin
(D) Abciximab
(E) Streptokinase

4. A 53-year-old obese woman is brought into the emergency room by her concerned husband approximately 1 hour after complaining of constant abdominal pain, nausea, and shortness of breath. An electrocardiogram (ECG) and cardiac enzyme tests indicate a moderate myocardial infarction (MI) due to occlusion of the left descending coronary artery. Which of the following would be the best course of treatment for this patient?

(A) Reteplase
(B) Heparin
(C) Eptifibatide
(D) Lovastatin

5. A young couple present to their primary care physician stating that they are trying to conceive. They would like to know if the future mom-to-be needs to be on any supplements. Along with recommending a multivitamin with folic acid, the doctor also suggests an iron supplement. Pregnant women develop iron deficiency anemia because of

(A) Increased bleeding tendency
(B) Increased dietary deficiency
(C) Malabsorption
(D) Increased iron demands
(E) Increased excretion

6. A 65-year-old diabetic man develops end-stage renal disease. His glomerular filtration capacity is now low enough to require dialysis. His nephrologist also explains that the patient will require weekly injections of synthetic erythropoietin (EPO), since this protein is normally produced by the kidney. What is the mechanism of action of EPO?

(A) It increases proliferation of erythroid precursor cells in the bone marrow
(B) It decreases the release of reticulocytes from the bone marrow
(C) It decreases hemoglobin synthesis
(D) It is independent of the amount of iron stored in the body
(E) It participates in the mitochondrial reaction that produces succinyl-CoA

7. A 47-year-old man with a history of alcohol abuse presents to the urgent care clinic complaining of lightheadedness and dyspnea on exertion. His laboratory studies indicate a low hemoglobin level. Peripheral smear shows increased number of spherocytes. What agent could be used to treat this patient's anemia?

(A) Iron supplements
(B) Erythropoietin
(C) Vitamin B_6
(D) Vitamin B_{12}
(E) Folic acid

8. A 40-year-old morbidly obese woman undergoes gastric bypass surgery to help her lose weight. Her surgeon reminds her that now she will have to get a monthly injection of vitamin B_{12}, since the part of her stomach responsible for production of intrinsic factor has been removed. Which of the following is true about vitamin B_{12}?

(A) Loss of vitamin B_{12} from the body is a rapid process
(B) The molecule of vitamin B_{12} contains copper
(C) Vitamin B_{12} is not required for fatty acid metabolism
(D) A deficiency results in impaired DNA replication
(E) Neurologic deficits are not seen with this kind of anemia

9. A 31-year-old pregnant woman presents to her obstetrician for a routine visit. She has several questions for her doctor, one of which has to do with the supplements that she was advised to take at her first prenatal visit. She stated she leads a very busy lifestyle and sometimes forgets to take all the pills she is supposed to take. She wants to know the purpose of folic acid supplementation in pregnancy.

(A) It increases oxygen-carrying capacity of the blood
(B) It decreases the risk of neural tube defects
(C) It aids in bone growth of the maturing fetus
(D) It stimulates myelopoiesis of erythroid progenitor cells
(E) It reduces blood viscosity during pregnancy

10. A 29-year-old African-American man presents to the emergency department with a chief complaint of severe pain in his arms and legs. Since this has happened to him before, he knows that what he is experiencing is a sickle crisis. He states that since he does not have medical insurance, he only comes to see a doctor when he experiences these "crises." Which pain medication is the emergency physician likely to prescribe?

(A) Indomethacin
(B) Hydrocodone
(C) Acetaminophen
(D) Celecoxib
(E) Hydroxyurea

11. A 74-year-old woman who is undergoing chemotherapy for advanced lung cancer presents to the infusion center for her next treatment. Before each treatment her white count, hemoglobin, and platelet counts are checked to make sure she is not experiencing chemotherapy-related cytotoxicity. Her blood sample is run in the analyzer, and her platelet count is reported to be at a dangerously low level. Which medication is her oncologist likely to prescribe in this situation, along with a platelet transfusion?

(A) Erythropoietin
(B) Oprelvekin
(C) Filgrastim
(D) Sargramostim
(E) Leucovorin

12. A 55-year-old woman undergoes an open cholecystectomy. She is admitted for postoperative observation and started on subcutaneous heparin treatment to prevent formation of deep venous thrombosis, a major risk factor for pulmonary embolism. Which of the following is true regarding the mechanism of action of heparin?

(A) Heparin increases activity of antithrombin
(B) Serine proteases of the clotting cascade are deactivated
(C) Heparin catalyzes clotting in vitro
(D) Heparin aids sequestration of lipoproteins
(E) Clotting factor is activated

13. A 63-year-old man has a history of atrial fibrillation. To reduce his risk of a stroke, his physician had given him an anticoagulant medication. This agent, while being of tremendous benefit to this patient, comes with its associated risks, such as spontaneous hemorrhage. To monitor the appropriateness of the current dosage of the medication, the patient comes in frequently to have the laboratory check his prothrombin level. Which medication must this patient be taking?

(A) Heparin
(B) Fragmin
(C) Lovenox
(D) Coumarin
(E) Protamine

14. A 75-year-old man is brought to the emergency department after being found on the floor of his room. His wife tells you that his medical history includes two prior strokes, for which he is now taking a "small pill that works on platelets." Your attending tells you that there are newer agents now that work by preventing platelet aggregation. He asks you if you know the names of any such agents. You are very excited, because you, in fact, had just reviewed your pharmacology. Which answer do you give?

(A) Heparin
(B) Coumarin
(C) Clopidogrel
(D) Alteplase
(E) Dextran

Answers and Explanations

1. **The answer is D.** After 6–7 days of parenteral feeding, vitamin K stores are depleted and clotting factor biosynthesis is impaired. Ticlopidine is an anticoagulant, and urokinase is a thrombolytic; both would be contraindicated in this circumstance. Folic acid would not improve the condition of the patient.

2. **The answer is A.** Erythropoietin (EPO) stimulates the production of erythrocytes, which are frequently diminished as a consequence of anticancer therapy and correct the patient's hematocrit level. Digoxin is a cardiac glycoside that can improve contractility in impaired myocardium but would not be used in this circumstance. Enalapril is an angiotensin-converting enzyme (ACE) inhibitor that would have little effect on the patient's condition.

3. **The answer is B.** The patient has symptoms consistent with a transient ischemic attack (TIA). Prophylactic antiplatelet therapy should be instituted while the diagnosis is confirmed. Heparin is not suitable for outpatient use. Anistreplase and streptokinase are thrombolytics that may be used within hours of a thrombotic stroke but not after 2 days after a possible TIA.

4. **The answer is A.** Thrombolytics such as the recombinant tissue plasminogen activator (tPA) reteplase reduce morbidity and mortality if used shortly after an acute myocardial infarction (AMI). Heparin might be used after resolution of the AMI. If the patient is above recommended levels of low-density lipoprotein (LDL) cholesterol, she should be treated with a cholesterol-lowering drug such as lovastatin.

5. **The answer is D.** Pregnancy and lactation are the states of increased iron demands. While increased bleeding tendency, dietary deficiency, and malabsorption are all true causes of iron deficiency anemia, they are not the culprits during pregnancy. Iron storage is regulated at the level of absorption, and very little of it is lost from the body.

6. **The answer is A.** Erythropoietin (EPO) increases the rate of proliferation and differentiation of erythroid precursor cells in the bone marrow. It increases the release of reticulocytes. It also increases hemoglobin synthesis. Erythropoietin requires adequate iron stores. Participation in the mitochondrial reaction that produces succinyl-CoA refers to the mechanism of action of one of the natural cobalamins, deoxyadenosylcobalamin.

7. **The answer is C.** Sideroblastic anemia may develop in alcoholics and patients undergoing antituberculin therapy. This condition is treated with vitamin B_6 supplements (pyridoxine). Iron supplements are used in iron deficiency anemia. Erythropoietin is used in anemia caused by AIDS, chemotherapy, and renal failure. Vitamin B_{12} and folic acid are used for megaloblastic anemias caused by depletion of the vitamin.

8. **The answer is D.** Deficiency of vitamin B_{12} results in impaired DNA replication. Loss of vitamin B_{12} is a very slow process, with hepatic stores being sufficient for up to 5 years. The molecule of vitamin B_{12} contains cobalt. Vitamin B_{12} is essential for normal fatty acid metabolism. Vitamin B_{12} deficiency causes irreversible neurologic disorders.

9. **The answer is B.** Folic acid supplementation has been shown to decrease the incidence of neural tube defects. Increasing the oxygen-carrying capacity of the blood refers to a possible role of iron supplements. Calcium is helpful in adding bone growth. Stimulating myelopoiesis of erythroid progenitor cells refers to the mechanism of action of erythropoietin. Finally, reduction of blood viscosity during pregnancy refers to pentoxifylline; however, this medication is not recommended during pregnancy.

10. **The answer is E.** Hydroxyurea increases the production of fetal hemoglobin and has been shown to be effective in reducing painful episodes of sickle crisis. Indomethacin is a nonsteroidal anti-inflammatory drug (NSAID) commonly used for pain associated with rheumatoid arthritis.

Hydrocodone is a narcotic pain reliever that is only recommended in cases of severe pain, such as that caused by surgery. Acetaminophen is unlikely to be helpful in this patient's situation, as this agent is useful for mild-to-moderate pain. Celecoxib is a COX-2 inhibitor used in a variety of inflammatory conditions.

11. **The answer is B.** Oprelvekin has been shown to reduce the need for platelet transfusions following myelosuppressive chemotherapy. Erythropoietin is used for anemia. Filgrastim and sargramostim are used for neutropenia. Leucovorin is used in patients undergoing treatment with methotrexate, to prevent some of its side effects.

12. **The answer is A.** Heparin increases the activity of antithrombin by 1,000-fold. Antithrombin, in turn, activates serine proteases of the clotting cascade. Heparin has a direct anticoagulant activity and can inhibit clotting in vitro. Heparin releases lipoprotein lipase from vascular beds, which accelerates clearing of lipoproteins from plasma. The clotting factor is inactivated, which releases heparin and allows it to be recycled.

13. **The answer is D.** Coumarin is commonly used in patients with atrial fibrillation for prevention of thromboembolic events, such as stroke. Prothrombin times should be frequently monitored in patients taking coumarin, as bleeding is a common adverse effect. Heparin is monitored with partial thromboplastin time. Fragmin and Lovenox are low-molecular-weight derivatives of heparin that do not require laboratory monitoring. Protamine is an agent used for heparin reversal.

14. **The answer is C.** Clopidogrel works by inhibiting platelet aggregation. Heparin works by increasing the activity of antithrombin. Coumarin interferes with γ-carboxylation of several clotting factors. Alteplase is a thrombolytic. Dextran impairs fibrin polymerization and platelet function.

chapter **8**

Drugs Acting on the Gastrointestinal Tract

I. ANTIEMETICS

A. Vomiting reflex

1. The vomiting reflex is a coordinated reflex controlled by a bilateral **vomiting center** in the dorsal portion of the lateral reticular formation in the medulla.
2. Pharmacologic intervention relies on inhibition of inputs or depression of the vomiting center. The vomiting center receives inputs from several sources:
   a. **Chemoreceptor trigger zone (CTZ)**
   b. **Vestibular apparatus**
   c. **Peripheral afferents** from the pharynx, gastrointestinal (GI) tract, and genitals
   d. **Higher cortical centers**
3. ***Serotonin (5-HT_3)-receptors***, which are the predominant mediators of the reflex, are present in the vomiting center, the CTZ, and in the periphery.

B. Vertigo

1. ***True (objective) vertigo***
   a. True vertigo is **hallucination of movement,** usually caused by a brain lesion or damage to cranial nerve (CN) VIII (cochlear nerve) or the labyrinthine system.
   b. Patients with **Ménière disease** have true vertigo as one of their symptoms.
2. ***Subjective vertigo*** is **prosyncopal light-headedness,** which may be caused by cochlear or vestibular ischemia.

C. Antiemetics are useful in the treatment of vomiting associated with motion sickness, chemotherapy-induced emesis (CIE), radiation-induced emesis (RIE), postoperative nausea and vomiting (PONV), and other causes.

1. ***Cholinoceptor antagonists***
   a. Cholinergic antagonists **reduce the excitability of labyrinthine receptors** and depress conduction from the vestibular apparatus to the vomiting center.
   b. Cholinergic antagonists are used to treat **motion sickness** and in **preoperative situations.** They are not useful in treating nausea caused by chemotherapy.
   c. Cholinergic antagonists produce adverse effects that include drowsiness, dry mouth, and blurred vision.
   d. **Scopolamine** (Trans-Scop) is preferred over atropine because it has a longer duration of action and a more pronounced central nervous system (CNS) action.
   e. Transdermal delivery of **scopolamine** via a skin patch decreases the incidence of adverse effects and produces relief for 72 hours.
2. ***Histamine H_1-receptor antagonists***
   a. Histamine H_1-receptor antagonists include **meclizine** (Antivert, Bonine), **cyclizine** (Marezine), **dimenhydrinate** (Dramamine), and **promethazine** (Phenergan).
   b. These agents most likely act by inhibiting histamine pathways, and cholinergic pathways (**receptor "crossover"**) of the vestibular apparatus.

c. Histamine H_1-receptor antagonists are used to treat **motion sickness and true vertigo.**
d. **Cyclizine** and **meclizine** are drugs of choice for nausea and vomiting associated with **pregnancy**.
e. These agents produce sedation and dry mouth and have anticholinergic side effects.

3. ***Dopamine receptor antagonists***
   a. **Metoclopramide** (Reglan)
      (1) Metoclopramide **blocks dopamine D_2-receptors within the CTZ.**
      (2) Metoclopramide increases the sensitivity of the GI tract to the action of acetylcholine (ACh); this **enhances GI motility and gastric emptying** and increases lower esophageal sphincter tone.
      (3) High doses of metoclopramide antagonize serotonin (5-HT_3)-receptors in the vomiting center and GI tract.
      (4) Metoclopramide is used to treat **nausea due to chemotherapy** (caused by agents such as cisplatin and doxorubicin) and **narcotic-induced vomiting.**
      (5) Metoclopramide produces sedation, diarrhea, **extrapyramidal effects,** and elevated prolactin secretion.
   b. **Phenothiazines and butyrophenones**
      (1) These agents include the phenothiazine **prochlorperazine** (Compazine), and the butyrophone **droperidol** (Inapsine), which is only available in an intravenous (IV) formulation.
      (2) These agents **block dopaminergic receptors in the CTZ** and appear to inhibit peripheral transmission to the vomiting center. They also **block alpha$_1$-adrenoceptors**. **Prochlorperazine** also **blocks muscarinic cholinoceptors.**
      (3) These agents are used to treat **CIE, RIE, and PONV.**
      (4) Adverse actions include anticholinergic effects such as drowsiness, dry mouth, and blurred vision (less pronounced with **droperidol**), **extrapyramidal effects,** and orthostatic hypotension. These agents are **contraindicated in Parkinson disease** because of their extrapyramidal effects.
      (5) **Droperidol** use is associated with **QT prolongation and torsade de pointes** and has a **black box warning.**
4. ***Serotonin 5-HT_3 antagonists***
   a. **Ondansetron** (Zofran), **dolasetron** (Anzemet), **granisetron** (Kytril), and **palonosetron** (Aloxi)
      (1) These agents are **serotonin (5-HT_3)-receptor antagonists.** Activation of these receptors in the CNS and GI tract is a key component in triggering vomiting.
      (2) These agents are very effective against **CIE** and **RIE** and are second-line agents for PONV. They are **not effective for motion-sickness**-induced nausea and vomiting.
      (3) All of these agents can be administered orally and parenterally, except **palonosetron** which is only available for parenteral administration.
      (4) **Palonosetron** has a long duration of action with a half-life ($t_{1/2}$) of 40 hours.
      (5) Dose reduction of **ondansetron** may be necessary for patients with hepatic insufficiency.
      (6) The most common adverse effects of these drugs are headache and mild constipation.
      (7) **Dolasetron** prolongs the QT interval.
   b. These agents are often combined with **corticosteroids such as dexamethasone** (Decadron) and **methylprednisolone** (Solu-Medrol) to produce an enhanced antiemetic effect that is possibly due to corticosteroid inhibition of prostaglandin synthesis.
5. ***Cannabinoids***
   a. **Dronabinol** (Marinol) is an oral preparation of Δ-9-tetrahydrocannabinol, the active cannabinoid in marijuana.
   b. This drug may act by **inhibiting the vomiting center through stimulation of CB_1-subtype of cannabinoid receptors.**
   c. This drug is alternative agent **used to control CIE.**
   d. Adverse effects include sedation, tachycardia, hypotension, and behavioral alterations similar to those associated with the use of marijuana (see V X F).
6. ***Benzodiazepines***
   a. Benzodiazepines include **lorazepam** (Ativan) and **diazepam** (Valium).
   b. Benzodiazepines act as anxiolytic agents to reduce **anticipatory emesis. Diazepam** is useful as a treatment of **vertigo,** and it controls symptoms in **Ménière disease** in 60%–70% of patients.

7. ***Neurokinin 1 (NK1) receptor antagonists***
   a. **Aprepitant** (Emend) is a **substance P neurokinin 1 (NK1) receptor antagonist** used to manage the **delayed phase of emesis caused by chemotherapy.** It is used in a combination with 5-HT_3 antagonists and corticosteroids.

II. ANOREXIGENICS AND APPETITE ENHANCERS

A. General characteristics of anorexigenics

1. Anorexigenics are drugs that **decrease appetite** or **promote satiety.** They are used for the **adjunct treatment of obesity.**
2. Prolonged use of some anorexigenics may lead to physical or psychologic **dependence.**

B. Amphetamines and amphetamine derivatives (selected)

1. ***Amphetamine, methamphetamine, dextroamphetamine, and phentermine*** (Adipex) **act centrally** and elevate the synaptic concentration of catecholamines and dopamine, producing a **reduction in food-seeking behavior.**
2. These agents are contraindicated in pregnancy.
3. These agents have a high risk of dependence.

C. Sibutramine (Meridia)

1. Sibutramine is a **monamine oxidase inhibitor** (MAOI) that interferes with the reuptake of norepinephrine, serotonin, and dopamine.
2. Sibutramine **reduces appetite** and may enhance energy expenditure.

D. Orlistat (Xenical)

1. Orlistat is a reversible lipase inhibitor used for the **management of obesity** and is also available over the counter. It **inactivates the enzymes,** thus making them unavailable to digest dietary fats. Orlistat **inhibits absorption of fats by approximately 30%.**
2. Orlistat should be used in conjunction with **reduced caloric intake.**
3. This agent is contraindicated in patients with **cholestasis** and **malabsorption syndromes.**
4. **Fat-soluble vitamins** should be supplemented when taking Orlistat.
5. Major side effects are GI: fecal spotting, flatulence, and diarrhea.

E. ***Dronabinol*** (Δ-9-tetrahydrocannabinol) (Marinol) **stimulates appetite,** among its other activities. For this reason it is used in patients with acquired immune deficiency syndrome (**AIDS**) **and cancer** who are malnourished due to lack of appetite.

F. ***Megestrol*** (Megace) is a progestational agent that has a side effect **increased appetite.** It can be used in liquid or, more commonly, a pill form. Use leads to **increased caloric intake and weight gain.** This agent is also used as a second- or third-line therapy for **breast cancer** patients who have progressed on tamoxifen (see Chapter 12).

III. AGENTS USED FOR UPPER GI TRACT DISORDERS

A. Goal of therapy for upper GI tract disorders (**peptic ulcers and gastroesophageal reflux disease [GERD]**) is to **reduce gastric acid production**, to **neutralize gastric H^+**, or **to protect the walls of the stomach** from the acid and pepsin released by the stomach.

B. Antacids

1. ***General characteristics***
   a. Antacids are **weak bases** that are taken orally and that **partially neutralize gastric acid, reduce pepsin activity, and stimulate prostaglandin production.**
   b. Antacids **reduce the pain** associated with ulcers and may promote healing.

c. Antacids have been largely **replaced for GI disorders by other drugs** but are still used commonly by patients as nonprescription remedies for dyspepsia.

2. ***Prototype agents***
   a. **Sodium bicarbonate** (Alka Seltzer)
      (1) Sodium bicarbonate is absorbed systemically and **should not be used for long-term treatment.**
      (2) Sodium bicarbonate is **contraindicated in hypertension, heart failure, and renal failure** because of its high sodium content.
   b. **Calcium carbonate** (TUMS, Os-Cal)
      (1) Calcium carbonate is partially absorbed from the GI tract and thus has some systemic effects. It **should not be used for long-term treatment.**
      (2) Calcium carbonate may stimulate gastrin release and thereby cause rebound acid production.
      (3) Calcium carbonate is **contraindicated in patients with renal disease.** It may cause nausea and belching.
   c. **Magnesium hydroxide**
      (1) Magnesium hydroxide is not absorbed from the GI tract and therefore produces **no systemic effects.** This agent can be used for long-term therapy.
      (2) The most frequent adverse effect associated with magnesium hydroxide is **diarrhea.**
   d. **Aluminum hydroxide**
      (1) Aluminum hydroxide is **not absorbed** from the GI tract; it has no systemic effects.
      (2) Aluminum hydroxide causes **constipation.**
   e. **Combination products** include various preparations (Maalox, Mylanta II, Gelusil) that **combine magnesium hydroxide** and **aluminum hydroxide** to achieve a balance between the agents' adverse effects on the bowel.

3. ***Drug interactions.*** Antacids alter the bioavailability of many drugs by the following mechanisms:
   a. The **increase in gastric pH** produced by antacids decreases the absorption of acidic drugs and increases the absorption of basic drugs.
   b. The **metal ion** in some preparations can **chelate other drugs** (e.g., **digoxin** and **tetracycline**) and **prevent** their **absorption.**

C. Inhibitors of gastric acid production (Fig. 8-1)

1. ***Histamine H_2-receptor antagonists***
   a. **Mechanism of action.** The H_2-receptor antagonists, **cimetidine** (Tagamet), **ranitidine** (Zantac), **famotidine** (Pepcid), and **nizatidine** (Axid) act as **competitive inhibitors of the histamine H_2-receptor on the parietal cell.** This results in a marked **decrease in histamine-stimulated gastric acid secretion.** Although other agents such as gastrin and acetylcholine may induce acid secretion, **histamine** is the predominant final mediator that **stimulates parietal acid secretion.** These drugs are rapidly absorbed, and effects are observed within **a few minutes to hours.**
   b. **Therapeutic uses**
      (1) Histamine H_2-receptor antagonists are used to treat **peptic ulcer disease** to promote the healing of gastric and duodenal ulcers. However, when they are used as sole agents, recurrence is observed in 90% of patients.
      (2) These agents are used to treat **GERD** and **Zollinger-Ellison syndrome.**
      (3) These drugs are used on an as-needed basis for rapid relief from **dyspepsia.**
      (4) These drugs are administered IV in intensive care settings to reduce the incidence of stress-related ulcers.
   c. **Adverse effects**
      (1) Histamine H_2-receptor antagonists are associated with a low incidence of mild GI upset, headache, and mental confusion, especially in the elderly. A rare adverse effect is **thrombocytopenia.**
      (2) The bioavailability of these agents is decreased by antacids.
      (3) **Cimetidine** is also an **androgen-receptor antagonist** and can induce gynecomastia and impotence.

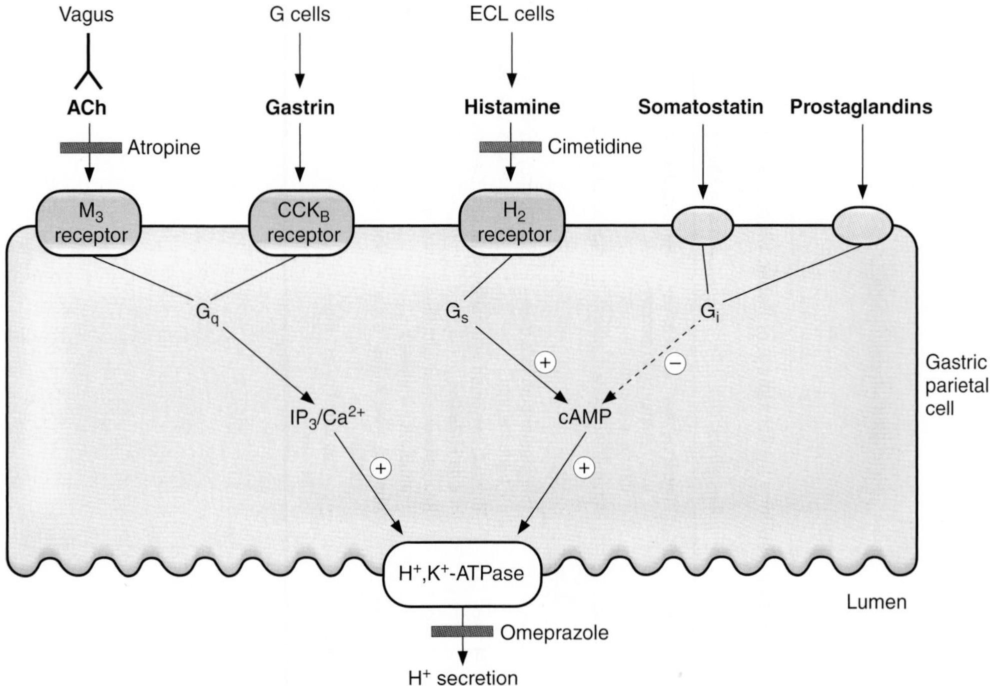

FIGURE 8-1. Site of action on parietal cells of three classes of antisecretory drugs. cAMP, cyclic adenosine monophosphate; H_2, histamine-2 receptor; M_1, muscarinic receptor.

(4) **Cimetidine** is a **competitive inhibitor of the cytochrome P-450** mixed-function oxidase system; it can **increase** the half-life of drugs that are metabolized by this system (e.g., **warfarin, theophylline, phenytoin,** and the **benzodiazepines**).

(5) **Cimetidine decreases** the absorption of **ketoconazole.**

(6) **Ranitidine, famotidine, and nizatidine do not bind to the androgen receptor;** their effect on drug metabolism is negligible.

2. ***Proton-pump inhibitors (PPIs)***
   a. **Omeprazole** (Prilosec), **lansoprazole** (Prevacid), **esomeprazole** (Nexium), **pantoprazole** (Protonix), and **rabeprazole** (Aciphex) are covalent, **irreversible inhibitors of the H^+/K^+-ATPase proton pump in parietal cells.** As lipophilic weak bases, these **prodrugs** concentrate in the acidic compartments of parietal cells where they are rapidly **converted to an active thiophilic sulfonamide cation.** The sulfonamide forms a covalent disulfide linkage to the H^+/K^+-ATPase proton pump that results in its inactivation, thereby blocking the transport of acid from the cell into the lumen.
   b. These agents **reduce both meal-stimulated and basal acid secretion.** Desired effects **may take 3–4 days** since not all proton pumps are inhibited with the first dose of these medications.
   c. These agents are the most effective drugs for treatment of all forms of **GERD.**
   d. These agents **reduce *Helicobacter pylori (H. pylori)*-associated ulcers** and gastric **damage induced by nonsteroidal anti-inflammatory drug (NSAID) therapy.** Proton pump inhibitors are more effective for this indication than histamine H_2-receptor blockers.
   e. These agents are useful in patients with **Zollinger-Ellison syndrome,** for **reflux esophagitis,** and for **ulcers refractory to H_2-receptor antagonists.** (See Table 8-1 for information on their use in ulcer treatment regimens.)
   f. **Parenteral (IV) formulations** are used for patients requiring **immediate acid secretion reduction.**
   g. Adverse effects include headaches and GI disturbances; the reduction in acid production may permit bacterial overgrowth with increased incidence of respiratory and enteric infections.

table 8-1 Combinations Approved by FDA or Recommended by the American College of Gastroenterology for Treatment of Peptic Ulcer Disease

Bismuth Compounds	Antibacterial 1	Antibacterial 2	Acid Inhibitor	Rx	Comments	Adverse Effects
Bismuth subsalicylate (Pepto Bismol), 4× daily	Metronidazole (Flagyl), 3× daily	Amoxicillin or tetracycline, 4× daily		14 days	"Triple therapy"; if not effective, resistance to metronidazole is assumed	Nausea, diarrhea, vomiting
Bismuth subsalicylate (Pepto Bismol), 4× daily	Clarithromycin (use when resistance to metronidazole occurs), 3× daily	Amoxicillin or tetracycline, 4× daily		14 days	Alternative "triple therapy"	Nausea, diarrhea, vomiting
Bismuth subsalicylate (Pepto Bismol), 4× daily	Metronidazole (Flagyl), 3× daily	Tetracycline, 4× daily	Omeprazole (Prilosec), 2× daily	7 days	15% greater cure rate than "triple therapy"	Significantly reduced incidence of GI side effects
Bismuth citrate, 2× daily	Clarithromycin (Biaxin), 3× daily		Ranitidine (Tritec), 2× daily	14 days	Bismuth combined with ranitidine (Tritec)	Nausea, diarrhea
Bismuth subsalicylate	Tetracycline plus metronidazole		Ranitidine or cimetidine	14 days	Bismuth combined with these antibiotics (Helidac)	Nausea, diarrhea, melena
	Clarithromycin, 3× daily	Metronidazole	Omeprazole	14 days	About as effective as "triple therapy"	Nausea, taste loss
	Clarithromycin, 3× daily	Amoxicillin	Omeprazole	14 days	About as effective as "triple therapy"	Nausea

D. Treatment of peptic ulcer disease

1. The most **common cause** of peptic and duodenal ulcers is **infection by** the **anaerobic bacteria *H. Pylori,*** which lives on the gastric mucosa under the mucous layer.
2. The most effective treatment is "**triple therapy,**" which consists of **two antibiotics** (usually clarithromycin and amoxicillin) and a **proton pump inhibitor,** and it may include colloidal **bismuth (Pepto Bismol)** (Table 8-1).
3. These treatments result in the cure of ulceration and the eradication of *H. pylori* in most cases. In refractory cases, antibacterial resistance or noncompliance should be assumed, and susceptibility testing should be undertaken.

E. Protective agents

1. ***Sucralfate (Carafate)***
   a. Sucralfate is a **polysaccharide complexed with aluminum hydroxide.** Gastric pH is low enough to produce extensive cross-linking and polymerization of sucralfate.
   b. Sucralfate has a particular affinity for exposed proteins in the crater of **duodenal ulcers;** it protects ulcerated areas from further damage and promotes healing. Sucralfate stimulates mucosal production of prostaglandins and inhibits pepsin. It is also used in critical care settings for **stress-related gastritis.**
   c. Sucralfate produces constipation and nausea.
2. ***Misoprostol (Cytotec),*** a **congener of prostaglandin E_1** that acts in the GI tract **to stimulate bicarbonate and mucus production,** is rarely used due to its adverse effect profile and its **dosing schedule of four times daily.**
3. **Bismuth subsalicylate** (Pepto Bismol)—see VI B 3.

IV. PROKINETIC AGENTS

A. Prokinetic drugs enhance the contractile force of the GI tract and increase transit of its contents.

B. Metoclopramide (Reglan)

1. Metoclopramide is a **dopamine-receptor antagonist.** In the GI tract, dopamine is **inhibitory;** blockade of dopamine receptors may allow stimulatory actions of ACh at muscarinic synapses to predominate.
2. This agent **increases lower esophageal tone, stimulates gastric emptying, and increases rate of transit through the small bowel.**
3. Metoclopramide is used to **treat reflux esophagitis, gastric motor failure,** and **diabetic gastroparesis;** it is also used to **promote advancement of nasoenteric feeding tubes** in critically ill patients.
4. This agent is also a useful **antiemetic** for nausea associated with chemotherapy.
5. Metoclopramide produces sedation, **extrapyramidal effects,** and increased prolactin secretion.
6. **Cisapride** (Propulsid), a seotoninin 5-HT_4-receptor antagonist that is chemically related to metoclopramide, is only available for compassionate use for motility disorders and GERD due to its high potential for serious adverse cardiac effects and numerous contraindications.

V. DRUGS USED TO DISSOLVE GALLSTONES

A. Ursodiol (Actigall)

1. Ursodiol is ursodeoxycholic acid, a minor **naturally occurring bile acid.**
2. Ursodiol is an oral agent; it requires administration for **months to reach** full effect.
3. This drug's conjugated form **reduces hepatic synthesis and secretion of cholesterol into bile, and its reabsorption by the intestine.** It effectively dissolves **cholesterol gallstones**, but not radiopaque stones.
4. Ursodiol may be combined with **sonic lithotripsy** to dissolve gallstone fragments.

5. This agent may be used for prevention of gallstones in patients who are undergoing **rapid weight loss,** such as gastric bypass patients.
6. Ursodiol has a low incidence of diarrhea.

VI. DIGESTIVE ENZYME REPLACEMENTS

A. General characteristics

1. Digestive enzyme replacements are preparations of **semipurified enzymes,** typically extracted from pig pancreas. They contain various mixtures of **lipase,** proteolytic enzymes such as **trypsin,** and **amylase.**
2. These agents include **pancrelipase** (Cotazym-S, Entolase, others) and **lactase** (LactAid).
3. Digestive enzyme replacements are used to treat **exocrine pancreatic insufficiency, cystic fibrosis,** and **steatorrhea.** Lactase is useful in **lactose-intolerant individuals.**

B. Adverse effects. Digestive enzyme replacements produce hyperuricemia, hyperuricosuria, allergic reactions, and GI upset.

VII. AGENTS THAT ACT ON THE LOWER GI TRACT

A. Laxatives (stool softeners, antidiarrheals) act primarily on the large intestine to **promote an increase in the fluid** accumulated in the bowel, **decrease net absorption of fluid** from the bowel, or **alter bowel motility.** These actions facilitate the evacuation of fecal material. Laxatives should not be used chronically as they may induce "laxative dependence."

1. ***Bulk-forming laxatives***
   a. Bulk-forming laxatives include **psyllium** (Metamucil, others), **methylcellulose** (Citrucel), and **polycarbophil** (Fibercon, Fiber Lax).
   b. Bulk-forming laxatives are hydrophilic **natural or semisynthetic polysaccharide or cellulose derivatives** that are poorly absorbed from the bowel lumen and **retain water in the bowel.** The increased luminal mass **stimulates peristalsis.**
   c. These agents are the treatment of choice for **chronic constipation.**
   d. Bulk-forming laxatives produce laxation after 2–4 days; adequate hydration is required.
   e. These agents may cause bloating and flatulence.
2. ***Osmotic agents*** include both salt-containing and salt-free agents.
   a. **Salt-containing osmotic laxatives (saline laxatives)**
      (1) Salt-containing osmotic laxatives include **magnesium sulfate, magnesium citrate, magnesium hydroxide, sodium phosphates,** and **mineral water.**
      (2) These agents are poorly absorbed ions that **retain water in the lumen by osmosis** and cause a **reflex increase in peristalsis.**
      (3) Salt-containing osmotic laxatives are taken orally. Sodium phosphates are also effective rectally. Onset of action typically occurs 3–6 hours after oral administration and 5–15 minutes after rectal administration. They require adequate hydration for effect.
      (4) These agents are used for **short-term evacuation of the bowel before surgery or diagnostic procedures** or for **elimination of parasites** after anthelmintic administration.
      (5) Some systemic effects are possible with these agents, especially in cases of renal dysfunction; these effects include hypermagnesemia and hypernatremia. In critically ill patients, caution should be used before administering these agents as they cause **intravascular volume depletion** and may lead to exacerbation of hypovolemic shock.
   b. **Salt-free osmotic laxatives**
      (1) Salt-free osmotic laxatives include **glycerin, lactulose** (Chronulac), and **polyethylene glycol-electrolyte solutions** (Colyte, Go-Lytely).
      (2) These agents may be administered rectally (glycerin) or orally (lactulose). Go-Lytely is used for **preoperative colon preparation.**

3. ***Irritant (stimulant) laxatives***
   a. Irritant laxatives include diphenylmethane derivatives such as **bisacodyl** (Modane, Dulcolax), the anthraquinone derivative **senna** (Senokot), and **castor oil.**
   b. Irritant laxatives **stimulate smooth muscle contractions resulting from their irritant action on the bowel mucosa.** Local bowel **inflammation also promotes accumulation of water and electrolytes.** The increased luminal contents stimulate reflex peristalsis, and the irritant action stimulates peristalsis directly.
   c. The onset of action occurs in 6–12 hours; these agents require adequate hydration.
   d. Chronic use of irritant laxatives may result in **cathartic colon,** a condition of **colonic distention,** and development of **laxative dependence.**
4. ***Stool softeners***
   a. Stool softeners include **docusate sodium** (Colace, others).
   b. Stool softeners have a **detergent action** that facilitates the mixing of water and fatty substances to **increase luminal mass.**
   c. These agents are marginally effective and are used to produce **short-term laxation** and to reduce straining at defecation. They are also used to **prevent constipation;** they are not effective in treating ongoing constipation.
5. ***Coating agents: mineral oil***
   a. Mineral oil, now seldom used clinically due to its potentially serious adverse actions, **coats fecal contents** and thereby inhibits absorption of water.
   b. Mineral oil **decreases absorption of fat-soluble vitamins. Lipoid pneumonia** can develop if mineral oil is aspirated.

B. **Antidiarrheal agents.** Antidiarrheal agents aim to decrease fecal water content by **increasing solute absorption and decreasing intestinal secretion and motility.** Increased transit time facilitates water reabsorption. Therapy with these drugs should be reserved for patients with significant and persistent symptoms of diarrhea.
1. ***Opioids* act directly on opioid μ-receptors** to decrease transit rate, stimulate segmental (nonpropulsive) contraction, and inhibit longitudinal contraction. They also **stimulate electrolyte absorption** (mediated by opioid μ- and δ-receptors).
   a. **Diphenoxylate** (Lomotil)
      (1) Diphenoxylate, a synthetic morphine analogue, and its active metabolite, **difenoxin** (Motofen), are used for the treatment of diarrhea and not analgesia.
      (2) Diphenoxylate is used as a combination product with **atropine** to reduce the potential for abuse.
      (3) At high doses this agent may produce CNS effects including nausea and vomiting, sedation, and constipation.
   b. **Loperamide** (Imodium)
      (1) Loperamide is an **opioid agonist** with **no CNS activity,** except at very high doses, but with marked effects on the intestine. It binds to opioid receptors in the GI tract.
      (2) Loperamide has a faster onset and longer duration of action than diphenoxylate.
      (3) Loperamide has fewer adverse effects than diphenoxylate. However, overdose can result in severe constipation, paralytic ileus, and CNS depression.
   c. **Other opioids** include **camphorated opium tincture** (Paregoric), **deodorized tincture of opium** (Laudanum), and **codeine.**
2. ***Adsorbents***
   a. Adsorbents include **kaolin** and **pectin** (Kaopectate).
   b. These agents **act by adsorbing fluid, toxins, and bacteria and are used for acute diarrhea.** They are less effective than other agents.
   c. These agents are not absorbed; they are nontoxic; may absorb other drugs if given within 2 hours of their administration.
3. ***Bismuth subsalicylate (Pepto Bismol)***
   a. The salicylate in this agent **inhibits prostaglandin and chloride secretion in the intestine to reduce the liquid content of the stools.** It is effective for both treatment and prophylaxis of **traveler's diarrhea** and other forms of diarrhea.
   b. Bismuth subsalicylate forms a protective coating in the GI tract and has **direct antimicrobial activity.** It is used to treat ***H. pylori* infection.**

c. Bismuth subsalicylate is also used effectively to **bind toxins produced by *Vibrio cholerae* and *Escherichia coli*.** The salicylate can be absorbed across the intestine.
d. Bismuth subsalicylate produces adverse effects that include **tinnitus.** It may also produce **black stools** and staining of the tongue.

4. ***Octreotide (Sandostatin)***
a. Octreotide is a synthetic 8-amino acid **analogue of somatostatin.** It is effective for treatment of diarrhea caused by **short-gut syndrome and dumping syndrome.**
b. Octreotide is used in cases of **severe diarrhea caused by excessive release of GI tract hormones,** including gastrin, motilin, vasoactive intestinal polypeptide, glucagon, and others. As such, octreotide is used in treatment of **carcinoids** and vasoactive intestinal polypeptide-secreting tumors (**VIPomas**).
c. This agent must be administered parenterally.
d. Octreotide causes mild GI dysfunction and pain at the site of injection.

5. ***Oral rehydration solutions***
a. Oral rehydration solutions include **WHO solution** and **Infalyte.**
b. Oral rehydration solutions are **balanced salt solutions** containing glucose, sucrose, or rice powder.
c. These solutions **increase water absorption** from the bowel lumen by increasing Na^+-substrate transport across intestinal epithelial cells.
d. Oral rehydration solutions can remedy 99% of acute cases of **childhood diarrhea.**

C. Agents used in inflammatory bowel disease (IBD): ulcerative colitis and Crohn disease

1. ***Mesalamine*** (Asacol, Pentasa), ***sulfasalazine*** (Azulfidine), ***olsalazine*** (Dipentum), and ***balsalazide*** (Colazal)
a. **Mesalamine (5-aminosalicylic acid or 5-ASA**), the active agent for treatment of IBD, is formulated as delayed-release microgranules (Penstasa), a pH-sensitive resin (Asacol), a suspension enema (Canasa), or wax suppository (Rowasa). **Sulfasalazine, olsalazine, and balsalazide** are dimers that **contain the active agent 5-ASA bound by an azo bond (N=N) to an inert compound or to another molecule of 5-ASA that prevent its absorption.** The azo bond is cleaved in the terminal ileum by bacterial enzyme. The released **5-ASA acts topically within the colon.** Although the exact mechanism of action of these agents is uncertain, these agents interfere with the production of inflammatory cytokines.
b. These agents are most effective for the treatment of **mild-to-moderate ulcerative colitis.**
c. **Sulfasalazine** is bound by an azo bond to **sulfapyridine** that when released and absorbed is responsible, due to the sulfa moiety, for a **high incidence of adverse effects** that include nausea, headaches, bone marrow suppression, general malaise, and **hypersensitivity. Slow acetylators** of sulfapyridine are most likely to experience adverse effects. The other agents are generally well tolerated. **Olsalazine** may cause a **secretory diarrhea.**

2. ***Glucocorticoids*** and other **drugs reacting on the immune system**
a. **Prednisone** is used most commonly in **acute exacerbation** of the disease, as well as in **maintenance therapy.**
b. **Budesonide** (Entocort) is an an analogue of prednisolone. It has low oral bioavailability, so enteric-coated, delayed-release formulations are more commonly used.
c. The mechanism of action for these agents involves **inhibition of proinflammatory cytokines.** Glucocorticoids carry a high incidence of **systemic side effects,** so their use in maintenance therapy is limited.
d. Up to **60% of patients with IBD are steroid-unresponsive** or have only a partial response.
e. Glucocorticoids **stimulate sodium absorption in the jejunum, ileum, and colon;** glucocoticoids such as budesonide and prednisone are also used to treat **refractory diarrhea** unresponsive to other agents (see VII B).

3. ***Azathioprine*** (Imuran) and ***6-mercaptopurine*** (Purinethol) are **purine antimetabolites** and thus immune suppressants. The onset of therapeutic action is **delayed by several weeks;** therefore these agents are **not used in an acute setting.** These agents are used for **maintenance and remission of IBD in patients who do not respond well to steroids.** Major side effect is **bone marrow depression.**

4. ***Methotrexate*** (Rheumatrex, Trexall) is another immune suppressant that acts via **inhibition of dihydrofolate reductase.** It is used to **induce and maintain remission in patients with Crohn disease who do not respond well to steroids** (it is also used to treat rheumatoid arthritis and cancer). **Bone marrow suppression** is a major side effect when this drug is used at higher doses.
5. ***Infliximab*** (Remicade) is a **monoclonal antibody that binds to and neutralizes TNF-α, a major cytokine that mediates the T_H1 immune response present during inflammation, specifically in Crohn disease.** It is administered only IV. Improvement of symptoms is observed in two-thirds of patients, and repeat infusions are required for maintenance of remission. Adverse effects include infection, including reactivation of tuberculosis.

D. Agents used in treatment of irritable bowel syndrome (IBS)

1. ***Alosetron*** (Lotronex) is a **5-HT_3 antagonist** that blocks receptors on enteric neurons, thereby **reducing distention and inhibiting colonic motility.** Its main use is in "**diarrhea predominant" IBS. Alosetron may cause severe constipation with ischemic colitis that requires its discontinuation.** Therefore, its **use is restricted** to patients who have not responded to other therapies and who are educated to its risk.
2. ***Tegaserod*** (Zelnorm), a **serotonin 5-HT_4 partial agonist** that results in **stimulation of peristalsis and enhancement of gastric emptying,** is used as to treat patients with chronic "**constipation predominant**" IBS. Tegaserod is a relatively safe agent.

DRUG SUMMARY TABLE

Antiemetics
Cholinoceptor, histamine receptor, and dopamine receptor antagonists
Scopolamine (Transderm Scop, Hyoscine)
Dimenhydrinate (Dramamine)
Cyclizine (Marezine)
Meclizine (Antivert, Bonine)
Prochlorperazine (Compazine)
Droperidol (Inapsine)
Metoclopramide (Reglan)
Serotonin receptor antagonists
Ondansetron (Zofran)
Granisetron (Kytril)
Dolasetron (Anzemet)
Palonosetron (Aloxi)
Cannabinoids
Dronabinol (Marinol)
Benzodiazepines
Lorazepam (Ativan)
Diazepam (Valium)
Neurokinin receptor antagonists
Aprepitant (Emend)

Anorexigenics and Appetite Enhancers
Amphetamines
Phentermine (Adipex)
Phenypropanolamine (Acutrim, Dexetrim)
Sibutramine (Meridia)
Orlistat (Xenical)
Dronabinol (Marinol)
Megestrol (Megace)

Agents Used for Upper GI
Antacids
Sodium bicarbonate (Alka Seltzer)
Calcium carbonate (TUMS, Os-Cal)
Magnesium and aluminum hydroxide (Maalox)
Histamine H_2-receptor antagonists
Cimetidine (Tagamet)
Ranitidine (Zantac)
Famotidine (Pepcid)
Nizatidine (Axid)
Proton pump inhibitors (PPIs)
Omeprazole (Prilosec)
Lansoprazole (Prevacid)
Pantoprazole (Protonix)
Rabeprazole (AcipHex)
Esomeprazole (Nexium)
Mucosal protective agents
Sucralfate (Carafate)
Misoprostol (Cytotec)

Drugs Acting on Lower GI
Laxatives: bulk forming agents
Psyllium (Metamucil)
Methylcellulose (Citrucel)
Polycarbophil (Fibercon, Fiber Lax)
Laxatives: osmotic agents
Magnesium salts, sodium phosphates
Mineral water
Lactulose (Chronulac)
PGE solutions (Colyte, Go-Lytely)
Glycerin
Laxatives: irritant agents
Bisacodyl (Dulcolax, Modane)
Senna (Senokot)
Castor oil
Stool softeners
Docusate (Colace)
Coating agents
Mineral oil
Antidiarrheal agents: opioids
Opium tincture (Paregoric)
Loperamide (Imodium)
Diphenoxylate (Lomotil)
Difenoxin (Motofen)
Antidiarrheal agents: adsorbents
Kaolin + pectin (Kaopectate)
Antidiarrheal agents: miscellaneous
Bismuth subsalicylate (Pepto Bismol)
Octreotide (Sandostatin)
WHO solution
Infalyte
Agents for inflammatory bowel disease (IBD)
Sulfasalazine (Azulfidine)
Mesalamine (Asacol, Pentasa)
Olsalazine (Dipentum)
Balsalazide (Colazal)
Budesonide (Entocort)
Prednisone
Azathioprine (Imuran)
6-Mercaptopurine (Purinethol)
Methotrexate (Rheumatrex, Trexall)
Infliximab (Remicade)
Agents for irritable bowel syndrome (IBS)
Alosetron (Lotronex)
Tegaserod (Zelnorm)

Prokinetic Agents
Metoclopramide (Reglan)
Cisapride (Propulsid)

Drugs Used to Dissolve Gallstones
Ursodiol (Actigal)

Digestive Enzyme Replacements
Pancrelipase (Cotazym-S, Entolase)
Lactase (LactAid)

Review Test for Chapter 8

Directions: Each of the numbered items or incomplete statements in this section is followed by answers or by completions of the statement. Select the ONE lettered answer or completion that is BEST in each case.

1. A 54-year-old man with a 75-pack/year history of tobacco abuse and alcohol abuse has developed carcinoma of the larynx. His treatment includes concurrent high-dose cisplatin and radiation therapy. He has developed significant nausea and vomiting. Which would be the best agent to treat these side effects?

(A) Metoclopramide
(B) Ondansetron
(C) Meclizine
(D) Promethazine
(E) Loperamide

2. Aprepitant is which of the following?

(A) Cholinergic antagonist
(B) Dopaminergic agonist
(C) Histamine H_1-receptor antagonist
(D) Serotonin 5-HT_3 antagonist
(E) Substance P antagonist

3. A 74-year-old man went on a cruise to celebrate his 50th wedding anniversary. Concerned about a history of motion sickness, the patient saw his primary care physician about a medication to take. He is now seen by the onboard physician with complaints of blurred vision, confusion, constipation, and urinary retention. Which of the following did the primary care physician likely prescribe?

(A) Scopolamine
(B) Metoclopramide
(C) Haloperidol
(D) Dronabinol
(E) Ondansetron

4. Which of the following drugs would be best to use to treat irritable bowel syndrome (IBS) in a 53-year-old woman?

(A) Infliximab
(B) Diphenoxylate
(C) Cimetidine
(D) Tegaserod
(E) Orlistat

5. A 35-year-old AIDS patient is admitted for the treatment of *Pneumocystis* pneumonia (PCP). He is obviously cachetic and has a poor appetite. He admits that he only feels like eating after he "smokes some weed." Because you can't legally prescribe marijuana, you decide to start therapy with what agent?

(A) Granisetron
(B) Sibutramine
(C) Dronabinol
(D) Phentermine
(E) Dextroamphetamine

6. As a gastroenterologist, you recommend the use of a histamine H_2-blocker for a patient who has a history of atrial fibrillation, for which he takes warfarin. Your office receives a call from his primary physician, who has admitted the patient for warfarin toxicity. Which of the following H_2-blockers has the patient likely been taking?

(A) Cimetidine
(B) Ranitidine
(C) Scopolamine
(D) Famotidine
(E) Nizatidine

7. A 34-year-old man is seen over multiple visits for complaints of "ulcers," despite the use of ranitidine. Further studies, finding elevated levels of gastrin and evidence of ulcers involving the jejunum, suggest a diagnosis of Zollinger-Ellison syndrome. Which of the following agents would be most useful in the management of this patient?

(A) Famotidine
(B) Lansoprazole
(C) Misoprostol
(D) Propantheline
(E) Pepto Bismol

8. A 63-year-old man with long-standing, poorly controlled diabetes is admitted for yet another episode of ketoacidosis. Now that he is out of the intensive care unit and beginning to eat, he complains of regurgitation of food following even small meals. You suspect the development of diabetic gastropathy, a consequence of his autonomic neuropathy. Which of the following might help his condition?

(A) Sucralfate
(B) Metoclopramide
(C) Scopolamine
(D) Misoprostol
(E) Pepto Bismol

9. A 78-year-old woman sees her primary care physician with complaints of "heartburn." Her history includes only hypertension. She lives on a fixed income and has no prescription coverage. Her doctor recommends over-the-counter antacids to be used regularly. Which of the following would be a good choice and why?

(A) Sodium bicarbonate because it is good for long-term use
(B) Calcium carbonate because it is good for long-term use and she could use the calcium
(C) Magnesium hydroxide for short-term use only because of her hypertension
(D) A combined agent to balance the constipation associated with magnesium hydroxide and the diarrhea associated with aluminum hydroxide
(E) A combined agent to balance the diarrhea associated with magnesium hydroxide and the constipation associated with aluminum hydroxide

10. An otherwise healthy 33-year-old man sees his physician for a routine physical. The patient has no complaints and is planning on vacationing in Mexico next month. However, he is afraid of developing traveler's diarrhea. You recommend that he take which of the following drugs for prophylaxis?

(A) Glucocorticoids
(B) Loperamide
(C) Bismuth subsalicylate
(D) Kaolin
(E) Diphenoxylate

11. A 72-year-old man with a 150-pack/year history of cigarette smoking presents for further work-up of a large mass seen on a recent chest x-ray. The patient reports a 50-lb unintentional weight loss over the last 3 months and a poor appetite. In addition to beginning chemotherapy, the oncologist decides to add which agent to promote his appetite?

(A) Aprepitant
(B) Ipecac
(C) Lorazepam
(D) Ondansetron
(E) Megestrol

12. A 65-year-old man presents to his family physician with a 3-month history of watery diarrhea. He is referred to a gastroenterologist, who finds that the patient is also hypokalemic and achlorhydric and has an elevated serum level of vasoactive intestinal peptide due to a pancreatic islet cell tumor (VIPoma). Which agent would be best to treat the patient's symptoms?

(A) Gastrin
(B) Octreotide
(C) Glucagon
(D) Bismuth subsalicylate
(E) Sulfasalazine

Answers and Explanations

1. **The answer is B.** Ondansetron is a 5-HT3 antagonist that is highly effective in the treatment of cisplatin-induced chemotherapy, better so than metoclopramide. Both meclizine and promethazine are antagonists of H_1-receptors used in the treatment of motion sickness, true vertigo, and pregnancy-associated nausea. Loperamide is an antidiarrheal agent.

2. **The answer is E.** Aprepitant is the first available substance P antagonist used for the prevention of both sudden and delayed chemotherapy-induced nausea and vomiting. It can be used synergistically with serotonin 5-HT_3 antagonists such as ondansetron. The other antagonists, cholinergic (i.e., scopolamine), histaminic (i.e., promethazine), and dopaminergic (i.e., metoclopramide), are used to treat nausea and vomiting, although not in this setting.

3. **The answer is A.** Scopolamine is a cholinergic antagonist that is likely associated with all the patient's new symptoms. Metoclopramide can cause extrapyramidal effects, as can haloperidol. Dronabinol can cause sedation, dry mouth, psychotic effects, and orthostatic hypotension. Ondansetron can cause mild headache.

4. **The answer is D.** Tegaserod has been shown to provide some relief of irritable bowel syndrome (IBS). Infliximab is a biologic agent used in the management of inflammatory bowel disease (IBD). Diphenoxylate is a morphine analogue used to treat diarrhea. Cimetidine is used to treat esophageal reflux. Orlistat is an agent used to manage obesity.

5. **The answer is C.** Dronabinol is used in the treatment of AIDS wasting, specifically to increase appetite. Dronabinol contains Δ-9-tetrahydrocannabinol, the active ingredient in marijuana. Granisetron is effective for nausea and vomiting in chemotherapy. The other agents, sibutramine, phentermine, and dextroamphetamine, are used to aid in weight loss.

6. **The answer is A.** Cimetidine is a competitive inhibitor of the P-450 system, which thereby increases the half-life of warfarin. This can lead to supratherapeutic levels of the drug and bleeding problems. The other H_2-blockers, including ranitidine, famotidine, and nizatidine, are not metabolized by the P-450 system.

7. **The answer is B.** Lansoprazole is an H^+/K^+-ATPase proton pump inhibitor useful in the treatment of patients who have failed histamine H_2-blocker therapy and patients with Zollinger-Ellison syndrome. Famotidine is a histamine H_2-blocker. Misoprostol is used to prevent ulcers in patients taking nonsteroidal anti-inflammatory drugs (NSAIDs). Propantheline is a cholinergic agent used in conjunction with other agents, and rarely alone. Ulcers associated with *Helicobacter pylori (H. pylori)* can be treated with Pepto Bismol.

8. **The answer is B.** Poor gastric emptying is a manifestation of the neuropathy that accompanies long-standing diabetes. Metoclopramide is a prokinetic agent used in the treatment of diabetic gastroparesis. Sucralfate, scopolamine, and misoprostol are use to treat gastric ulcers. Pepto Bismol is added in the case of peptic ulcers due to *Helicobacter pylori (H. pylori).*

9. **The answer is E.** Both sodium bicarbonate and calcium carbonate are not for long-term use. In addition, sodium bicarbonate is contraindicated in patients with hypertension. A combined agent like Maalox or Mylanta II provides a balance between the diarrhea associated with magnesium hydroxide and the constipation associated with aluminum hydroxide.

10. **The answer is C.** Bismuth subsalicylate is effective for both the treatment and prophylaxis of traveler's diarrhea, most often due to *Escherichia coli (E. coli)*-contaminated water. Loperamide and diphenoxylate are good to treat diarrhea, but generally are not used for prophylaxis. Glucocorticoids are for diarrhea refractory to normal treatment.

11. **The answer is E.** Megestrol acetate is used as an appetite stimulant and results in weight gain in some patients with cancer. Aprepitant, lorazepam, and ondansetron, while having different mechanisms, are all used for nausea and vomiting, which he may experience eventually with his chemotherapy. Ipecac is proemetic.

12. **The answer is B.** Octreotide is used in the treatment of endocrine tumors such as gastrinomas, glucagonomas, and VIPomas to help alleviate the diarrhea. Bismuth subsalicylate is used to treat traveler's diarrhea, and sulfasalazine is used treat such inflammatory bowel disease, such as Crohn disease. Gastrin is a GI hormone.

chapter 9

Drugs Acting on the Pulmonary System

I. INTRODUCTION TO PULMONARY DISORDERS

In **asthma, chronic bronchitis,** and **rhinitis,** the effective diameter of the airways is decreased. The goal of therapy is to decrease airway resistance by increasing the diameter of the bronchi and decreasing mucus secretion or stagnation in the airways.

A. Asthma

1. ***Asthma is characterized by acute episodes of bronchoconstriction caused by underlying airway inflammation.*** A hallmark of asthma is bronchial hyperreactivity to numerous kinds of endogenous or exogenous stimuli. In asthmatic patients, the response to various stimuli is amplified by persistent inflammation.
2. ***Antigenic stimuli trigger the release of mediators*** (leukotrienes, histamine, and many others) that cause a bronchospastic response, with smooth muscle contraction, mucus secretion, and recruitment of inflammatory cells such as eosinophils, basophils, and macrophages (early-phase response).
3. Late-phase response (which may occur in hours or days) is an inflammatory response; levels of histamine and other mediators released from inflammatory cells rise again and may induce bronchospasm. Eventually fibrin and collagen deposition and tissue destruction occur.
4. Nonantigenic stimuli (cool air, exercise, nonoxidizing pollutants) can trigger nonspecific bronchoconstriction after early-phase sensitization.

B. Chronic bronchitis

1. Chronic bronchitis is characterized by pulmonary obstruction caused by excessive production of mucus due to hyperplasia and hyperfunctioning of mucus-secreting goblet cells.
2. Chronic bronchitis is often induced by an irritant.

C. Rhinitis

1. Rhinitis is a decrease in nasal airways due to thickening of the mucosa and increased mucus secretion.
2. Rhinitis may be caused by allergy, viruses, vasomotor abnormalities, or rhinitis medicamentosa.

II. AGENTS USED TO TREAT ASTHMA AND OTHER BRONCHIAL DISORDERS (TABLE 9-1)

Treatment of asthma is based on the severity of the disease and response to individual agents.

A. Adrenergic agonists

1. ***General characteristics***
   a. Adrenergic agonists stimulate β_2-adrenoceptors, resulting in relaxation of bronchial smooth muscle. These agents also inhibit the release of mediators and stimulate mucociliary clearance.

table 9-1 Recommendations for Management of Asthma

Severity	Symptoms	Recommended Treatment (Short Term)	Recommended Treatment (Long Term)
Mild intermittent	Symptoms (wheezing, etc.) <2 a week; nighttime symptoms <2 a month	Short-acting inhaled β_2 agonists	No daily medication required
Mild persistent	Symptoms >2 a week, <1 a day; nighttime symptoms >2 a month	Short-acting β_2 agonist	Daily inhaled low-dose corticosteroid, alternative cromolyn, or nedocromil, or theophilline
Moderate persistent	Symptoms daily; nighttime symptoms >1 a week	Short-acting β_2 agonist	Inhaled corticosteroid (medium dose) and long-acting inhaled β_2-agonist
Severe persistent	Continual symptoms; frequent	Short-acting inhaled β_2 agonist	Inhaled corticosteroid (high dose), inhaled long-acting β_2 agonist, and oral corticosteroids

Modified from Expert Panel Report III: Guidelines for the Diagnosis and Management of Asthma, National Asthma Education and Prevention Program, 2007.

b. Adrenergic agonists are useful for the treatment of the acute bronchoconstriction (exacerbations) of asthma.

c. Depending on biologic half-life of the drug, these agents are used both for quick relief and for long-term control.

d. The use of short-acting, inhaled β_2-adrenoceptor agonists on a daily basis, with increasing necessity of use, indicates the need for additional long-term pharmacotherapy.

2. *Short-acting β_2-adrenoceptor agonists*

a. Albuterol, levalbuterol, pirbuterol, metaproterenol

(1) These agents have enhanced β_2-receptor selectivity.

(2) These agents are generally administered by inhalation and their onset of action is 1–5 minutes. Some preparations are available for oral administration.

(3) Long-term use of these agents for the treatment of chronic asthma has been associated with diminished control, perhaps due to β-receptor down-regulation.

b. Nonselective agents

(1) Isoproterenol is a relatively nonselective β-receptor agonist and a potent bronchodilator. Isoproterenol is most effective in asthmatic patients when administered as an inhalant. During an acute attack, dosing every 1–2 hours is typically required; oral preparations are administered 4 times daily (qid).

(2) Epinephrine is available over the counter (OTC) and acts as a β_1-, β_2-, and α_1-adrenoceptor agonist. Epinephrine can be administered as an inhalant or subcutaneously (in emergency circumstances); onset of action occurs within 5–10 minutes, and duration is 60–90 minutes.

3. *Long-acting β_2-adrenoceptor agonists*

a. Salmeterol (Serevent), formoterol (Foradil)

(1) These agents are administered as inhalants but have a slower onset of action and a longer duration of action than the short-acting preparations. Both have very lipophilic side chains that slow diffusion out of the airway.

(2) These agents are very effective for prophylaxis of asthma but should not be used to treat an acute attack.

b. Terbutaline is a moderately specific β_2-agonist that is currently available for injection or as a tablet. As with the other mixed β-adrenoceptor agonists, systemic use is cardiostimulatory.

4. *Adverse effects of adrenergic agonists*

a. The adverse effects of adrenergic agonists are based on receptor occupancy.

b. These adverse effects are minimized by inhalant delivery of the adrenergic agonists directly to the airways.

(1) Epinephrine and isoproterenol have significant β_1-receptor activity and can cause cardiac effects, including tachycardia and arrhythmias, and the exacerbation of angina.

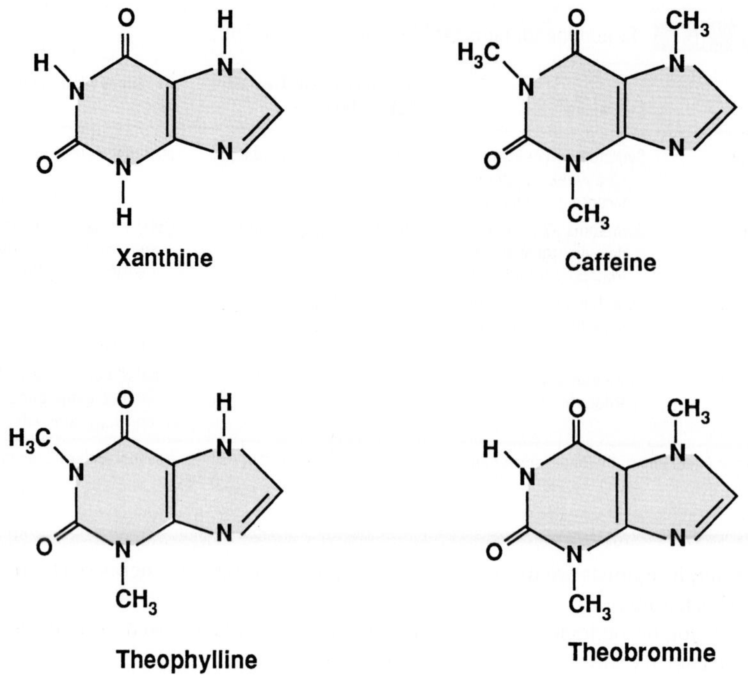

FIGURE 9-1. Structures of methylxanthines, including xanthine, caffeine, theophylline, and theobromine.

(2) The most common adverse effect of β_2-adrenoreceptor agonists is skeletal muscle tremor.

(3) The adverse effects of α-adrenoceptor agonists include vasoconstriction and hypertension.

(4) Tachyphylaxis, a blunting in the response to adrenergic agonists on repeated use, can be countered by switching to a different agonist or by adding a methylxanthine or corticosteroid to the regimen.

B. Methylxanthines (Fig. 9-1)

1. *General characteristics*

a. For asthma, the most frequently administered methylxanthine is theophylline (1,3-dimethylxanthine). Additional members of this family include theobromine and caffeine.

b. Because of the limited solubility of theophylline in water, it is complexed as a salt, as in aminophylline and oxtriphylline.

2. *Mechanism of action*

a. Methylxanthines cause bronchodilation by action on the smooth muscles in the airways. The exact mechanism remains controversial; some data suggest that it is an adenosine-receptor antagonist (adenosine causes bronchoconstriction and promotes the release of histamine from mast cells). In addition, these drugs may decrease the entry and mobilization of cellular Ca^{2+} stores. However, theophylline analogues that lack adenosine-antagonist activity maintain bronchodilator activity.

b. Theophylline also has some anti-inflammatory properties and reduces airway responsiveness to agents such as histamine and to allergens.

c. Theophylline is effective in reducing the synergistic effect of adenosine and antigen stimulation on histamine release.

d. Theophylline inhibits phosphodiesterase (leading to increased cyclic adenosine monophosphate (cAMP)), but this effect requires very high doses, and its contribution to bronchodilation remains to be established.

3. *Pharmacologic effects*

a. Respiratory system. Methylxanthines affect a number of physiologic systems, but they are most useful in the treatment of asthma because of the following:

(1) These agents produce rapid relaxation of bronchial smooth muscle.
(2) Methylxanthines decrease histamine release in response to reaginic (immunoglobulin E) stimulation.
(3) These agents stimulate ciliary transport of mucus.
(4) Methylxanthines improve respiratory performance by improving the contractility of the diaphragm and by stimulating the medullary respiratory center.

b. Other systems
(1) Methylxanthines have positive chronotropic and inotropic actions on the heart.
(2) These agents cause pulmonary and peripheral vasodilation but cerebral vasoconstriction.
(3) Methylxanthines cause an increase in alertness and cortical arousal at low doses; at high doses, this can proceed to severe nervousness and seizures due to medullary stimulation.
(4) These agents stimulate gastric acid and pepsinogen release.
(5) Methylxanthines cause diuresis.

4. ***Pharmacologic properties***
a. Methylxanthines are almost completely absorbed after oral administration.
b. Methylxanthines are readily permeable into all tissue compartments; these agents cross the placenta and can enter breast milk.
c. Methylxanthines are metabolized extensively in the liver and are excreted by the kidney.

5. ***Prototype drug: theophylline***
a. Theophylline is available in a microcrystalline form for inhalation and as a sustained-release preparation; it can be administered intravenously (IV).
b. **Theophylline has a very narrow therapeutic index;** blood levels should be monitored on the initiation of therapy.
c. Theophylline has a variable half-life ($t_{1/2}$), approximately 8–9 hours in adults, but shorter in children. Clearance of theophylline is affected by diet, drugs, and hepatic disease.

6. ***Therapeutic uses***
a. Methylxanthines are considered adjuncts to inhaled corticosteroids and are used to treat acute or chronic asthma that is unresponsive to inhaled corticosteroids or β-adrenoceptor agonists; they can be administered prophylactically.
b. These agents are used to treat chronic obstructive lung disease and emphysema.
c. Methylxanthines are used to treat apnea in preterm infants (based on stimulation of the central respiratory center); usually, caffeine is the agent of choice for this therapy.

7. ***Adverse effects***
a. The adverse effects of methylxanthines include arrhythmias, nervousness, vomiting, and gastrointestinal bleeding.
b. Methylxanthines may cause behavioral problems in children.
c. The combined use of these agents with β_2-adrenoceptor agonists is now suspected to be responsible for recent rises in asthma mortality.

C. Muscarinic antagonists

1. Muscarinic antagonists include **ipratropium bromide** (Atrovent) and atropine.
2. Muscarinic antagonists are competitive antagonists of acetylcholine (ACh) at the muscarinic receptor. They inhibit ACh-mediated constriction of bronchial airways. Anticholinergics also decrease vagal-stimulated mucus secretion.
3. These agents are somewhat variable in their effectiveness as bronchodilators in asthma, but they are useful in patients who are refractory to, or intolerant of, sympathomimetics or methylxanthines.
4. Ipratropium, a quaternary amine that is poorly absorbed and does not cross the blood-brain barrier, is administered as an aerosol; its low systemic absorption limits adverse effects.
5. **Tiotropium (Spiriva)** is a long-acting muscarinic antagonist approved for maintenance of chronic obstructive pulmonary disease (COPD).
6. **Atropine** is readily absorbed into the systemic circulation. The adverse effects of atropine include drowsiness, sedation, dry mouth, and blurred vision; these effects limit its use as an antiasthmatic.

D. Chromones

1. *Cromolyn sodium (Intal)*

a. Cromolyn sodium is disodium cromoglycate, a salt of very low solubility in aqueous solutions.

b. The precise mechanism of action of these drugs is unclear, but they inhibit the release of mediators from mast cells; suppress the activation of neutrophils, eosinophiles, and monocytes; and inhibit cough reflexes. These activities may be due to inhibition of chloride channels. They do not cause relaxation of bronchial smooth muscle.

c. Cromolyn sodium is poorly absorbed. It must be administered by inhalation; it is available as a microparticulate powder or as an aerosol.

d. Cromolyn sodium is used prophylactically in asthma; it does not reverse an established bronchospasm. It is the only antiasthmatic that inhibits both early- and late-phase responses.

e. Cromolyn sodium produces generally localized adverse effects, which include sore throat, cough, and dry mouth. It may infrequently cause dermatitis, gastroenteritis, nausea, and headache.

2. *Nedocromil sodium (Tilade)*

a. Nedocromil sodium is similar in action to cromolyn.

b. This agent appears to be more effective than cromolyn in blocking bronchospasm induced by exercise or cold air.

c. Nedocromil sodium is administered as an inhalant.

E. Glucocorticoids

1. Glucocorticoids include beclomethasone (Beclovent, Vanceril), triamcinolone acetate (Azmacort), budesonide (Rhinocort), flunisolide (AeroBid), and fluticasone propionate (Flovent).

2. Glucocorticoids produce a significant increase in airway diameter, probably by attenuating prostaglandin and leukotriene synthesis via inhibition of the phospholipase A_2 reaction and by generally inhibiting the immune response. They increase responsiveness to sympathomimetics and decrease mucus production.

3. Glucocorticoids are available as oral, topical, and inhaled agents.

   a. Use of inhaled glucocorticoids is recommended for the initial treatment of asthma, with additional agents added as needed. They are used prophylactically rather than to reverse an acute attack. The most common adverse effects of inhaled glucocorticoids are hoarseness and oral candidiasis; the most serious adverse effects are adrenal suppression and osteoporosis.

   b. Inhaled glucocorticoids are partially absorbed.

   c. Because of their systemic adverse effects, **oral glucocorticoids** (see Chapter 10) are usually reserved for patients with severe persistent asthma.

F. Leukotriene inhibitors

1. *Zafirlukast (Accolate) and montelukast (Singulair)*

a. Zafirlukast and montelukast are antagonists of the leukotriene receptor LT_1. This blocks the action of the cys-leukotrienes C_4, D_4, and E_4 (LTC_4, LTD_4, LTE_4, respectively).

b. The drugs reduce bronchoconstriction and inflammatory cell infiltration.

c. Most studies with this class of drugs have been done with mild persistent asthma, and they appear to be moderately effective.

d. These drugs are recommended as an alternative to medium-dose inhaled glucocorticoids in moderate and severe persistent asthma.

e. Adverse effects of zafirlukast include headache and elevation in liver enzymes.

f. Zafirlukast and montelukast are administered orally, 1–2 times per day.

g. Zafirlukast inhibits the metabolism of warfarin.

2. *Zileuton (Zyflo)*

a. Zileuton inhibits 5-lipoxygenase, the rate-limiting enzyme in leukotriene biosynthesis.

b. Zileuton causes an immediate and sustained 15% improvement in forced expiratory volume in patients with mild persistent asthma.

c. This agent relieves bronchoconstriction from exercise.

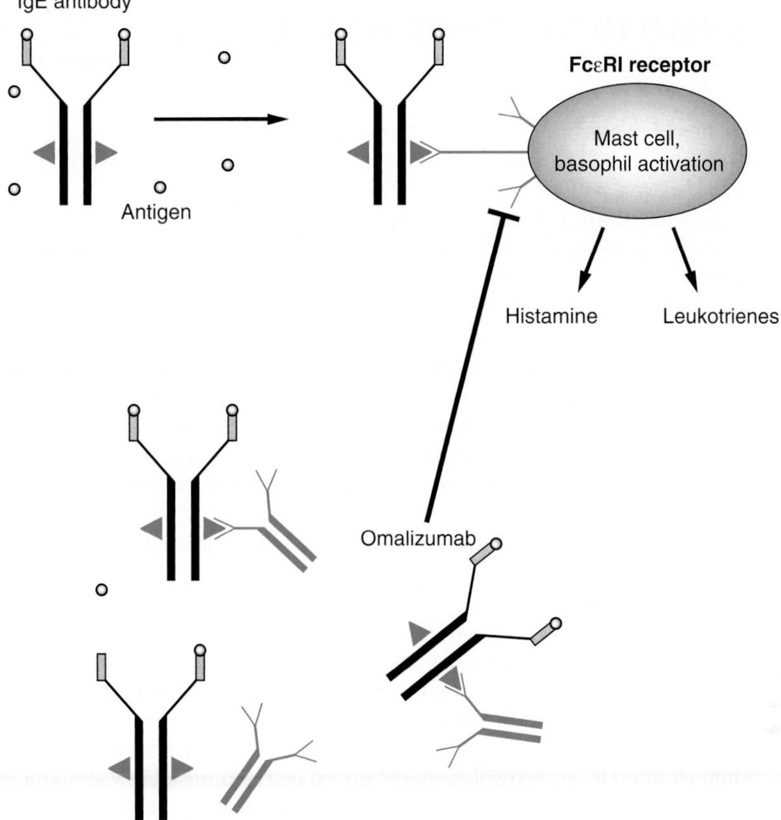

FIGURE 9-2. The mechanism of action of anti-IgE antibodies.

d. Zileuton is administered orally, usually 4 times per day.

e. Zileuton may cause liver toxicity; hepatic enzymes should be monitored; elderly women appear to be at highest risk. Zileuton may cause flulike symptoms: chills, fatigue, fever.

f. Zileuton inhibits microsomal P-450s and thereby decreases the metabolism of terfenadine, warfarin, and theophylline.

G. α_1-Proteinase inhibitor (Prolastin, Aralast)

1. α_1-Proteinase inhibitor is used to treat emphysema caused by a deficiency in α_1-proteinase, a peptide that inhibits elastase. In patients with the deficiency, elastase destroys lung parenchyma.
2. This agent is administered by weekly IV injection to treat patients homozygous for this deficiency.

H. Anti-IgE antibody (Fig. 9-2)

1. **Omalizumab binds to human IgE's high-affinity Fc receptor (FcεRI),** blocking the binding of IgE to mast cells and basophils and other cells associated with the allergic response. It also lowers free serum IgE concentrations by as much as 90% and, since it does not block the allergen–antibody reaction, leads to a reduction in allergen concentrations.
2. These activities reduce both the early-phase degranulation reaction of mast cells and the late-phase release of mediators.
3. Omalizumab is approved for treatment of asthma in patients over 12 years old who are refractory to inhaled glucocorticoids and those asthmatic patients with allergies.
4. The drug is administered by subcutaneous injection every 2–4 weeks.

III. DRUGS USED TO TREAT RHINITIS AND COUGH

A. Rhinitis

1. ***Characteristics of rhinitis***
   - a. Congestion is caused by increased mucus production, vasodilation, and fluid accumulation in mucosal spaces.
   - b. Mucus production, vasodilation, and parasympathetic stimulation and airway widening are produced by inflammatory mediators (histamine, leukotrienes, prostaglandins, and kinins).
2. ***Selected drugs***
   - a. **Antihistamines** (see Chapter 6)
     - (1) Antihistamines are histamine$_1$ (H_1)-receptor antagonists; they include diphenhydramine, brompheniramine, chlorpheniramine, and loratadine, which are useful in allergic rhinitis but have little effect on rhinitis associated with colds.
     - (2) Antihistamines reduce the parasympathetic tone of arterioles and decrease secretion through their anticholinergic activity. Anticholinergics might be more effective in rhinitis, but the doses required produce systemic adverse effects. **Ipratropium bromide** (Atrovent), a poorly absorbed ACh antagonist administered by nasal spray, is approved for rhinorrhea associated with the common cold or with allergic or nonallergic seasonal rhinitis.
   - b. **α-Adrenoceptor agonists**
     - (1) α-Adrenoceptor agonists act as nasal decongestants.
     - (2) These agents include epinephrine and oxymetazoline, which are administered as nasal aerosols; pseudoephedrine, which is administered orally; and phenylephrine, which may be administered orally or as a nasal aerosol.
     - (3) α-Adrenoceptor agonists may be administered as nasal aerosols or as oral agents. Administration as an aerosol is characterized by rapid onset, few systemic effects, and an increased tendency to produce rebound nasal congestion. Oral administration results in longer duration of action, increased systemic effects, and less potential for rebound congestion and dependence.
     - (4) These agents reduce airway resistance by constricting dilated arterioles in the nasal mucosa.
     - (5) α-Adrenoceptor agonists produce adverse effects that include nervousness, tremor, insomnia, dizziness, and rhinitis medicamentosa (chronic mucosal inflammation due to prolonged use of topical vasoconstrictors, characterized by rebound congestion, tachyphylaxis, dependence, and eventual mucosal necrosis).
   - c. **Inhaled corticosteroids**
     - (1) Topical corticosteroids include beclomethasone (Beconase, Vancenase) and flunisolide (Nasalide).
     - (2) Topical corticosteroids are administered as nasal sprays to reduce systemic absorption and adverse effects.
     - (3) These agents require 1–2 weeks for full effect.
   - d. **Cromolyn and nedocromil**
     - (1) Cromolyn and nedocromil are antiasthma agents with anti-inflammatory activity; they may also be used to treat rhinitis.
     - (2) These drugs are administered several times daily by aerosol spray or nebulizer.

B. Cough

1. ***Characteristics of cough.*** **Cough is produced by the cough reflex, which is integrated in the cough center in the medulla.** The initial stimulus for cough probably arises in the bronchial mucosa, where irritation results in bronchoconstriction. "Cough" receptors, specialized stretch receptors in the trachea and bronchial tree, send vagal afferents to the cough center and trigger the cough reflex.
2. ***Selected drugs***
   - a. Antitussive agents

(1) Codeine, hydrocodone, and hydromorphone
  (a) Codeine, hydrocodone, and hydromorphone are opiates that decrease sensitivity of the central cough center to peripheral stimuli and decrease mucosal secretions. Antitussive actions occur at doses lower than those required for analgesia.
  (b) These agents produce constipation, nausea, and respiratory depression.
(2) **Dextromethorphan**
  (a) Dextromethorphan is the l-isomer of an opioid; it is active as an antitussive, but it is devoid of analgesic action or addictive liability.
  (b) Dextromethorphan is less constipating than **codeine.**
(3) Benzonatate (Tessalon)
  (a) Benzonatate is a glycerol derivative chemically similar to **procaine** and other ester-type anesthetics.
  (b) Benzonatate reduces the activity of peripheral cough receptors and also appears to reduce the threshold of the central cough center.
(4) Diphenhydramine
  (a) Diphenhydramine is an H_1-receptor antagonist; however, antitussive activity is probably not mediated at this receptor.
  (b) Diphenhydramine acts centrally to decrease the sensitivity of the cough center to afferents.

b. Expectorants stimulate the production of a watery, less-viscous mucus; they include **guaifenesin.**
(1) Guaifenesin acts directly via the gastrointestinal tract to stimulate the vagal reflex.
(2) Near-emetic doses of guaifenesin are required for beneficial effect; these doses are not attained in typical OTC preparations.

c. Mucolytics: **Acetylcysteine**
(1) Acetylcysteine reduces the viscosity of mucus and sputum by cleaving disulfide bonds.
(2) Acetylcysteine is delivered as an **inhalant** and modestly reduces COPD exacerbation rates by roughly 30%.

DRUG SUMMARY TABLE

Short-Acting β_2-Adrenoceptor Agonists
Albuterol (Proventil, Ventolin)
Levalbuterol (Xopenex)
Pirbuterol (Maxair)
Metaproterenol (Alupent)
Epinephirine (Primatine Mist, Bronkaid Mist)
Isoproterenol (Isuprel)

Long-Acting β_2-Adrenoceptor Agonists
Salmeterol (Serevent)
Formoterol (Foradil)
Terbutaline (generic)

Other Adrenoceptor Agonists for Asthma
Epinephrine (Asthmahaler, Epifrin, others)
Isoproterenol (Isuprel)
Ephedrine (Broncholate, Primatene)

Methylxanthines
Theophylline (Elixophyllin, others)

Muscarinic Antagonists
Ipratropium bromide (Atrovent)
Tiotropium (Spirva)
Atropine (generic)

Chromones
Cromolyn sodium (Intal)
Nedocromil sodium (Tilade)

Inhaled Glucocorticoids
Beclomethasone (Beclovent, Vanceril)
Triamcinolone acetate (Azmacort)
Budesonide (Rhinocort)
Flunisolide (AeroBid)
Fluticasone propionate (Flovent)
Ciclesonide (Alvesco)
Mometasone (Flovent)

Leukotriene Inhibitors
Zafirlukast (Accolate)
Montelukast (Singulair)
Zileuton (Zyflo)

Enzyme Inhibitors
α_1-Proteinase inhibitor (Prolastin, Aralast)

Anti-IgE Antibody
Omalizumab (Xolair)

Antihistamines (selected H_1-receptor antagonists, see Chapter 6)
Diphenhydramine (Benadryl, Compose, generic)
Loratadine (Claritin)
Fexofenadine (Allegra)
Chlorpheniramine (generic)
Brompheniramine (generic)

α-Adrenoceptor Agonists (selected, see Chapter 2
Oxymetazoline (Afrin, others)
Phenylephrine (Neo-Synephrine, others)
Pseudoephedrine (Sudafed, Afrinol, others)

Antitussives
Codeine (generic)
Hydrocodone (Tussigon, Hycodan, others)
Hydromorphone (Dilaudid)
Dextromethorphan (generic)
Benzonatate (Tessalon)

Expectorants
Guaifenesin (Extussive, Fenesin, others)

Mucolytics
Acetylcysteine (Acetadote, Mucomyst)

Review Test for Chapter 9

Directions: Each of the numbered items or incomplete statements in this section is followed by answers or by completions of the statement. Select the ONE lettered answer or completion that is BEST in each case.

1. A 17-year-old patient is brought to your allergy practice complaining of chronic cough that gets quite severe at times. The condition occurs about twice a week and is beginning to interfere with his studies. Which of the following would be most appropriate treatment for this patient?

(A) Oral prednisone
(B) Omalizumab
(C) Diphenhydramine
(D) Inhaled budesonide
(E) Theophylline

2. A woman who has asthma and is recovering from a myocardial infarction is on several medications including a baby aspirin a day. She complains of large bruises on her arms and legs and some fatigue. A standard blood panel reveals markedly elevated alanine aminotransferase (ALT). Which of the following is most likely responsible for the increase in liver enzymes?

(A) Heparin
(B) Zileuton
(C) Zafirlukast
(D) Albuterol
(E) Aspirin

3. A 20-year-old college student participates in several intramural athletic programs but is complaining that his asthma, which you have been treating for 5 years, is getting worse. In the last month, he has used his albuterol inhaler at least 20 times following baseball practice, but he has not been waking much at night. You elect to change his treatment regimen. Which of the following would be the best change in treatment for this patient?

(A) Oral triamcinolone
(B) Zileuton
(C) Salmeterol
(D) Nedocromil

4. Which of the following statements regarding the pharmacokinetics of theophylline is correct?

(A) It is primarily metabolized by the kidney
(B) Its metabolism depends on age
(C) It is poorly absorbed after oral administration
(D) It has a wide therapeutic index

5. Which of the following statements correctly describes the action of theophylline?

(A) It stimulates cyclic AMP phosphodiesterase
(B) It is an adenosine-receptor antagonist
(C) It does not cross the blood–brain barrier
(D) It blocks the release of ACh in the bronchial tree

6. Which of the following statements regarding opiate action is correct?

(A) It triggers a vagal reflex to suppress cough
(B) It can cause diarrhea
(C) Its expectorant action is caused by stimulation of mucus production
(D) It acts centrally to suppress the medullary cough center

7. Which of the following statements about the mechanism of action of ipratropium is correct?

(A) It acts centrally to decrease vagal ACh release
(B) It inhibits pulmonary ACh receptors
(C) It decreases mast cell release of histamine
(D) It blocks the action of histamine at H_1 receptors

8. Zileuton is useful in the treatment of asthma because it

(A) Inhibits prostaglandin biosynthesis
(B) Inhibits leukotriene synthesis
(C) Inhibits leukotriene receptors
(D) Inhibits 12-lipoxygenase

Answers and Explanations

1. **The answer is D.** This is a fairly classical presentation of asthma, which should be confirmed with further pulmonary testing. Mild persistent asthma can be treated several ways (Table 9-1), but inhaled glucocorticoids are very effective. Oral prednisone has many side effects, especially in a young person. Omalizumab is for patients who are refractory to other treatments and those with allergies. Antihistamines such as diphenhydramine are poorly effective in asthma, and theophylline is only moderately effective.

2. **The answer is B.** Zileuton is a leukotriene synthesis inhibitor that can cause increases in hepatic enzymes and altered liver function. It decreases the rate of heparin metabolism, leaving patients prone to easy bruising. Zafirlukast and albuterol are antiasthmatic agents but do not alter liver enzymes. Aspirin might cause bleeding disorders, but the low dose this patient is taking is unlikely to be responsible for the liver enzyme abnormalities.

3. **The answer is C.** The patient's asthma is worsening, especially in response to exercise or increased allergen exposure, and the excessive of short-acting β_2-agonists requires a change in medication. The best choice would be a long-acting β_2-agonist like salmeterol. Oral glucocorticoids have many adverse effects, and zileuton and nedocromil are unlikely to be sufficiently efficacious in the worsening asthma.

4. **The answer is B.** The metabolism of theophylline depends on age; the half-life of the drug in children is much shorter than in adults. The methylxanthines are all well absorbed and are metabolized in the liver.

5. **The answer is B.** Theophylline may have several mechanisms of action, but its adenosine-receptor antagonist activity and the inhibition of phosphodiesterase are the best understood.

6. **The answer is D.** Opioids act centrally to decrease the sensitivity of the cough center; they also decrease propulsion in the bowel.

7. **The answer is B.** Ipratropium is an ACh-receptor antagonist; it is poorly absorbed, so most of its effect is in the lung. It does not cross the blood–brain barrier and does not block mediator release or H_1-receptors.

8. **The answer is B.** By inhibiting 5-lipoxygenase, zileuton reduces leukotriene biosynthesis; it does not inhibit (and in fact it might increase) prostaglandin synthesis.

chapter 10

Drugs Acting on the Endocrine System

I. HORMONE RECEPTORS

All known hormones, and drugs that mimic hormones, act via one of **two basic receptor systems:** membrane-associated receptors and intracellular receptors (see Chapter 1).

A. Membrane-associated receptors

1. Membrane-associated receptors bind hydrophilic hormones (which penetrate the plasma membrane poorly), such as insulin, adrenocorticotropic hormone (ACTH), and epinephrine, outside the cell.
2. Membrane-associated receptors transmit signals into the cell by a variety of "second messenger" mechanisms, including the following:
   a. Changes in cyclic adenosine monophosphate (cAMP) or cyclic guanosine monophosphate (cGMP) caused by changes in the activity of cyclases
   b. Increased phosphoinositide turnover via increased phosphoinositide kinase activity
   c. Increased intracellular Ca^{2+} by action on Ca^{2+} channels
   d. Increased tyrosine phosphorylation on specific proteins by the action of tyrosine kinases

B. Intracellular receptors

1. Intracellular receptors bind hydrophobic hormones (which penetrate the plasma membrane easily) such as cortisol, retinol, and estrogen inside the cell—either in the cytoplasm or the nucleus.
2. Intracellular receptors modulate the transcription rate of specific target genes to change the levels of cellular proteins.

II. THE HYPOTHALAMUS

A. Agents affecting growth hormone

1. Growth hormone-releasing hormone (GHRH)
   a. GHRH is an active peptide of 44 amino acids released by the hypothalamus and arcuate nucleus.
   b. GHRH binds to specific membrane GHRH receptors on pituitary somatotrophs.
   c. GHRH rapidly elevates serum growth hormone (somatotropin) levels with high specificity.
   d. A GHRH analogue composed of the amino-terminal 24 residues, sermorelin, was available for use to diagnose pituitary responsiveness and growth hormone secretory capacity but has been removed from the U.S. market.
   e. GHRH release from the arcuate nucleus is also modulated by "GH secretagogues" via a unique GH secretagogue receptor. The endogenous ligand for this receptor is ghrelin, a peptide secreted by the stomach in response to fasting. Ghrelin also stimulates appetite.

2. ***Somatotropin release-inhibiting hormone (SST, somatostatin)***
   a. Somatotropin release-inhibiting hormone has two forms, a 14-amino acid peptide and a 28-amino acid peptide that are produced by differential proteolysis from the same precursor. These peptides are produced in the hypothalamus and other areas of the brain and by pancreatic D cells, as well as by other cells in the gastrointestinal (GI) tract.
   b. SST binds to specific somatostatin receptors in the plasma membrane of target tissues.
   c. At least five different isoforms of somatostatin receptors (SSTR1–SSTR5) are expressed, with marked differences in their tissue distribution.
   d. Somatostatin inhibits the release of growth hormone and thyroid-stimulating hormone (TSH) from the pituitary and the release of glucagon and insulin from the pancreas. Somatostatin also inhibits secretion of a number of gut peptides such as vasoactive intestinal polypeptide (VIP), and it inhibits growth and proliferation of many cell types. It also inhibits the secretion of vasodilator hormones, especially within the gut.
   e. Octreotide is an octapeptide SST analogue available for use in the United States It is administered by subcutaneous (SC), intramuscular (IM), or intravenous (IV) injection.
   f. Octreotide is used to treat acromegaly; severe diarrhea associated with hypersecretory states such as vasoactive intestinal polypeptide-secreting tumors (VIPomas); variceal and upper GI bleeding; and TSH-secreting adenomas.
   g. Adverse effects of octreotide include nausea, cramps, and increased gallstone formation. Both hypo- and hyperglycemia have been reported following its use.

B. Gonadotropin-releasing hormone (GnRH) and analogues

1. Endogenous GnRH is a 10-amino acid peptide secreted from the hypothalamus. It binds to specific receptors on pituitary gonadotrophs.
2. Short-term or pulsatile administration of GnRH agonists increases the synthesis and release of both luteinizing hormone (LH) and follicle-stimulating hormone (FSH). This occurs by modulating the function of the hypophyseal–pituitary gonadal axis (Fig. 10-1, left side).
3. Long-term administration (2–4 weeks) of GnRH inhibits the release of both LH and FSH by causing a reduction in the number of GnRH receptors.
4. **GnRH analogues have two main uses**
   a. **Chemical castration,** which is useful in the treatment of hormone-dependent cancers and hyperplasias such as prostate cancer, breast cancer, endometriosis, and fibroids
   b. **Treatment of infertility**
5. Adverse effects include a transient worsening of symptoms, hot flashes, and induction of ovarian cysts in the first months of long-term treatment.
6. GnRH analogues are listed in Table 10-1
   a. **Gonadorelin hydrochloride or acetate**
      (1) Decapeptide identical in sequence to endogenous GnRH
      (2) The hydrochloride is used in the diagnosis of hypogonadism; the acetate is used for treatment of infertility.
   b. Nafarelin acetate
      (1) Nafarelin acetate is a synthetic decapeptide of GnRH with one modified amino acid. It is about 200 times more potent than GnRH and is administered as a nasal spray.
      (2) Nafarelin is used for the management of endometriosis and central precocious puberty.
   c. Triptorelin (Trelstar Depot), a decapeptide that is more potent than GnRH
   d. **Goserelin**
      (1) Goserelin acetate contains two amino acid substitutions that increase its half-life compared with that of endogenous GnRH.
      (2) This peptide is injected either SC, as a long-acting implant, or by IV infusion. The half-life of the peptide is approximately 10–20 minutes following IV administration. Peak response is achieved 15 minutes after IV administration and 30–60 minutes after SC injection. The therapeutic effectiveness of the implant is 28 days.
   e. **Leuprolide acetate**
      (1) Leuprolide acetate is synthetic 9-amino acid GnRH analogue with increased potency.
      (2) Leuprolide is administered parenterally, and a long-acting (up to 6 months) controlled release preparation is available.

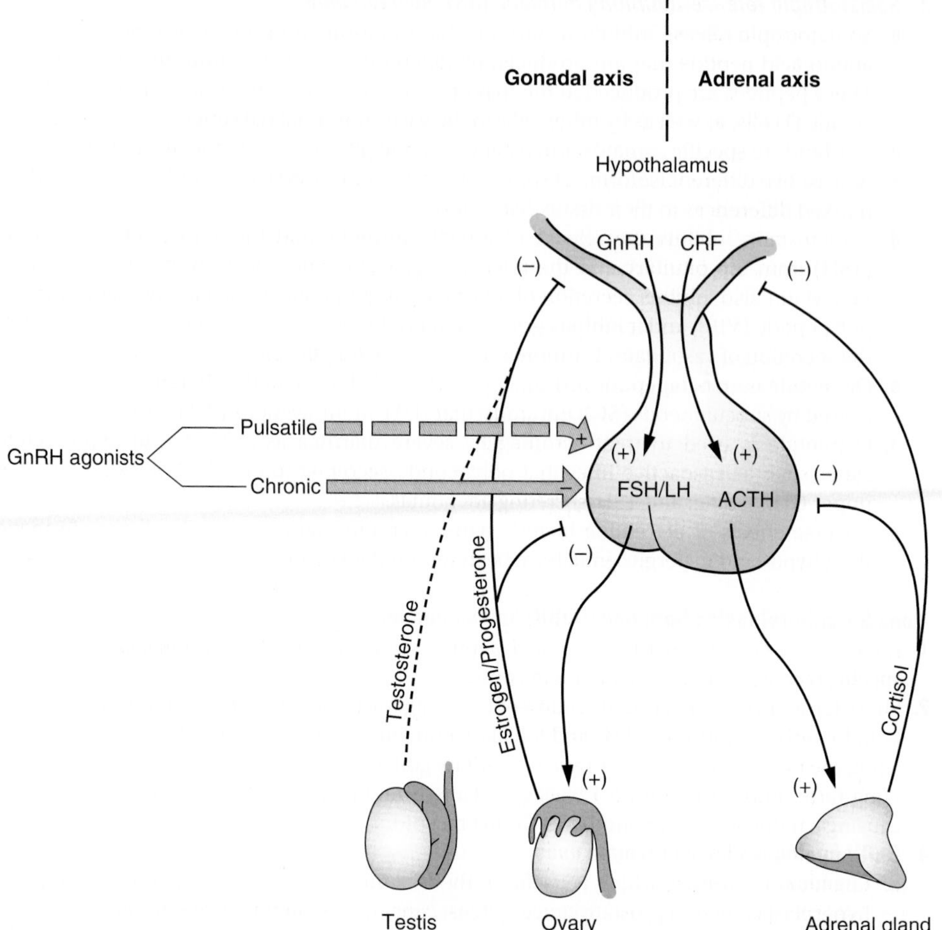

FIGURE 10-1. The hypothalamic–pituitary axis. The pituitary releases trophic hormones such as follicle-stimulating hormone *(FSH)* and luteinizing hormone *(LH)* or adrenocorticotropic hormone *(ACTH)* in response to releasing hormones produced in the hypothalamus. The trophic hormones act on peripheral organs such as the ovary or testis to increase the production of gonadal steroids. Gonadal steroids in turn exert negative feedback on the hypothalamus and pituitary. *CRF,* corticotropin-releasing factor; *GnRH,* gonadotropin-releasing hormone.

table 10-1 Gonadotropin Analogues

Drug	Administration	Uses
GnRH Receptor Agonists		
Leuprolide (Lupron, Eligard)	SC, IM, implant	PC, BC, Endo, Fibro, PP
Gonadorelin (Factrel, Lutrepulse)	IV, SC	DA, Fert
Triptorelin (Trelstar)	IM	Fert, Endo, PC, H
Nafarelin (Synarel)	Intranasal	PP, Endo, Fibr, H
Goserelin (Zoladex)	SC implant	PC, BC, Endo, Fib
Histrelin (Vantas)	SC implant	PC
GnRH Receptor Antagonists		
Ganirelix (Antagon)	SC	Fert
Abarelix (Plenaxis)	IM	PC
Cetrorelix (Cetrotide)	SC	Fert

PC, prostate cancer; BC, breast cancer; Endo, endometriosis; Fibr, fibroids; Fert, fertility; PP, precocious puberty; DA, diagnostic agent; H, hirsutism.

(3) Leuprolide acetate may be used to treat prostate cancer, prostatic hypertrophy, breast cancer, endometriosis, and fibroids.

f. Histrelin is a nonpeptide GNRH analogue; implant delivers drug continuously for 1 year.

g. GnRH antagonists

(1) Cetrorelix and ganirelix are class of GnRH analogues that act as pure antagonists; they do not cause a surge of testosterone or estradiol on initiation of therapy.

(2) All are decapeptides and administered SC or IM.

(3) An advantage of the GnRH antagonists over the GnRH agonists (e.g., leuprolide) is a reduction in the required fertility therapy cycle from several weeks (i.e., 3 weeks with leuprolide) to only several days. Secondarily, the effects of GnRH antagonists start and reverse rapidly, allowing pituitary function to return to baseline within 1–4 days after drug discontinuation.

(4) These drugs are used as part of an assisted reproductive technology procedure for endometriosis and benign prostatic hyperplasia.

C. Prolactin-releasing factor (PRF) and prolactin-inhibiting factor (PIF). Secretion of **prolactin** from the pituitary is controlled by both **inhibition** (mediated by PIF, which is dopamine) and **stimulation** (mediated by PRF).

1. *PRF*

a. Several peptides, including thyrotropin-releasing hormone (TRH), that increase the synthesis and release of prolactin have been identified in the hypothalamus and placenta; however, their physiologic role is unclear.

b. Drugs that reduce central nervous system (CNS) dopaminergic activity cause an increase in prolactin secretion, as will dopamine antagonists. These include

(1) Antipsychotics, including chlorpromazine and haloperidol

(2) Antidepressants, including imipramine

(3) Antianxiety agents, including diazepam

c. Various hormones also stimulate prolactin secretion; these include testosterone, estrogen, TRH, and VIP.

d. Drugs that promote prolactin secretion are used to treat lactation failure.

2. *PIF*

a. Inhibition of prolactin secretion can be produced by a number of dopamine agonists.

(1) Bromocriptine acts as an agonist of dopamine D_2-receptors and an antagonist of D_1-receptors.

(2) Cabergoline is a potent D_2 agonist with greater D_2 selectivity. It is more effective in reducing hyperprolactinemia than bromocriptine and has a long half-life that permits twice-weekly dosing.

b. Therapeutic uses of these agents include the inhibition of prolactin secretion in amenorrhea, galactorrhea, and prolactin-secreting tumors; the correction of female infertility secondary to hyperprolactinemia; and the treatment of Parkinson disease.

D. Corticotropin-releasing hormone (CRH), corticorelin

1. CRH is a 41-amino acid peptide found in the hypothalamus and in the gut; it is isolated from ovine hypothalamus (Corticorelin) for diagnostic use.

2. CRH stimulates ACTH synthesis and release in pituitary corticotrophs by binding to specific membrane receptors.

3. CRH is subject to rapid proteolysis; it must be given IV.

4. Corticorelin is ovine CRH and is used diagnostically to discriminate between pituitary or ectopic sources of ACTH production and to differentiate between hypothalamic–hypophyseal or primary adrenal disease.

E. Thyrotropin-releasing hormone (TRH)

1. TRH is a tripeptide (Glu-His-Pro) found in the hypothalamus and other locations in the brain.

2. TRH binds to specific membrane receptors and stimulates the secretion of TSH from the pituitary and induces prolactin secretion.

3. TRH is no longer available in the United States.

III. THE ANTERIOR PITUITARY

A. Growth hormone agonists (GH, somatotropin), methionyl-growth hormone **(somatrem), and antagonists (Pegvisomant)**

1. ***Structure***
   - **a.** Growth hormone is a 191-amino acid protein produced in the anterior pituitary.
   - **b.** Secretion of GH is controlled by hypothalamic factors: GHRH and SST (see above).
2. ***Actions and pharmacologic properties***
   - **a.** The effects of GH are mediated by specific membrane receptors. GH has two independent receptor interaction domains, and one molecule of GH tethers two GH receptors together and the homodimer activates a tyrosine kinase, Jak2.
   - **b.** GH has both direct actions and indirect actions mediated by the induction of insulin-like growth factor-1 (IGF-1) synthesis in and release from liver and kidney.
     - **(1)** Direct actions of GH include
       - **(a)** Antagonism of the action of insulin
       - **(b)** Stimulation of triglyceride hydrolysis in adipose tissue
       - **(c)** Increased hepatic glucose output
       - **(d)** Positive calcium balance
       - **(e)** Renal reabsorption of sodium and potassium
       - **(f)** Production of somatomedins or IGFs in the liver and other tissues
     - **(2)** Indirect actions of GH mediated by IGF-1 include
       - **(a)** Longitudinal growth of bones and growth of soft tissue
       - **(b)** Increased amino acid transport, DNA and RNA synthesis, and proliferation of many tissues
       - **(c)** Increased protein synthesis and positive nitrogen balance
   - **c.** GH is administered by IM or SC injection. Peak blood levels are obtained in 2–4 hours; activity persists for 36 hours after administration, because of the relatively long half-life of somatomedins. A depot preparation (Nutropin Depot) composed of microspheres of somatropin embedded in biodegradable polyactide–coglycodide (PLG) microspheres is designed to decrease the number of injections required.
3. ***Therapeutic uses***
   - **a.** GH is used for replacement therapy in children with GH deficiency before epiphyseal closure.
   - **b.** GH stimulates growth in patients with Turner syndrome.
   - **c.** Other approved uses include long-term replacement of GH deficiency in adults, treatment of cachexia and acquired immune deficiency syndrome (AIDS) wasting, positive nitrogen balance in patients with severe burns, Prader-Willi syndrome in children, and short bowel syndrome.
4. ***Adverse effects and contraindications***
   - **a.** In about 2% of patients, anti-GH antibodies develop. Edema, metabolic disturbances, and injection site reactions have been reported with GH treatment.
   - **b.** Administration of GH is contraindicated in obese patients, patients with closed epiphyses who do not have GH deficiency, and patients with neoplastic disease.

B. GH antagonists, pegvisomant

1. Pegvisomant is a GH receptor antagonist. It is a recombinant GH that contains nine mutations that allow it to bind to one GH receptor, but it fails to bind a second GH receptor. This blocks the action of endogenous GH.
2. Used specifically for the treatment of acromegaly
3. Pegvisomant is administered SC.

C. Gonadotropins

1. ***Luteinizing hormone (LH) and follicle-stimulating hormone (FSH)***
   - **a.** Structure

(1) LH and FSH are glycoproteins found in the anterior pituitary.

(2) LH, FSH, and TSH are all composed of an identical α subunit and a β subunit unique to each hormone.

b. Actions and pharmacologic properties

(1) The activity of LH and FSH is mediated by specific membrane receptors that cause an increase in intracellular cAMP.

(2) In women, LH increases estrogen production in the ovary and is required for progesterone production by the corpus luteum after ovulation. FSH is required for normal development and maturation of the ovarian follicles.

(3) In men, LH induces testosterone production by the interstitial (Leydig) cells of the testis. FSH acts on the testis to stimulate spermatogenesis and the synthesis of androgen-binding protein.

c. Therapeutic uses. FSH and LH of pituitary origin are not used pharmacologically. Rather, the menopausal and chorionic gonadotropins described below are used as the source of biologically active peptides.

2. ***Human menopausal gonadotropins (menotropins) and human chorionic gonadotropin (hCG)***

a. **Menotropins** are isolated from the urine of postmenopausal women and contain a mixture of LH and FSH. Urofollitropin (Bravelle) is immunologically purified FSH from the urine of pregnant women.

b. **hCG** is produced by the placenta and can be isolated and purified from the urine of pregnant women. hCG is nearly identical in activity to LH, but it differs in sequence and in carbohydrate content.

c. Recombinant human FSH (follitropin-α and follitropin-β are available). They have less batch-to-batch variability than preparations derived from urine. Recombinant LH is also available (Lutropin alpha).

d. Menotropins and hCG must be administered parenterally.

e. Therapeutic uses

(1) Menotropins are used in concert with hCG to stimulate ovulation in women with functioning ovaries; approximately 75% of women treated with these peptides ovulate.

(2) hCG can be used in both men and women to stimulate gonadal steroidogenesis in cases of LH insufficiency.

(3) hCG can be used to induce external sexual maturation and spermatogenesis in men with secondary hypogonadism, but this may require months of treatment.

(4) In the absence of an anatomic block, hCG can also promote the descent of the testes in cryptorchidism.

f. Adverse effects and contraindications

(1) Menotropins and hCG cause ovarian enlargement in about 20% of treated women.

(2) Menotropins and hCG may cause ovarian hyperstimulation syndrome in up to 1% of patients, resulting in acute respiratory distress, ascites, hypovolemia, and shock.

D. Thyroid-stimulating hormone (TSH, thyrotropin α) (Thyrogen)

1. TSH is a 211-amino acid glycoprotein with two subunits that is secreted from the anterior pituitary.
2. TSH stimulates the production and release of triiodothyronine (T_3) and thyroxine (T_4) from the thyroid gland. The effect is mediated by stimulation of specific TSH receptors in the plasma membrane, thereby increasing intracellular cAMP.
3. Thyrotropin-α is available for use in diagnosing the cause of thyroid deficiency.

E. Adrenocorticotropic hormone (ACTH, corticotropin) and cosyntropin

1. ***Structure***

a. ACTH is a 39-amino acid peptide secreted from the anterior pituitary. The N-terminal 24-amino acid portion of the peptide has full biologic activity.

b. The N-terminal 13-amino acids of ACTH are identical to those in α-melanocyte-stimulating hormone (α-MSH).

2. ***Actions and pharmacologic properties***
   a. ACTH stimulates the adrenocortical secretion of glucocorticoids and, to a lesser extent, mineralocorticoids and androgens. Effects are mediated by specific membrane-bound ACTH receptors coupled to an increase in intracellular cAMP.
   b. Excess ACTH levels may produce hyperpigmentation because of activity of the intrinsic α-MSH portion of the peptide.
   c. ACTH is available in both human and bovine purified preparations, as well as synthetic 1-24-ACTH (cosyntropin).
   d. All preparations of ACTH are administered parenterally.
3. ***Therapeutic uses***
   a. ACTH is used in the evaluation of primary or secondary hypoadrenalism.
   b. ACTH may be used in special circumstances when an increase in glucocorticoids is desired. However, the direct administration of steroids is usually preferred.
4. ***Adverse effects and contraindications***
   a. The adverse effects associated with ACTH are similar to those of glucocorticoids.
   b. Allergic reactions, acne, hirsutism, and amenorrhea have also been reported.

IV. THE POSTERIOR PITUITARY

A. Antidiuretic hormone (ADH, vasopressin)

1. ***Structure***
   a. ADH is a 9-amino acid peptide synthesized in the hypothalamus and stored in the posterior pituitary.
   b. ADH is released in response to increasing plasma osmolarity or a fall in blood pressure.
2. ***Actions***
   a. The actions of ADH are mediated by three types of specific receptors: V_{1a}, located in vascular smooth muscle, myometrium, and kidney; V_{1b}, located in the central nervous system and adrenal medulla; and V_2, located in renal tubules. V_1 receptors are coupled to increased inositide turnover and increased intracellular Ca^{2+}; V_2 receptors are coupled to an increase in cAMP.
   b. ADH causes the permeability to water to increase in renal tubules because of the insertion of water channels composed of the protein aquaporin-2 into the apical and basolateral membranes. ADH also increases the transport of urea in the inner medullary collecting duct, which increases the urine-concentrating ability of the kidney.
   c. ADH causes vasoconstriction (via V_{1a} receptors) at higher doses.
   d. ADH stimulates the hepatic synthesis of coagulation factor VIII and von Willebrand factor.
3. ***Pharmacologic properties of ADH preparations***
   a. Aqueous vasopressin (Pitressin), a short-acting preparation that acts on both V_1 and V_2 receptors, is administered parenterally and lasts 2–6 hours.
   b. Desmopressin acetate (DDAVP, Stimate) is a longer-lasting (10–20 h) preparation administered intranasally, parenterally, or orally.
4. ***Therapeutic uses***
   a. Desmopressin is the most effective treatment for severe diabetes insipidus because its V_2 activity is 3,000 times greater than its V_1 activity; but it is not effective in the nephrogenic form of the disease.
   b. Vasopressin is included in the advanced cardiac life support (ACLS) protocol as a substitute for epinephrine in cardiac arrest with asystole. It has been useful in treating some types of GI bleeding, specifically esophageal variceal bleeding and bleeding caused by colonic diverticula, but this use is no longer approved.
5. Adverse effects. ADH preparations produce headache, nausea, and cramps, and they may cause constriction of coronary arteries.
6. ***Drug interactions***
   a. Clofibrate increases secretion of ADH from the pituitary and can be used to treat mild forms of diabetes insipidus.

b. Chlorpropamide and tricyclic antidepressants increase the sensitivity of the tubular cells to ADH.
c. Li^+ inhibits the synthesis of aquaporin.

B. Oxytocin

1. ***Structure***
   a. Oxytocin is a 9-amino acid peptide synthesized in the hypothalamus and secreted by the posterior pituitary.
   b. Oxytocin differs from ADH by only two amino acids.
2. ***Actions and pharmacologic properties***
   a. Elicits milk ejection from the breast
   b. Stimulates contraction of uterine smooth muscle
   c. Oxytocin has been associated with parental, mating, and social behaviors.
   d. Is infused IV, administered IM, or delivered intranasally. The plasma $t_{1/2}$ of oxytocin is 5–10 minutes.
3. ***Therapeutic uses***
   a. Is used for induction and maintenance of labor
   b. Stimulates milk ejection from the breast
   c. Is sometimes used to control postpartum uterine bleeding (more readily controlled with ergot alkaloids)
4. ***Adverse effects and contraindications***
   a. Oxytocin can produce hypertension and water intoxication (ADH activity).
   b. Oxytocin can cause uterine rupture and should not be used after uterine surgery or if signs of fetal distress are present.

V. DRUGS ACTING ON THE GONADAL AND REPRODUCTIVE SYSTEM

A. Estrogens

1. ***Structure***
   a. Natural estrogens (Fig. 10-2)
      (1) Natural estrogens include 17β-estradiol, estrone, and estriol, each of which contains 18 carbon atoms. The most potent natural estrogen is 17β-estradiol.
      (2) Natural estrogens are produced by the metabolism of cholesterol; testosterone is the immediate precursor of estradiol. Conversion of testosterone to 17β-estradiol is catalyzed by the enzyme aromatase.
      (3) Estrone and estriol are produced in the liver and other peripheral tissues from 17β-estradiol and are frequently conjugated by esterification to sulfates.
      (4) Equilin, an estrone derivative, is a pharmacologically useful estrogen purified from horse urine.
   b. Synthetic estrogens
      (1) A variety of synthetic estrogens have been produced.
      (2) Frequently used synthetic estrogens include the steroidal agents ethinyl estradiol and mestranol and the nonsteroidal compounds diethylstilbestrol (DES) and dienestrol.
2. ***Mechanism of action.*** Estrogens bind to specific intracellular receptors. The hormone- receptor complex interacts with specific DNA sequences and alters the transcription rates of target genes (Figure 1-1F) by recruiting coactivators and corepressors. They may also affect the half-life of specific messenger RNAs. These events lead to a change in the synthesis of specific proteins within a target cell. There are two estrogen receptors: ER-α, the "classical" estrogen receptor, and ER-β, that differ in their tissue distribution; while both receptors have about the same affinity for 17β-estradiol, they have differential affinities for other ligands and affect target genes in a differential manner.

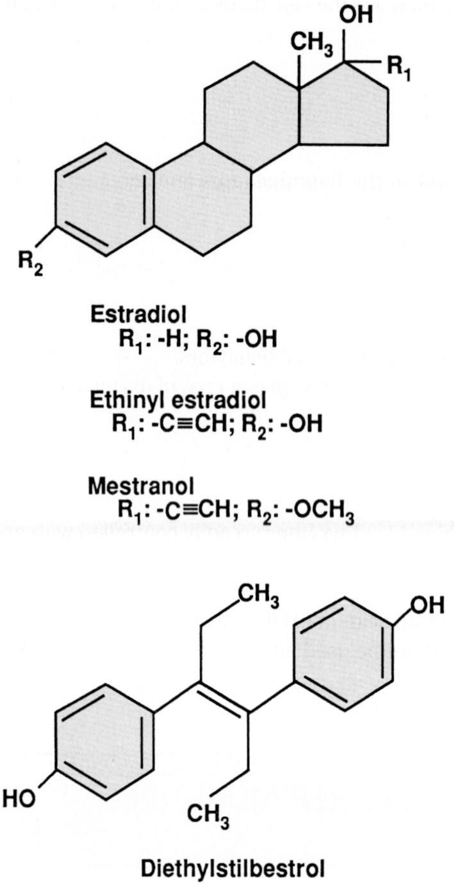

Estradiol
R_1: -H; R_2: -OH

Ethinyl estradiol
R_1: -C≡CH; R_2: -OH

Mestranol
R_1: -C≡CH; R_2: -OCH_3

Diethylstilbestrol

FIGURE 10-2. Structures of estrogens.

3. ***Metabolism***
   - **a.** 17β-Estradiol is extensively (98%) bound to sex steroid–binding globulin (SSBG) and to serum albumin.
   - **b.** Estrone sulfate, when combined with α-equilin or with other estrogenic sulfates, is effective orally, but natural estrogens are subject to a large first-pass effect. Synthetic estrogens may be administered orally, topically, transdermally, or by injection.
   - **c.** All estrogens are extensively metabolized in the liver and are conjugated with either glucuronic acid or sulfate, hydroxylated or O-methylated. Most metabolites are excreted in the urine, with approximately 10% undergoing enterohepatic circulation and eventual elimination in the feces.
4. ***Actions***
   - **a.** Growth and development
     - **(1)** Estrogens are required for the development and maturation of female internal and external genitalia, growth of the breasts, linear bone growth at puberty, and closure of the epiphyses. Typical female distribution of subcutaneous fat and pubic and axillary hair is also influenced by estrogens.
     - **(2)** Estrogens are required in the uterus for growth of myometrium and for growth and development of the endometrial lining. Continuous exposure can lead to endometrial hyperplasia and bleeding.
   - **b.** Menstrual cycle. Estrogens are required for ovarian follicular development and regulation of the menstrual cycle.
   - **c.** Systemic metabolism

(1) Estrogens promote a positive nitrogen balance, increase plasma triglycerides, and tend to decrease serum cholesterol by decreasing low-density lipoprotein (LDL) and increasing high-density lipoprotein (HDL) concentrations.

(2) Estrogens decrease total serum proteins but increase levels of transferrin, steroid- and thyroid-binding globulins, plasminogen, fibrinogen, and coagulation factors II, VII, VIII, IX, and X. Antithrombin III, protein C, and protein S levels are decreased.

(3) Estrogens decrease bone resorption, with little effect on bone formation.

d. Influence libido and mood

5. *Therapeutic uses*

a. Hypogonadism. Estrogens are used for estrogen replacement therapy in ovarian failure or after castration.

b. Menstrual abnormalities

c. Menopausal therapy

(1) Menopausal hormone therapy (MHT) can be achieved with oral, parenteral, topical (intravaginal), or transdermal estrogens, in various combinations with or without progestins.

(2) Postmenopausal therapy improves hot flashes, sweating, and atrophic vaginitis.

(3) Postmenopausal therapy slows the rate of bone loss.

(4) Estrogens are usually administered in a cyclical manner to avoid long periods of continuous exposure.

(5) Concomitant use of estrogen therapy with a progestin reduces the incidence of endometrial carcinoma.

(6) Transdermal delivery of 17β-estradiol using a skin patch is effective and long-lasting in treating menopausal symptoms.

d. Oral contraception (see V E 1)

e. Androgen-dependent prostatic tumors are effectively treated by diethylstilbestrol (DES).

6. *Adverse effects and contraindications*

a. Estrogens are associated with nausea, headaches, cholestasis, and gallbladder disease.

b. Estrogens present an increased risk (5–15 times) of endometrial cancer that is dose and duration dependent. Risk is reduced by periodic withdrawal of estrogen therapy and replacement by progestin treatment.

c. Estrogen therapy is the major cause of postmenopausal bleeding and may mask bleeding due to endometrial cancer.

d. DES is associated with adenocarcinoma of the vagina; incidence in women exposed in utero to DES is 1:1000; genital malformation is much more common.

e. Estrogens are contraindicated in the presence of estrogen-dependent or estrogen-responsive carcinoma, liver disease, or thromboembolic disease.

f. Recent large clinical trials indicate that some regimens of MHT are associated with increased risk of myocardial infarction, stroke, breast cancer, and dementia. Whether this risk is solely attributable to the estrogenic component and whether or not all estrogenic preparations at all doses share these liabilities are unresolved.

B. Antiestrogens interfere with the binding of estrogen with its specific receptor, and they may also alter the conformation of the estrogen receptor such that it fails to activate target genes. This class of compounds is distinguished from progestins and androgens, which also possess physiologic antiestrogenic activity.

1. *Clomiphene, fulvestrant*

a. Clomiphene and fulvestrant are nonsteroidal agents.

b. Clomiphene and fulvestrant bind competitively to the estrogen receptor and may also reduce levels of some mitogens. Clomiphene has partial agonist activity in some tissues including the ovary and endometrium; fulvestrant appears to be an antagonist is all tissues.

c. These agents eventually reduce the number of functional receptors available for endogenous estrogens and diminish estrogen action both along the hypothalamic–pituitary axis and in peripheral tissues.

d. Clomiphene is used to treat infertility in cases of anovulation in women with an intact hypothalamic–pituitary and sufficient production of estrogen. Fulvestrant is used to treat women with progressive breast cancer after tamoxifen (see below).

e. These agents may cause ovarian enlargement, hot flashes, nausea, and vomiting.

2. ***Danazol***

a. Danazol is a testosterone derivative with antiandrogen and antiestrogenic activities.

b. Danazol inhibits several of the enzymes involved in steroidogenesis; may also bind to estrogen and androgen receptors; and inhibits gonadotropin release in both men and women.

c. Danazol is used to treat endometriosis and fibrocystic disease of the breast.

d. This agent may cause edema, masculinization (deepening of the voice and decreased breast size) in some women, headache, and hepatocellular disease.

e. Danazol is contraindicated in pregnant women or in patients with hepatic disease.

C. Selective estrogen receptor modulators (SERMS) (Fig. 10-3)

1. SERMs are ligands for the estrogen receptor that have agonist activity in one tissue but may have antagonist activity or no activity in another tissue. The response of a tissue is determined by the conformation that the ligand confers upon the estrogen receptor, and the set of coactivators that are expressed in that tissue (Fig 10-4). Currently, there are three SERMs approved for use in the United States.: tamoxifen, raloxifene, and toremifene; many others are in clinical trial.

a. Tamoxifen is an estrogen antagonist in the breast and in the brain but is an agonist in the uterus and in bone. It is used in the treatment of advanced breast cancer and for primary prevention of breast cancer in women at high risk of the disease. Tamoxifen increases the risk of endometrial cancer.

b. Raloxifene is an agonist in bone but has no effect on the uterus or breast and is an estrogen antagonist in the brain. It is used for the treatment and prevention of osteoporosis and for uterine fibroids. Raloxifen has been shown to reduce the risk of estrogen-receptor positive invasive breast cancer by 66%–76%.

c. Toremifene is used to treat metastatic breast cancer.

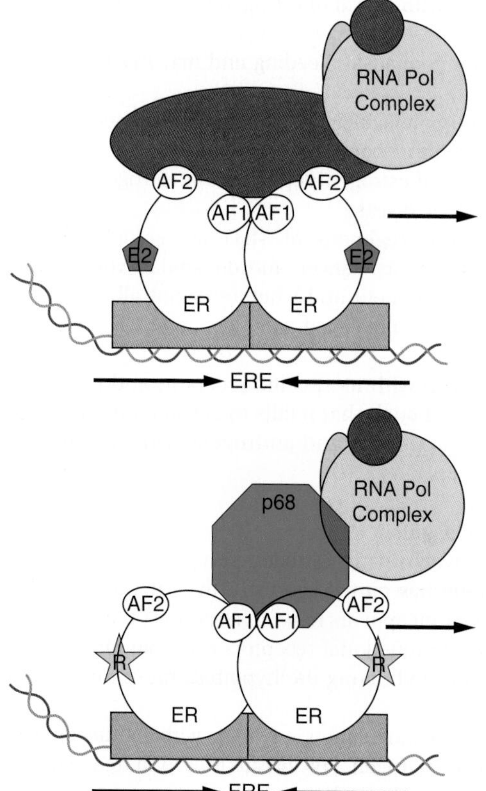

FIGURE 10-3. Mechanism of action of SERMs. Two cell types, uterine and breast epithelia, are illustrated. *Top:* 17β-estradiol binds to the estrogen receptor (ER) and induces a conformational change. Some coactivators *(blue shapes)* can interact with this conformation and thus increase transcription of specific genes *(arrow).* Both cell types express a coactivator that can respond to the 17β-estradiol-induced conformation. *Bottom:* Tamoxifen induces a different conformation of ER. Uterine epithelia expresses coactivator that increases transcription; breast epithelia do not express such coactivators.

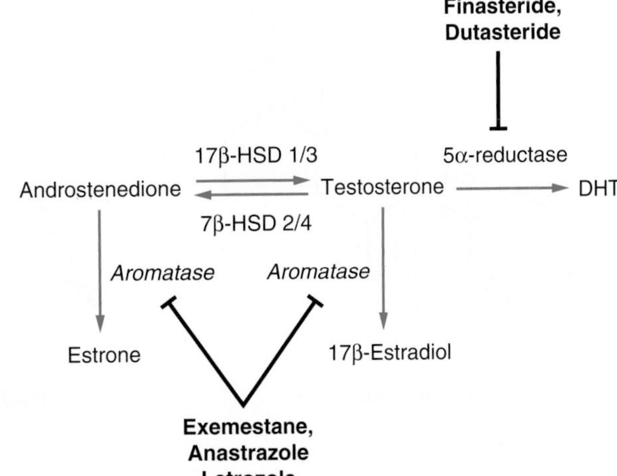

FIGURE 10-4. Enzymatic conversion of androgens to estrogens and dihydrotestosterone. 17β-HSD is hydroxysteroid dehydrogenase. There are 5 isoforms of this enzyme: types 1 and 3 catalyze reactions that make more-active steroids; types 2 and 4 make less active metabolites.

2. Common adverse effects of SERMs are edema, hot flashes, nausea, vomiting, vaginal bleeding, and vaginal discharge. There is an increase in thromboembolemic events with raloxifene but not with tamoxifen.

D. Aromatase inhibitors (see Fig. 10-4)

1. Aromatase is the enzyme that catalyses the final step in the production of estrogens from androgenic precursors within the ovary or in peripheral tissues.
2. Aromatase inhibitors are a new class of oral estrogen synthesis inhibitors.
   a. **Exemestane** is a steroidal, irreversible aromatase inhibitor. It is approved for use in the treatment of breast cancer. Testolactone is another irreversible aromatase inhibitor. Major adverse effects include hot flashes, fatigue, and CNS effects such as insomnia, depression, and anxiety.
   b. **Anastrazole** and **letrozole** are nonsteroidal competitive inhibitors of aromatase. These drugs are used as first- or second-line agents in the treatment of breast cancer. Adverse effects include hot flashes, vaginal bleeding, insomnia, bone pain, and GI disturbances.

E. Progestins

1. ***Structure***
   a. The most important natural progestin is progesterone, which is synthesized by the ovaries, testes, and adrenals.
   b. Synthetic progestins include the 19-nor compounds, such as norethindrone, norgestrel, and levonorgestrel. All of these agents are potent oral progestins derived from testosterone; some have androgenic activity (Fig. 10-5).
   c. Several synthetic derivatives of progesterone have progestin activity, including megestrol (Megace), medroxyprogesterone acetate (Amen, Provera, others), and hydroxyprogesterone caproate. Gonanes include norgestimate and desogestrel; these agents have reduced androgenic activity. Drospirenone is a spironolactone analog with antimineralocorticoid, antiandrogenic, and progestational activity.
2. ***Actions and pharmacologic properties***
   a. Progestins bind to intranuclear receptors that alter transcription of target genes. There are two isoforms of the progesterone receptor PR-A and PR-B. Both are derived from the same gene. Progestins slow the mitotic activity of the estrogen-stimulated uterus, cause vascularization of the endometrium, and induce a more glandular appearance and function.
   b. Progestins slightly decrease triglycerides and HDL, and they slightly increase LDL, depending on preparation and dose. Progestins also increase lipoprotein lipase.
   c. Progestins increase basal and stimulated insulin secretion.

Progesterone

Medroxyprogesterone acetate

Testosterone

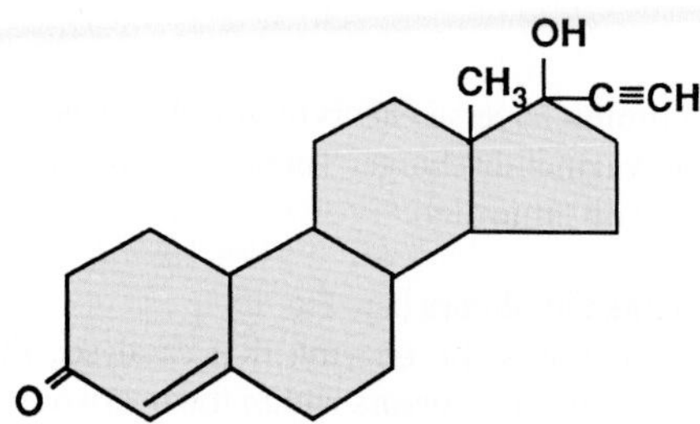

Norethindrone

FIGURE 10-5. Structures of some progestins and androgens.

- **d.** Progesterone is extensively bound to corticosteroid-binding globulin in the plasma and is not administered orally because of rapid hepatic metabolism.
- **e.** Progestins are eliminated by hydroxylation to pregnanediol and conjugation with glucuronic acid and subsequent urinary excretion.

3. *Therapeutic uses*

- **a.** Progestins are used for contraception, alone or combined with estrogens.
- **b.** Progestins may be administered orally, by depot injection, as a vaginal gel, and as a slow-release intrauterine device.
- **c.** These agents are used in the treatment of endometrial cancer and endometrial hyperplasia.
- **d.** Progestins control abnormal uterine bleeding.
- **e.** Progestins are used to delay menstruation for surgical or postoperative reasons.
- **f.** Megace is used to stimulate appetite in patients with cancer or AIDS.
- **g.** These agents are used diagnostically to evaluate endometrial function in amenorrhea.

F. Antiprogestins, mifepristone (RU-486)

- **a.** Mifepristone is a norethindrone derivative with potent antiprogestin and antiglucocorticoid activities.
- **b.** Mifepristone acts as a competitive antagonist of the progesterone and glucocorticoid receptors.
- **c.** Mifepristone has been approved for use to induce medical abortion in the first trimester.
  - **(1)** Mifepristone is combined with a parenteral or intravaginal application of a prostaglandin 48 hours after the antiprogestin to induce abortion.
  - **(2)** Mifepristone causes myometrial contractions and blastocyst detachment and expulsion.
  - **(3)** This combination is approximately 99% effective.

d. Mifepristone is used as an emergency postcoital contraceptive and is very effective if used within 72 hours of intercourse.

e. Relatively infrequent side effects of mifepristone include bleeding, nausea, and abdominal pain.

G. Hormonal contraceptives

1. *Oral contraceptives* represent the primary use of estrogens and progestins.

a. Types of oral contraceptives

(1) Combination pills

(a) Combination pills contain mixtures of estrogens and a progestin. The estrogen component (20–50 μg/day) is either **ethinyl estradiol** or **mestranol** (mestranol is metabolized to ethinyl estradiol); it is combined with a progestin (0.05–2.5 mg/day), such as **norethindrone, norgestrel, levonorgestrel, norethindrone acetate, ethynodiol diacetate, drospirenone, or desogestrel.**

(b) Combination pills reduce the level and cyclicity of both LH and FSH, resulting in a failure to ovulate.

(c) Combination pills are typically taken continuously for 21 days, followed by a 7-day withdrawal (or placebo) period to induce menses. Biphasic and triphasic formulations, which try to mimic the endogenous ratio of estrogen/progestin, are available.

(d) "Continuous dosage products" are available that contain ethinyl estradiol and levonorgestrel and are taken every day for 84 days followed by 7 days of inert tablets (Sesonale) or 7 days of low-dose ethinyl estradiol (Seasonique), thus producing four menstrual periods per year. Lybrel contains the same hormones taken continuously for 365 days to suppress menstruation.

(e) These pills also affect the genital tract in ways that are unfavorable for conception: thickening cervical mucus, speeding ovum transport through the fallopian tubes, and making the endometrium less favorable for implantation.

(2) Progestin-only preparations ("mini pills")

(a) Progestin-only preparations contain **norethindrone.**

(b) These preparations are taken daily on a continuous schedule.

(c) Progestin-only preparations do not completely suppress ovulation, resulting in irregular fertile periods. They are not as effective as the combination preparations.

(d) The mechanism of contraception is unclear, but it is likely due to the formation of a relatively atrophic endometrium (which impairs implantation) and viscous cervical mucus.

b. Adverse effects

(1) Cardiovascular

(a) Oral contraceptives are associated with a twofold to fourfold increase in morbidity and mortality due to myocardial infarction.

(b) The incidence of hypertension is three to six times higher among women taking oral contraceptives.

(c) Oral contraceptives produce a marked increase (up to 50%) in triglyceride levels, depending on the relative doses of estrogens and progestins in the individual preparation.

(d) The risk of cardiovascular complications increases markedly in women over age 35 and in women who smoke.

(2) Thromboembolic disease

(a) The risk of stroke is 2–10 times higher in individuals taking oral contraceptives.

(b) Estrogens increase levels of fibrinogen and coagulation factors II, VII, VIII, IX, and X, while decreasing concentrations of antithrombin III.

(3) Genitourinary tract. Oral contraceptives may reduce the incidence of ovarian and endometrial cancers.

(4) Hepatobiliary system. Oral contraceptives increase the incidence of gallbladder disease and gallstones.

(5) Other adverse effects of oral contraceptives include weight gain, edema, breast tenderness, headache, mood alteration, breakthrough bleeding, and amenorrhea on discontinuation.

c. Oral contraceptives are contraindicated in cardiovascular disease, thromboembolic disease, estrogen-dependent or estrogen-responsive cancer, impaired liver function, undiagnosed bleeding, and migraine.

2. ***Progestin injections***

a. Medroxyprogesterone acetate (Depo-Provera) is available as a suspension for SC or IM injections. This preparation provides contraception for 3 months.

3. ***Subcutaneous progestin implants***

a. Implanon is a synthetic progestin, etonogestrel, surrounded by a biomatrix skin. A single rod is placed under the skin and provides effective contraception for up to 3 years. Actual effectiveness is superior to that of combination oral contraceptives. Rods must be removed after 3 years.

b. Adverse effects are dominated by menstrual and bleeding irregularities.

4. ***Intrauterine devices (IUDs)***

a. Levonorgestrel-containing IUDs are available as a means of contraception.

b. Contraception is achieved mostly by local actions on the endometrium with hypotrophic glands and pseudodeciduilization. Ovulation occurs in about 50% of menstrual cycles.

c. These devices should be administered by a trained physician.

5. ***Postcoital (emergency) oral contraceptives***

a. Plan A (Yuzpe regimen): 100–120 μg of ethinyl estradiol with 0.5–0.75 mg of levonorgestrel, taken twice, 12 hours apart, has been found very effective if taken within 72 hours of coitus. At least 18 oral contraceptive preparations contain these two drugs.

b. Plan B: 0.750 mg of levonorgestrel, within 72 hours after unprotected intercourse, one dose taken as soon as possible, a second dose must be taken 12 hours after the initial dose. Women 18 and over can obtain Plan B through a pharmacist, younger women will need a prescription.

c. Nausea and vomiting are common with the use of postcoital oral contraceptives and can be severe. The risk of cancer in female offspring precludes this treatment if pregnancy is suspected.

H. Androgens and anabolic steroids

1. ***Testosterone***

a. Testosterone is synthesized primarily in the Leydig cells of the testis under the influence of LH. Testosterone is metabolized to the more potent 5α-dihydrotestosterone by 5α-reductase. There are two isoforms of this enzyme: type I, which is expressed in skin and liver; and type II, which is expressed in prostate, seminal vesicles, and hair follicles.

b. Testosterone is extensively bound (98%), mostly to SSBG and also to albumin.

c. Natural testosterone can be administered transdermally or parenterally (IM).

2. ***Synthetic androgens***

a. The 17-substituted testosterone esters (testosterone propionate, testosterone enanthate, and testosterone cypionate) are administered by injection, usually as a depot in oil.

b. 17-Alkyl testosterone derivatives include methyltestosterone, fluoxymesterone, and oxymetholone. Absorption of these oral agents is greater if they are administered sublingually, thus avoiding the large hepatic first-pass effect.

c. Nandrolone (Hybolin, Deca-Durabolin) and oxandrolone (Oxandrine, others) are testosterone derivatives with about a 5- to 10-fold higher anabolic-to-androgenic ratio than testosterone itself. Nandrolone is administered parenterally; oxandrolone is an oral agent.

3. ***Actions.*** Androgens form a complex with a specific intracellular receptor (a member of the nuclear-receptor family) and interact with specific genes to modulate differentiation, development, and growth. (See Fig. 1-1F.)

a. Androgenic actions

(1) Androgens stimulate the differentiation and development of Wolffian structures, including the epididymis, seminal vesicles, prostate, and penis.

(2) Androgens stimulate the development and maintenance of male secondary sexual characteristics.

b. Anabolic actions

(1) Anabolic steroids cause acceleration of epiphyseal closure, and they result in linear growth at puberty.

(2) Anabolic steroids cause an increase in muscle mass and lead to a positive nitrogen balance.
(3) Behavioral effects of anabolic steroids include aggressiveness and increased libido.

4. ***Uses***
   a. Prepubertal and postpubertal hypogonadism. Androgens promote linear growth and sexual maturation and maintain male secondary sexual characteristics, libido, and potency.
   b. Anemia
      (1) Androgens stimulate secretion of erythropoietin.
      (2) Androgens have largely been supplanted by recombinant erythropoietin (epoetin) for anemia, but they may be effective in some cases of bone marrow hypoplasia.
   c. Estrogen-dependent breast cancers
   d. Wasting disorders in AIDS or after severe burns
   e. Illicit use by athletes. Large doses of androgens increase the extent and rate of muscle formation and may increase the intensity of training.
   f. Hereditary angioedema. Androgens are used to treat hereditary angioedema based on androgen-dependent increases in C_1 complement inhibitor.
   g. The combination of testosterone or methyltestosterone with estrogens (either esterified estrogens or estradiol) may be used for menopausal hormone therapy when estrogens alone have not provided adequate therapeutic responses.
5. ***Adverse effects and contraindications***
   a. Androgens and anabolic steroids produce decreased testicular function, edema, and altered plasma lipids (increased LDL and decreased HDL levels).
   b. These agents cause masculinization in women.
   c. Androgens increase plasma fibrinolytic activity, causing severe bleeding with concomitant anticoagulant therapy.
   d. 17-Alkyl substituted androgens (but not testosterone ester preparations) are associated with increases in hepatic enzymes, hyperbilirubinemia, and cholestatic hepatitis, which may result in jaundice. Long-term use is associated with liver tumors.
   e. Androgens and anabolic steroids are contraindicated in pregnant women and in patients with carcinoma of the prostate or hepatic, renal, or cardiovascular disease.

I. **Antiandrogens** are agents that impair the action or synthesis of endogenous androgens.

1. ***Flutamide, bicalutamide, nilutamide***
   a. Flutamide is a steroidal oral antiandrogen that acts as a competitive androgen-receptor antagonist. Nilutamide and bicalutamide are nonsteroidal androgen-receptor antagonists with better specificity for the androgen receptor and have a longer half-life that permits once-a-day dosing rather than three times a day for finasteride.
   b. These drugs are useful in the treatment of prostatic carcinoma and are highly efficacious when combined with long-term GnRH agonist therapy.
   c. Adverse effects include gynecomastia, elevation in liver enzymes, chest pain, and GI disturbances.
2. ***Finasteride (Proscar)***
   a. Finasteride inhibits type II 5α-reductase, thereby reducing the production of the potent androgen 5α-dihydrotestosterone.
   b. Finasteride is used to treat benign prostatic hypertrophy (BPH) and male pattern baldness.
   c. Finasteride decreases prostate volume and increases urine flow.
3. ***Dutasteride***
   a. Dutasteride inhibits both type I and II 5α-reductase and is more potent than finasteride. Serum dihydrotachysterol (DHT) levels can be reduced by more than 90% in 2 weeks.
   b. Dutasteride is used to treat BPH and baldness.
4. ***Ketoconazole***
   a. Ketoconazole is an antifungal agent that blocks multiple P-450–dependent steps in steroidogenesis.
   b. Ketoconazole can be used to treat precocious puberty and hirsutism.

5. ***Spironolactone***
   a. Spironolactone antagonizes the binding of both androgen and aldosterone at their respective receptors; it also decreases the activity of the steroidogenic enzyme 17-hydroxylase.
   b. Spironolactone is used as a diuretic and to treat hirsutism in women (usually in combination with estrogen).

VI. THE ADRENAL CORTEX

A. Corticosteroids

1. ***Natural adrenocortical steroids***
   a. Glucocorticoids are synthesized under the control of ACTH (Fig. 10-6). Cortisol (hydrocortisone) is the predominant natural glucocorticoid in humans. The 3-keto and 11-hydroxyl groups are important for biologic activity.
   b. The major mineralocorticoid of the adrenal cortex is aldosterone. 11-Deoxycorticosterone, an aldosterone precursor, has both mineralocorticoid and glucocorticoid activity.
   c. The adrenals also synthesize various androgens, predominantly dehydroepiandrosterone and androstenedione.
2. ***Synthetic adrenocortical steroids***
   a. A wide array of steroid compounds with various ratios of mineralocorticoid to glucocorticoid properties has been synthesized. The most important of these compounds are listed in Table 10-2.

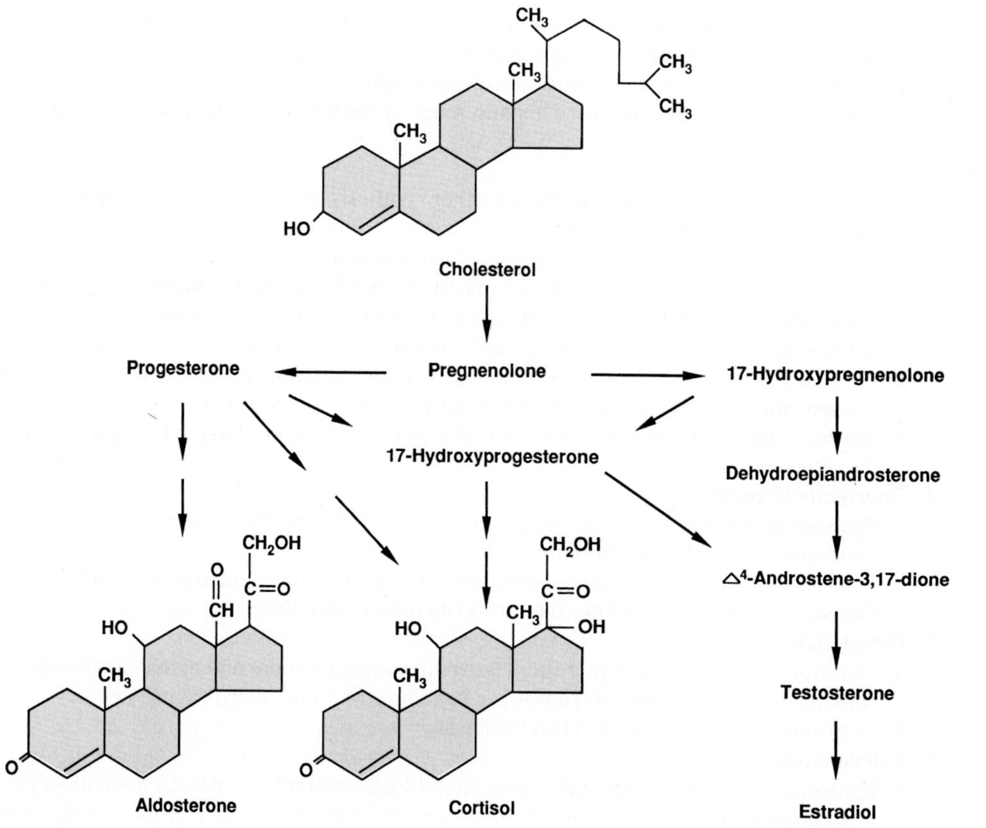

FIGURE 10-6. Biosynthesis of adrenal steroids.

table 10-2 Properties of Adrenocortical Steroids

Agent	Equivalent Dose (mg)	Metabolic Potency	Anti-Inflammatory Potency	Sodium-retaining Potency
Oral Glucocorticoids				
Cortisol	20	20	1	1
Cortisone	25	20	1	1
Prednisone	5	5	4	0.5
Prednisolone	5	5	4	0.5
Dexamethasone	0.75	1	30	0.05
Betamethasone	0.6	1.0–1.5	25–40	0.05
Triamcinolone	4	4	5	0.1
Aldosterone		0.3		3000
Fludrocortisone	0.01	0.1		125–250
Topical Glucocorticoids				
Betamethasone	Highest potency			
Clobetasol	Highest potency			
Halobetasol	Highest potency			
Amcinonide	High potency			
Fluocinonide	High potency			
Triamcinolone	High potency			
Beclomethasone	Medium potency			
Fluticasone	Medium potency			
Hydrocortisone	Medium potency			
Dexamethasone	Low potency			
Desonide	Low potency			

b. Cortisone acetate and prednisone are 11-keto steroids that are converted to 11-hydroxyl groups by the liver to give cortisol and prednisolone, respectively.

c. A C_1–C_2 double bond, as in prednisolone and prednisone, increases glucocorticoid activity without increasing mineralocorticoid activity.

d. The addition of a 9α-fluoro group (e.g., dexamethasone or fludrocortisone) increases activity.

e. Methylation or hydroxylation at the 16α position abolishes mineralocorticoid activity with little effect on glucocorticoid potency.

3. ***Mechanism of action.*** The effects of mineralocorticoids and glucocorticoids are mediated by two separate and **specific intracellular receptors**, the MR (mineralocorticoid receptor) and GR (glucocorticoid receptor), respectively. Natural and synthetic steroids enter cells rapidly and interact with these intracellular receptors. The resulting complexes modulate the transcription rate of specific genes and lead to an increase or decrease in the levels of specific proteins.

4. ***Pharmacologic properties***

a. Plasma binding

(1) 80% of circulating cortisol is bound to corticosteroid-binding globulin (CBG); 10% is bound to plasma albumin.

(2) Some of the potent synthetic glucocorticoids, such as dexamethasone, do not bind to CBG, leaving all of the absorbed drug in a free state.

b. Both natural and synthetic steroids are excreted by the kidney following reduction and formation of glucuronides or sulfates.

c. All of the steroids listed in Table 10-2 (except aldosterone) may be administered orally. A variety of glucocorticoids, including cortisol, prednisolone, and dexamethasone, can be injected IM or SC. Various glucocorticoid preparations are available for otic, rectal, or topical administration. As discussed in Chapter 9, glucocorticoids administered as inhalants are used to treat asthma.

d. Agents with the longest half-life tend to be the most potent.
   (1) Short-acting agents such as cortisol are active for 8–12 hours.
   (2) Intermediate-acting agents such as prednisolone are active for 12–36 hours.
   (3) Long-acting agents such as dexamethasone are active for 39–54 hours.

e. Drug administration attempts to pattern the circadian rhythm: A double dose is given in the morning, and a single dose is given in the afternoon.

f. Alternate-day therapy relieves clinical manifestations of the disease state while causing less severe suppression of the adrenal–hypothalamic–pituitary axis. In this therapy, large doses of short-acting or intermediate-acting glucocorticoids are administered every other day.

g. Patients removed from long-term glucocorticoid therapy must be weaned off the drug over several days, using progressively lower doses to allow recovery of adrenal responsiveness.

5. *Glucocorticoids*

a. Actions. Glucocorticoids affect virtually all tissues. Therapeutic actions and adverse effects are extensions of these physiologic effects.
   (1) Physiologic effects
      (a) The physiologic effects of glucocorticoids are mediated by increased protein breakdown, leading to a **negative nitrogen balance.**
      (b) Glucocorticoids **increase blood glucose levels** by stimulation of gluconeogenesis.
      (c) These agents **increase** the **synthesis** of several **key enzymes** involved in glucose and amino acid metabolism.
      (d) Glucocorticoids **increase plasma fatty acids** and **ketone body formation** via increased lipolysis and decreased glucose uptake into fat cells and redistribution of body fat.
      (e) These agents **increase kaliuresis** via increasing renal blood flow and GFR; increased protein metabolism results in release of intracellular potassium.
      (f) Glucocorticoids decrease intestinal absorption of Ca^{2+}.
      (g) Glucocorticoids promote Na^{+} and water retention.
   (2) Anti-Inflammatory effects. The anti-inflammatory effects of glucocorticoids are produced by the inhibition of all of the classic signs of inflammation (erythema, swelling, soreness, and heat). Specific effects include:
      (a) Inhibition of the antigenic response of macrophages and leukocytes
      (b) Inhibition of vascular permeability by reduction of histamine release and the action of kinins
      (c) Inhibition of arachidonic acid and prostaglandin production by inhibition of phospholipase A_2
      (d) Inhibition of cytokine production, including IL-1, IL-2, IL-3, IL-6, tumor necrosis factor (TNF)-α, and granulocyte–macrophage colony-stimulating factor (GM-CSF)
   (3) Immunologic effects
      (a) Glucocorticoids decrease circulating lymphocytes, monocytes, eosinophils, and basophils.
      (b) Glucocorticoids increase circulating neutrophils.
      (c) Long-term therapy results in involution and atrophy of all lymphoid tissues.
   (4) Other effects
      (a) Inhibition of plasma ACTH and possible adrenal atrophy
      (b) Inhibition of fibroblast growth and collagen synthesis
      (c) Stimulation of acid and pepsin secretion in the stomach
      (d) Altered CNS responses, influencing mood and sleep patterns
      (e) Enhanced neuromuscular transmission
      (f) Induction of surfactant production in the fetal lung at term

b. Therapeutic uses
   (1) Glucocorticoids are used in replacement therapy for primary or secondary insufficiency (Addison disease); this therapy usually requires the use of both a mineralocorticoid and a glucocorticoid.
   (2) Inflammation and immunosuppression
      (a) Glucocorticoids are used to treat the following disorders: rheumatoid arthritis, bursitis, lupus erythematosus, and other autoimmune diseases; asthma; nephrotic syndrome; ulcerative colitis; and ocular inflammation.

(b) These agents are also used in hypersensitivity and allergic reactions.
(c) Glucocorticoids can reduce organ or graft rejection.
(3) Sarcoidosis
(4) Dermatologic disorders
(5) Idiopathic nephrosis of children
(6) Neuromuscular disorders, such as Bell's palsy
(7) Shock
(8) Adrenocortical hyperplasia
(9) Stimulation of surfactant production and acceleration of lung maturation in a preterm fetus
(10) Neoplastic diseases, including adult and childhood leukemias
(11) Diagnosis of Cushing syndrome (dexamethasone suppression test)

c. Adverse effects and contraindications
(1) Most of the adverse effects of glucocorticoids are exaggerated physiologic effects leading to a state of iatrogenic Cushing disease.
(2) Certain glucocorticoids have mineralocorticoid activity, potentially causing sodium retention, potassium loss, and eventual hypokalemic, hypochloremic alkalosis.
(3) Adverse effects of glucocorticoids include the following:
(a) Adrenal suppression
(b) Hyperglycemia and other metabolic disturbances including steroid-induced diabetes mellitus and weight gain
(c) Osteoporosis
(d) Peptic ulcer
(e) Cataracts and increased intraocular pressure leading to glaucoma
(f) Edema
(g) Hypertension
(h) Increased susceptibility to infection and poor wound healing
(i) Muscle weakness and tissue loss

6. *Mineralocorticoids*

a. Actions
(1) Mineralocorticoids primarily affect the kidney, regulating salt and water balance and increasing sodium retention and potassium loss.
(2) Fludrocortisone (Florinef) is the agent of choice for long-term mineralocorticoid replacement.
(3) Adverse effects include sodium retention and hypokalemia, edema, and hypertension.

b. Therapeutic uses. Mineralocorticoids are used in replacement therapy to maintain electrolyte and fluid balance in hypoadrenalism.

B. Adrenocortical antagonists

1. *Mitotane (o,p′-DDD)*

a. Mitotane causes selective atrophy of the zona fasciculata and zona reticularis and can reduce plasma cortisol level in Cushing syndrome produced by adrenal carcinoma.
b. Mitotane use is limited to adrenal carcinomas when other therapies are not feasible.
c. Severe adverse effects of mitotane are not unusual and may include GI distress, mental confusion, lethargy, and dermal toxicity.

2. *Aminoglutethimide*

a. Aminoglutethimide blocks the conversion of cholesterol to pregnenolone and reduces adrenal production of aldosterone, cortisol, and androgens. The reduction in plasma cortisol triggers a compensatory increase in ACTH that antagonizes the effect of aminoglutethimide. ACTH release may be prevented by coadministration of a glucocorticoid such as cortisol.
b. Aminoglutethimide is useful in treating hyperadrenalism due to adrenal carcinoma or congenital adrenal hyperplasia.
c. Adverse effects of aminoglutethimide include drowsiness, rashes, and nausea.

3. *Metyrapone*

a. Metyrapone blocks the activity of 11-hydroxylase, thereby reducing cortisol production.
b. Metyrapone is used diagnostically to assess adrenal and pituitary function.

4. *Ketoconazole*

a. Ketoconazole is an antifungal agent that, at high doses, is a potent inhibitor of several of the P-450 enzymes involved in steroidogenesis in the adrenals and gonads.

b. Ketoconazole is useful in treating hirsutism and Cushing syndrome.

VII. THE THYROID

A. Thyroid hormone receptor agonists

1. *Synthesis of natural thyroid hormones*

a. Natural thyroid hormones are formed by the iodination of tyrosine residues on the glycoprotein thyroglobulin. A tyrosine residue may be iodinated at one (monoiodotyrosine, MIT) or two (diiodotyrosine, DIT) positions. Two iodinated tyrosines are then coupled to synthesize triiodothyronine (T_3; formed from one molecule each of MIT and DIT) or thyroxine (T_4; formed from two DIT molecules). T_4 synthesis exceeds T_3 synthesis five-fold. Eighty percent of circulating T_3 is derived from deiodination of T_4.

b. Biosynthesis is stimulated by TSH, which acts by a membrane-associated receptor that increases follicular cell cAMP.

c. I^- is a potent inhibitor of thyroid hormone release.

2. *Thyroid hormone preparations*

a. Thyroid hormone preparations include the following:

(1) **Levothyroxine** sodium, a synthetic sodium salt of T_4 that maintains normal T_4 and T_3 levels

(2) **Liothyronine** sodium, a synthetic sodium salt of T_3

(3) **Liotrix**, a 4:1 mixture of the above T_4 and T_3 preparations

(4) **Thyroid USP**, which is prepared from dried and defatted animal thyroid glands and contains a mixture of T_4, T_3, MIT, and DIT

b. The potency of thyroid hormone preparations can vary.

c. Given the availability of synthetics, thyroid USP is not recommended for initial therapy.

3. *Mechanism of action.* Thyroid hormones interact with specific receptor proteins located in the nucleus of target cells and alter the synthesis rate of specific mRNAs, leading to increased production of specific proteins, including Na^+/K^+-ATPase. Increased ATP hydrolysis and oxygen consumption contribute to the effects of thyroid hormones on basal metabolic rate and thermogenesis. T_3 is the most important ligand for the thyroid receptor; T_4 binds very weakly. Thyroid hormones affect virtually all tissues.

4. *Pharmacologic properties*

a. More than 99% of circulating T_4 is bound to plasma proteins; only 5%–10% of T_3 is protein bound. Most T_3 and T_4 are bound to thyroid-binding globulin (TBG). T_4 also binds to prealbumin, and both T_4 and T_3 bind weakly to albumin.

b. T_3 has a $t_{1/2}$ of approximately 1 day; T_4 has a $t_{1/2}$ of approximately 5–7 days.

c. Levothyroxine sodium and liothyronine sodium can be administered orally or IV. Oral absorption rates range from 30% to 65%. Levothyroxine sodium is preferred to liothyronine because it has better oral absorption, has a longer $t_{1/2}$, and produces a favorable T_4:T_3 ratio.

d. Metabolism

(1) T_3 and T_4 are inactivated by deiodination.

(2) Conjugation of T_3 and T_4 with glucuronic acid or sulfate occurs in the liver, and these metabolites are secreted in the bile.

(3) Some enterohepatic circulation of the metabolites occurs; 20%–40% of T_4 is eliminated in the feces.

5. *Actions*

a. Thyroid hormones are essential for normal physical and mental development of the fetus. Linear growth of the long bones, growth of the brain, and normal myelination depend on thyroid hormone. Hypothyroidism in infants leads to cretinism (myxedema with physical and mental retardation).

b. These agents increase the basal metabolic rate and blood sugar levels. They also increase the synthesis of fatty acids and decrease plasma cholesterol and triglyceride levels.

c. Thyroid hormones increase the heart rate and peripheral resistance.

d. These agents inhibit TRH and TSH release from the hypothalamus and pituitary, respectively.

e. Thyroid hormones exert maintenance effects on the CNS, reproductive tract, GI tract, and musculature.

6. *Therapeutic uses*

a. Primary, secondary, or tertiary hypothyroidism caused by

(1) Hashimoto disease

(2) Myxedema

(3) Simple goiter (thyroid gland enlargement without hyperthyroidism)

(4) Following surgical ablation of the thyroid gland

b. TSH-dependent carcinomas of the thyroid may be treated with thyroid hormones if other therapies are not feasible.

7. *Adverse effects*

a. Thyroid hormones produce iatrogenic hyperthyroidism, nervousness, anxiety, and headache.

b. These agents induce arrhythmias, angina, or infarction in patients with underlying cardiovascular disease.

c. Thyroid hormones should be used cautiously in the elderly.

B. Antithyroid drugs

1. *Thioamides*

a. Thioamides include **propylthiouracil** (PTU) and **methimazole**; methimazole is approximately 10 times more potent than PTU.

b. Thioamides interfere with the **organification and coupling of iodide by inhibiting the peroxidase enzyme**. PTU inhibits the conversion of T_4 to T_3.

c. Thioamides remain active after oral administration; 50%–80% is absorbed.

d. These agents have a $t_{1/2}$ of approximately 1–2 hours; they are concentrated in the thyroid gland and inhibit thyroid hormone biosynthesis for 6–24 hours. They do not affect T_3/T_4 already within the thyroid; attaining euthyroid status when initiating therapy may take 2–4 months.

e. Thioamides are eliminated in the urine as glucuronides.

f. Thioamides treat hyperthyroidism from a variety of causes, including Graves disease and toxic goiter. Thioamides are also used to control hyperthyroidism prior to thyroid surgery.

g. These agents commonly cause rashes, headache, or nausea; they may also induce leukopenia or agranulocytosis.

2. *Anion inhibitors of thyroid function*

a. Anion inhibitors of thyroid function include thiocyanate, perchlorate, and fluoborate.

b. These agents are monovalent anions with a hydrated radius similar in size to that of iodide.

c. Anion inhibitors competitively inhibit the transport of iodide by the thyroid gland.

d. These agents are limited by severe toxicities (including fatal aplastic anemia) to occasional diagnostic use for thyroid function.

3. *Iodide*

a. In high intracellular concentrations, iodide inhibits several steps in thyroid hormone biosynthesis, including iodide transport and organification (Wolff-Chaikoff effect).

b. Iodide inhibits the release of thyroid hormone.

c. Iodide is usually combined with a thioamide; it is rarely used as sole therapy.

d. This agent is used before thyroid surgery, causing firming of thyroid tissues and decreased thyroid vascularity, and in the treatment of spirotrichosis.

e. Iodide may cause angioedema, rash, a metallic taste on administration, and hypersensitivity reactions.

4. *Radioactive iodine ^{131}I*

a. Radioactive iodine ^{131}I emits beta particles and x-rays and has a radioactive $t_{1/2}$ of approximately 8 days. ^{131}I is transported and concentrated in the thyroid like the nonradioactive isotope. High-energy radioiodine emissions are toxic to follicular cells.

b. Radioactive iodine ^{131}I treats hyperthyroidism via nonsurgical ablation of the thyroid gland or reduction of hyperactive thyroid gland without damage to surrounding tissue.
c. This agent is helpful (in low doses) in the diagnosis of hyperthyroidism, hypothyroidism, and goiter; it may be used to assess thyroid responsiveness.
d. Overdosage of this agent commonly induces hypothyroidism.

VIII. THE PANCREAS AND GLUCOSE HOMEOSTASIS

A. Insulin

1. *Structure and synthesis*

a. Insulin is a polypeptide hormone produced by the pancreatic β cell. Insulin consists of two chains, A and B, linked by two disulfide bridges.
b. Human insulin contains 51 amino acids. Bovine insulin differs from human insulin at three amino acid sites; porcine insulin differs in only one amino acid.
c. Insulin is stored as a complex with Zn^{2+}; two molecules of zinc complex six molecules of insulin.
d. Insulin synthesis and release are modulated by the following:
   (1) The most important stimulus is glucose. Amino acids, fatty acids, and ketone bodies also stimulate release.
   (2) The islets of Langerhans contain several cell types besides β cells that synthesize and release peptide humoral agents (including glucagon and somatostatin) that can modulate insulin secretion.
   (3) α-Adrenergic pathways inhibit secretion of insulin; this is the predominant inhibitory mechanism.
e. β-Adrenergic stimulation increases insulin release.
f. Elevated intracellular Ca^{2+} acts as an insulin secretagogue.

2. *Mechanism of action*

a. Insulin binds to specific high-affinity receptors with tyrosine kinase activity located in the plasma membrane. Specific tyrosine residues of the insulin receptor become phosphorylated (autophosphorylation); other substrates for phosphorylation include IRS-1–4 (insulin receptor substrates-1 to -4). The increase in glucose transport in muscle and adipose tissue is mediated by the recruitment of hexose transport molecules (GLUT-1 and GLUT-4) into the plasma membrane.
b. Insulin alters the phosphorylation state of key metabolic enzymes, leading to enzymatic activation or inactivation.
c. Insulin induces the transcription of several genes involved in increasing glucose catabolism and specifically inhibits transcription of other genes involved in gluconeogenesis.

3. *Actions.* Insulin promotes systemic cellular K^+ uptake.

a. Liver
   (1) Inhibits glucose production and increases glycolysis
   (2) Inhibits glycogenolysis and stimulates glycogen synthesis
   (3) Increases the synthesis of triglycerides
   (4) Increases protein synthesis
b. Muscle
   (1) Increases glucose transport and glycolysis
   (2) Increases glycogen deposition
   (3) Increases protein synthesis
c. Adipose tissue
   (1) Increases glucose transport
   (2) Increases lipogenesis and lipoprotein lipase
   (3) Decreases intracellular lipolysis

4. *Pharmacologic properties*

a. Insulin has a $t_{1/2}$ of 5–10 minutes.
b. Insulin is degraded by hepatic glutathione–insulin transhydrogenase, which reduces the disulfide linkages between the A and B chains, producing two biologically inactive peptides.

table 10-3 Pharmacologic Properties of Agents Used for Long-Term Management of Hyperglycemia

Agent	Route of Administration	Onset of Action	Duration of Action
Insulins			
Rapid acting			
Insulin glulisine	SC	20 min	1–2 h
Insulin aspart	SC	15 min	3–5 h
Insulin lispro	SC	15 min	3–5 h
Short acting			
Regular	SC, IM, IV	15 min	2–5 h
Intermediate acting			
Isophane	SC	2 h	24 h
Slow acting			
Insulin glargine	SC	1.5	24 h
Insulin detemir	SC	1.5	12–20 h
Ultralente	SC	4 h	36 h
Sulfonylureas			
Tolbutamide	Oral	20 min	6–10 h
Acetohexamide	Oral	20 min	12–20 h
Tolazamide	Oral	20 min	10–14 h
Glipizide	Oral	30 min	16–24 h
Glyburide	Oral	1–2 h	24 h
Glimepiride	Oral	1–2 h	24 h
Chlorpropamide	Oral	1–2 h	>24 h
Biguanines			
Metformin	Oral	~2 h	6 h
Meglitinides			
Repaglinide	Oral	20 min	1 h
Nateglinide	Oral	30 min	1–2 h
α-Glucosidase inhibitors			
Acarbose	Oral	30 min	2 h
Miglitol	Oral		
Thiazolidinediones			
Pioglitazone	Oral	3 h	12 h
Rosaglitazone	Oral	3 h	12–18 h
Incretins			
Exenatide	SC	1 h	2–3 h
DPP-IV inhibitor			
Sitagliptin	Oral	2 h	12 h
Amylin analog			
Pramlintide	SC	30 min	3 h

5. ***Insulin preparations*** (Table 10-3)
   a. Historically, insulin preparations were derived from bovine and porcine glands. Bovine insulin was removed from the U.S. market due to concern about "mad cow" disease; preparation of porcine insulin was stopped in 2005. Human insulin is prepared by recombinant DNA techniques to produce the human peptide in bacteria.
   b. Insulin preparations are often mixed to control blood sugar levels: A single morning injection of a lente or ultralente form is typically supplemented with preprandial injections of a rapid-acting product. Dosage regimens must be individualized.
      (1) Rapid acting. **Insulin glulisine**, **insulin aspart**, and **insulin lispro** are human insulins that have been modified at 1–2 amino acids in the B chain to increase their solubility. These

insulins dissociate into monomers almost instantly upon SC injection. They provide better postprandial control of glucose levels than regular insulin.

(2) Short acting. **Regular insulin** is prepared as a recombinant human protein.

(3) Intermediate acting. **Isophane insulin (or Neutral Protamine Hagedorn, NPH)** is prepared by precipitating insulin–zinc complexes with protamine, a mixture of basic peptides. This slows absorption and extends the duration of action.

(4) Long acting

(a) **Ultralente insulin** has a larger particle size than lente products.

(b) **Glargine insulin** has a single amino acid in the A chain and two additional amino acids in the B chain that differ from regular insulin. This causes it to form a stable, slowly dissolving precipitate upon injection.

(c) **Detemir** insulin has a 14-carbon fatty acid (myristic acid) added to the A chain and an amino acid removed from the B chain; this also causes it to form a stable, slowly dissolving precipitate.

6. ***Therapeutic uses.*** Insulin is used to treat all of the manifestations of hyperglycemia in **both type I (insulin-dependent)** and **type II (non-insulin-dependent) diabetes mellitus**. Most type II diabetics are treated with dietary changes and oral hypoglycemic agents. In serious cases of type II diabetes in which these treatments are inadequate to control blood glucose levels, insulin may be required.

7. ***Adverse effects***

a. Hypoglycemia may occur from insulin overdose, insufficient caloric intake, strenuous exercise, or when combined with ethanol. Sequelae include tachycardia, sweating, and sympathetic and parasympathetic actions that can progress to coma.

b. Hypokalemia

c. Anaphylactoid reaction

d. Lipodystrophy or hypertrophy of subcutaneous fat at the injection site

e. Weight gain

B. Oral hypoglycemic agents

1. ***Sulfonylureas***

a. Structure

(1) **First-generation** compounds include **tolbutamide, acetohexamide, tolazamide,** and **chlorpropamide.**

(2) Second-generation compounds include glyburide and glipizide; they are up to 200 times more potent than first-generation agents.

(3) Third-generation **compounds, such as glimepiride,** may be used in conjunction with insulin. These compounds may interact with different cellular proteins than other sulfonylureas.

(4) All of the sulfonylureas are well absorbed after oral administration and bind to plasma proteins, notably albumin.

b. Mechanism of action

(1) Sulfonylureas cause an increase in the amount of insulin secreted by the β cells in response to a glucose challenge. Sulfonylureas block K^+ channels in β cells, leading to depolarization, increased Ca^{2+} entry via voltage-dependent calcium channels, and increased secretion.

(2) These agents increase sensitivity to insulin, perhaps by increasing the number of insulin receptors. However, sulfonylureas do not decrease the insulin requirements of patients with type I diabetes.

(3) Sulfonylureas decrease serum glucagon, which opposes the action of insulin.

c. Pharmacologic properties (see Table 10-3). Pharmacologic failure with oral antidiabetic agents is common, initially affecting 15%–30% of patients and as many as 90% after 6–7 years of therapy.

(1) Short-acting agents

(a) Short-acting sulfonylureas include **tolbutamide.**

(b) Short-acting sulfonylureas are rapidly absorbed; absorption is not affected if taken with food.

(c) As with all sulfonylureas, **hypoglycemia** is a potentially dangerous adverse effect of these short-acting agents. Other adverse effects include dermatologic disorders and GI disturbances, including nausea and heartburn.

(2) Intermediate-acting agents

(a) **Acetohexamide**

(i) Acetohexamide is rapidly absorbed.

(ii) Acetohexamide is metabolized to hydrohexamide, which is biologically active and has a $t_{1/2}$ of 6 hours.

(iii) Acetohexamide has uricosuric properties, making it useful in diabetic patients with gout.

(b) **Tolazamide**

(i) Tolazamide is slowly absorbed.

(ii) Tolazamide is about 5 times more potent on a milligram basis than tolbutamide

(iii) Tolazamide exerts a **mild diuretic effect.**

(c) **Glipizide**

(i) Glipizide is rapidly absorbed, but absorption can be delayed by food.

(ii) Glipizide becomes highly protein-bound in the plasma.

(d) **Glyburide**

(i) Glyburide is rapidly absorbed.

(ii) Glyburide inhibits hepatic glucose production.

(iii) Glyburide exerts a **mild diuretic effect.**

(3) Long-acting agents

(a) Long-acting sulfonylureas include **chlorpropamide** and **glimepiride.**

(b) Long-acting sulfonylureas are rapidly absorbed.

(c) These agents are extensively reabsorbed in the kidney; reabsorption is slowed under basic pH conditions.

(d) Long-acting sulfonylureas cause adverse effects more frequently than other sulfonylureas. Water retention is common, and alcohol consumption produces a **disulfiram-like reaction** in some patients.

(e) These agents are contraindicated in elderly patients, in whom toxicities seem to be exacerbated.

d. Therapeutic uses

(1) Sulfonylureas are very useful in treating type II diabetes mellitus but are not effective against type I diabetes.

(2) Sulfonylureas should not be used in patients with renal or liver disease.

2. ***Biguanine hypoglycemics*** include metformin.

a. Metformin reduces hepatic glucose production and intestinal absorption of glucose; it does not alter insulin secretion. These effects are believed to be due to an increase in the activity of AMP kinase, a key intracellular regulator of energy homeostasis.

b. Metformin increases peripheral insulin sensitivity.

c. Metformin may be used alone or in combination with sulfonylureas and thiazolidinediones.

d. Metformin has been found useful in the treatment of polycystic ovary syndrome (PCOS); it lowers serum androgens and restores normal menstrual cycles and ovulation.

e. Metformin rarely causes hypoglycemia or weight gain.

f. Adverse effects of metformin include lactic acidosis.

3. ***Meglitinides: repaglinide and nateglinide***

a. These agents are oral insulin secretagogues that act by blocking ATP-dependent K^+ channels, leading to increased insulin secretion by pancreatic β-cells.

b. Nateglinide has a more rapid onset of action and is more specific for pancreatic K^+ channels than repaglinide.

c. These drugs are metabolized by the liver and should not be used in patients with hepatic insufficiency.

d. The major adverse effect of these drugs is hypoglycemia.

4. ***α-Glucosidase inhibitors*** include acarbose and miglitol.

a. Acarbose and miglitol are oligosaccharides or oligosaccharide derivatives.

b. They act as competitive, reversible inhibitors of pancreatic α-amylase and intestinal α-glucosidase enzymes; they act in the lumen of the intestine.
c. Inhibition of α-glucosidase prolongs digestion of carbohydrates and reduces peak plasma glucose levels.
d. Miglitol is a more potent inhibitor of sucrase and maltase than is acarbose. Unlike acarbose, miglitol does not inhibit pancreatic α-amylase but does inhibit isomaltose.
e. These drugs are usually combined with a sulfonylurea or another oral hypoglycemic agent.
f. α-Glucosidase inhibitors rarely cause hypoglycemia.

5. ***Thiazolidinediones*** include pioglitazone and rosiglitazone.
a. Thiazolidinediones are a new class of oral hypoglycemic agents that act by increasing tissue sensitivity to insulin.
b. These drugs bind to a specific intracellular receptor (PPAR-γ), a member of the nuclear-receptor family. Rosiglitazone has about 10-fold higher affinity for PPAR-γ than does pioglitazone.
c. Thiazolidinediones predominantly affect liver, skeletal muscle, and adipose tissue.
(1) In the liver, thiazolidinediones decrease glucose output and decreases insulin levels.
(2) In muscle, thiazolidinediones increase glucose uptake.
(3) In adipose tissue, these drugs increase glucose uptake and decrease fatty acid release and may increase the release of hormones such as adiponectin and resistin.
d. The actions of these drugs require the presence of insulin.
e. Thiazolidinediones reduce plasma glucose and triglycerides.
f. Thiazolidinediones do not cause hypoglycemia.

6. ***Incretin mimetics***
a. Endogenous human incretins, such as glucagon-like peptide-1 (GLP-1) are released from the gut and enhance insulin secretion.
b. Exenatide is a 39-amino acid GLP-1 agonist isolated from the salivary gland venom of the lizard *Heloderma suspectum* (Gila monster). It also reduces appetite.
c. Exenatide decreases glucagon secretion, slows gastric emptying, reduces food intake, and promotes β-cell proliferation.
d. SC injection of exenatide may improve glycemic control in patients with type II diabetes mellitus who have not achieved adequate glycemic control on metformin, a sulfonylurea, or a combination of metformin and a sulfonylurea.

7. ***Dipeptidyl peptidase 4 (DPP-IV) inhibitors***
a. **Sitagliptin** is the first in a new class of antidiabetic agents that act by inhibiting dipeptidyl peptidase 4, a serine protease.
b. Dipeptidyl peptidase 4 is responsible for the proteolysis of th eincretins, including GLP-1 and glucose-dependent insulinotropic peptide (GIP).
c. **Sitagliptin** may also improve β-cell function.
d. In monotherapy or in combination with metformin, sitagliptin decreased fasting and post-prandial plasma glucose concentrations and plasma HbA1c concentration.
e. Administered orally; most common side effect was headache.

8. ***Amylin analogs.*** **Pramlintide** is a synthetic amylin analog. Amylin is a polypeptide stored and secreted by β-cells of the pancreas, and it acts in concert with insulin to reduce blood sugar.
a. Pramlintide acts to slow gastric emptying, decrease glucagon secretion, and decreases appetite.
b. Administered SC, typically with insulin. Common side effects are hypoglycemia and nausea.

C. Agents that increase blood glucose (hyperglycemics)

1. ***Glucagon***
a. Structure and synthesis
(1) Glucagon is a single-chain polypeptide of 29 amino acids produced by the α cells of the pancreas.
(2) Glucagon shares a structural homology with secretin, VIP, and gastric inhibitory peptide.

(3) Secretion of glucagon is inhibited by elevated plasma glucose, insulin, and somatostatin.
(4) Secretion of glucagon is stimulated by amino acids, sympathetic stimulation, and sympathetic secretion.

b. Actions and pharmacologic properties
(1) Membrane-bound receptors are most abundant in the liver; response is coupled to an increase in cAMP.
(2) Glucagon stimulates the use of glycogen stores and gluconeogenesis; in general, its actions oppose those of insulin.
(3) Large doses produce marked relaxation of smooth muscle.
(4) Glucagon is extensively degraded in the liver and kidney and is also subject to hydrolysis in plasma. Plasma $t_{1/2}$ of glucagon is approximately 3–5 minutes.

c. Therapeutic uses
(1) Glucagon produces rescue from hypoglycemic crisis. Glucagon rapidly increases blood glucose in insulin-induced hypoglycemia if hepatic glycogen stores are adequate.
(2) Glucagon provides intestinal relaxation prior to radiologic examination.
(3) Glucagon causes β-cell stimulation of insulin secretion; it is used to assess pancreatic reserves.

d. Adverse effects. The adverse effects of glucagon are minimal; there is a low incidence of nausea and vomiting.

2. ***Diazoxide (Proglycem)***
a. Diazoxide is a nondiuretic thiazide that promptly increases blood glucose levels by direct inhibition of insulin secretion.
b. Diazoxide is useful in cases of insulinoma or leucine-sensitive hypoglycemia.
c. Diazoxide may cause sodium retention, GI irritation, and changes in circulating white blood cells.

IX. THE CALCIUM HOMEOSTATIC SYSTEM

A. **Calcium** is the major extracellular divalent cation, primarily (40%–50%) existing as free ionized Ca^{2+} (the biologically active fraction). Approximately 40% of serum Ca^{2+} is bound to plasma proteins, especially albumin, with the remaining 10% complexed to such anions as citrate.

B. Drugs affecting Ca^{2+} homeostasis

1. ***Parathyroid hormone (PTH)***
a. Structure
(1) PTH is an 84-amino acid peptide secreted by the parathyroid glands in response to low serum ionized Ca^{2+}.
(2) Agents such as β-adrenoceptor agonists, which increase cAMP in the parathyroid gland, cause an increase in PTH secretion.

b. Actions and pharmacologic properties
(1) Activity in the kidney and in bone is mediated by specific PTH receptors, which are in turn coupled to an increase in cAMP. Significant quantities of cAMP are found in the urine after PTH stimulation.
(2) In bone, PTH can increase both the rate of bone formation and the rate of bone resorption. This is mediated by cytokines produced by osteoblasts that regulate the number and activity of osteoclasts.
(a) Continuous exposure to PTH results in net bone resorption.
(b) Pulsatile exposure results in net bone formation.
(3) In the kidney, PTH increases the reabsorption of Ca^{2+} and Mg^{2+}, and it increases production of 1,25-$(OH)_2D_3$ from 25-$(OH)D_3$. PTH also decreases reabsorption of phosphate, bicarbonate, amino acids, sulfate, sodium, and chloride.

(4) In the GI tract, PTH increases intestinal absorption of Ca^{2+} indirectly through an increase in 1,25-$(OH)_2D_3$.

(5) PTH is rapidly degraded ($t_{1/2}$ is 2–5 min) by renal and hepatic metabolism.

c. Teriparatide

(1) Teriparatide is recombinant human PTH 1-34 which behaves as a full PTH agonist.

(2) Teriparatide is administered parenterally once a day, and this intermittent exposure results in net bone formation.

(3) Teriparatide is used in the treatment of osteoporosis.

(4) Teriparatide is also used as a diagnostic agent to distinguish pseudohypoparathyroidism from true hypoparathyroidism.

(5) Major adverse effects are hypercalcemia and hypercalciurea. Infrequent adverse effects include dizziness, depression, pain, headache, and leg cramps.

2. *Calcitonin*

a. Structure. Calcitonin is a 32-amino acid peptide secreted by perifollicular cells of the thyroid gland in response to elevated plasma Ca^{2+}. Gastrin, glucagon, cholecystokinin, and epinephrine can also increase calcitonin secretion.

b. Actions. Calcitonin antagonizes the actions of PTH through an independent mechanism:

(1) Calcitonin interacts with specific receptors on osteoclasts to decrease net reabsorption of Ca^{2+}. Calcitonin may also stimulate bone formation.

(2) Calcitonin increases renal excretion of Ca^{2+}, Na^{+}, and phosphate.

c. Pharmacologic properties

(1) Synthetic salmon calcitonin (Fortical, Miacalcin) differs from human calcitonin at 13 of 32 amino acids and has a longer half-life.

(2) Currently approved products are administered parenterally or as a nasal spray.

(3) Decreases in plasma Ca^{2+} are seen in 2 hours and persist for 6–8 hours.

d. Therapeutic uses

(1) Calcitonin reduces hypercalcemia due to **Paget disease,** hyperparathyroidism, idiopathic juvenile hypercalcemia, vitamin D intoxication, osteolytic bone disorders, and osteoporosis.

(2) Patients frequently (20%) become refractory to chronic administration, possibly because of the production of anticalcitonin antibodies

3. *Vitamin D and vitamin D metabolites* (Table 10-4)

a. Structure. The calciferols, vitamin D_3 (cholecalciferol) and vitamin D_2 (ergocalciferol), are secosteroid members of the steroid hormone family.

b. Synthesis

(1) Vitamin D_3 is produced in the skin from cholesterol; this synthesis requires exposure to ultraviolet light.

(2) 25-$(OH)D_3$ (calcifediol)

(a) Calcifediol is produced in the liver by hydroxylation of vitamin D_3.

(b) Calcifediol is the most abundant calciferol metabolite in the plasma.

(3) 1,25-$(OH)_2D_3$ (calcitriol)

table 10-4 Pharmacologic Properties of Vitamin D Preparations

Agent	Metabolic Route	Onset of Action	Half-life
Ergocalciferol (D2)	Hepatic, renal	10–14 days	30 days
Cholecalciferol (D3)	Hepatic, renal	10–14 days	30 days
Calcifediol	Renal	8–10 days	20 days
Calcitriol	None	10 h	15 h
Calcipotriene	Hepatic, renal	10 days	30 days
Doxercalciferol	Hepatic	5–8 h	36 h
Paricalcitol	None	Minutes (IV)	15 h

(a) Calcitriol is produced in the kidney by further hydroxylation of 25-(OH)D_3 by 1α-hydroxylase. Regulation of 1α-hydroxylase activity determines the serum levels of **calcitriol.** Enzymatic activity is increased by PTH, estrogens, prolactin, and other agents, and it is decreased by 1,25-$(OH)_2D_3$ and phosphate (direct effect).

(b) Calcitriol is the most active metabolite of vitamin D.

(4) Vitamin D_2 (ergocalciferol)

(a) Vitamin D_2 is derived from plant metabolism of ergosterol and has a slightly different side chain, which does not alter its biologic effects in humans.

(b) In humans, vitamin D_2 is metabolized in the same manner as vitamin D_3 and appears to be bioequivalent.

(5) Paricalcitrol (1,25-$(OH)_2$-19 norvitamin D_2) is a 1,25-hydroxylated vitamin D_2 derivative that reduces serum PTH levels without affecting serum Ca^{2+} or PO_4^{2-} levels. It is approved to treat hyperparathyroidism in patients with renal failure who are on dialysis. It is administered by infusion.

(6) 22-Oxacalcitrol (maxacalcitrol) is a 1,25-$(OH)_2D_3$ derivative containing an oxygen instead of a carbon at position 22 in the side chain. Compared with 1,25-D_3, it binds with low affinity to the serum vitamin D-binding globulin. It is a potent suppressor of PTH and is useful in patients with secondary (to renal failure) or primary hyperparathyroidism.

(7) Doxercalciferol (1α-(OH) vitamin D_2) is administered orally or IV for hyperparathyroidism secondary to renal failure. It does not increase intestinal Ca^{2+} absorption and does not cause hypercalcemia.

(8) Calcipotriene

(a) Calcipotriene is a 1,24-$(OH)_2D_3$ derivative for topical administration for the treatment of skin disorders such as psoriasis.

(b) Calcipotriene has reduced effects on calcium homeostasis.

c. Actions and pharmacologic properties (Table 10-4)

(1) Calcitriol increases plasma levels of both Ca^{2+} and phosphate by acting on several organ systems:

(a) **Intestine:** Increases Ca^{2+} absorption from the GI tract

(b) **Bone:** Mobilizes Ca^{2+} and phosphate, probably by stimulation of calcium flux out of osteoblasts

(c) **Kidney:** Increases reabsorption of both Ca^{2+} and phosphate

(2) All vitamin D metabolites bind to a specific plasma-binding protein, vitamin D-binding protein (DBP).

(3) Vitamin D, calcifediol, and calcitriol are all administered orally; calcitriol may be administered parenterally.

d. Therapeutic uses

(1) Elevate serum Ca^{2+}. Vitamin D and vitamin D metabolites are used to treat hypocalcemia caused by a number of diseases, including vitamin D deficiency (nutritional rickets), hypoparathyroidism, renal disease, malabsorption, and osteoporosis.

(2) Reduce cellular proliferation

(a) Recent evidence has shown that 1,25-$(OH)_2D_3$ can block differentiation and proliferation of many cell types. For this reason, the drug has been successfully used in the treatment of certain **leukemias.**

(b) **Topical calcipotriene** has been approved for the treatment of **psoriasis;** it reduces fibroblast proliferation and induces differentiation of epidermal keratinocytes.

4. *Bisphosphonates*

a. Chemistry and pharmacokinetics. Bisphosphonates (P-C-P) are analogues of pyrophosphate (P-O-P) that bind directly to hydroxyapatite crystals in bone and impair reabsorption.

(1) **First-generation bisphosphonate: etidronate disodium**

(2) **Second-generation** bisphosphonates contain a nitrogen, are called aminobisphosphonates, and include **alendronate, ibandronate, and pamidronate.** They are at least 10 times more potent than first-generation agents.

(3) **Third-generation bisphosphonates, risedronate and zoldronic acid,** have a nitrogen within a heterocyclic ring and are 10,000 times more potent than first-generation agents.

(4) After oral administration, all bisphosphonates have very poor (1%–3%) oral absorption. Etidronate, especially, is associated with esophageal irritation and erosion. Recommendation is to administer on an empty stomach with a full glass of water and remain standing for 30 minutes.

b. **Etidronate,** the first bisphosphonate discovered

(1) Mechanism of action. The nonnitrogenous bisphosphonates are internalized by osteoclasts and converted into an ATP analogue that cannot be hydrolyzed. This metabolite impairs various functions and induces apoptosis in osteoclasts.

(2) Can be administered IV or orally

c. **Aminobisphosphonates**

(1) Mechanism of action is inhibition of farnesyl diphosphate synthase, part of the cholesterol biosynthetic pathway. This impairs posttranslational modification of a number of regulator proteins critical for osteoclast function including Ras, Rho, and Rac. There is recent evidence that aminobisphosphonates also induce a unique ATP analogue that induces osteoclast apoptosis.

(2) Oral administration only; poorly absorbed

(3) Aminobisphosphonates are not associated with the problems of reflux and osteomalacia.

d. Uses

(1) Paget disease—given orally, clinical symptoms improve relatively slowly (1–3 months)

(2) Effective in 60%–70% of cases; normalization of serum Ca^{2+} levels in 2–8 days

(3) Heterotopic ossification

(4) Aminobisphosphonates are approved for the prevention of osteoporosis

e. **Adverse effects.** GI disturbances include GI bleeding and diarrhea; arthralgia; and nonspecified chest pain. When used for prolonged periods (years), etidronate can interfere with mineralization of bone (osteomalacia).

5. ***Calcium sensor sensitizers—calcimimetics***

a. The parathyroid gland senses Ca^{2+} via the action of the protein **CaSR.** Activation of CaSR reduces the amount of PTH synthesized and released by the gland.

b. **Cinacalcet (Sensipar)** is an oral agent that acts like Ca^{2+} on the CaSR; this reduces serum PTH.

c. Cinacalcet is approved for use in patients with hyperparathyroidism secondary to renal disease.

d. Hypocalcemia is the major adverse effect of cinacalcet.

6. ***Secondary agents affecting Ca^{2+} homeostasis***

a. Thiazide diuretics reduce the renal excretion of Ca^{2+} and the incidence of kidney stone formation in patients with idiopathic hypercalciuria.

b. Loop diuretics. Agents such as furosemide increase renal excretion of Ca^{2+}.

c. Glucocorticoids increase bone resorption and reduce intestinal absorption of Ca^{2+} by interfering with 1,25-$(OH)_2D_3$. The net effect is to reduce plasma Ca^{2+} levels.

d. Estrogens

(1) Estrogens indirectly impair the action of PTH on bone and in the kidney.

(2) Estrogens are used in the treatment of osteoporosis.

C. Calcium supplements

1. Calcium supplements are available in a variety of Ca^{2+} concentrations and in parenteral and oral formulations.
2. Calcium supplements are useful as dietary supplements for the treatment or prevention of osteoporosis and for the immediate treatment of acute hypocalcemia and hypocalcemic tetany.
3. Calcium supplements may cause hypercalcemia with long-term use.

X. RETINOIC ACID AND DERIVATIVES

A. Structure. Retinol (vitamin A) is a prohormone that is converted by intracellular enzymes to activate the active agents **all-*trans*-retinoic acid** and **9-*cis*-retinoic acid.** Other retinol metabolites are biologically active.

B. Action

1. **The actions of retinoids are mediated via intracellular receptors of two main classes: RAR (retinoic acid receptor) and RXR (retinoid X receptor). Rexinoids are ligands that interact specifically with the RXRs.**
   a. Each of these classes has at least three distinct isoforms (α,β,γ with unique biologic properties).
   b. The retinoid receptors are members of the nuclear receptor family and act by modulating transcription of specific genes.
2. **Retinoids are morphogens, playing important roles during embryonic development,** including the regulation of cellular proliferation and differentiation, and the modulation of immune function and cytokine production. They cause severe fetal malformations and must be used with extreme caution in females of childbearing age.

C. Tretinoin

1. ***Tretinoin is all-trans-retinoic acid,*** a naturally occurring metabolite of vitamin A. Tretinoin as a topical preparation used for the treatment of acne and photoaged skin, as an oral agent it is used in the treatment of acute promyelocytic leukemia (APL), and may be used in the treatment of Kaposi sarcoma.
2. Adverse effects of tretinoin include tenderness, erythema, and burning. There is also an increased risk of sunburn. Oral administration is associated with a syndrome of hypervitaminosis A, which includes headache, fever, bone pain, nausea, vomiting, and rash.

D. Isotretinoin

1. Isotretinoin is an oral agent used for the treatment of severe acne and the symptomatic management of keratinization disorders. It reversibly reduces the size of sebaceous glands and hence the production of sebum. It is the 13-*cis* isomer of tretinoin.
2. Adverse effects of isotretinoin include inflammation of mucous membranes (most often the lips), rash, and alopecia. Less common adverse effects include arthralgia and myalgia. Retinoids tend to inhibit lipoprotein lipase, which leads to an increase in serum triglycerides.
3. Isotretinoin is teratogenic.

E. Acitretin (Soriatane)

1. Acitretin is an oral agent approved for the treatment of psoriasis and other disorders of keratinization. In addition, acitretin has been studied in cutaneous T-cell lymphoma and for the prevention of skin cancers following solid organ transplantation.
2. Adverse effects of acitretin include **skin and nail abnormalities.**
3. Acitretin is teratogenic.

F. **Alitretinoin (Panretin)** is a synthetic version of 9-*cis*-retinoic acid. It is a topical cream approved for use in the skin disorders associated with Kaposi syndrome.

G. Tazarotene (Avage)

1. Following topical application, tazarotene undergoes esterase hydrolysis to the active form, tazarotenic acid, which binds to all three members of the RAR family, with some specificity for β and γ subtypes.
2. It is used to treat psoriasis, photoaging (fine wrinkles), and acne vulgaris.
3. The most common adverse effects seen with tazarotene are skin related: rash, desquamation, and pruritus.

H. **Adapalene** is a topical retinoid-like drug for the treatment of mild-to-moderate acne vulgaris. It is a naphtholic acid derivative that binds to RARs.

I. Bexarotene

1. Bexarotene is a synthetic oral and topical rexinoid with selectivity for the retinoid X-receptor.
2. It is used in the treatment of cutaneous T-cell lymphoma, Kaposi sarcoma, and breast and lung cancers. It has also been used to treat psoriasis.
3. Its major adverse effects are hyperlipidemias, both hypertriglyceridemia and hypercholesterolemia. Other serous adverse effects include acute pancreatitis and hepatic dysfunction.

DRUG SUMMARY TABLE

Hypothalamic/Pituitary Agents
Octreotide (Sandostatin)
Gonadorelin (Factrel, Leutrepulse)
Nafarelin acetate (Synarel)
Triptorelin (Trelstar Depot)
Goserelin (Zoladex)
Leuprolide acetate (Lupron, Eligard)
Histrelin (Vantas)
Cetrorelix (Cetrotide)
Ganirelix (Antagon)
Abarelix (Plenax)
Bromocriptine (Parlodel)
Cabergoline (Dostinex)
Pergolide (Permax)
Corticorelin (Acthrel)
Somatotropin, rhGH, (Humatrope, others)
Somatrem (Protropin)
Pegvisomant (Somavert)
Thyrotropin α (Thyrogen)
Corticotrophin, ACTH (H.P. Acthar)
Cosyntropin (Cortrosyn)
Oxytocin (Pitocin, Syntocinon)
Vasopressin (Pitressin)
Desmopressin acetate (DDAVP, Stimate)

Gonadotropins
Menotropins (Pergonal, Repronex)
Urofollitropin (Bravelle)
hCG (Pregnyl, Novarel, others)
Follitropin α (Gonal F)
Follitropin β (Puregon, Follistim)

Estrogens
17β-estradiol (generic)
Estrone (Primestrin, Estra AQ)
Equilin (Premarin)
Ethinyl estradiol (Estinyl, Feminone, others)
Mestranol
Diethylstilbestrol (Stilphostrol)
Dienestrol (DV, Estraguard)

Anti-Estrogens
Clomiphene (Clomid, Milophene, Serophene)
Fulvestrant (Faslodex)
Danazol (Danocrine)

SERMs
Tamoxifen (Novaldex, generic)
Raloxifene (Evista)
Toremifene (Fareston)

Thyroid Hormones
Thyroid USP (Armour Thyroid, Dathroid)
Liotrix (Thyrolar)
Liothyronine sodium (Cytomel)
Levothyroxine sodium (Levothroid, Synthroid, others)

Antithyroid Preparations
Methimazole (Tapazole)
Propylthiouracil (PTU)
Iodine (Lugol's Solution)
Sodium Iodide (I^{131}) (Iodotope, Megatope)

Insulin Preparations
Insulin glulisine (Apidra)
Insulin aspart (NovoLog)
Insulin lispro (Humalog)
Regular (human) (Humulin R, Novilin-R, others)
Lente (human) (Humulin L, Novilin-L)
Isophane (human) (Humulin N, Novilin-N
Insulin Glargine (Lantus)
Insulin Detemir (Levemir)
Ultralente (human) (Humulin U)
Protamine-zinc (human) (Humalog Mix 75/25, others)

Oral Hypoglycemics
Sulfonylureas
Tolbutamide (Orinase, Tol-Tab, generic)
Acetohexamide (Dymelor, generic)
Tolazamide (Tolinase, generic)
Glipizide (Glucotrol, generic)
Glyburide (Dibeta, Micronase, generic)
Glimepiride (Amaryl, generic)
Chlorpropamide (Diabinase, generic)
Biguanines
Metformin (Fotamet, generic)
Meglitinides
Repaglinide (Prandin)
Nateglinide (Starlix)
α-Glucosidase Inhibitors
Acarbose (Precose)
Miglitol (Glyset)
Thiazolidinediones
Pioglitazone (Actos)
Rosaglitazone (Avandia)
Incretins
Exenatide (Byetta)
Glucagon (Glucagen, generic)

Aromatase Inhibitors
Exemestane (Aromasin)
Anastrazole (Arimidex)
Letrozole (Femara)

Progestins
Hydroxyprogesterone caproate (Delalutin, others)
Megestrol (Megace)
medroxyprogesterone acetate (Amen, Provera, others)
Norethindrone (Norlutin, Micronor, others)
Norgestrel (Ovrette)
Norgestimate
Levonorgestrel (Mirena, Plan B)

Anti-Progestins
Mifepristone (RU-486) (Mifeprex)

Androgens
Testosterone (generic, Testoderm)
Testosterone propionate (Testex)
Testosterone enanthate (Andryl, Delatestryl, others)
Testosterone cypionate (Depo-Testosterone)
Methyltestosterone (Metandren, Android, others)
Fluoxymesterone (Halotestin, others)
Oxymetholone (Anadrol, Anapolon)
Nandrolone (Hybolin, Deca-Durabolin)
Oxandrolone (Oxandrine)

Anti-Androgens
Flutamide (Eulexin)
Bicalutamide (Casodex)
Nilutamide (Niladron)
Finasteride (Proscar)
Dutasteride (Avodart)
Ketoconazole (Nizoral)
Spironolactone (Aldactone)

Corticosteroids
Cortisol (hydrocortisone) (generic)
Cortisone (Cortone)
Prednisone (Deltason, Predone, others)
Prednisolone (Prelone, generic)
Dexamethasone (Decadron, Corta-stat, others)
Betamethasone (Betastat)
Triamcinolone (Triamcot, others)
Aldosterone
Fludrocortisone (Florenif)
Clobetasol (Clobevate, Clovex, others)
Halobetasol (Ultravate)
Amcinonide (Cyclocort, generic)
Fluocinonide (Lidex, Vanos)
Beclomethasone (Beconase, Qvar)
Fluticasone (Cutivate, Flonase)
Desonide (Desowen, LoKara)

Adrenocortical Antagonists
Mitotane (Lysodren)
Aminoglutethimide (Cytadren)
Metyrapone (Metopirone)

Agents Affecting Ca^{2+} Homeostasis
Teriparatide (Forteo)
Calcitonin (salmon) (Fortical, Miacalcin)
Ergocalciferol (Calciferol, Ergo G, generic)
Calcifediol (Calderol)
Dihydrotachysterol (DHT)
Calcitriol (Rocaltrol, Calcijex, generic)
Calcipotriene (Dovonex)
Doxercalciferol (Hectorol)
Alfacalcidol (One-Alpha)
Paricalcitrol (Zemplar)
Maxacalcitol (Oxarol)

Bisphosphonates
Etidronate disodium (Didronel)
Alendronate (Fosamax)
Ibandronate (Boniva)
Pamidronate (Aredia)
Risedronate (Actonel)
Zoldronic acid (Zolmeta)

Calcimimetics
Cinacalcet (Sensipar)

Retinoids
Tretinoin (Retin A, Renova, ATRA)
Isotretinoin (Accutane)
Acitretin (Soriatane)
Alitretinoin (Panretin)
Tazarotene (Avage)
Adapalene (Differin)

Rexinoids
Bexarotene (Targretin)

Review Test for Chapter 10

Directions: Each of the numbered items or incomplete statements in this section is followed by answers or by completions of the statement. Select the ONE lettered answer or completion that is BEST in each case.

1. A 49-year-old woman complains of sweating profusely nearly every night. She had a transvaginal hysterectomy 5 years ago but has intact ovaries. Upon physical examination you note that she has a BMI of 22, but all her vital signs are normal. Which of the following would best treat her condition?

(A) Conjugated estrogens
(B) Levonorgestrel
(C) Raloxifene
(D) Calcitriol

2. A patient who has recently undergone a kidney transplant is immunosuppressed with dexamethasone and sirolimus. He is involved in a serious car accident. Besides the necessary treatment of the trauma, which of the following actions would be necessary?

(A) Begin low-dose fludrocortisone therapy
(B) Increase the dose of dexamethasone
(C) Discontinue use of the sacrolimus
(D) Begin treatment with methyltestosterone

3. A male patient is diagnosed with a large, benign prostatic mass, and he has the urge to urinate frequently. He is begun on leuprolide acetate therapy. He returns to your office 3 days later complaining that his urge to urinate has increased, not decreased. What accounts for this action?

(A) Direct effect of leuprolide on the prostate
(B) Reduction of the conversion of testosterone to dihydrotachysterol (DHT)
(C) Transient agonist action (''flare'') of leuprolide causing a temporary increase in androgen production
(D) Prostatic resistance to leuprolide

4. A 16-year-old female patient enters your dermatology clinic complaining of a rash. She is not taking any medications and is well dressed and groomed. You diagnose a mild case of acne vulgaris and notice that the girl's skin and hair appear unusually oily. Which of the following would be the best treatment for the acne?

(A) Calcipotriene
(B) Topical dexamethasone
(C) Isotretinoin
(D) Bexarotene

5. A 36-year-old woman complains of hot flashes, feelings of weakness, and increased appetite. You observe that she is tachycardic and has a prominent pulse pressure. Results of a test for anti-TSH antibodies are positive. Which of the following would be the most appropriate treatment for this patient?

(A) Methimazole
(B) Liotrix
(C) Thyrotropin α
(D) Ketoconazole

6. A 45-year-old female patient has fasting glucose levels of 147 mg/dL, and with a glucose tolerance test, you have confirmed the diagnosis of type II diabetes. You begin therapy with metformin, but her fasting glucose levels remain above 100 mg/dL. You elect to change her therapy to glyburide. This drug acts to

(A) Increase insulin secretion
(B) Decrease glucocorticoid levels
(C) Decrease tissue sensitivity to insulin
(D) Decrease insulin half-life

7. A 55-year-old woman complains of worsening pain in her back that is not alleviated by NSAIDs. You suspect a bone-related condition and order a series of x-rays and a magnetic resonance image (MRI) of the spine. These studies indicate an advanced case of osteosarcoma. You admit the patient, and later that evening she becomes unresponsive and moribund. Her electrolytes are normal except for Ca^{2+}, which is elevated at 4.2 mM. Which of the following would be most appropriate choice for treating this condition?

(A) Furosemide
(B) Thiazides
(C) Vitamin D
(D) Parathyroid hormone (PTH)

8. A cab driver with a 10-year history of alcoholism presents with ictarus and yellow sclera; serum bilirubin levels are elevated and liver function tests are all abnormal. In addition, his serum calcium at 2.0 mM is abnormally low. You elect to use a vitamin D derivative to correct his calcium level. Which of the following would be most appropriate for his patient?

(A) Ergosterol
(B) Dihydrotachysterol
(C) Calcitriol
(D) Cholecalciferol

Answers and Explanations

1. **The answer is A.** Vasomotor symptoms are the most common complaint of perimenopausal women. Estrogen is the only effective treatment of these symptoms. Since there is no concern of endometrial cancer, a progestin is not indicated. Raloxifene makes hot flashes worse; and while a vitamin D analogue might help maintain Ca^{2+}, it would not have any effect on the vasomotor symptoms.

2. **The answer is B.** Patients taking glucocorticoids long term have suppressed pituitary–adrenal function and do not respond to trauma with increased cortisol biosynthesis. It is necessary to increase the dose of glucocorticoid in this circumstance. A mineralocorticoid would not be beneficial.

3. **The answer is C.** Leuprolide and the other GnRH agonists typically cause a transient increase in gonadal steroid production before down-regulation of receptors occurs. This is called a "flare."

4. **The answer is C.** Isotretinoin is a retinoid that is especially useful in treating acne; it reduces oil production in the skin. Calcipotriene is used to treat psoriasis. Bexarotene is a rexinoid used to treat skin disorders, but not acne.

5. **The answer is B.** The patient has hyperthyroidism due to activating anti-TSH antibodies. Methimazole blocks the initial oxidation of iodine as well as the coupling of monoiodotyrosine (MIT) and diiodotyrosine (DIT) into the mature T_4. Liotrix is a thyroid hormone preparation and would be contraindicated. Ketoconazole inhibits a number of P-450–catalyzed reactions but not the production of thyroid hormone.

6. **The answer is A.** Sulfonylureas such as glyburide increase the release of insulin from the pancreas. They also may cause an increase in insulin receptors, which increases tissue sensitivity to insulin. They do not slow insulin clearance, and they do not decrease glucocorticoid levels.

7. **The answer is A.** Thiazides and loop diuretics have opposite effects on Ca^{2+} excretion; loop diuretics like furosemide increase Ca^{2+} excretion and hence reduce hypercalcemia. Vitamin D and parathyroid hormone (PTH) both increase serum Ca^{2+}.

8. **The answer is C.** Calcitriol would be the most effective agent for hypocalcemia in a patient with impaired liver function. The liver provides the required 25-hydroxylation of dihydrotachysterol (DHT), cholecalciferol, and ergosterol.

chapter 11

Drugs Used in Treatment of Infectious Diseases

I. INFECTIOUS DISEASE THERAPY

Infectious disease therapy is based on the principle of selective toxicity: Destroy the infecting organism without damage to the host by exploiting basic biochemical and physical differences between the two organisms.

A. Choice of appropriate antibacterial agent

1. The drug of choice is usually the most active drug against the pathogen or the least toxic of several alternative drugs.
2. An antibacterial agent is often used prophylactically against single microorganisms (e.g., to prevent endocarditis in patients undergoing procedures that lead to bacteremia, such as dental work).
3. The choice of drug depends on the effectiveness of host defense mechanisms in controlling the infection. The drug selected for use may be either a **bactericidal** agent (causing the death of the microorganism) or **bacteriostatic** agent (temporarily inhibiting the growth of the microorganism).
4. Drug choice is related to the mechanism of drug action in one of the following general categories:
   a. Inhibits bacterial cell wall biosynthesis
   b. Inhibits bacterial protein synthesis
   c. Inhibits bacterial metabolism
   d. Inhibits bacterial nucleic acid synthesis

B. Host determinants include history of drug reactions; site of infection; renal, hepatic, and immune status; age; pregnancy and lactation; metabolic abnormalities; pharmacokinetic factors; preexisting organ dysfunction; and genetic factors.

C. Bacterial determinants include **intrinsic resistance,** escape from antibiotic effect, and **acquired resistance,** which can occur as a result of the following:

1. ***Spontaneous, random chromosomal mutations,*** which occur at a frequency of 10^{-12} to 10^{-5}. These mutations are commonly due to a change in either a structural protein receptor for an antibiotic or a protein involved in drug transport.
2. Extrachromosomal transfer of drug-resistant genes
   a. **Transformation** is transfer of naked DNA between cells of the same species.
   b. **Transduction via R plasmids** is asexual transfer of plasmid DNA in a bacterial virus between bacteria of same species.
   c. **Conjugation** is the passage of genes from bacteria to bacteria via direct contact through a sex pilus or bridge. Conjugation occurs primarily in gram-negative bacilli, and it is the principal mechanism of acquired resistance among enterobacteria.
   d. **Transpositions** occur as a result of movement or "jumping" of **transposons** (stretches of DNA containing insertion sequences at each end) from plasmid to plasmid or from plasmid to chromosome and back; this process is independent of bacterial recombination.

II. ANTIBACTERIALS

A. Inhibitors of bacterial cell wall biosynthesis

1. *Penicillins*

a. Structure and mechanism of action

(1) Penicillins are analogues of alanine dipeptide (Fig. 11-1).

(2) Penicillins consist of a thiazolidine ring attached to a **β-lactam ring.** Integrity of the β-lactam ring is required for antibacterial activity. Modifications of the R-group side-chain (attached to the β-lactam ring) alter the pharmacologic properties and resistance to β-lactamase.

(3) Penicillins **inactivate bacterial transpeptidases** and prevent the cross-linking of peptidoglycan polymers that is essential for bacterial cell wall integrity. This results in **loss of rigidity and a susceptibility to rupture.** Penicillins also bind to, and **inactivate, penicillin-binding proteins (PBPs)** involved in cell wall synthesis. Autolysin's action in the presence of penicillin further weakens the cell wall.

(4) Penicillins are **bactericidal** for growing cells. **Gram-positive bacteria** with thick external cell walls are particularly susceptible.

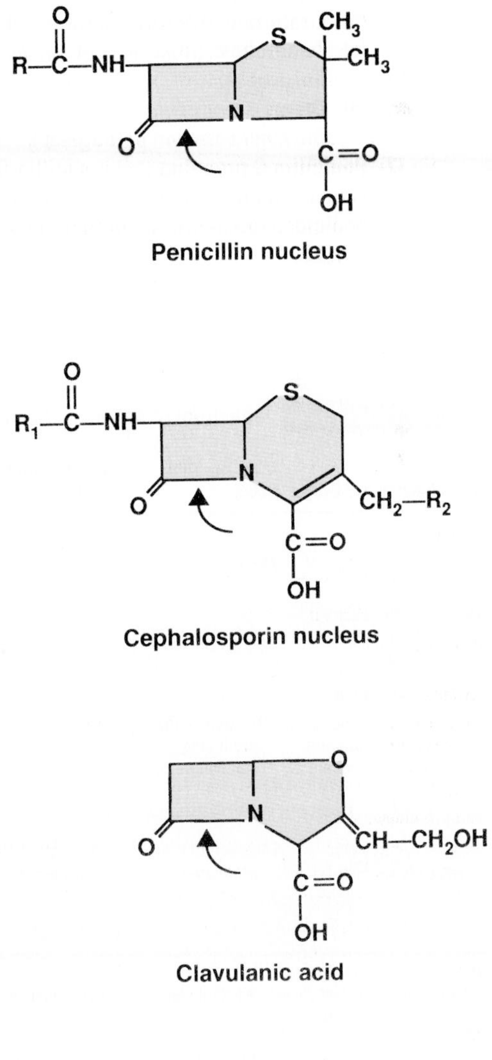

Penicillin nucleus

Cephalosporin nucleus

Clavulanic acid

FIGURE 11-1. Structures of penicillin, cephalosporin, and clavulanic acid nuclei. *Arrows* indicate bond attacked by β-lactamases.

(5) The major cause of **resistance** is the production of **β-lactamases (penicillinases).** The genes for β-lactamases can be transmitted during conjugation or as small plasmids (minus conjugation genes) via transduction. Common organisms capable of producing penicillinase include *Staphylococcus aureus, Escherichia coli, Pseudomonas aeruginosa, Neisseria gonorrhoeae,* and *Bacillus, Proteus,* and *Bacteroides* species.

(6) Resistance may also occur because bacteria lack receptors or other penicillin-binding proteins, are impermeable to penicillins, lack cell walls, or are metabolically inactive.

b. Pharmacologic properties

(1) Penicillins are absorbed rapidly after enteral administration, although erratically, and parenteral administration, and are distributed throughout body fluids; they penetrate the cerebrospinal fluid (CSF) and ocular fluid to a significant extent only during inflammation.

(2) Gastrointestinal (GI) absorption of penicillins may be decreased in the presence of food.

c. Selected drugs and their therapeutic uses (Table 11-1)

(1) **Penicillin G and penicillin V** are mainly used to treat infections with the following organisms (resistant strains of bacteria are being isolated more frequently):

(a) **Gram-positive cocci** (aerobic): Pneumococci, streptococci (except *S. faecalis*), and non-penicillinase-producing staphylococci

(b) **Gram-positive rods** (aerobic): *Bacillus* species, also *Clostridium perfringens, C. diphtheriae,* and *Listeria* spp., although the use of these agents is declining due to availability of better drugs.

(c) **Gram-negative aerobes:** Gonococci (non-penicillinase-producing) and meningococci

(d) Gram-negative rods (aerobic): None

(e) **Anaerobes:** Most, except *Bacteroides fragilis.* These agents are used against oral anaerobes.

(f) **Other:** *Treponema pallidum* (syphilis) and *Leptospira* spp. This group represents the **most common pathogens** for which first-generation penicillins are used today.

(2) **Penicillin G procaine** and **penicillin G benzathine** (Bicillin) are suspensions of penicillin G that prolong its half-life (30 min) allowing a reduced the frequency of injections. **Probenicid**, a uricosuric agent that blocks renal secretion of penicillin, is used rarely for this purpose.

table 11-1 Spectrum of Activity of Penicillins

Classification and Drugs	Gram-positive Cocci	Gram-positive Rods	Gram-negative Cocci	Gram-negative Rods	Anaerobes
Prototype					
Penicillin G, penicillin V	**Most**	*Bacillus*	Gonococci and meningococci[a]	None	Most (except *B. fragilis*)
Penicillinase resistant					
Nafcillin, oxacillin, dicloxacillin	**Staphylococci**[b]	—	—	—	—
Extended spectrum					
Ampicillin, amoxicillin, ampicillin/sulbactam, amoxicillin/clavulanic acid	Most penicillinase-producing staphylococci[b]	*Bacillus*	Gonococci and meningococci[c]	***Salmonella, H. influenzae, Proteus,*** and ***enterococci***	—
Antipseudomonal					
Ticarcillin/clavulanic acid, piperacillin	Less potent than prototypes	Less potent than prototypes	Less potent than prototypes	*Proteus, E. coli, Salmonella, Pseudomonas, Enterobacter,* and *Klebsiella*	—

[a]Non-penicillinase-producing.
[b]Not effective against methicillin-resistant staphylococcal infections.
[c]Penicillinase producing.

(3) **Penicillinase-resistant penicillins** (**oxacillin**, **dicloxacillin**, and **nafcillin**) are used predominantly for penicillinase-producing **staphylococcal infections.** The use of these agents, which are administered orally, is declining due to the increased incidence of so-called **methicillin-resistant *Staphylococcus aureus* (MRSA)** that also confers resistance to cephalosporins.

(4) **Extended-spectrum penicillins**

(a) Extended-spectrum penicillins are inactivated by β-lactamases.

(b) These agents have a broadened **gram-negative** coverage. Resistance has become a more common problem.

(i) **Ampicillin.** Ampicillin is useful for infections caused by *Haemophilus influenzae, Streptococcus pneumonia, Streptococcus pyrogenes, Neisseria meningitides, Proteus mirabilis,* and *Enterococcus faecalis.*

(ii) **Amoxicillin** (Amoxil) is similar to **ampicillin,** but it has **better oral absorption.** Amoxicillin is commonly used for endocarditis prophylaxis before major procedures.

(iii) **Piperacillin** has good activity against *Pseudomonas* spp. and *Enterobacter* spp.

(5) **Clavulanic acid**

(a) Clavulanic acid is structurally related to **penicillin** (see Figure 11-1), but it has **no antimicrobial properties** of its own.

(b) Clavulanic acid **irreversibly inhibits β-lactamase;** when administered with penicillins, clavulanic acid exposes penicillinase-producing organisms to therapeutic concentrations of penicillin.

(c) Clavulanic acid is used in combination products **amoxicillin/clavulanic acid** (Augmentin) and **ticarcillin/clavulanic acid** (Timentin) for oral and parenteral administration, respectively.

(6) **Sulbactam, tazobactam**

(a) These agents are **β-lactamase inhibitors** structurally related to **penicillin.**

(b) Sulbactam is marketed in the combination product **ampicillin/sulbactam** (Unasyn). **Tazobactam** is used in combination with **piperacillin** under the name **Zosyn.**

(c) **Ampicillin/sulbactam** is used parenterally and provides coverage similar to that provided by amoxicillin/clavulanic acid. It is most commonly used for **gram-negative** bacteria as well as most **anaerobes. Piperacillin/tazobactam** is effective against most **gram-negative** organisms, including ***Pseudomonas*** spp.

d. **Adverse effects**

(1) Penicillins cause **hypersensitivity** reactions in nearly 10% of patients. All types of reactions, from a simple rash to anaphylaxis, can be observed within 2 minutes or up to 3 days following administration.

(2) Other adverse effects result from direct irritation or pain on injection, GI upset, or superinfection.

e. **Endocarditis prophylaxis**

(1) Endocarditis prophylaxis is indicated for patients with **prosthetic heart valves;** those who have **previously been diagnosed with endocarditis;** patients **born with cyanotic heart disease;** and **patients with surgically constructed systemic pulmonary shunts.** Patients with intermediate risk for endocarditis are those who were born with other congenital cardiac abnormalities; those with acquired valvular dysfunction; and patients with hypertrophic cardiomyopathy.

(2) Endocarditis prophylaxis is recommended for the above patients who are planning to undergo **major dental procedures; procedures involving the respiratory tract,** such as bronchoscopy and tonsillectomy; and **operations and procedures involving the GI and genitourinary tracts.**

(3) Agents most commonly used for endocarditis prophylaxis are **amoxicillin or ampicillin.** Those who are allergic to penicillins can take **clindamycin or azithromycin**

2. ***Cephalosporins*** (Table 11-2)

a. **Structure and mechanism of action**

(1) Cephalosporins consist of a 7-aminocephalosporanic acid nucleus and a β-lactam ring linked to a dihydrothiazine ring (see Fig. 11-1). Substitutions at R_1 determine antibacterial activity. Substitutions at R_2 determine pharmacokinetics.

(2) Cephalosporins have the same mechanisms of action as penicillins.

table 11-2 Properties of Cephalosporins

Drugs and Route of Administration[a]	Spectrum of Activity	Enters CNS	Resistance to β-Lactamase	
			Plasmid	*Chromosomal*
First generation				
Cephalexin (O) Cefadroxil (O) Cefazolin (P)	Gram-positive and some gram-negative organisms Use: ***E. coli, Klebsiella, Proteus mirabilis,*** penicillin- and sulfonamide-resistant **UTI, surgical prophylaxis**	No	Yes	No
Second generation				
Cefaclor (O) Cefotetan (P) Cefoxitin (P) Cefuroxime (P,O)	Spectrum extends to indole-positive ***Proteus,*** and **anaerobes** Use: **UTI, respiratory tract infections, surgical prophylaxis**	No	Yes	Relatively
Third and fourth generation				
Ceftizoxime (P) Cefotaxime (P) Ceftriaxone (P) Cefdinir (P) Ceftazidime (P) Cefixime (O) Cefoperazone (P) Cefepime (P)	Reduced gram-positive activity; ***Pseudomonas*** (cefoperazone and ceftazidime only), *N. gonorrhoeae, N. meningitidis, H. influenza, Enterobacter, Salmonella,* indole-positive *Proteus, Serratia, E. coli;* moderate **anaerobe** activity Use: Serious **nosocomial infections, gonorrhea, meningitis**	Yes, especially ceftriaxone (but not cefoperazone)	Yes	Relatively (most)
Other agents				
Aztreonam	**Gram-negative** organisms (no cross-sensitivity)	Yes	Yes	Yes
Imipenem/cilastatin	Use: **Broad-spectrum**			

[a]O, oral administration; P, parenteral administration.

b. Pharmacologic properties

(1) Cephalosporins are widely distributed in body fluids; selected agents (**cefuroxime** [Ceftin, Zinacef], **cefotaxime** [Claforan], and **ceftizoxime** [Cefizox]) penetrate CSF.

(2) Probenecid slows secretion of cephalosporins.

(3) Each newer generation of cephalosporins is increasingly **resistant to penicillinases.** Third-generation cephalosporins are sensitive to another class of β-lactamase, the **cephalosporinases** (genes are generally located on chromosomes as opposed to plasmids).

c. Selected drugs and their therapeutic uses. Cephalosporins are categorized by their antibacterial spectrum. All are inactive against enterococci and methicillin-resistant staphylococci.

(1) First-generation cephalosporins

(a) First-generation cephalosporins include **cephalexin** (Keflex), **cefazolin** (Ancef, Kefzol), and **cefadroxil** (Duricef).

(b) These agents have good activity against **some gram-positive organisms** (streptococci) **and some gram-negative** organisms. First-generation cephalosporins are used mainly for ***E. coli, Klebsiella*** infections, and penicillin- and sulfonamide-resistant **urinary tract infections.** They are also used **prophylactically in various surgical procedures.**

(c) These agents **do not penetrate CSF.**

(2) Second-generation cephalosporins

(a) Second-generation cephalosporins include **cefoxitin** (Mefoxin), **cefaclor** (Ceclor), **cefuroxime** (Zinacef, Ceftin), **cefotetan** (Cefotan), **and cefprozil** (Cefzil).

(b) These agents have a somewhat broader spectrum of activity than first-generation drugs. They are used in treatment of **streptococcal** infections as well as infections caused by ***E. coli, Klebsiella,*** and ***Proteus*** **spp.** Most **anaerobes** (with exception of *C. difficile*) are covered as well.

(c) Second-generation cephalosporins are used primarily in the management of **urinary and respiratory tract, bone, and soft-tissue infections** and prophylactically in various **surgical procedures.**

(d) Second-generation agents have, to a great extent, been supplanted by third-generation agents.

(e) With the exception of cefuroxime, these agents do not penetrate CSF.

(3) **Third-generation cephalosporins**

(a) Third-generation cephalosporins include **cefdinir** (Omnicef), **cefixime** (Suprax), **cefotaxime** (Clarofan), **ceftizoxime** (Cefizox), **ceftazidime** (Fortaz, Tazicef), **ceftriaxone** (Rocephin), and **cefoperazone** (Cefobid).

(b) These agents have **enhanced activity against gram-negative** organisms. They demonstrate high potency against *Haemophilus influenzae,* ***N. gonorrhoeae, N. meningitides, Enterobacter, Salmonella,*** **indole-positive** ***Proteus, and Serratia*** spp., **and** ***E. coli;*** and **moderate activity against anaerobes. Cefoperazone** and **ceftazidime** have excellent activity against ***P. aeruginosa.*** **Ceftriaxone** is used for sexually transmitted infections caused by ***gonorrhea***, as well as in empiric therapy for community-acquired **meningitis.**

(c) With the exception of cefoperazone, third-generation cephalosporins **penetrate the CSF.**

(d) These agents are excreted by the kidney, except **cefoperazone** and **ceftriaxone,** which are excreted through the biliary tract, thus enabling the use of these agents for **infections of the biliary tree.**

(e) Third-generation cephalosporins are used to treat gonorrhea, Lyme disease, meningitis, and serious **hospital-acquired gram-negative infections,** alone or in combination with an aminoglycoside.

(4) **Fourth-generation cephalosporins. Cefepime** (Maxipime) has a powerful coverage against ***Pseudomonas*** spp., as well as other **gram-negative** bacteria.

d. **Adverse effects and drug interactions**

(1) Cephalosporins most commonly cause **hypersensitivity reactions** (2%–5%); 5%–10% of penicillin-sensitive persons are also hypersensitive to cephalosporins.

(2) Alcohol intolerance **(disulfiram-like)** is seen with **cefamandole and ceftriaxone.**

(3) Cephalosporins may cause **bleeding disorders;** these disorders can be prevented by vitamin K administration.

(4) Cephalosporins may be **nephrotoxic** when administered with diuretics.

(5) These agents may cause **superinfection with gram-positive organisms or fungi.** Cephalosporins are the number one cause of **hospital-acquired** ***C. difficile*** **colitis,** a potentially life-threatening infection.

3. ***Other Beta-lactam drugs***

a. **Aztreonam (Azactam)**

(1) Aztreonam is a naturally occurring monobactam lacking the thiazolidine ring that is **highly resistant to β-lactamases.**

(2) Aztreonam has **good activity against gram-negative** organisms, but it lacks activity against anaerobes and gram-positive organisms.

(3) This agent demonstrates **no cross-reactivity with penicillins or cephalosporins** for hypersensitivity reactions.

(4) Aztreonam is administered parenterally.

(5) Aztreonam is useful for various types of infections caused by ***E. coli, Klebsiella pneumoniae, H. influenzae, P. aeruginosa, Enterobacter*** spp., ***Citrobacter*** spp., and ***Proteus mirabilis.***

b. **Carbapenems (imipenem-cilastatin** [Primaxin], **ertapenem** [Invanz], **meropenem** [Merrem IV], **aztreonam** [Azactam])

(1) Carbapenems are derivatives of thienamycin that have a **broad spectrum** of antibacterial activity.

(2) Imipenem is marketed in the combination product **imipenem/cilastatin** (Primaxin); **cilastatin** is an inhibitor of renal dehydropeptidase I (which inactivates imipenem).

(3) Carbapenems are relatively **resistant to β-lactamases.**

(4) Carbapenems demonstrate **no cross-resistance** with other antibiotics.

(5) These agents are useful for infections caused by ***penicillinase-producing S. aureus, E. coli, Klebsiella*** spp., ***Enterobacter*** spp., and ***H. influenzae,*** among others. They are powerful agents used for ***Pseudomonas*** infections.

(6) Nausea, vomiting, diarrhea, and skin rashes, and at higer doses, seizures, are their most common adverse effects, particularly for **imipenem**.

4. *Other inhibitors of bacterial cell wall biosynthesis*

a. Vancomycin (Vancocin, Vancoled)

(1) Vancomycin is a tricyclic glycopeptide that **binds to the terminal end of growing peptidoglycan to prevent further elongation and cross-linking;** this results in decreased cell membrane activity and increased cell lysis.

(2) Vancomycin is active against **gram-positive organisms;** resistant strains have been reported.

(3) Vancomycin is synergistic with aminoglycosides, but it is ototoxic and nephrotoxic.

(4) Vancomycin is not absorbed from GI tract. It is administered intravenously (IV).

(5) This agent is used in **serious MRSA infections,** in patients allergic to penicillins and cephalosporins, and to treat **antibiotic-associated enterocolitis** (*C. difficile* colitis).

(6) Vancomycin penetrates CSF only during inflammation.

(7) Vancomycin is administered by slow IV infusion, except in the treatment of enterocolitis, when it is given orally. Rapid infusion may cause anaphylactoid reactions and "**red neck" syndrome** (flushing caused by release of histamine).

(8) Vancomycin demonstrates **no cross-resistance** with other antibiotics.

(9) High levels of vancomycin may cause **ototoxicity** with permanent auditory impairment.

b. Bacitracin

(1) Bacitracin inhibits dephosphorylation and reuse of the phospholipid required for acceptance of *N*-acetylmuramic acid pentapeptide, the building block of the peptidoglycan complex.

(2) Bacitracin is most active against **gram-positive** bacteria.

(3) Bacitracin is **used only topically** in combination with **neomycin or polymyxin** for minor infections (Neosporin).

c. Cycloserine (Seromycin)

(1) Cycloserine is an amino acid analogue that inhibits alanine racemase and the incorporation of alanine into the peptidoglycan pentapeptide.

(2) Cycloserine is active against **mycobacteria and gram-negative bacteria.**

(3) This agent is used only as a second-line drug for treatment of urinary tract infection and tuberculosis (TB).

(4) Cycloserine may cause severe central nervous system (CNS) toxicity, including seizures and acute psychosis.

d. Daptomycin (Cubicin)

(1) Daptomycin is a bactericidal agent that binds to and depolarizes the cell membrane resulting in loss of membrane potential and rapid cell death.

(2) Daptomycin has antibacterial actions similar to vancomycin.

(3) It is active against vancomycin-resistant strains.

e. Fosfomycin (Monural)

(1) Fosfomycin inhibits the enzyme **enolpyruvate transferase** and therby interferes downstream with the formation of bacterial cell wall specific N-acetylmuramic acid.

(2) This oral agent is active against both gram-positive and gram-negative organisms. It is used to treat simple lower **urinary tract infection.**

B. Inhibitors of bacterial protein synthesis

1. *Aminoglycosides* (Fig. 11-2)

a. Structure and mechanism of action

(1) Aminoglycosides are amino sugars in glycosidic linkage to a hexoseaminocyclitol.

(2) Aminoglycosides **inhibit bacterial protein synthesis;** they are **bacteriocidal** against most **gram-negative aerobic bacteria.**

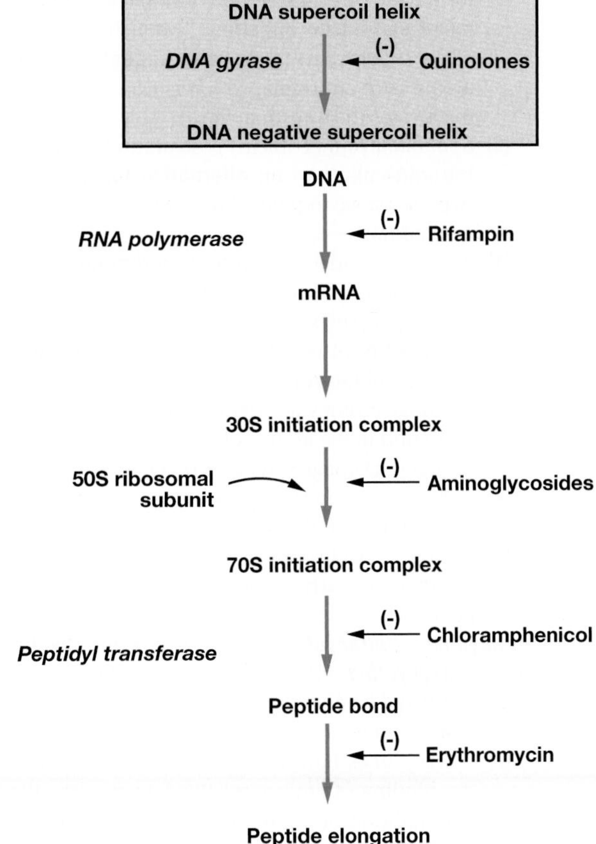

FIGURE 11-2. Antimicrobial action on bacterial nucleic acid and protein synthesis.

(3) Aminoglycosides are polycations that initially passively diffuse via **porin channels** through the outer membrane of gram-negative aerobes bacteria. Transport across the inner membrane requires active uptake that is dependent on electron transport (**gram-negative aerobes only**), the so-called **energy dependent phase I transport.**

(4) Inside the cell, these agents interact with receptor proteins on the **30S ribosomal subunit.** This "freezes" the initiation complex and leads to a buildup of monosomes; it also causes translation errors.

(5) Resistance generally results from bacterial enzymes that inactivate the drugs. The resistance contained on plasmids is transmitted by conjugation.

b. Pharmacologic properties. These agents do not penetrate CSF.

c. Selected drugs and their therapeutic uses

(1) The role for aminoglycosides has decreased substantially due to their **narrow spectrum of activity and toxicity**, and the availability of other agents.

(2) **Streptomycin** is currently used only for **plague** *(Yersinia pestis),* for **severe cases of brucellosis,** and as an adjunct to the treatment of recalcitrant **mycobacterial infections.**

(3) **Gentamicin** (Garamycin), **tobramycin** (Nebcin)

(a) Gentamicin and tobramycin are active against ***Enterobacter,* indole-positive *Proteus, Pseudomonas, Klebsiella,* and *Serratia*** spp., among other gram-negative organisms.

(b) These agents are **often used in combination with β-lactam antibiotics** for serious infections that require broad coverage.

(4) **Amikacin** (Amikin) is used in the treatment of **severe gram-negative infections,** especially those resistant to gentamicin or tobramycin.

(5) **Neomycin** (Mycifradin) **and kanamycin** (Kantrex, Klebcil) are **administered topically for minor soft-tissue infections** (often in combination with **bacitracin** and **polymyxin**) or orally (neomycin) for **hepatic encephalopathy** (GI bacteria by-products result in large amounts of ammonia, which is normally cleared by liver; use of neomycin temporarily inactivates the intestinal flora).

(6) **Spectinomycin** (Tobicin) is structurally related to aminoglycosides and is administered intramuscularly as an **alternative for the treatment of acute gonorrhea** or in patients hypersensitive to penicillin or for gonococci resistant to penicillin.

d. Adverse effects

(1) Aminoglycosides have a **narrow therapeutic index;** it may be necessary to monitor serum concentrations and individualize the dose.

(2) Aminoglycosides are **ototoxic,** affecting either vestibular (**streptomycin, gentamicin,** and **tobramycin**) or cochlear auditory (**neomycin, kanamycin, amikacin** [Amikin], **gentamicin,** and **tobramycin**) function.

(3) Aminoglycosides are **nephrotoxic;** they produce acute tubular necrosis that leads to a reduction in the glomerular filtration rate and a rise in serum creatinine and blood urea nitrogen. Damage is usually reversible.

(4) At high doses, these agents produce a curare-like neuromuscular blockade with respiratory paralysis. Calcium gluconate and neostigmine are antidotes.

(5) Aminoglycosides rarely cause hypersensitivity reactions, except **spectinomycin** and **neomycin,** which, when applied topically, can cause contact dermatitis in as many as 8% of patients.

2. *Tetracyclines (tetracycline* *[Sumycin]*, oxytetracycline *[Terramycin]*, *demeclocycline* *[Declomycin]*, *doxycycline* *[Vibramycin]*, *minocycline* *[Minocin]*, *tigecycline* *[Tygacil])*

a. Structure and mechanism of action

(1) Tetracyclines are derivatives of naphthacene carboxamide.

(2) Tetracyclines bind reversibly to the **30S subunit** of bacterial ribosomes. This prevents the binding of aminoacyl tRNA to the acceptor site on the mRNA-ribosome complex and addition of amino acids to the growing peptide, thus **inhibiting bacterial protein synthesis;** these agents are **bacteriostatic.**

(3) Resistance is plasmid-mediated and results primarily from a decreased ability to accumulate in the bacteria and from the production of an inhibitor of the binding site for tetracyclines. Resistance to one tetracycline confers resistance to some, but not all, congeners.

b. Pharmacologic properties

(1) Tetracyclines are variably, but adequately, absorbed from the GI tract; they can also be administered parenterally; **tigecycline,** an exception, is only administered IV. Absorption is impaired by stomach contents, especially milk and antacids.

(2) Tetracyclines are distributed throughout body fluids; therapeutic concentrations in the brain and CSF can be achieved with minocycline.

(3) The primary route of elimination for most tetracyclines is the kidney.

(4) Many tetracyclines undergo **enterohepatic recirculation. Doxycycline** is excreted almost entirely via bile into the feces and hence is the **safest tetracycline** to administer to individuals **with impaired renal function.**

c. Spectrum and therapeutic uses

(1) Tetracyclines are active against **both gram-negative and gram-positive organisms,** but the use of these agents is declining because of increased resistance and the development of safer drugs.

(2) Tetracyclines are used predominantly for the treatment of **rickettsial infections,** including Rocky Mountain spotted fever, **cholera, Lyme disease, and infections caused by *Chlamydia* spp. and *Mycoplasma pneumoniae.*** These agents may be useful for the treatment of **inflammatory acne vulgaris.** They are also used in combination regimens for elimination of infections caused by ***Helicobacter pylori.***

(3) **Demeclocycline** is used in refractory cases of **"syndrome of inappropriate secretion of antidiuretic hormone" (SIADH).** It interferes with action of ADH at the renal collecting duct by impairing generation and action of cyclic AMP.

(4) **Tigecycline**, a derivative of minocycline, has a broad spectrum of activity and has activity against many tetracycline-resistant organisms.

d. **Adverse effects**

(1) Tetracyclines produce GI upset, including nausea, vomiting, and diarrhea.

(2) At high doses, tetracyclines can cause **hepatic damage,** particularly in pregnant women.

(3) When exposed to strong ultraviolet light, as in sunlight, these agents, **demeclocycline** in particular, can cause **dermatologic reactions.**

(4) Tetracyclines can complex with calcium in bone. Children age 6 months to 5 years receiving tetracycline therapy can develop **tooth discolorations.** These agents can also **retard bone growth in neonates.**

(5) Tetracyclines can cause superinfection by resistant staphylococci or clostridia as a result of altered GI ecology; this condition can be life threatening.

3. ***Chloramphenicol***

a. **Structure and mechanism of action** (see Fig. 11-2)

(1) Chloramphenicol contains a nitrobenzene moiety and is a derivative of dichloroacetic acid.

(2) Chloramphenicol **inhibits bacterial protein synthesis.**

(3) This agent binds to the bacterial **50S ribosomal subunit** to block the action of peptidyl transferase and thus prevents amino acid incorporation into newly formed peptides. High concentrations inhibit eukaryote mitochondrial protein synthesis.

(4) Resistance results from the production of a plasmid-encoded **acetyltransferase** capable of inactivating the drug.

b. **Pharmacologic properties**

(1) Chloramphenicol is absorbed rapidly and distributed throughout body fluids.

(2) Therapeutic levels can be obtained in the CSF.

(3) An inactive pro-drug, **chloramphenicol succinate**, is used for parenteral administration. On absorption it is hydrolyzed by plasma esterases.

(4) Chloramphenicol inhibits cytochrome P-450 isozymes (CYP).

c. **Therapeutic uses**

(1) Chloramphenicol is a **broad-spectrum antibiotic** used to treat most **gram-negative organisms,** many **anaerobes, clostridia, chlamydia, mycoplasma, and rickettsia.** However, because of the potential for **severe and sometimes fatal adverse effects,** use of this agent is limited to the treatment of infections that cannot be treated with other drugs; these infections include **typhoid fever** (although resistance is increasingly a problem), **meningitis** due to *H. influenzae* in patients allergic to penicillins and the newer cephalosporins, and some instances of infections caused by **ampicillin-resistant strains.**

(2) Chloramphenicol may also be used for the treatment of certain **anaerobic infections of the brain** (especially *B. fragilis*) in combination with **penicillin,** and as an alternative to **tetracycline** in the treatment of **rickettsial** disease.

d. **Adverse effects**

(1) Chloramphenicol causes dose-related **bone marrow suppression,** resulting in pancytopenia that may lead to **irreversible aplastic anemia.** This effect has low incidence (1:30,000) but a **high mortality rate.** Also, chloramphenicol causes **hemolytic anemia** in patients with low levels of **glucose 6-phosphate dehydrogenase.**

(2) Chloramphenicol causes **reticulocytopenia,** perhaps as a result of the inhibition of mitochondrial protein synthesis.

(3) Neonates given large doses of chloramphenicol develop **gray baby syndrome.** This syndrome results from the inadequacy of both cytochrome P-450 and glucuronic acid conjugation systems to detoxify the drug. Elevated plasma chloramphenicol levels cause a shocklike syndrome and a reduction in peripheral circulation; the incidence of fatalities is high (40%).

(4) Chloramphenicol inhibition of cytochrome P-450 isozymes can result in elevated and toxic levels of other drugs.

4. ***Erythromycin, clarithromycin*** *(Biaxin),* ***azithromycin*** *(Zithromax),* ***telithromycin*** *(Ketek)*

a. **Structure and mechanism of action** (see Fig. 11-2)

(1) Erythromycin is a **macrolide** antibiotic composed of a multimembered lactone ring attached to deoxysugars.
(2) Erythromycin **inhibits protein synthesis** by binding irreversibly to the bacterial **50S ribosomal subunit.** It inhibits aminoacyl translocation and the formation of initiation complexes. It is usually bacteriostatic, but at higher concentrations can be bactericidal.
(3) Resistance is plasmid-encoded and is prevalent in most strains of staphylococci and, to some extent, in streptococci. It is due primarily to increased **active efflux** or **ribosomal protection** by increased methylase production.

b. **Pharmacologic properties**
(1) Erythromycin is inactivated by stomach acid and is therefore administered as an **enteric-coated tablet.**
(2) Erythromycin **distributes** into all **body fluids** except the brain and CSF.

c. **Therapeutic use**
(1) Erythromycin is active against **gram-positive organisms.**
(2) This agent is useful as a penicillin substitute in **penicillin-hypersensitive patients.**
(3) Erythromycin is the most effective drug for **Legionnaires disease** *(Legionella pneumophila)*; it is also useful for the treatment of **syphilis, *Mycoplasma pneumoniae,* corynebacterial infections (e.g., diphtheria), and *Bordetella pertussis* disease (whooping cough).** Azithromycin is commonly used for **community-acquired "walking" pneumonia and sinusitis.**
(4) Clarithromycin or azithromycin are effective in the multidrug-regimen treatment of disseminated ***Mycobacterium* avium-intracellulare complex infections in AIDS patients.**

d. **Adverse effects**
(1) Erythromycin and other macrolides cause GI dysfunction (clarithromycin less so) but rarely produce serious adverse effects; the oral form of erythromycin may cause **allergic cholestatic hepatitis,** which is readily reversible by cessation of the drug.
(2) Erythromycin has a high incidence of **thrombophlebitis** when administered IV.
(3) Erythromycin inhibits hepatic **cytochrome P-450–mediated metabolism** of **warfarin, phenytoin,** and others, possibly leading to toxic accumulation.

5. ***Clindamycin*** *(Cleocin)*
a. Clindamycin acts like erythromycin.
b. Clindamycin can be administered orally and is well distributed throughout body fluids, except for the CNS.
c. Use of clindamycin is limited to alternative therapy for abscesses associated with infections caused by anaerobes, such as *B. fragilis.* It is used in dental patients with valvular heart disease for **prophylaxis of endocarditis.** Topical preparations of the drug are used for treatment of acne.
d. Clindamycin produces **diarrhea,** which is observed in up to 20% of individuals. Potential severe **pseudomembranous colitis** occurs as a result of superinfection by resistant clostridia.

C. Inhibitors of bacterial metabolism

1. ***Sulfonamides: sulfadoxine/pyrimethamine*** *(Fansidar)*, ***sulfisoxazole, sulfadiazine, silver sulfadiazine*** *(Silvadene)*, ***sulfasalazine*** *(Azaline, Azulfidine)*, ***trimethoprim*** *(Proloprim)*, ***and trimethoprim/sulfamethoxazole*** *(Bactrim, Septra)*
a. **Structure and mechanism of action** (Fig. 11-3)
(1) Sulfonamides are structural analogues of *para*-aminobenzoic acid (PABA).
(2) They prevent the synthesis of **dihydrofolic acid,** which, following its reduction to tetrahydrofolic acid by dihydrofolate reductase, is essential for the production of nucleic acid (purines and pyrimidines) and amino acids, and thus bacterial growth. Sulfonamides are **bacteriostatic.**

b. **Pharmacologic properties.** Most sulfonamides are well absorbed from the GI tract and readily penetrate CSF.

c. **Spectrum and therapeutic uses**
(1) Sulfonamides inhibit both **gram-negative and gram-positive** organisms. They are used to treat **urinary tract infections (*E. coli*), nocardiosis (*Actinomyces* spp.),** and **toxoplasmosis** and as bacterial prophylaxis for **recurrent otitis media.** Their use has diminished due to development of resistant strains.

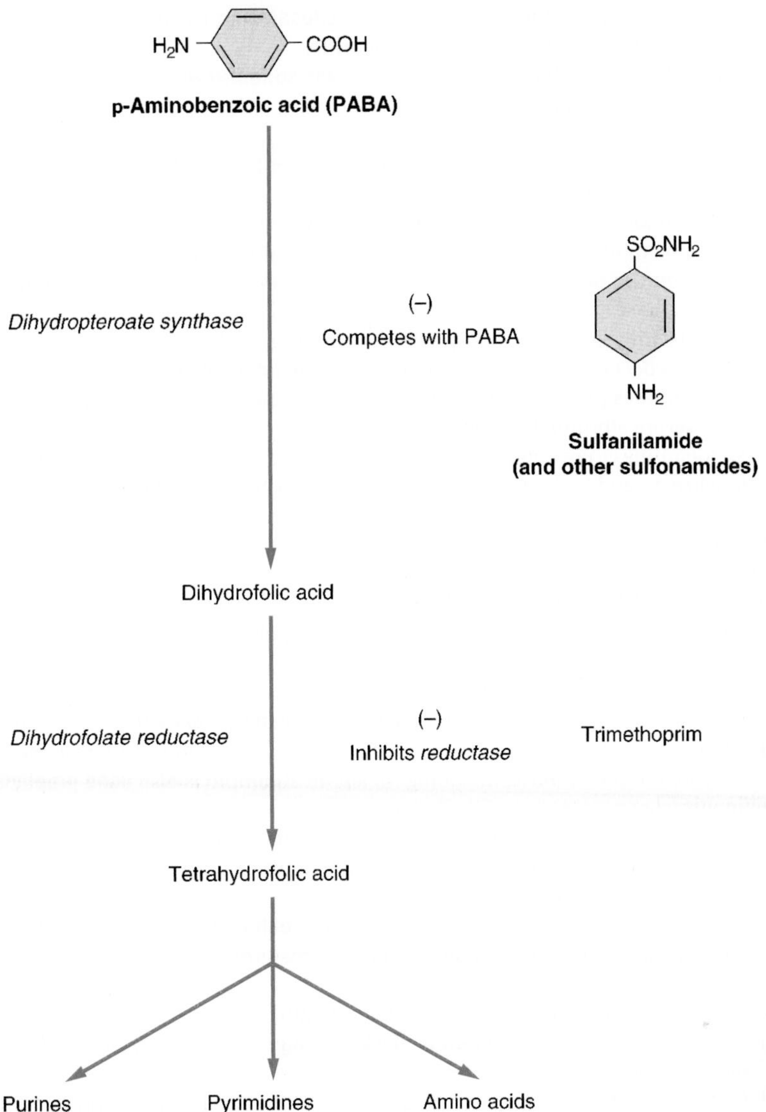

FIGURE 11-3. Sulfonamides and trimethoprim inhibition of tetrahydrofolic acid synthesis.

(2) However, because **sulfamethoxazole,** a competitive inhibitor of the activity of bacterial dihydropteroate synthase, and **trimethoprim,** a competitive inhibitor of microbial dihydrofolate reductase, inhibit two different enzymes of the same metabolic pathway, their actions are **synergistic,** and they are used as a combination product (Bactrim, Septra).

(3) This combination agent is used to treat **uncomplicated urinary tract infections,** especially those associated with the use of indwelling catheters; bacterial **prostatitis; GI infections (particularly shigellosis); and traveler's diarrhea.**

(4) Bactrim is also used for **prophylaxis of PCP** (*Pneumocystis jirovecii,* formerly known as *Pneumocystis carinii* pneumonia) in patients with HIV/AIDS, and in patients who are on immune-suppressive therapy. It is also used for actual **treatment of PCP** at higher doses.

(5) Long-acting sulfonamides include **sulfadoxine,** which is marketed in the combination **sulfadoxine/pyrimethamine** (Fansidar). Pyrimethamine is an inhibitor of parasitic dihydrofolate reductase. The combination is used in the **treatment of malaria** caused by chloroquine-resistant *Plasmodium falciparum.*

(6) **Poorly absorbed sulfonamides** such as **sulfasalazine** (Azaline, Azulfidine) are used to treat **ulcerative colitis** and **regional enteritis.**

(7) **Topically used sulfonamides** such as **silver sulfadiazine** (Silvadene) are used for the treatment of **wound and burn infections.**

d. **Adverse effects**

(1) Sulfonamides produce **hypersensitivity** reactions (rashes, fever, eosinophilia) in approximately 3% of individuals receiving oral doses.

(2) Sulfonamides rarely cause **Stevens-Johnson syndrome,** an infrequent but fatal form of erythema multiforme associated with lesions of skin and mucous membranes.

(3) Sulfonamides produce nausea and vomiting; also, they occasionally produce photosensitivity and serum sickness reactions.

(4) Patients with glucose-6-phosphate dehydrogenase deficiency are more susceptible to adverse effects (manifested primarily as **hemolytic aplastic anemia**).

(5) Sulfonamides produce **kernicterus** in neonates because of the displacement of bilirubin from serum albumin binding sites.

(6) Sulfonamides may potentiate the effects of other drugs, such as oral anticoagulants, sulfonylureas, and hydantoin anticonvulsants, possibly by displacement from albumin.

D. Inhibitors of bacterial nucleic acid synthesis

1. *Rifampin* (*Rifadin, Rimactane*)

a. Rifampin is an **RNA synthesis inhibitor.**

b. Rifampin inhibits bacterial DNA-dependent RNA polymerase by binding to the β- subunit of the polymerase (see Fig. 11-2).

c. It is widely distributed, including to CSF.

d. Rifampin is active against **most gram-positive organisms, *Neisseria* spp.,** and **mycobacteria,** including *M. tuberculosis.* It is used in combination with other drugs for the treatment of most **atypical mycobacteria,** including *M. leprae.* Rifampin is also **used prophylactically for meningitis** from meningococci or *H. influenzae.*

e. Resistance develops rapidly because of decreased affinity of RNA polymerase.

f. Adverse effects of rifampin include nausea and vomiting, dermatitis, and red-orange discoloration of feces, urine, tears, and sweat.

g. Rifampin induces liver microsomal enzymes and **enhances the metabolism of other drugs** such as anticoagulants, contraceptives, and corticosteroids.

2. *DNA-binding agents*

a. **Nitrofurantoin** (Furadantin, Macrobid, Macrodantin)

(1) Nitrofurantoin causes **bacterial DNA damage** by an unknown mechanism; it is **bacteriostatic.**

(2) **Nitrofurantoin** is concentrated in urine and is used solely as a **urinary tract antiseptic** against *E. coli.* Other urinary tract gram-negative bacteria are often resistant.

(3) Adverse effects of nitrofurantoin include nausea and vomiting, headache, hemolytic anemia in glucose-6-phosphatase deficient patients, and acute pneumonitis; this agent turns urine brown.

b. **Fluoroquinolones**

(1) These agents, **ciprofloxacin** (Cipro), **norfloxacin** (Noroxin), **ofloxacin** (Floxin), **levofloxacin** (Levaquin), **moxifloxacin** (Avelox), **lomefloxacin** (Maxaquin), and **gemifloxacin** (Factive), are fluorinated analogs of **nalidixic acid** (NegGram), which is now used infrequently.

(2) Fluoroquinolones inhibit bacterial **DNA gyrase (topoisomerase II),** and therefore, DNA supercooling in **gram-negative bacteria**. They also inhibit **topoisomerase IV** in **gram-positive organisms** and thereby interfere with separation of replicated chromosomal DNA.

(3) **Ciprofloxacin, ofloxacin, levofloxacin,** and **lomefloxacin** are highly active against gram-negative bacteria and moderately active against gram-positive bacteria. **Moxifloxacin** and **gemifloxacin** have even greater activity against gram-positive organisms.

(4) Quinolones are concentrated in urine; thus, they are used as a **urinary tract antiseptic.** These agents are useful against urinary tract infections and against infections caused by

N. gonorrhoeae or **methicillin-resistant staphylococci,** as well as for upper and lower respiratory tract infections resulting from infections with **mycoplasma**, **legionella**, and **chlamydia**, among others. **Ofloxacin** is used for **otitis media** in a topical (otic drop) form. **Ciprofloxacin** can be used against ***Bacillus anthracis.***

(5) Resistance is due to point mutations in the target enzyme or to changes in the organism's permeability to the drugs.

(6) Adverse effects include nausea and vomiting, GI pain, rashes, and fever. Cartilage toxicity has been reported, and thus these agents should not be used in children and young adults.

E. Polymyxins, Mupirocin (Bactroban)

1. Polymyxin is a cationic basic polypeptide that acts as a detergent to **disrupt the cell membrane** functions of **gram-negative** bacteria (bactericidal).
2. This agent is poorly absorbed and is poorly distributed to tissues.
3. Polymyxin has substantial **nephrotoxicity** and **neurotoxicity** and is therefore only for ophthalmic, otic, or topical use.
4. Polymyxin B often is applied as a topical ointment in mixture with bacitracin or neomycin, or both (Neosporin).
5. ***Mupirocin*** is a natural product produced by *Pseudomonas fluorescens.* It is used topically and prophylactically for ***S. aureus*** infections.

F. Metronidazole (Flagyl)

1. Metronidazole, a prodrug, is **bactericidal** against most **anaerobic bacteria**, as well as other organisms, including **anaerobic protozoal parasites.**
2. Its mechanism of action is unclear, but it has been proposed that an intermediate in the reduction of metronidazole, produced only in anaerobic bacteria and protozoa, is bound to DNA and electron-transport proteins, thus **inhibiting nucleic acid synthesis.**
3. This agent is used for many anaerobic infections (e.g., ***T. vaginalis, C. difficile*** **colitis**), alone, or as part of a multicoverage regimen.
4. Metronidazole has a **disulfiram-like effect;** therefore, alcohol should be avoided. Use of this agent should also be avoided in the **first trimester of pregnancy.**

G. Agents used against vancomycin-resistant organisms

1. ***Daptomycin*** *(Cubicin)* is a very powerful cyclic lipopeptide bactericidal agent that has a spectrum of activity similar to vancomycin. It is used to treat complicated infections caused by **MRSA, VRE** (vancomycin-resistant *enterococci*), **MRSE (*S. epidermidis*),** and ***Streptococcus pyogenes.*** It can cause myopathy.
2. ***Linezolid*** *(Zyvox)* is an oxazolidinone used to treat severe infections caused by **MRSA and VRE,** as well as **multidrug-resistant *S. pneumoniae.*** It has been successfully used for **Staphylococcus osteomyelitis.** Myelosuppression and pseudomembranous colitis can occur with the use of this agent.
3. ***Synercid*** is a combination product of two **streptogranins, quinupristin** and **dalfopristin,** that is administered IV to treat severe infections caused by **VRE, MRSA,** and **multidrug-resistant streptococci.** The streptogranins **bind the 50S ribosomal subunit** and are **bactericidal** for most organisms. They inhibit CYP 3A4. Adverse effects include pain at the infusion site and arthralgias and myalgias.

III. ANTIMYCOBACTERIAL AGENTS (TABLE 11-3)

A. First-line drugs used in the treatment of TB

1. *Isoniazid (INH)*

a. Structure and mechanism of action

(1) INH is an analogue of pyridoxine (vitamin B_6).

table 11-3 Major Uses of Antibacterial and Antifungal Drugs

Drug	Major Organisms	Alternative Drugs
Penicillin	All aerobic gram-positive cocci (except penicillinase-producing and methicillin-resistant staphylococci, penicillinase-producing gonococci, and *Streptococcus faecalis*); *Leptospira*; ***Treponema*** (syphilis, yaws); all gram-positive anaerobes (peptococci, peptostreptococci, clostridia) and gram-negative anaerobes (except *B. fragilis*)	Ampicillin or tetracycline, amoxicillin/clavulanic acid, ticarcillin/clavulanic acid, chloramphenicol, or erythromycin[a]
Penicillinase-resistant penicillins	Penicillinase-producing staphylococci	Vancomycin or cephalosporin
Vancomycin	Methicillin-resistant staphylococci	Daptomycin
Ampicillin	Penicillinase-producing staphylococci, *N meningitides, H influenzae*	Penicillin and aminoglycoside or vancomycin
Aminoglycosides	Coliforms (*E. coli, Klebsiella, Enterobacter, Serratia, Proteus*)	Third-generation cephalosporin, trimethoprim/ sulfamethoxazole, or extended-spectrum penicillin[a]
Aminoglycoside and extended-spectrum penicillin **(double coverage)**	*Pseudomonas aeruginosa*	Third-generation cephalosporin
Tetracycline	*Brucella, Campylobacter, Yersinia pestis* (plague), *Francisella tularensis* (tularemia), *Vibrio, Pseudomonas pseudomallei* and *mallei, Borrelia* (relapsing fever), *Mycoplasma pneumoniae,* chlamydiae, and rickettsiae	Streptomycin, erythromycin, chloramphenicol, or trimethoprim/ sulfamethoxazole
Chloramphenicol	*Salmonella, Haemophilus* spp.	Trimethoprim/sulfamethoxazole, ampicillin, or third-generation cephalosporin
Erythromycin	*Legionella* spp.	
Trimethoprim/ sulfamethoxazole	*E coli,* PCP	
Sulfonamides	*Nocardia*	
Metronidazole	*B. fragilis, C. difficile*	
Isoniazid (and rifampin and/or ethambutol)	*M. tuberculosis* and atypical *Mycobacterium* spp.	
Dapsone (and rifampin)	*M. leprae*	
Amphotericin B	*Candida, Torulopsis,* coccidioidomycosis, histoplasmosis, aspergillosis, and mucormycosis	
Amphotericin B and flucytosine	*Cryptococcus neoformans*	
Ketoconazole	Blastomycosis, paracoccidioidomycosis, and sporotrichosis	

[a]Choice of particular drug depends on sensitivity of the individual organism.

(2) INH is a **prodrug** whose active metabolite inhibits synthesis of the **mycobacterial cell wall.** It does so by inhibiting the enzyme enoyl-ACP reductase required for the synthesis of mycolic acid which is unique to mycobacteria.

b. Pharmacologic properties

(1) INH **penetrates most body fluids and accumulates in caseated lesions.** It enters host cells and has access to intracellular forms of mycobacteria.

(2) INH is the most active drug against ***Mycobacterium tuberculosis*** and possibly *M. kansasii,* but it is not active against most atypical mycobacteria.

(3) INH demonstrates no cross-resistance with other first-line antitubercular drugs.

(4) INH is acetylated in the liver; acetylisoniazid is eliminated faster than isoniazid. Metabolism of INH is genetically determined. Acetylation of INH is genetically determined (**"rapid acetylators"** and **"slow acetylators"**).

c. **Therapeutic use**

(1) INH is administered **in combination** with one and sometimes two or more other first-line drugs to avoid the development of resistance (see below) most often due to mutations that result in its decreased conversion to the active metabolite.

(2) For **prophylaxis,** INH is used alone.

d. **Adverse effects**

(1) INH may produce allergic reactions, including rash or fever, in up to 2% of patients.

(2) The metabolites of INH may be hepatotoxic; fast acetylators are more susceptible. **Hepatotoxicity** with jaundice is observed in up to 3% of individuals over age 35.

(3) INH can inhibit mammalian pyridoxal kinase. High serum concentrations of this agent may result in **peripheral neuropathy;** slow acetylators are more susceptible. This effect is minimized by coadministration of **pyridoxine.**

(4) Isoniazid inhibits the metabolism of other drugs, especially diphenylhydantoin.

2. ***Rifampin*** *(Rifadin, Rimactane)*

a. **Structure and mechanism of action**

(1) Rifampin is a semisynthetic derivative of the antibiotic rifamycin.

(2) Rifampin selectively inhibits the β-subunit of the DNA-dependent RNA polymerase of microorganisms to suppress the initiation of **RNA synthesis.** Most **atypical mycobacteria** are sensitive. Resistance, a change in affinity of the polymerase, develops rapidly when the drug is used alone.

(3) Rifampin is used in combination with **isoniazid** and **pyrizinamide** (see below) and also **prophylactically** for exposure to **meningococci and *H. influenzae.***

(4) **Rifapentine** (Priftin), an analogue of rifampin, is used once weekly generally after sputum cultures convert to negative (during the continuation phase after ~2 months of therapy). Its pharmacology is similar to rifampin.

(5) **Rifabutin** (Ansamycin), an analogue of rifampin, is a less potent inducer of cytochrome P-450 enzymes that is used to treat TB-infected HIV patients receiving antiretroviral therapy with drugs that are substrates for cytochrome P-450 (e.g., protease inhibitors).

b. **Pharmacologic properties**

(1) Rifampin is absorbed orally. It enters enterohepatic circulation and induces hepatic microsomes **to decrease the half-lives of other drugs,** such as **anticonvulsants.**

(2) Adverse effects are minor; they include nausea and vomiting, fever, and jaundice.

3. ***Ethambutol*** *(Myambutol)*

a. **Structure and mechanism of action**

(1) Ethambutol inhibits **arabinosyl transferases** involved in cell wall biosynthesis.

(2) Ethambutol is specific for ***M. tuberculosis*** and *M. kansasii.*

b. **Therapeutic use.** Ethambutol is administered orally in **combination** with isoniazid to avoid development of resistance.

c. **Adverse effects**

(1) Ethambutol produces **visual disturbances,** resulting from reversible retrobulbar neuritis, and minor GI disturbances. Dose adjustment may be necessary in cases of renal failure.

(2) Ethambutol decreases urate secretion and may precipitate gout.

4. ***Streptomycin*** on occasion is administered parenterally in **combination with other antimycobacterial agents;** it may be part of multidrug regimens to treat resistant strains of TB.

5. ***Pyrazinamide***

a. Pyrazinamide is an analogue of nicotinamide that **inhibits mycolic acid synthesis.**

b. Pyrazinamide is inactive at neutral pH, but it inhibits tubercle bacilli in the acidic (pH 5) phagosomes of macrophages.

c. **Hepatotoxicity** is the major adverse effect, with occasional jaundice and (rarely) death. Pyrazinamide inhibits urate excretion and can precipitate acute episodes of gout.

d. Pyrazinamide acts primarily on **extracellular tubercle bacilli.**

B. Second-line drugs used in the treatment of tuberculosis

1. ***Aminosalicylic acid (PAS)***

a. Aminosalicylic acid is an analogue of PABA; it works like sulfonamides but only **penetrates mycobacteria.**

b. Aminosalicylic acid produces GI disturbances.

2. ***Ethionamide*** *(Trecator-SC)*
   a. Ethionamide is an analogue of isoniazid.
   b. Ethionamide, a prodrug, blocks the **synthesis of mycolic acid.** Resistance develops rapidly, but there is no cross-resistance to INH.
   c. Ethionamide is **poorly tolerated;** it commonly produces severe GI disturbances. Without concomitant pyridoxine peripheral, neuropathies may occur. Hepatotoxicity is not uncommon.
3. ***Cycloserine (Seromycin, Pulvules)***
   a. Cycloserine is an analogue of d-alanine that **inhibits cell wall biosynthesis.**
   b. Cycloserine causes **CNS toxicity,** including seizures and peripheral neuropathy; alcohol increases the possibility of seizures.
4. ***Other agents.*** Parenterally and/or orally administered agents include **fluoroquinolones, kanamycin, amikacin,** and **capreomycin** (Capastat Sulfate), protein synthesis inhibitors.
5. ***Guidelines for anti-TB therapy*** include **PPD skin tests** that are interpreted 24–48 hours after injection. The size of induration (5–15 mm) is noted, and patients are treated according to the risk-stratification category.
   a. A **5-mm induration** is considered a positive result in HIV-positive patients, recent contacts of patients with active TB, patients whose chest x-ray shows fibrotic changes indicating old TB infection, and immune-suppressed patients.
   b. A **10-mm induration** is considered a positive result in persons who recently moved from a high-prevalence country, injection drug users, residents and employees of high-risk congregate settings (this includes healthcare workers), persons with certain medical conditions that put them at high risk (e.g., diabetes or cancer), and children.
   c. A **15-mm induration** is a positive result in persons who have no risk factors for TB.
6. ***Commonly used drug regimens for TB.*** In general, **6-month regimens** are used for patients with culture-positive TB. The regimen consists of **INH, rifampin, pyrazinamide, and ethambutol.** All four agents are used for the initial 2 months. The continuation phase is 4 months and consists of the first two agents only. This phase is extended an additional 3 months for patients who had cavitary lesions at presentation or on a follow-up chest x-ray, or are culture positive at the 2-month point. **Second-line agents** (e.g., fluoroquinolones, cycloserine, amikacin) can be used when there is resistance to first-line agents.

C. Drugs used in the treatment of infections caused by *Mycobacterium leprae* (leprosy)

1. Dapsone
   a. Dapsone is a sulfone structurally related to sulfonamides; it competitively **inhibits dihydropteroate synthase to prevent folic acid biosynthesis.**
   b. Dapsone is more effective against ***M. leprae*** than against *M. tuberculosis;* it is also used as a **second-line** agent to treat ***Pneumocystis* pneumonia** in AIDS patients.
   c. Treatment may require **several years to life;** dapsone is often used **in combination with rifampin** to delay the development of resistance. Dapsone may be used alone to provide **prophylaxis** for family members.
   d. Dapsone produces hemolysis, methemoglobinemia, nausea, rash, and headache.
2. ***Rifampin*** is also effective, but it is often used in combination with **dapsone** to decrease the risk of resistance.
3. ***Clofazimine*** *(Lamprene)* is used with dapsone and rifampin for **sulfone-resistant leprosy** or in patients intolerant to sulfones; it may also be effective against atypical mycobacteria. The mechanism of action is unknown.

D. Drugs used against atypical mycobacteria

1. Atypical mycobacteria include ***M. kansasii, M. marinum, M. avium* complex, *M. scrofulaceum,*** and **others.** These account for about 10% of mycobacterial infections in the U.S.
2. ***MAC (M. avium complex)*** includes *M. avium* and *M. intracellulare.* This is an important pathogen that causes disseminated disease in **late stages of AIDS,** usually when **CD4 counts fall below 50** per microliter. A combination of agents is used to prevent emergence of resistance. **Rifabutin** may be used for patients with **CD4 counts below 200** to reduce the incidence of MAC

bacteremia, but the survival advantage has not been proven. The treatment for this infection is usually **life-long**. Isoniazid and pyrazinamide are not used to treat MAC infections.

3. Most commonly used agents for this group of pathogens include **ciprofloxacin, azithromycin, clarithromycin, amikacin, doxycycline, and TMP-sulfa.** Most agents are used in combination to prevent development of resistance. **MAC** is usually treated with a combination of **clarithromycin or azithromycin and ethambutol, with addition of ciprofloxacin in some cases.**

IV. ANTIFUNGAL AGENTS (SEE TABLE 11-3)

A. Drugs that affect fungal membranes

1. *Amphotericin B*

a. Structure and mechanism of action. Amphotericin B is an antibiotic that binds to ergosterol, a major component of fungal cell membranes. It is believed to form "amphotericin pores" that alter membrane stability and allow **leakage of cellular contents.** Bacteria are not susceptible because they lack ergosterol. Amphotericin B binds to mammalian cholesterol with much lower affinity, but this action may explain some adverse effects.

b. Pharmacologic properties

(1) Amphotericin B is poorly absorbed from the GI tract; it is effective by this route only on GI fungal infections. Amphotericin B is usually administered IV as a lipid formulation, but it can be administered intrathecally; it has poor penetration into the CNS.

(2) Amphotericin B is 90% bound to plasma proteins.

c. Therapeutic uses

(1) Amphotericin B is used to treat **most severe fungal infections,** including those caused by ***Candida albicans, Histoplasma capsulatum, Cryptococcus neoformans, Coccidioides immitis, Blastomyces dermatitidis, Aspergillus*** **spp., and** ***Sporothrix schenckii,*** especially in immunocompromised patients.

(2) This agent is the most effective antifungal agent and is usually the drug of choice for major systemic infections. **Liposome-encapsulated amphotericin B** is less toxic.

(3) In some cases, combination therapy with **flucytosine** is advantageous, particularly for the treatment of *Candida* infections, cryptococcal meningitis, and systemic candidiasis.

d. Adverse effects

(1) The adverse effects of amphotericin B are significant; this agent causes **chills and fever** in 50% of patients and **impaired renal function** in 80%.

(2) Amphotericin B may also produce anaphylaxis, thrombocytopenia, severe pain, and seizures.

2. *Itraconazole, ketoconazole, miconazole, fluconazole, clotrimazole, voriconazole, and others*

a. General properties

(1) These agents are imidazoles or triazoles that **inhibit the cytochrome P-450–mediated sterol demethylation of lanosterol to ergosterol** in fungal membranes. The affinity of the mammalian P-450–dependent enzyme is significantly lower; however, these agents **can inhibit cortisone and testosterone synthesis.**

(2) These agents are **broad-spectrum** antifungals; they also inhibit many gram-positive bacteria and some protozoa.

b. Itraconazole (Sporonox), **ketoconazole** (Nizoral)

(1) Itraconazole has replaced ketaconazole for treatment of all mycoses except when cost is a factor.

(2) Itraconazole can be administered orally or topically. It is also used systemically for certain mycoses.

(3) Itraconazole does not penetrate CSF.

(4) Itraconazole is the drug of choice for **disseminated blastomycosis;** it is very useful for the treatment of **histoplasmosis** and also for **paracoccidioidomycosis.** Ketoconazole is used **topically for dermatophyte infections** and mucocutaneous candidiasis and as a shampoo for **seborrheic dermatitis.**

(5) **Inhibition of cytochrome P-450 metabolism (CYP3A4)** increases or decreases metabolism of many drugs, which may lead to serious toxicities.
(6) Itraconazole most commonly causes **gastric upset** (3%–20% of patients). Itching, rashes, and headaches are observed in 1% of patients.
(7) Itraconazole may cause (rarely) hepatic failure.

c. **Miconazole** (Monistat)
(1) Miconazole is available for **topical** application, which is associated with a high incidence of burning and itching. This agent can be used for **tinea pedis, ringworm, and cutaneous and vulvovaginal candidiasis.**
(2) Miconazole is available for IV administration, but this is associated with a high incidence of adverse effects (phlebitis, pruritus, nausea, and anemia). It is generally used only when amphotericin B is contraindicated.

d. **Clotrimazole** (Lotrimin, Mycelex), **econazole** (Spectazole), **oxiconazole** (Oxistat), **sulconazole** (Exelderm), **sertaconazole** (Ertaczo), **butoconazole** (Gynazole-1), **terconazole** (terazol-3)
(1) These agents are available for **topical** application and are useful for many **dermatophyte infections.**
(2) **Clotrimazole-betamethasone** (Lotrisone) is available as a topical antifungal- corticosteroid combination.

e. **Fluconazole** (Diflucan)
(1) Fluconazole is available for IV or oral administration.
(2) Fluconazole is useful for oropharyngeal, isopharyngeal, and systemic **candidiasis.** Fluconazole also penetrates the CSF and is the drug of choice for short-term and maintenance therapy of **cryptococcal meningitis** and for the treatment of disseminated **histoplasmosis** and **coccidioidomycosis.**
(3) Adverse effects include nausea and vomiting, diarrhea, and reversible alopecia.
(4) Fluconazole **inhibits CYP34A and CYP2C9** to increase plasma levels of numerous other drugs.

f. **Voriconazole** (Vfend)
(1) Voriconazole is approved for primary treatment of **acute invasive aspergillosis** and salvage therapy for rare but serious fungal infections caused by the pathogens ***Scedosporium apiospermum*** and ***Fusarium*** **spp.**
(2) Voriconazole **inhibits** several **cytochrome P-450 liver enzymes** to significantly decrease the clearance of numerous drugs.

3. ***Nystatin*** *(Mycostatin)*
a. Nystatin is a polyene antibiotic that is similar in structure and mechanism of action to **amphotericin B.**
b. Nystatin is **too toxic for systemic administration.** It is not absorbed from the GI tract; oral preparations can be used for **infections of the mouth.**
c. Nystatin is used only for ***Candida*** **infections of the skin, mucous membranes, and intestinal tract.**

B. Other antifungal agents

1. ***Griseofulvin*** *(Fulvicin, Grisactin)*
a. Griseofulvin binds to microtubules and **prevents spindle formation and mitosis in fungi.** It also binds filament proteins such as keratin. The drug **accumulates in skin, hair, and nails.**
b. Griseofulvin is administered as oral therapy for **dermatophyte infections.**
c. Griseofulvin is used for long-term therapy of **hair and nail infections.**
d. Griseofulvin is generally well tolerated (GI distress and rash); rare CNS effects and hepatotoxicity occur (blood checks should be conducted during therapy).

2. ***Flucytosine*** *(Ancobon)*
a. Flucytosine is actively transported into fungal cells and is converted to **5-fluorouracil** and subsequently to **5-fluorodeoxyuridylic acid,** which inhibits thymidylate synthetase and thus pyrimidine and **nucleic acid synthesis.** Human cells lack the ability to convert large amounts of flucytosine to the uracil form.
b. Resistance develops rapidly and limits its use; flucytosine is rarely used as a single drug, but it is often used in **combination with other antifungal agents.**

c. Flucytosine is relatively nontoxic; the major adverse effects of this agent are **depression of bone marrow function** at high doses and hair loss. **Uracil** administration can limit bone marrow effects.

3. ***Tolnaftate*** *(Aftate, Tinactin),* ***naftifine*** *(Naftin),* ***terbinefine*** *(Lamisil),* ***butenafine*** *(Lotrimin),* ***cyclopirox*** *(Loprox).* These drugs are used topically for **dermatophyte infections.**
4. ***Caspofungin*** *(Cancidas)* is a large cyclic peptide that inhibits fungal cell wall. It is used for **salvage therapy in patients with severe aspergillosis** who failed therapy with amphotericin B. It may also be useful in systemic candidal infections.
5. ***Trimethoprim-sulfa*** *(Bactrim, Septra)* is used for **PCP,** an opportunistic infection caused by ***Pneumocystis jirovecii,*** frequently encountered in immune-compromised patients, such as those with AIDS or kidney transplant recipients. The combination is also used for prevention of this infection. Patients allergic to sulfa products can use **pentamidine** or a combination **TMP-dapsone.**

V. ANTIPARASITIC DRUGS

A. Agents active against protozoal infections

1. *Antimalarials*

a. Malaria

(1) In the primary state of infection, sporozoites are injected into the host by the female mosquito (or a contaminated needle). In this **preerythrocytic stage,** the sporozoites are resistant to drug therapy. The sporozoites migrate to the liver (**primary exoerythrocytic stage**) and then sporulate (*Plasmodium vivax* and *P. ovale* may not develop to mature liver stages for up to 2 years [**hypnozoites**]). The merozoites that emerge infect erythrocytes (**erythrocytic stage**), where asexual division leads to cell lysis and causes clinical symptoms. The merozoites released can reinfect other red blood cells, reinfect the liver (*P. vivax* and *P. ovale;* secondary erythrocytic stage), or differentiate into sexual forms (gametocytes) that can reproduce in the gut of another female mosquito.

(2) *P. malariae* and *P. falciparum* differ from the other plasmodia in that the merozoites cannot reinfect the liver to produce a secondary exoerythrocytic stage. The lack of a tissue reservoir makes therapy somewhat easier.

b. Therapy rationale (see www.cdc.gov/travel)

(1) Chloroquine (Aralen), **hydroxychloroquine** (Plaquenil)

(a) Chloroquine, and the equivalent hydroxychloroquine, concentrates in acidic parasite vacuoles, raising their pH and **inhibiting activity of heme polymerase,** which converts host hemoglobin toxic by-products to nontoxic polymerized material.

(b) Chloroquine is used for control of **acute, recurrent attacks,** but it is not radically curative. **Chloroquine** is effective against all plasmodia (*P. falciparum, P. vivax, P. malariae, P. ovale*). For chloroquine-resistant plasmodia **quinine sulfate is** used. **Pyrimethamine/sulfadoxine, doxycycline, quinidine,** or **clindamycin** may be used as adjunctive therapy.

(c) In prophylaxis, chloroquine is used to suppress erythrocytic forms either before or during exposure; **primaquine** is added after exposure to treat exoerythrocytic forms. In regions with chloroquine-resistant strains, **mefloquine** or **atovaquone/proguanil** (Malarone) is used for prophylaxis. Doxycycline, an antibiotic, is used when multidrug resistance to *P. falciparum* is prevalent.

(d) Chloroquine is also occasionally used in **rheumatoid arthritis** for anti-inflammatory action and as an alternative with emetine for **amebiasis.**

(e) Many species of ***P. falciparum*** **are resistant** to chloroquine.

(f) Hemolysis can develop in glucose-6-phosphate dehydrogenase-deficient persons.

(g) Rapid parenteral administration or a single high dose (~ 30mg/kg) may be fatal.

(2) Primaquine (8-aminoquinoline)

(a) Primaquine is **used after exposure to *P. vivax* or *P. malaria* for terminal prophylaxis and (radical) cure** from malaria, usually in combination with chloroquine. It is not used for prophylaxis before exposure (casual prophylaxis).

(b) Primaquine is not given parenterally because of **severe hypotension.**

(c) Primaquine may result in **intravascular hemolysis or methemoglobinemia** in African Americans and dark-skinned Caucasians with glucose-6-phosphate dehydrogenase deficiency. Use of this agent is not advised during the first trimester of **pregnancy.**

(3) **Quinine, quinidine**

(a) Quinine is active against the **erythrocytic stage.** It is used primarily to treat **chloroquine-resistant *P. falciparum,*** often in combination with **pyrimethamine/sulfadoxine.**

(b) Quinine has a **low therapeutic index.** This agent produces **curare-like effects** on skeletal muscle, and it can cause headache, nausea, visual disturbances, dizziness, and tinnitus (**cinchonism**). **Hypoglycemia, which can be fatal,** and (rarely) **hypotension** may also occur.

(c) Quinine is associated with "**blackwater fever**" in previously sensitized patients; blackwater fever has a **fatality rate of 25%** due to intravascular coagulation and renal failure.

(d) Quinidine is more toxic than quinidine

(4) **Mefloquine** (Lariam)

(a) Mefloquine is useful for **prophylaxis and treatment of chloroquine-resistant *P. falciparum*** and with chloroquine for **prophylaxis against *P. vivax* and *P. ovale.***

(b) Mefloquinine causes GI disturbances at therapeutic doses. Seizures and other CNS manifestations are also seen.

(c) Use of mefloquine is **contraindicated** in patients with epilepsy or psychiatric disorders, in children under 2 years, in patients using drugs that alter cardiac conduction, and in women during pregnancy or not practicing birth control.

(5) **Atovaquone** (Mepron), **atovaquone/proguanil** (Malarone)

(a) Atovaquone inhibits electron transport to reduce the membrane potential of mitochondria. Resistance develops rapidly.

(b) Co-administration of **atovaquone with proguanil** (a fixed dose) is effective for **treatment and prophylaxis of *P. falciparum.*** The mechanism of antimalarial action of proguanil is uncertain. Its metabolite (cycloguanil) selectively inhibits plasmodia **dihydofolate reductase/ thymidylate synthetase** to inhibit DNA synthesis.

(c) These drugs are generally well tolerated. Adverse effects include GI dysfunction, headache, and rash.

(d) Atovaquone is used an alternative treatment for *P. jirovici* pneumonia.

(6) **Pyrimethamine** (Daraprim)

(a) Pyrimethamine **inhibits dihyrofolate reductase** of plasmodia at concentrations less than that for needed to inhibit the host enzyme.

(b) Pyrimethamine is used in combination with **sulfadoxine,** a sulfonamide with similar pharmacologic properties, in the combination product Fansidar.

(c) Pyrimethamine is associated with **megaloblastic anemia and folate deficiency** (at high doses).

c. **Antibacterial agents**

(1) **Sulfonamides and sulfones** are particularly important in the **prophylaxis of chloroquine-resistant strains.**

(2) **Tetracyclines** and **doxycycline** are used as short-term prophylactic agents in areas with multiresistant strains of plasmodia.

d. **Artemisinins** and analogs

(1) Artemisin (quinghaosu) is the active agent of an herbal medicine. It and its major synthetic analogs (artensuate, artemether), which are usually used in combination treatments (mefloquine), are rapidly metabolized to dihydroartemisinin that has good activity for the initial treatment of *P. falciparum* infections.

(2) Although not FDA approved, they are widely available

2. ***Agents active against amebiasis*** (Fig. 11-4)

a. **Amebiasis.** The major infecting organism is *Entamoeba histolytica,* which is ingested in cyst form, divides in the colon, and can invade the intestinal wall to cause severe dysentery.

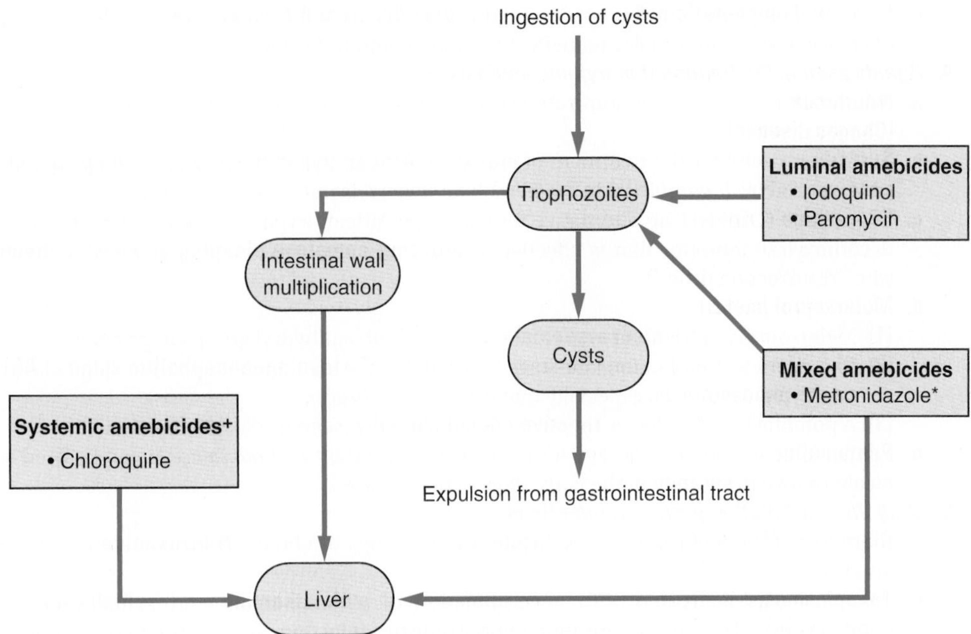

FIGURE 11-4. Agents active against amebiasis.

b. **General drug characteristics.** The tissue amebicide **metronidazole** is active against organisms in the intestinal wall, liver, and other **extraintestinal tissues.** Metronidazole is only partially effective against organisms in the intestinal lumen. The luminal amebicides, **iodoquinol, paromomycin**, and **nitazoxanide** act effectively in the **intestinal lumen.**

c. **Metronidazole** (Flagyl)
   (1) Metronidazole is used for **intestinal amebiasis** as well as for **amebic liver abscesses,** generally in combination with **iodoquinol** or **paromycin** to eradicate luminal disease. This agent is also active against ***Giardia intestinalis*** (formerly *G. lamblia*) and ***Trichomonas vaginalis.*** Metronidazole shows activity against many **anaerobic bacteria.**
   (2) Metronidazole has a **disulfiram-like effect;** therefore, alcohol should be avoided.
   (3) Use of this agent should be avoided in the **first trimester of pregnancy.**

d. **Iodoquinol (Yodoxin)**
   (1) Iodoquinol is active against both **trophozoite and cyst forms in the intestinal lumen** but not in the intestinal wall or extraintestinal tissues.
   (2) Iodoquinol produces adverse effects, sometimes irreversible at higher than recommended doses or duration of administration, which include **optic atrophy and visual defects** and subacute myelooptic neuropathy (**SMON syndrome**).

e. **Paromomycin** (Humatin) is a broad-spectrum antibiotic related to neomycin and streptomycin that is useful as an alternative treatment of **mild-to-moderate luminal infections** or in **asymptomatic carriers** in place of iodoquinol.

3. ***Agents active against leishmaniasis***
   a. **Stibogluconate sodium (Pentostam)**
      (1) Stibogluconate sodium is a **pentavalent antimonial.**
      (2) This agent is effective against all ***Leishmania;*** therapy is a 10-day or 30-day course and may need to be repeated.
   b. **Pentamidine (Pentam)** is administered intramuscularly to treat ***L. donovani*** **infections** when antimonials have failed or are contraindicated. However, adverse effects are numerous and include severe and dangerous **nephrotoxicity** and **hypoglycemia.**

c. **Liposomal amphotericin B** is used to treat ***L. braziliensis* and *L. mexicana.*** It is also the drug of choice when antimonials are ineffective or are contraindicated.

4. ***Agents used in the treatment of trypanosomiasis***
   a. **Nifurtimox** is used to treat South American trypanosomiasis caused by *Trypanosoma cruzi* **(Chagas disease).**
   b. **Suramin** is useful for the treatment of end-stage **African trypanosomiasis,** or **sleeping sickness**, caused by *T. gambiense* in the hemolytic stage; it is not effective against *T. cruzi.*
   c. **Eflornithine** (Ornidyl), an alternative for late-stage African trypanosomiasis, is an ornithine decarboxylase inhibitor that is effective in **arousing comatose sleeping sickness patients** (the ''resurrection drug'').
   d. **Melarsoprol (mel B)**
      (1) Melarsoprol is a **trivalent arsenical** that reacts with sulfhydryl groups in proteins.
      (2) This agent is useful in the late-stage treatment of the **meningoencephalitic stage of African trypanosomiasis,** especially that caused by *T. brucei.*
      (3) A potentially fatal effect is **reactive encephalopathy** (seen in 1%–5% of patients).
   e. **Pentamidine** is standard therapy for the disease caused by *T. rhodesiense*; it can be used as an alternative to **suramin** in the early stage of the disease.
5. ***Drug therapy for other protozoal infections***
   a. **Giardiasis. Metronidazole** and **tindazole** are the drugs of choice. **Nitazoxanide** (Alinia) is also used.
   b. **Toxoplasmosis** is treated with a combination of **pyrimethamine** and **sulfadiazine** (or **clindamycin**). This is a common opportunistic infection in immune-compromised patients.

B. Agents active against metazoan infections (anthelmintics)

1. ***Agents effective against nematode (roundworm) infections***
   a. **Mebendazole** (Vermox) **and albendazole** (Albenza)
      (1) Mebendazole and albendazole are benzimidazole carbamates that **bind with high affinity to parasite free B-tubulin** to inhibit its polymerization and microtubule assembly. These agents also irreversibly **inhibit glucose uptake by nematodes;** the resulting glycogen depletion and decreased ATP production **immobilizes the intestinal parasite,** which is then cleared from the GI tract.
      (2) Albendazole is used to treat **cysticercosis and cystic hydatid disease,** for which it is the drug of choice.
      (3) Mebendazole and albendazole are used to treat **roundworm infections** caused **by *Ascaris lumbricoides, Capillaria philippinensis, Enterobius vermicularis* (pinworm),** *Necator americanus* **(hookworm),** and ***Trichuris trichiura* (whipworm).** It is also recommended for infections caused by the **cestodes *Echinococcus granulosus* and *E. multilocularis.***
      (4) Mebendazole and albendazole are embryo toxic and **teratogenic.**
      (5) **Thiabendazole** (Mintezol) has been used to treat a wide variety of nematodes, but, due to its toxicity, its clinical use has declined sharply.
   b. **Pyrantel pamoate** (Antiminth)
      (1) Pyrantel pamoate selectively produces **depolarizing neuromuscular blockade and inhibition of acetylcholinesterase (AChE)** of the worm, resulting in **paralysis;** intestinal nematodes are flushed from the system.
      (2) Pyrantel pamoate is useful for the treatment of infections caused by **roundworm, hookworm, and pinworm.**
   c. **Piperazine citrate** (Vermizine)
      (1) Piperazine citrate **blocks the response to ACh,** which results in altered parasite membrane permeability and **paralysis.**
      (2) Piperazine citrate is absorbed from the GI tract; adverse effects are minimal.
      (3) Piperazine citrate provides effective treatment of **ascariasis** and **enterobiasis.**
   d. **Diethylcarbamazine** (Hetrazan)
      (1) This agent decreases microfilariae **muscular activity,** causing their dislocation, and it also **disrupts their membranes,** making them susceptible to host defense mechanisms.

(2) Diethylcarbamazine is the drug of choice to treat **loiasis,** despite host response-induced toxicity, and it is a first-line agent for the treatment of **lymphatic filariasis and tropical pulmonary eosinophilia caused by *Wucheria bancrofti* and *Brugia malayi.***

(3) Host destruction of parasites results, depending on the parasite, in **severe but reversible reactions,** including leukocytosis, retinal hemorrhages and ocular complications, tachycardia, rash, fever, encephalitis, and lymph node enlargement and swelling.

e. **Ivermectin** (Mectizan)

(1) Ivermectin causes **paralysis of the organism's musculature** by activation of **invertebrate-specific glutamate-gated Cl^- channels.**

(2) This agent is the drug of choice for the treatment of **onchocerciasis,** and it is a first-line agent for the treatment of **lymphatic filariasis** and **tropical pulmonary eosinophilia** caused by ***W. bancrofti* and *B. malayi.***

2. ***Agents effective against cestode (tapeworm) and trematode (fluke) infections***

a. **Praziquantel** (Biltricide)

(1) Praziquantel causes muscle contraction, with **paralysis** of the worm; it also causes **tegmental damage,** with host-defense activation and destruction of the worm.

(2) Praziquantel is the most effective drug against all types of **fluke infections,** including blood fluke infections (**schistosomiasis**), intestinal and liver fluke infections, and lung fluke infections (**paragonimiasis**). It is also useful in the treatment of **tapeworm infections.**

(3) Use of this agent is contraindicated in ocular cysticercosis because of host-defense–induced **irreversible eye damage.**

b. **Bithionol inhibits parasite respiration.** It is recommended for ***Fasciola hepatica*** (sheep liver fluke infection) and as an alternative to **praziquantel** for **acute paragonimiasis.**

VI. ANTIVIRAL DRUGS

A. Antiherpesvirus drugs

1. ***Acyclovir*** *(Zovirax)*

a. Acyclovir is a **purine analogue** that needs to be converted to nucleoside triphosphate for activity.

b. Acyclovir **requires viral thymidine kinase** to be converted to monophosphate; it then uses cellular enzymes to be converted to a triphosphate form that competitively **inhibits the activity of viral DNA polymerase;** acyclovir triphosphate is also incorporated into viral DNA, where it acts to compete with deoxy GTP for viral DNA polymerase and as a chain terminator. Acyclovir **does not eradicate latent virus;** it has good CSF penetration.

c. **Valacyclovir** (Valtrex), a prodrug, is converted rapidly and completely to acyclovir, **increasing its oral bioavailability** to 50%. It is used similarly to acyclovir. In addition, this agent can be used for **prevention of cytomegalovirus (CMV) reactivation** in immune-compromised patients.

d. This agent is active against **herpes simplex virus (HSV)** types I and II, **Epstein-Barr virus, varicella-zoster virus (VZV),** and **CMV.** Chronic oral administration provides suppression and **shortening of duration of symptoms** in recurrent genital herpes. It is also used in herpes zoster in immunocompromised patients; ophthalmic application is used to treat **herpes simplex dendritic keratitis;** and topical application is used for **mucocutaneous herpetic infections** in immunosuppressed patients. The agent is also used in immune-compromised patients for **prevention of reactivation of HSV** infection.

e. In up to 5% of patients, reversible renal insufficiency due to **crystalline nephropathy,** or **neurotoxicity,** including tremor, delirium, and seizures, develop.

f. Resistance generally develops due to decreased viral thymidine kinase activity or an alteration in DNA polymerase.

g. **Famciclovir** (Famvir) is a prodrug that is well absorbed and then converted by deacetylation to **penciclovir,** which has activity similar to that of acyclovir except that it does not cause chain termination.

2. ***Ganciclovir*** *(Cytovene)*
   a. Ganciclovir is a deoxyguanosine analogue that, as the triphosphate (like acyclovir), **inhibits replication of CMV** (also HSV but not as well); monophosphorylation in CMV is catalyzed by a viral phosphotransferase (in HSV by a viral thymidine kinase).
   b. Ganciclovir is used to treat **CMV retinitis, colitis,** or **esophagitis** in immunocompromised patients; it is also used for the **prevention or suppression of CMV infection in renal transplant patients.** It can also be used in combination therapy with **Foscarnet,** which is shown to be more effective. Ganciclovir is also used for **CMV pneumonitis** in combination with IV CMV Ig.
   c. **Resistance** is primarily the result of impaired phosphorylation due to a point mutation or a deletion in the **viral phosphotransferase.**
   d. The dose-limiting toxicity is **reversible neutropenia** and **thrombocytopenia.**
   e. **Valganciclovir** is an ester prodrug that is converted to ganciclovir by intestinal enzymes. Its uses are similar to those of ganciclovir.
3. ***Foscarnet*** *(Foscavir)*
   a. Foscarnet inhibits **viral DNA polymerase** directly by reversibly but noncompetitively binding to the pyrophosphate binding site.
   b. **Resistance** is due to point mutations in **viral DNA polymerase;** foscarnet is **not cross-resistant** with most other antivirals.
   c. Foscarnet is approved for use in the treatment of **CMV retinitis** and **acyclovir-resistant HSV infections.** When used with ganciclovir, the two agents act synergistically.
   d. The therapeutic efficacy of foscarnet is limited by nephrotoxicity and hypocalcemia-related symptoms, including paresthesia, arrhythmias, and seizures.
4. ***Trifluridine*** *(Viroptic)*
   a. Trifluridine replaces thymidine in viral DNA and causes **fraudulent base pairing;** it also **inhibits viral DNA polymerase** and enzymes in the dTTP pathway.
   b. Adverse effects of these agents include edema around the eyes or eyelids with pain, pruritus, and inflammation.
   c. Trifluridine is used topically for **herpetic infections of the eye (HSV keratitis).**
5. ***Vidarabine*** *(Vira-A)*
   a. Vidarabine is phosphorylated to the triphosphate by cellular enzymes and then **inhibits viral DNA polymerase** with inhibition of DNA synthesis; it may act also as a chain terminator.
   b. It is administered ophthalmically for **herpetic eye infections.**
6. ***Fomivirsen*** *(Vitravene)* inhibits CMV replication through an **antisense mechanism directed against CMV mRNA.** It is used **intravitreally** for **CMV retinitis.**
7. ***Cidofovir*** *(Vistide)* is a **cytosine analogue active against CMV.** It does not require viral enzymes for phosphorylation. This agent is used for **CMV retinitis.** It must be **administered IV with probenecid** to reduce **nephrotoxicity.**
8. ***Docosanol*** (Abrevia), ***Penciclovir*** (Denavir)—These drugs are over-the-counter topical agents used to treat **herpes labialis.** Docosanol prevents viral penetration of cells by inhibiting cell-cell fusion.

B. Anti-influenza agents

1. ***Amantadine*** *(Symmetrel)* ***and rimantadine*** *(Flumadine)*
   a. Amantadine and rimantadine **inhibit the endosome-mediated uncoating of single-stranded RNA viruses prior to transcription and replication;** they may prevent the release of viral nucleic acid into the cell.
   b. Amantadine and rimantadine are used to treat orthomyxovirus (**influenza A**) infections when **administered within the first 48 hours of symptoms,** and as **prophylaxis during flu season.** These agents do not suppress the immune response to the influenza A vaccine.
   c. These agents cause **mild CNS effects** (insomnia, nervousness) and some GI dysfunction. Patients with a history of epilepsy require close monitoring.
2. ***Ribavirin*** *(Virazole)*
   a. Ribavirin **inhibits inosine monophosphate dehydrogenase and viral DNA and RNA polymerases;** the mechanism of action is not clear.

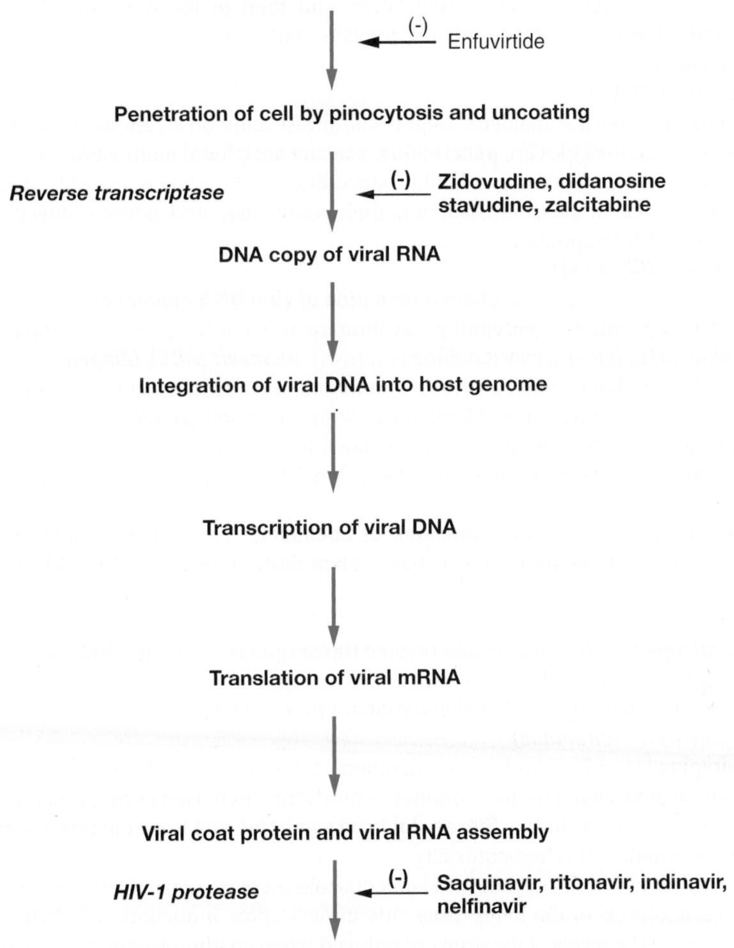

FIGURE 11-5. Sites of action of anti-AIDS drugs.

b. Ribavirin is administered as an aerosol to treat **respiratory syncytial virus.** An IV formulation is used for the treatment of **Lassa fever.** This agent may also be beneficial against **measles pneumonitis,** as well as severe respiratory **influenza** infections.
c. Bronchial irritation is a common adverse effect.

3. ***Zanamivir*** *(Relenza)* **and *Oseltamivir*** *(Tamiflu)* are **neuraminidase inhibitors.** They are used for treatment of **acute uncomplicated influenza infection.** The agents are effective against both **influenza A and B.**

C. **Antiretroviral drugs** (Fig. 11-5)—**nucleoside reverse transcriptase inhibitors (NRTIs)**

1. NRTIs act by competitively **inhibiting HIV-encoded RNA-dependent DNA polymerase (reverse transcriptase)** to cause chain termination that decreases viral DNA synthesis and virus replication. They prevent infection but do not clear cells already infected.
2. NRTIs must first **undergo intracellular phosphorylation** to be active.
3. Combination therapy of NRTIs with drugs from the other three classes of antiretroviral agents is most effective, both for treatment and to reduce the likelihood of the development of resistance.
4. ***Zidovudine (AZT)*** (Retrovir)
   a. The adverse effects of zidovudine, a pyrimidine analogue, include headache, diarrhea, and fever; **dose-limiting toxicities** are **granulocytopenia** and **anemia.**

b. AZT reduces the **rate of progression of HIV.** When given to pregnant women starting in the second trimester, then during labor, and then to the newborn, the **vertical transmission of HIV** is reduced by up to 25%. This agent is also used for **postexposure prophylaxis.**

5. ***Didanosine (ddI)*** *(Videx)*
   a. Didanosine, a purine analogue, requires administration on an empty stomach.
   b. Dose-limiting toxicities are **pancreatitis, sensory peripheral neuropathy,** and **optic neuritis.**
6. ***Stavudine*** *(Zerit).* Except for acid lability, stavudine, a thymidine nucleoside analogue, is similar to **didanosine** in pharmacokinetics, therapeutic use, and adverse effects that typically resolved with discontinuation.
7. ***Zalcitabine (ddC)*** *(Hivid)*
   a. Zalcitabine may also cause **chain termination of viral DNA elongation.**
   b. **Reversible peripheral neuropathy** may limit the use of this agent in 30% of patients.
8. ***Lamivudine (3TC) (Epivir),*** **emtricitabine** (Emtriva), ***abacavir (ABC), (Ziagen)***
   a. Side effects of **lamivudine,** a **cytosine analogue,** include headache and GI upset. **Emtricitabine** is a fluorinated analog of lamivudine with a long half-life that allows for once-daily dosing. Its adverse effect profile is similar to laivudine.
   b. **Abacavir** is a **guanosine analogue.** Occasional fatal hypersensitivity reactions have been reported.
9. ***Tenofovir (TDF)*** *(Viread)* is an **analogue of adenosine.** This agent is more convenient than older antiretroviral agents in that it has a **once-daily** dosing schedule. Most common side effects are GI.

D. Antiretroviral agents—non-nucleoside reverse transcriptase inhibitors (NNRTIs)

1. NNRTIs act similarly to NRTIs (see above).
2. These agents **do not require phosphorylation** for their activity.
3. ***Nevirapine (NVP) (Viramune)***
   a. **Nevirapine** is used in combination regimens. It has also recently been shown to **reduce vertical transmission** of HIV from mother to newborn when used as monotherapy.
   b. Severe reactions, including **Steven-Johnson syndrome and toxic epidermal necrolysis,** have been reported, as has hepatotoxicity.
   c. Concurrent use of nevirapine and ketoconazole increase plasma levels of the former, while decreasing levels of the latter drugs due to nevirapine induction of **CYP3A** metabolism by nevirapine. The levels of the drug are reduced when coadministered with rifampin.
4. ***Delavirdine (DLV)*** *(Rescriptor),* ***Efavirenz (EFV)*** *(Sustiva)*
   a. These agents are used in combination regimens.
   b. Side effects of **DLV** include rash and GI upset. The drug is metabolized by **CYP3A** system. Drug interaction should be monitored.
   c. **EFV** is dosed **once daily.** It is also metabolized by **CYP3A.** Main side effects of this agent are dizziness, insomnia, confusion, amnesia, nightmares, and other **CNS effects.** These are observed in up to 50% of patients and usually abate with time.

E. HIV-1 protease inhibitors (**PIs**; see Fig. 11-5)

1. ***HIV-1 protease inhibitors*** competitively **inhibit viral-induced Gag-Pol polyprotein cleavage by HIV-1 protease,** a step necessary for virion maturation; this leads to clearance of the immature virion.
2. ***These agents are*** used in combination **with nucleoside analogues to delay and possibly reverse the clinical progression of AIDS.**
3. These drugs are frequently associated with **development of lipodystrophy** and also significant drug interactions due to **inhibition of CYP3A4.**
4. ***Resistance*** due to changes in the protease gene has been described; different modifications may be responsible for resistance to some protease inhibitors. Resistance is more common when patients are noncompliant or take drug "holidays" or when inhibitors are used as monotherapy or are given at subtherapeutic doses.
5. HIV-1 protease inhibitors include the following:
   a. **Saquinavir** (Invirase)

(1) The bioavailability of this agent is reduced by other drugs that increase **liver microsomal enzyme activity;** it is increased by drugs that inhibit enzyme activity.
(2) Saquinavir is well tolerated, but because of its **limited bioavailability** due to extensive first-pass metabolism, it has only a modest effect. Therefore, for greater efficacy, it is often **co-administered with ritonavir**, a protease inhibitor (see below).
(3) The most common adverse effects include GI disturbances and rash.

b. **Ritonavir** (Norvir)
(1) Ritonavir extensively **inhibits many liver cytochrome P-450 enzymes,** leading to accumulation of many drugs that are metabolized by this system (including saquinavir). It also **induces** some forms of **cytochrome P-450 enzymes**, leading to reduced bioavailability of other drugs. Close monitoring of other agents patients are using is recommended.
(2) Ritonavir has an adverse effect profile that includes moderate GI disturbances, headache, fatigue, taste disturbances, and perioral paresthesia.
(3) **Lopinavir–ritonavir** (Kaletra) combination is shown to enhance efficacy of both drugs while reducing toxicity.

c. **Indinavir** (Crixivan)
(1) Like ritonavir, it **interferes with liver microsomal enzyme metabolism,** but not to the same extent, and it inhibits the metabolism of some drugs and vice versa.
(2) Indinavir is well tolerated. Mild GI symptoms and reversible **nephrolithiasis** can develop due to precipitation in the renal collecting duct system; these effects can be prevented with attention to hydration. Indirect **hyperbilirubinemia** is also common.

d. **Nelfinavir** (Viracept), **Amprenavir** (Agenerase), **Fosamprenavir** (Lexiva)
(1) These agents exhibit drug interactions similar to those of **indinavir.**
(2) Moderate diarrhea and fatigue have been reported.
(3) **Amprenavir** may cause **severe rashes.** Therefore, it is usually **coadministered with ritonavir. Fosamprenavir** is a prodrug of amprenavir that allows for reduced daily dosing.

e. **Atazanavir** (Reataz)
(1) Common adverse effects of atazanavir include GI disturbances and indirect hyperbilirubinemia with jaundice.
(2) **Atazanavir**, like other PIs, **inhibits CYP3A4 and CYP 2C9** with a great likelihood of drug-drug interactions.

f. **Tipranavir** (Aptivus)
(1) Tipranavir, whose bioavailability is increased with a high-fat meal, undergoes extensive **first-pass metabolism** and, therefore, is **co-administered with ritonavir**.
(2) Its most common adverse effects are **GI disturbances** and **rash** (it contains a sulfonamide moiety). Its use is also associated with development of **hepatic dysfunction** (black box warning).

F. **Anti-HIV agents—fusion inhibitors. Enfuvirtide (Fuzeon)** blocks entry of virus into the cell by **binding to viral gp41 glycoprotein.** This drug is administered **subcutaneously,** with injection site reactions being the most common side effect. It is used in **combination** therapies.

G. **Highly active antiretroviral therapy (HAART)**—HAART refers to highly successful **combination drug regimens,** usually 3–4 agents from several different classes, that are used in treatment of HIV/AIDS to **prevent development of resistance.**

H. **Antihepatitis agents**

1. ***Lamivudine*** *(Epivir)* is a cytosine analogue used for **HBV** infections, providing effective and rapid response in most patients. This agent **slows progression to liver fibrosis.** It has an excellent safety profile at doses used for HBV infections.
2. ***Adefovir*** *(Hepsera)* is also used for treatment of **HBV.** This agent is a **nucleotide analogue.** Adefovir demonstrates dose-related **nephrotoxicity.**
3. ***Interferon alpha*** *(Intron),* ***peginterferon alfa*** *(pegylated interferon alpha),* and **Interferon-alfacon1** (Infergen) are agents that are capable of **inhibiting both RNA** and **protein synthesis** by initiating a series of reactions, including **activation of the JAK-Stat pathway**, that eventually lead to inhibition of viral replication. These agents are used for both **HBV** and **HCV.**

Combination with **ribavirin** leads to synergistic effects. Pegylated agents allow for once-weekly dosing. Adverse effects include an **influenza-like syndrome** after injection that resolves soon thereafter, **thrombocytopenia and granulocytopenia,** as well as **neuropsychiatric effects.**

4. **Ribavirin.** An oral dose of ribavirin is used to treat hepatitis C.

I. Other antivirals

1. ***Palivizumab (Synagis)*** is a **monoclonal antibody** directed against the F glycoprotein on the surface of respiratory syncytial virus (RSV). It is used for prevention of **RSV** in high-risk infants and children, specifically those with bronchopulmonary dysplasia.
2. ***Imiquimod (Aldara)*** is a **topical** agent used for **anal and genital warts** caused by human papilloma virus **(HPV).** The exact mechanism of action is not well elucidated.
3. **Ribavirin, in combination** with parenteral **pegylated interferon alfa,** is administered orally for **HCV infection.**

DRUG SUMMARY TABLE

Penicillins
Penicillin G
Penicillin V
Penicillin G benzathine (Bicillin)
Penicillin G procaine
Oxacillin
Dicloxacillin
Nafcillin
Ampicillin
Amoxicillin (Amoxil)
Piperacillin
Carbenicillin (Geocillin)
Amoxicillin/clavulanic acid (Augmentin)
Ticarcillin/clavulanic acid (Timentin)
Ampicillin/sulbactam (Unasyn)
Piperacillin/tazobactam (Zosyn)

Cephalosporins
First-generation
Cephalexin (Keflex)
Cefazolin (Ancef, Kefzol)
Cefadroxil (Duricef)
Second-generation
Cefoxitin (Mefoxin)
Cefaclor
Cefuroxime (Zinacef, Ceftin)
Cefotetan
Cefprozil (Cefzil)
Third- and fourth-generation
Cefdinir (Omnicef)
Cefixime (Suprax)
Cefotaxime (Clarofan)
Ceftizoxime (Cefizox)
Ceftazidime (Fortaz, Tazicef)
Ceftriaxone (Rocephin)
Cefoperazone (Cefobid)
Cefepime (Maxipime)
Cefditoren (Spectracef)
Cefpodoxime proxetil (Vantin)
Ceftibutin (Cedax)
Ceftizoxime (Cefizox)

Other Beta-lactams
Aztreonam (Azactam)
Imipenem-cilastatin (Primaxin)
Ertapenem (Invanz)
Meropenem (Merrem IV)

Other Cell Wall Inhibitors
Vancomycin (Vancocin)
Bacitracin
Cycloserine (Seromycin)
Daptomycin (Cubicin)
Fosfomycin (Monurol)

Aminoglycosides
Streptomycin
Gentamicin
Tobramycin
Amikacin (Amikin)
Neomycin
Kanamycin (Kantrex)
Spectinomycin (Tobicin)

Tetracyclines
Tetracycline (Sumycin)
Demeclocycline (Declomycin)
Doxycycline (Vibramycin)
Minocycline (Minocin)
Oxytetracycline (Terramycin)
Tigecycline (Tygacil)

Chloramphenicol
Erythromycins
Erythromycin
Clarithromycin (Biaxin)
Azithromycin (Zithromax)
Telithromycin (Ketek)
Clindamycin (Cleocin)

Sulfonamides
Sulfadoxine/pyrimethamine (Fansidar)
Sulfisoxazole
Sulfadiazine, Silver sulfadiazine (Silvadene)
Sulfasalazine (Azulfidine)
Trimethoprim/Sulfamethoxazole (Bactrim, Septra)

Nucleic Acid Inhibitors
Rifampin (Rifadin, Rimactane)
Nitrofurantoin (Furadantin, Macrobid, Macrodantin)

Quinolones
Nalidixic acid (NegGram)
Norfloxacin (Noroxin)
Ciprofloxacin (Cipro)
Ofloxacin (Floxin)
Levofloxacin (Levaquin)
Gatifloxacin (Tequin)
Moxifloxacin (Avelox)
Gemifloxacin (Factive)
Lomefloxacin (Maxaquin)

Polymyxin B
Mupirocin (Bactroban)
Metronidazole (Flagyl)

Agents for Highly Resistant Organisms
Daptomycin (Cubicin)
Linezolid (Zyvox)
Quinupristin/dalfopristin (Synercid)

Antimycobacterial Agents
Isoniazid (INH)
Rifampin (Rifadin)
Rifapentine (Priftin)
Rifabutin (Asamycin)
Ethambutol (Myambutol)
Streptomycin
Pyrazinamide
Aminosalicylic acid (PAS)
Ethionamide (Trecator-SC)
Cycloserine (Seromycin)

Drugs for *Mycobacteria leprae*
Dapsone
Clofazimine (Lamprene)

Antifungal Agents
Amphotericin B (Fungizone)
Ketoconazole (Nizoral)
Miconazole (Monistat)
Clotrimazole (Lotrimin)
Econazole (Spectazole)
Oxiconazole (Oxistat)
Fluconazole (Diflucan)
Voriconazole (Vfend)
Itraconazole (Sporonox)
Sertaconazole (Ertaczo)
Butoconazole (Gynazole-1)
Terconazole (terazol-3)
Nystatin (Mycostatin)

Griseofulvin (Fulvicin, Grisactin)
Flucytosine (Ancobon)
Tolnaftate (Aftate, Tinactin)
Naftifine (Naftin),
Terbinefine (Lamisil
Butenafine (Lotrimin)
Cyclopirox (Loprox)
Caspofungin (Cancidas)
TMP-Sulfa (Bactrim, Septra)

Antiparasitic Agents
Chloroquine (Aralen), Hydroxychloroquine (Plaquenil)
Primaquine
Quinine, Quinidine
Mefloquine (Lariam)
Atovaquone (Mepron), Atavaquone/Proguanil (Malarone)
Pyrimethamine/sulfadoxine (Fansidar)
Chloroguanide (Proguanil)
Metronidazole (Flagyl)
Tindazole (Tindamax)
Nitazoxanide (Alinia)
Iodoquinol (Yodoxin)
*Stibogluconate sodium (Pentostam)
Pentamidine (Pentam)
*Nifurtimox (Lamprit)
*Suramin (Belganyl)
Eflornithine (Ornidyl)
*Melarsoprol (Mel B)
Mebendazole (Vermox)
Albendazole (Albenza)
Thiabendazole (Mintezol)
Pyrantel pamoate (Antiminth)
Piperazine citrate (Vermizine)
Diethylcarbamazine (Hertazan)
Ivermectin (Mectizan)
Praziquantel (Biltricide)
Bithionol (Bitin)
Available from the CDC.

Antivirals—antiherpetic
Acyclovir (Zovirax)
Valacyclovir (Valtrex)
Famciclovir (Famvir)
Ganciclovir (Cytovene)
Idoxuridine (Herplex)
Valganciclovir (Valcyte)
Foscarnet (Foscavir)
Trifluridine (Viroptic)
Vidarabine (Vira-A)
Fomivirsen (Vitravene)
Cidofovir (Vistide)
Penciclovir (Denavir)
Docosanol (Abreva)

Antivirals—anti-influenza
Amantadine (Symmetrel)
Rimantadine (Flumadine)
Ribavirin (Virazole)
Zanamivir (Relenza)
Oseltamivir (Tamiflu)

Antivirals—antiretroviral
Zidovudine (Retrovir)
Didanosine (Videx)
Stavudine (Zerit)
Zalcitabine (Hivid)
Lamivudine (Epivir)
Abacavir (Ziagen)
Tenofovir (Viread)
Emtrictabine (Emtriva)
Nevirapine (Viramune)
Delavirdine (Rescriptor)
Efavirenz (Sustiva)
Saquinavir (Invirase)
Atazanavir (Reataz)
Tipranavir (Aptivus)
Ritonavir (Norvir)
Indinavir (Crixivan)
Nelfinavir (Viracept)
Amprenavir (Agenerase)
Fosamprenavir (Lexiva)
Enfuvirtide (Fuzeon)

Antivirals—antihepatitis
Lamivudine (Epivir)
Adefovir (Hepsera)
Interferon alpha (Intron, Rebetron, Alferon-N, Roferon-A)
Interferon alphacon1 (Infergen)
Pegylated interferon alfa (Pegasys, PEG-Intron)

Antivirals—other
Palivizumab (Synagis)
Imiquimod (Aldera)

Review Test for Chapter 11

Directions: Each of the numbered items or incomplete statements in this section is followed by answers or by completions of the statement. Select the ONE lettered answer or completion that is BEST in each case.

1. A 27-year-old man presents with complaints of a painless ulcer on his penis. He admits to having unprotected intercourse with a woman he met in a bar during a conference 2 weeks ago. A scraping of the lesion, visualized by dark field microscopy, demonstrates spirochetes, and a diagnosis of syphilis is made. Which of the following is the treatment of choice assuming the patient has no known allergies?

(A) Benzathine penicillin G
(B) Penicillin G
(C) Penicillin V
(D) Doxycycline
(E) Bacitracin

2. A 19-year-old military recruit living in the army barracks develops a severe headache, photophobia, and a stiff neck, prompting a visit to the emergency room. A lumbar puncture reveals a diagnosis of bacterial meningitis. Which of the following cephalosporins is likely to be given to this patient?

(A) Cefazolin
(B) Cefuroxime axetil
(C) Ceftriaxone
(D) Cefoperazone
(E) Cefepime

3. A 27-year-old intravenous drug abuser is admitted for fever and shortness of breath. Multiple blood cultures drawn demonstrate *S. aureus*. The cultures further suggest resistance to methicillin. The attending physician also orders a transesophageal echocardiogram that shows tricuspid vegetations consistent with endocarditis. Which of the following is an appropriate antibiotic?

(A) Aztreonam
(B) Imipenem
(C) Gentamicin
(D) Vancomycin
(E) Ceftriaxone

4. A 57-year-old chronic alcoholic develops hepatic encephalopathy. In an attempt to decrease his ammonia levels, you decide to sterilize his intestines, knowing that the gastrointestinal flora is responsible for the ammonia that his liver can no longer detoxify. Which antibiotic, given orally, will accomplish this?

(A) Neomycin
(B) Vancomycin
(C) Erythromycin
(D) Ciprofloxacin
(E) Nitrofurantoin

5. A 12-year-old boy presents with a rash on the palms and the soles of his feet as well as fever and headache. He was camping last weekend and admits to being bitten by a tick. His Weil-Felix test result is positive, suggesting Rocky Mountain spotted fever. What antibiotic should be given?

(A) Streptomycin
(B) Bacitracin
(C) Ciprofloxacin
(D) Doxycycline
(E) Erythromycin

6. A 27-year-old African American woman is seen in the emergency room with complaints of urinary frequency, urgency, and dysuria. A urinary analysis demonstrates bacteria and white blood cells, and she is given trimethoprim/sulfamethoxazole. She now returns with sores and blisters around her mouth and on the inside of her mouth. Given her history and findings, what should you include in the differential of her current complaint?

(A) Glucose-6-phosphate dehydrogenase deficiency
(B) Steven-Johnson syndrome
(C) Red man syndrome
(D) Aplastic anemia
(E) Disseminated *M. avium-intracellulare* infection

7. A 43-year-old HIV-positive woman with a $CD4^+$ count of 150 presents with shortness of breath. An arterial blood gas determination indicates hypoxia, and a chest x-ray shows bilateral interstitial infiltrates. A suspected diagnosis of *Pneumocystis carinii* pneumonia (PCP) is confirmed with bronchoscopy and silver staining of bronchial washings. Which of the following therapies should be started?

(A) Isoniazid
(B) Clindamycin
(C) Azithromycin
(D) Miconazole
(E) Trimethoprim/sulfamethoxazole

8. A 35-year-old diabetic woman presents to the emergency room with signs and symptoms of urinary tract infection, including fever, dysuria, and bacteriuria. Given that she is diabetic, she is admitted for treatment with intravenous ciprofloxacin. What is the mechanism of this drug?

(A) Inhibition of the 30s ribosome
(B) Inhibition of the 50s ribosome
(C) Inhibition of bacterial cell wall synthesis
(D) Inhibition of RNA synthesis
(E) Inhibition of DNA gyrase

9. A 35-year-old Mexican-American man presents to his family physician because his mother has been visiting from Mexico and was found to have tuberculosis (TB). The family physician places a purified protein derivative (PPD), which has negative results, but recommends prophylaxis against TB. Which of the following is indicated for TB prophylaxis in exposed adult patients?

(A) Rifampin
(B) Ethambutol
(C) Isoniazid
(D) Streptomycin
(E) Pyrazinamide

10. A 19-year-old woman has been under the care of an allergist and immunologist since she learned she had a deficiency of C5–9 (the membrane attack complex) of the complement cascade. Her roommate at college recently developed meningitis due to *Neisseria meningitides.* Upon learning this, her physician recommends that she begin taking what antibiotic for prophylaxis?

(A) Ceftriaxone
(B) Isoniazid
(C) Rifampin
(D) Dapsone
(E) *para*-Aminosalicylic acid (PAS)

11. A 12-year-old girl has undergone a bone marrow transplant for the treatment of acute lymphoblastic leukemia (ALL). Five days later, she develops fever, and blood cultures reveal *Candida albicans* in her blood. Which of the following antifungals would be appropriate to use immediately?

(A) Nystatin
(B) Miconazole
(C) Clotrimazole
(D) Ketoconazole
(E) Amphotericin

12. A 23-year-old AIDS patient develops fever, neck pain, and photophobia. He is seen in the emergency room, where a lumbar puncture is performed. The cerebrospinal fluid (CSF) reveals *Cryptococcus neoformans* on India ink stain. Which of the following agents is preferred for the treatment of cryptococcal meningitis?

(A) Tolnaftate
(B) Fluconazole
(C) Griseofulvin
(D) Cycloserine
(E) Flucytosine

13. A 23-year-old recent college graduate has plans to go to Africa to work for a year in the Peace Corps before returning to start medical school. He visits his family physician for a prescription for appropriate malarial prophylaxis. He brings a map from the Centers for Disease Control (CDC) that shows that the area he will be in has a high incidence of chloroquine resistance. Which antimalarial should he take?

(A) Primaquine
(B) Doxycycline
(C) Mefloquine
(D) Pyrimethamine
(E) Quinine

14. A 14-year-old boy returns from a Boy Scout backpack trip with foul-smelling watery diarrhea. On further questioning, he admits to drinking water from a mountain brook without first boiling it. Stool is sent for ova and parasites, confirming the diagnosis of *Giardia lamblia* infection. Which of the following drugs is appropriate treatment?

(A) Metronidazole
(B) Nifurtimox
(C) Suramin
(D) Mebendazole
(E) Thiabendazole

15. A 42-year-old AIDS patient presents to the emergency room with mental status changes and a headache. A computed tomography (CT) scan is ordered and demonstrates a ring enhancing lesion. You decide to treat him empirically due to the possibility of *Toxoplasmosis gondii* abscess. Which agent should be included in his treatment?

(A) Ivermectin
(B) Praziquantel
(C) Pyrimethamine
(D) Niclosamide
(E) Pyrantel pamoate

16. A 23-year-old immunocompetent woman sees her family physician with painful "bumps" on her labia and vulva. On examination, there are vesicles in the described region. You suspect herpes simplex infection on clinical grounds and recommend which of the following?

(A) Amantadine
(B) Valacyclovir
(C) Vidarabine
(D) Foscarnet
(E) Rimantadine

17. A 23-year-old HIV-positive woman presents to the obstetrician. The patient admits to missing her last two menstrual periods, and a urinary human chorionic gonadotropin (hCG) indicates that she is indeed pregnant. Which agent is used to decrease the risk of transmission of HIV to the unborn child?

(A) Idoxuridine
(B) Didanosine
(C) Saquinavir
(D) Zidovudine
(E) Interferon α

18. A 37-year-old woman presents with fever, malaise, and right upper quadrant pain. Blood tests reveal that she has an increase in her liver enzymes. In addition, hepatitis serology indicates that she has hepatitis B virus (HBV). Which of the following agents can be used in the management of this virus?

(A) Lamivudine
(B) Zidovudine
(C) Ribavirin
(D) Interferon α
(E) Acyclovir

Answers and Explanations

1. **The answer is A.** Patients with primary syphilis require a single intramuscular dose of benzathine penicillin G. Oral preparations of Pen G or Pen V are insufficient. Doxycycline for 14 days is an alternative treatment in penicillin-allergic patients. Bacitracin is only topical and insufficient for syphilis.

2. **The answer is C.** Ceftriaxone is a third-generation cephalosporin that has excellent CNS penetration. All the third-generation cephalosporins, except cefoperazone, enter the CNS. The first- and second-generation agents, cefazolin and cefuroxime, respectively, do not enter the CNS. There are limited data on the effectiveness of the fourth-generation agent, cefepime, in meningitis.

3. **The answer is D.** Vancomycin is the drug of choice for serious infections due to methicillin-resistant *S. aureus* (MRSA). In the case of endocarditis, the treatment is usually 6 weeks. MRSA's resistance is often due to altered penicillin-binding proteins, not β-lactamases, so aztreonam, imipenem, and ceftriaxone would not be useful. Gentamicin is often used in conjunction with penicillins in a non-MRSA setting.

4. **The answer is A.** Neomycin is used to sterilize the bowel, as it is not well absorbed from the gut. It is potentially nephrotoxic and ototoxic due to low (1%–3%) absorption. Vancomycin is typically used intravenously, although orally available, and does not provide adequate coverage for bowel sterilization. Although orally available, erythromycin, nitrofurantoin, and ciprofloxacin also do not have adequate coverage.

5. **The answer is D.** Doxycycline, a tetracycline (30S ribosome inhibitor), is the antibiotic of choice to treat Rocky Mountain spotted fever, a rickettsial disease. Streptomycin can be used to treat plague and brucellosis. Bacitracin is only used topically. Ciprofloxacin can be used to treat anthrax, and erythromycin is the most effective drug for the treatment of Legionnaires disease.

6. **The answer is B.** Steven-Johnson syndrome is a form of erythema multiforme, rarely associated with sulfonamide use. Patients with glucose-6-phosphate dehydrogenase deficiency are at risk of developing hemolytic anemia. Red man syndrome is associated with vancomycin. Aplastic anemia is a rare complication of clindamycin use. Disseminated *Mycobacterium avium-intracellulare* infection, more common in AIDS patients, is treated with macrolides.

7. **The answer is E.** Trimethoprim/sulfamoxazole is not only the treatment for *Pneumocystis carinii* pneumonia (PCP) but also should be considered for prophylaxis in patients undergoing immunosuppressive therapy or with HIV. Azithromycin can be use in Mycobacterium avium-intracellulare (MAC complex) in AIDS patients. Isoniazid is used for tuberculosis (TB), yet another illness more common in AIDS patients. Miconazole is an antifungal used for vulvovaginal candidiasis.

8. **The answer is E.** Ciprofloxacin is a quinolone, a group of antibiotics that inhibit bacterial topoisomerase II (DNA gyrase). The antibiotic classes that inhibit the 30S ribosome include aminoglycosides and tetracycline. Inhibitors of the 50S ribosome include chloramphenicol, erythromycin, and clindamycin. Bacterial cell wall inhibitors include penicillins, cephalosporins, and vancomycin. Rifampin inhibits DNA-dependent RNA polymerase (RNA synthesis).

9. **The answer is C.** Isoniazid can be used alone for the prophylaxis of tuberculosis (TB) in the case of such exposure. All the other agents are important in the treatment of known TB infection and are often used in combination with isoniazid. Often rifampin, ethambutol, streptomycin, isoniazid, and pyrazinamide are used for months together, as many strains are multidrug resistant.

10. **The answer is A.** Patients with increased risk of *Neisseria meningitides* infection can be given rifampin for prophylaxis. Ceftriaxone is often used in the case of confirmed meningitis. Isoniazid

is used for single-agent prophylaxis in the case of tuberculosis (TB) exposure. Dapsone and *para*-Aminosalicylic acid (PAS) are used in the treatment of leprosy.

11. **The answer is E.** Amphotericin is used in the treatment of severe disseminated candidiasis, sometimes in conjunction with flucytosine. It is often toxic and causes fevers and chills on infusion, the "shake and bake." Toxicity has been decreased with liposomal preparations. Nystatin is used as a "swish and swallow" treatment for oral candidiasis. Miconazole and clotrimazole are topical antifungals. Ketoconazole is good for mucocutaneous candidiasis.

12. **The answer is B.** Fluconazole is the best agent to treat cryptococcal meningitis and has good central nervous system (CNS) penetration. Flucytosine penetrates the CNS and is often used with other antifungals, as resistance to flucytosine commonly develops. Tolnaftate and griseofulvin are topical agents used in dermatophyte infections. Cycloserine is an alternative drug used for mycobacterial infections and is both nephrotoxic and causes seizures.

13. **The answer is C.** Mefloquine is the primary agent used for prophylaxis in chloroquine-resistant areas. Primaquine is not used for prophylaxis before exposure. Doxycycline is used with quinine for acute malarial attacks due to multiresistant strains. Pyrimethamine is used for suppressive care and not even for acute attacks.

14. **The answer is A.** Metronidazole is used to treat protozoal infections due to *Giardia, Entamoeba,* and *Trichomonas* spp. Nifurtimox is used to treat Chagas disease (due to *Trypanosoma cruzii*). Suramin is used to treat African trypanosomiasis. Mebendazole is used to treat round worm infections, and thiabendazole is used to treat *Strongyloides* infection.

15. **The answer is C.** Toxoplasmosis is treated with a combination of pyrimethamine and sulfadiazine. Ivermectin is used to treat filariasis, whereas praziquantel is used to treat schistosomiasis. Niclosamide can be used to treat tapeworm infections, and pyrantel pamoate is used to treat many helminth infections.

16. **The answer is B.** Valacyclovir is related to acyclovir, both of which are used for the treatment of oral and genital herpes in immunocompetent individuals. Vidarabine is used in more severe infections in neonates as well as in the treatment of zoster. Both amantadine and rimantadine are used in the treatment of influenza. Foscarnet is used in the treatment of cytomegalovirus (CMV) retinitis and acyclovir-resistant herpes simplex virus (HSV) infection.

17. **The answer is D.** Zidovudine is the only agent approved to prevent fetal transmission of HIV as it crosses the placenta. Idoxuridine is used in the treatment of herpes simplex virus (HSV) keratitis. Didanosine is used to treat HIV in children as young as 6 months. Saquinavir is used to treat HIV and is a protease inhibitor. Interferon α works best against single-stranded RNA viruses.

18. **The answer is A.** Lamivudine, a reverse transcriptase inhibitor of the HIV reverse transcriptase, also has activity against the reverse transcriptase of hepatitis B virus (HBV). Zidovudine does not display such cross-activity. Ribavirin and interferon α can be used in the treatment of hepatitis C, an RNA virus. Acyclovir is only effective against the herpes family DNA polymerase.

chapter 12

Cancer Chemotherapy

I. PRINCIPLES OF CANCER CHEMOTHERAPY

A. Therapeutic effect of anticancer agents

1. Because cancer may potentially arise from a single malignant cell, the therapeutic goal of cancer chemotherapy may require **total tumor cell kill,** which is the elimination of all neoplastic cells.
2. Early treatment is critical because the greater the tumor burden, the more difficult it is to treat the disease.
3. Achievement of a **therapeutic effect** often involves drugs that have a narrow **therapeutic index** (TI); it may require combinations of several drugs with different mechanisms of action, dose-limiting toxicities, or cross-resistance to minimize the adverse effects on nonneoplastic cells (Fig. 12-1).
4. A therapeutic effect is usually achieved by killing **actively growing cells,** which are most sensitive to this class of agents. Because normal cells and cancer cells have similar sensitivity to chemotherapeutic agents, adverse effects are mostly seen in normally dividing nonneoplastic cells, such as **bone marrow stem cells, gastric and intestinal mucosa, and hair follicles.**
5. Achievement of the therapeutic effect may involve the use of drugs, sometimes sequentially, that act only at **specific stages in the cell cycle** (e.g., the S phase and the M phase; Fig. 12-2).

B. Resistance

1. ***Primary resistance***
   a. Primary resistance is seen in tumor cells that **do not respond to initial therapy** using currently available drugs.
   b. Primary resistance is related to the **frequency of spontaneous mutation** (10^{-5}–10^{-10}). There is less likelihood that a small tumor burden has resistant cells. The probability that any tumor population has primary resistance to two non–cross-resistant drugs is even less likely (approximately the product of the two individual probabilities).
2. ***Acquired resistance***
   a. Acquired resistance **develops or appears during therapy.**
   b. Acquired resistance can result from the **amplification of target genes** (e.g., the gene for dihydrofolate reductase, which is the target for **methotrexate**). Gene amplification also occurs in the **multidrug resistance phenotype** (*MDR1* gene). In this case, cells overproduce cell surface glycoproteins (***P*-glycoproteins**) that actively transport bulky, natural product agents out of cells (Table 12-1). As a result, the cell fails to accumulate toxic concentrations of several different types of drugs.
3. ***Pharmacologic sanctuaries.*** Resistance may occur due to the inability of chemotherapeutic agents to reach sufficient "kill" levels in certain tissues (e.g., brain, ovaries, testes).

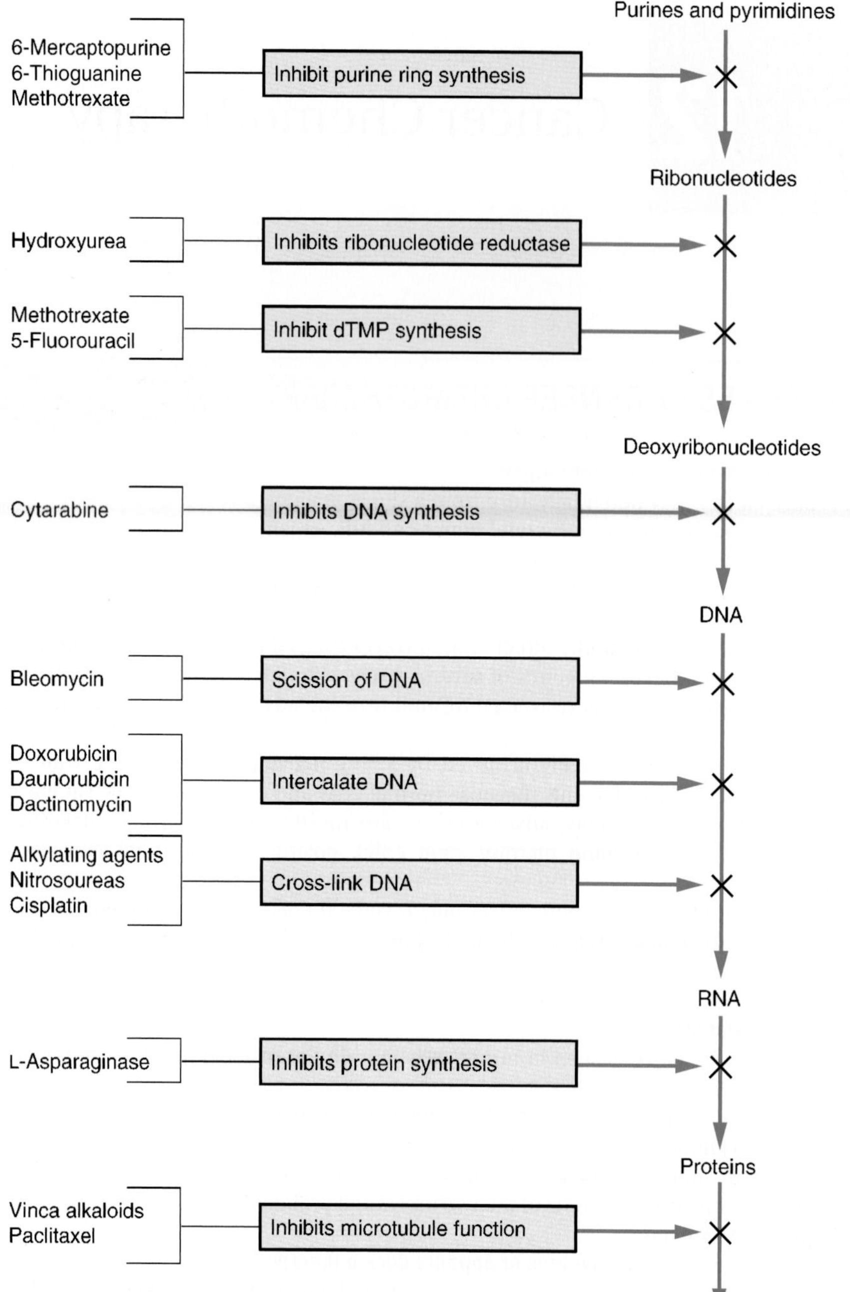

FIGURE 12-1. Sites of action for cancer chemotherapeutic drugs.

II. ALKYLATING AGENTS

A. Structure and mechanism

1. Clinically useful alkylating agents have a **nitrosourea,** ***bis*****-(chloroethyl)amine,** or **ethylenimine** moiety. The **electrophilic center** of these agents becomes covalently linked to the nucleophilic centers of target molecules. Nitrosoureas can also cause **carbamylation.**

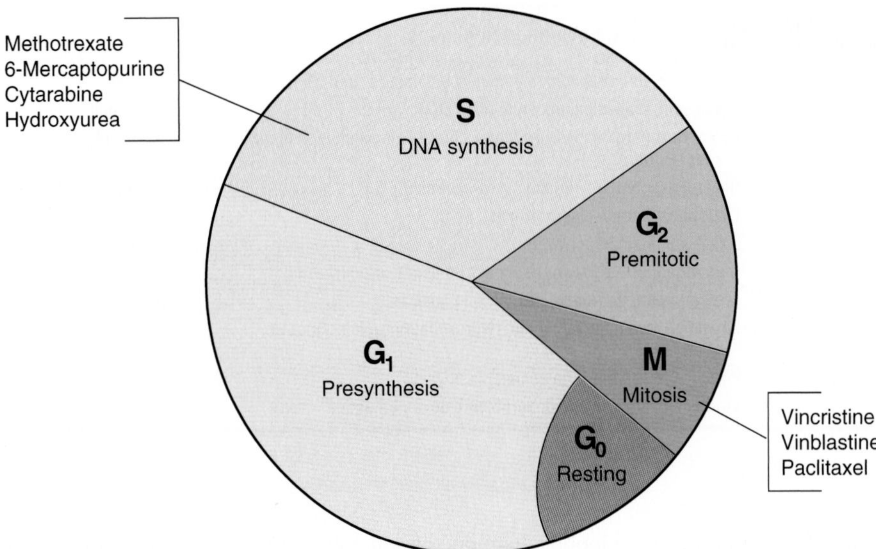

FIGURE 12-2. Cell-cycle specificity of some antitumor drugs. *S* is the phase of DNA synthesis; G_2 is the premitotic phase for synthesis of essential components for mitosis; *M* is the phase of mitosis in which cell division occurs; G_1 is the phase for synthesis of essential components for DNA synthesis; G_0 is a "resting" phase that cells may enter when they do not divide.

2. Alkylating agents target the **nitrogens (especially the N-7 of guanine)** and **oxygens of purines and pyrimidines** in DNA. This may lead to abnormal base pairing, depurination (followed by DNA chain scission), ring cleavage, and DNA strand crosslinks. These agents also target **other critical biologic moieties**—including carboxyl, imidazole, amino, sulfhydryl, and phosphate groups—which become alkylated.
3. These agents can act at all stages of the cell cycle, but cells are most susceptible to alkylation in **late G_1 to S phases.**
4. ***Acquired resistance*** can involve increases in DNA repair processes, reduction in cellular permeability to the drug, increased metabolism, and the production of glutathione (and other molecules containing thiols), which neutralizes alkylating agents by a conjugation reaction that is enzymatically catalyzed by glutathione S-transferase.

table 12-1 The Multidrug Resistance (*MDR*) Gene: Drug Specificity and Tissue Distribution

Drugs Affected by *MDR*	Drugs Not Affected by *MDR*
Adriamycin	Methotrexate
Daunomycin	6-Thioguanine
Dactinomycin	Cytarabine
Plicamycin	Cyclophosphamide
Etoposide	BCNU
Vinblastine	Bleomycin
Vincristine	Cisplatin
VP-16	
Tissues with High *MDR* Expression	**Tissues with Low *MDR* Expression**
Colon	Bone marrow
Liver	Breast
Pancreas	Ovary
Kidney	Skin
Adrenal	Central nervous system

table 12-2 Common Combination Regimens

ABVD	Adriamycin (doxorubicin), bleomycin, vinblastine, dacarbazine	Hodgkin
BEP	Bleomycin, etoposide, platinum (cisplatin)	Testicular
CHOP	Cyclophosphamide, hydroxydaunorubicin, Oncovin (vincristine), prednisone	Non-Hodgkin
CAF	Cyclophosphamide, adriamycin (doxorubicin), 5-FU	Breast
CMF	Cyclophosphamide, methotrexate, 5-FU	Breast
FOLFOX	5-FU, oxaliplatin, leucovorin	Colon
MOPP	Mustargen, Oncovin (vincristine), prednisone, procarbazine	Hodgkin
M-VAC	Methotrexate, vinblastin, doxorubicin, cisplatin	Bladder
R-CHOP	Rituximab, cyclophosphamide, Hydroxydaunorubicin, Oncovin, prednisone	Hodgkin
PVB	Platinum (cisplatin), vinblastine, bleomycin	Testicular
VAD	Vincristine, adriamycin (doxorubicin), dexamethasone	Multiple myeloma

5. With the exception of cyclophosphamide, parenterally administered alkylating agents are **direct vesicants** and can damage tissue at the injection site.
6. Some degree of **leucopenia** occurs at adequate therapeutic doses with all oral alkylating agents.
7. The dose-limiting toxicity is **bone marrow suppression.** Alkylating agents are also highly toxic to dividing **mucosal cells,** causing oral and gastrointestinal (GI) ulcers. Most of these agents also cause nausea and vomiting, which can be minimized by pretreatment with **5-HT$_3$ antagonists.** Most alkylating agents can cause **sterility,** and **alopecia** is common.
8. Patients with **xeroderma pigmentosa** are hypersensitive to alkylating agents.
9. Alkylating agents are **mutagenic** and can cause **secondary cancer** (e.g., leukemia) and sterility later in life.

B. Nitrogen mustards: bifunctional alkylating agents

1. ***Mechlorethamine (Mustargen)***
   a. Mechlorethamine is extremely hygroscopic and **unstable.** The active drug is present only for minutes.
   b. Mechlorethamine is administered intravenously (IV); it causes severe **local reactions.**
   c. This agent is used primarily in the **MOPP regimen** (Table 12-2) to treat **Hodgkin disease** and other lymphomas.
   d. **Leukopenia** and **thrombocytopenia** are dose-limiting toxicities; repeat courses of treatment are given only after marrow function has recovered. Nausea and vomiting generally occur.
2. ***Cyclophosphamide (Cytoxan) and ifosfamide (Ifex)***
   a. Cyclophosphamide may be administered orally, IV, or intramuscularly. It is metabolically activated to 4-hydroxycyclophosphamide, which in turn is nonenzymatically cleaved to aldophosphamide. In tumor cells aldophospamide is cleaved to **phosphoramide mustard,** which is toxic to tumor cells, and **acrolein,** the agent suspected to cause hemorrhagic cystitis.
   b. Cyclophosphamide is used to treat lymphomas, leukemias, mycosis fungoides, multiple myeloma, retinoblastoma, breast and ovarian carcinoma, and small cell lung cancer. It is a component of many combination treatments for a variety of cancers (Table 12-2).
   c. Cyclophosphamide has less incidence of thrombocytopenia than **mechlorethamine,** but **immunosuppression** is still the most important toxic effect. The metabolite acrolein may result in **hemorrhagic cystitis;** this effect can be prevented by coadministration of the sulfhydryl compound 2-mercaptoethanesulfonate **(MESNA),** which neutralizes acrolein at acidic pH in the urine. Reversible alopecia often occurs; nausea and vomiting are common.
   d. This agent is also used in some autoimmune conditions, such as lupus nephritis, and arteritis.

e. **Ifosfamide (Ifex)** is a cyclophosphamide analog with less potential to cause hemorrhagic cystitis. Central nervous system (CNS) and urinary tract toxicity limit its use to special applications (testicular cancer, stem cell rescue).

3. ***Melphalan (Alkeran) and chlorambucil (Leukeran)***
   a. Melphalan and chlorambucil are derivatives of **nitrogen mustard** that contain phenylalanine and an aromatic ring, respectively. Their pharmacology is similar to mechlorethamine.
   b. These agents are administered **orally.**
   c. **Melphalan** is often used to treat **multiple myeloma** and **carcinoma of the ovary.**
   d. The toxicity of mephalan is related mostly to myelosupression. Nausea and vomiting are infrequent; there **is no alopecia.**
   e. **Chlorambucil** is the slowest-acting nitrogen mustard and is the agent of choice in the treatment of **chronic lymphocytic leukemia, some lymphomas, and Hodgkin disease.** It produces less severe marrow suppression than other nitrogen mustards.

C. **Alkyl sulfonates: busulfan (Myleran)**

1. Busulfan is selectively myelosuppressive, inhibiting **granulocytopoiesis.**
2. Busulfan is administered orally to treat **chronic myelogenous leukemia** and other myeloproliferative disorders.
3. Busulfan produces adverse effects related to **myelosuppression.** It only occasionally produces nausea and vomiting. In high doses, it produces a rare but sometimes fatal **pulmonary fibrosis,** "busulfan lung."

D. **Nitrosoureas**

1. ***Carmustine (BiCNU, Gliadel), lomustine (CeeNU),*** *and* ***semustine (methyl-CCNU)***
   a. Carmustine, lomustine, and semustine are highly lipophilic; they **cross the blood–brain barrier.** Nitrosurea can carbamylate intracellular molecules.
   b. These agents are given orally except for **carmustine,** which is administered **IV.**
   c. Carmustine, lomustine, and semustine are useful in **Hodgkin disease** and other lymphomas, as well as in **tumors of the brain.**
   d. These agents are markedly **myelosuppressive,** but with delayed effect, possibly up to 6 weeks. Use of these agents may also result in **renal failure.**
   e. The use of these agents for various brain cancers has been declining since the introduction of **temozolomide** (see below).
2. ***Streptozocin (Zanosar)***
   a. Streptozocin is a natural **antibiotic** that is composed of **methylnitrosourea** linked to the 2-carbon of glucose.
   b. It is useful for the treatment of **pancreatic islet cell carcinoma** and **carcinoid.**
   c. This agent is **not myelosuppressive.** Nausea and vomiting almost always occur. **Renal toxicity** is the dose-limiting effect.

E. **Ethylenimine: thiotepa (triethylene thiophosphoramide)** is converted rapidly by liver mixed-function oxidases to its active metabolite triethylenephosphoramide (TEPA); it is used for high-dose chemotherapy regimens; it is active in ovarian cancer. Myelosupression is a major toxicity.

F. **Triazines: dacarbazine (DTIC-Dome) and tetrazines: temozolomide (Temodar)**

1. ***Dacarbazine*** is activated in the liver to a cell killing methylating metabolite.
2. Dacarbazine is administered IV primarily as a component of the **ABVD** regimen (adriamycin, bleomycin, vinblastine, and dacarbazine) to treat **Hodgkin disease, malignant melanoma,** and **soft tissue sarcomas.**
3. Dacabazine is moderately **myelosuppressive.** Nausea and vomiting occur in 90% of patients. Flu-like symptoms also occur.
4. ***Temozolomide*** acts similarly to dacarbazine. It is administered orally and is primarily used to treat refractory **anaplastic astrocytoma,** such as **glioblastoma multiforme**; **malignant melanoma;** and **uterine leiomyosarcoma.**
5. ***Temozolomide*** toxicities are mainly hematologic and gastrointestinal.

III. ANTIMETABOLITES

A. General characteristics

1. Antimetabolites are **S-phase–specific** drugs that are **structural analogues of essential metabolites** and that interfere with DNA synthesis.
2. ***Myelosuppression*** is the dose-limiting toxicity for all drugs in this class.

B. Methotrexate (Trexall)

1. ***Mechanism of action*** (Fig. 12-3)
   a. Methotrexate (MTX) is a **folic acid analogue** that **inhibits dihydrofolate reductase (DHFR).** This reduces the pool of tetrahydrofolate required for the conversion of deoxyuridylic acid (dUMP) to deoxythymidylic acid (dTMP), and consequently, N^5,N^{10}-methylenetetrahydrofolate is not formed. The net result is **indirect inhibition of DNA synthesis.** Methotrexate also inhibits RNA and protein synthesis.
   b. This agent also inhibits enzymes involved in **folate metabolism,** including dihydrofolate reductase.
   c. **Resistance** results from transport defects and also amplification or alterations in the gene for dihydrofolate reductase.
2. ***Pharmacologic properties***
   a. Methotrexate is administered orally, IV, intramuscularly, or intrathecally.
   b. Methotrexate is transported into cells by folate carriers and activated to various forms of polyglutamate.
   c. Methotrexate is poorly transported across the blood–brain barrier. Therapeutic concentrations in the CNS occur only with high-dose therapy or by **intrathecal** administration, such as to treat or prevent leukemic meningitis.
3. ***Therapeutic uses***
   a. Methotrexate is an important agent in **childhood acute lymphoblastic leukemia, choriocarcinoma,** and other trophoblastic tumors in women.
   b. This agent is also useful in combination with other drugs in the treatment of **Burkitt's lymphoma and other non-Hodgkin lymphomas, osteogenic sarcoma,** lung carcinoma, and head and neck carcinomas.
   c. Methotrexate can be used for treatment of **severe psoriasis** and has been used for immunosuppression following transplantation or in the management of a variety of **immune disorders,** including refractory rheumatoid arthritis, Crohn disease, Takayasu arteritis, and Wegener granulomatosis. It is also used for **therapeutic abortion.**
4. ***Adverse effects***
   a. Methotrexate is **myelosuppressive,** producing severe leukopenia, bone marrow aplasia, and thrombocytopenia. Dose monitoring and **leucovorin (folinic acid) "rescue"** are important adjuncts to successful therapy (leucovorin is converted to an essential cofactor for thymidylate sythetase).
   b. This agent may produce severe **GI disturbances.** Other adverse effects can occur in most body systems; alopecia, headache, and mucositis are common.
   c. **Renal toxicity** may occur because of precipitation (crystalluria) of the 7-OH metabolite of methotrexate.

C. Pemetrexed (Alimta)

1. ***Mechanism of action:*** The primary action of pemetrexed is inhibition of **thymidylate synthetase** (Fig. 12-3).
2. ***Pharmacologic properties:*** Like methotrexate, it is transported into cell by folate carriers and activated to various forms of polyglutamate.
3. ***Therapeutic uses:*** It is approved for use with cisplatin to treat **mesothelioma.**
4. ***Adverse effects:*** Myelosupression is its main adverse effect.

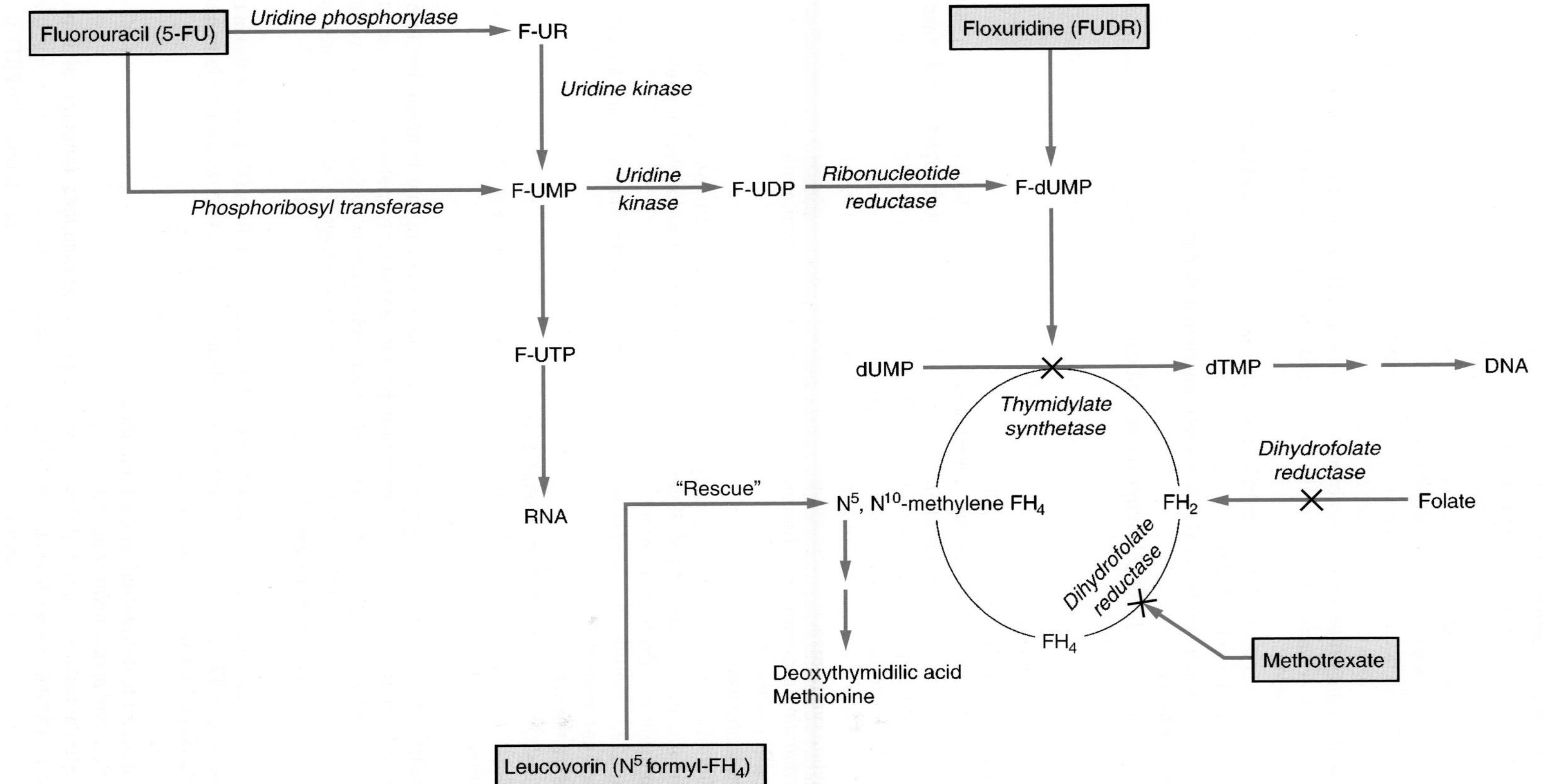

FIGURE 12-3. Mechanism of action of fluorouracil, floxuridine, methotrexate, and leucovorin (*5-FU,* 5-fluorouracil; *dUMP,* deoxyuridine monophosphate; FH_2, dihydrofolate; FH_4, tetrahydrofolate).

D. Cytarabine (ara-C) (Cytosar-U)

1. ***Structure and mechanism of action***
   a. Cytarabine is a **pyrimidine antagonist** that is an analogue of 2′-deoxycytidine. Accumulation of one of its metabolites inhibits the activity of **DNA polymerases** and, if incorporated into DNA, results in altered function of newly replicated DNA.
   b. Cytarabine is most active in the **S phase** of the cell cycle.
2. ***Resistance*** can occur via changes in any of the **enzymes** required for conversion of the nucleoside to the various phosphorylated forms.
3. ***Pharmacologic properties.*** Cytarabine is administered **IV,** generally by continuous infusion, or **intrathecally,** because absorption after oral administration is poor and unpredictable.
4. ***Therapeutic uses***
   a. Cytarabine is useful for the induction of remission in **acute leukemia,** especially acute myelogenous leukemia (AML).
   b. Cytarabine can also be used in the treatment of **non-Hodgkin** lymphoma.
5. ***Adverse effects***
   a. Cytarabine is highly **myelosuppressive** and can produce severe leukopenia, thrombocytopenia, and anemia.
   b. This agent also produces many other toxic effects, most frequently involving GI disturbances.

E. Fluorouracil (5-FU) (Adrucil)

1. ***Mechanism of action*** (see Fig. 12-3)
   a. Fluorouracil is a **pyrimidine antagonist** that needs to be converted to 5-fluoro-2′-deoxyuridine-5′-monophosphate, F-dUMP, which inhibits **thymidylate synthetase** and thus the production of dTMP and DNA, by forming a ternary complex between itself, N^5,N^{10}-methylenetetrahydrofolate, and the enzyme.
   b. **Resistance** is usually due to decreased conversion to F-UMP or altered or amplified thymidylate synthetase.
2. ***Pharmacologic properties.*** Fluorouracil is administered **parenterally;** it is also administered **topically** to treat skin cancers.
3. ***Therapeutic uses***
   a. Fluorouracil is useful in certain types of solid carcinomas; the major use of this agent is in the treatment of **breast and GI carcinomas** and **metastatic colon carcinomas,** sometimes by infusion into the hepatic artery.
   b. Applied **topically,** fluorouracil is used to treat **premalignant keratoses** and **superficial basal cell carcinomas.**
4. ***Adverse effects***
   a. This agent is markedly **myelosuppressive.**
   b. Fluorouracil produces GI disturbances, alopecia, and neurologic manifestations, along with other toxic effects.

F. ***Capecitabine*** (Xeloda) is a fluoropyrimidine carbamate prodrug that is **converted to 5-FU** once ingested. It is an **oral** agent used for **metastatic breast cancer** when patients are resistant to paclitaxel/anthracycline therapy and for **metastatic colorectal cancer.** Dermatitis and myelosuppression are common with the use of this agent. Hepatic enzymes should be monitored, as capecitabine may elevate **bilirubin** levels.

G. ***Gemcitabine*** (Gemzar) is another **pyrimidine antagonist** that inhibits DNA synthesis via **chain termination.** It is an **IV** agent used for **pancreatic cancer** as well as **non–small-cell lung cancer** and **bladder cancer.** Myelosuppression is the main limiting effect.

H. 6-Mercaptopurine (Purinethol) and 6-thioguanine

1. ***Structure and mechanism of action***
   a. 6-Mercaptopurine and 6-thioguanine are **purine antagonists (analogs of hypoxanthine and guanine,** respectively). They must be converted to ribonucleotides by the salvage pathway enzyme hypoxanthine-guanine phosphoribosyltransferase (**HGPRT**) to produce 6-thioguanosine-5′-phosphate (6-thioGMP) and 6-thioinosine-5′-phosphate (T-IMP).

b. 6-thioGMP can be further phosphorylated and is incorporated into DNA. This appears to be its major site of action, although the precise mechanism of cytotoxicity is unknown.
c. T-IMP accumulates and **inhibits nucleotide metabolism** at several steps. It can be converted into **thioguanine** derivatives and can also be incorporated into DNA.

2. ***Resistance*** is generally due to **deficiency in tumor cells of HGPRT.**
3. **6-*Mercaptopurine***
   a. 6-Mercaptopurine can be administered orally. This agent is incorporated into DNA and causes **base mispairing.**
   b. This agent is useful in the treatment of **ALL** and **AML**. It is also occasionally used for **Crohn disease.**
   c. **Bone marrow depression** is the dose-limiting toxicity. GI disturbances occur, including anorexia, nausea, and vomiting.
4. ***6-Thioguanine***
   a. 6-Thioguanine is administered **orally,** although absorption is incomplete.
   b. 6-Thioguanine is used for remission reduction and maintenance of **AML.**
   c. **Bone marrow depression** is the dose-limiting toxicity. GI disturbances are less severe than with 6-mercaptopurine.

I. **Cladribine** (Leustatin), a purine **antagonist**, is an **adenosine analogue** that is resistant to adenosine deaminase. It causes **DNA strand breaks** and **loss of NAD.** This agent is used for **hairy cell leukemia** and **non-Hodgkin lymphoma.** Cladribine causes **decreased CD4 and CD8 counts;** however, this effect is transient. It is administered **IV.**

J. **Fludarabine** (Fludara), a **purine antagonist**, interferes with **DNA synthesis** and induces cellular **apoptosis.** This agent is used for chronic lymphocytic leukemia (**CLL**) and **non-Hodgkin lymphoma.** It is an **IV** agent whose main side effect is **myelosuppression.**

K. Tretinoin (Vesanoid)

1. Tretinoin is a natural metabolite of **retinoid,** a vitamin A derivative. The agent induces **terminal differentiation of several precursor lines.** One target of tretinoin is the ***PML/RARα* gene,** which is involved in AML.
2. Tretinoin is used for refractory **acute promyelocytic leukemia,** M3 classification.
3. Cardiac **dysrhythmias** as well as dermatologic side effects are observed. This agent is also commonly used for treatment of acne and wrinkles.

IV. NATURAL PRODUCTS

A. Vinca alkaloids

1. ***Mechanism of action***
   a. Vinca alkaloids are derived from periwinkle plants. They **bind to β-tubulin** heterodimers and block polymerization with α-tubulin into microtubules, thus **disrupting microtubule assembly and the formation of the mitotic spindle.**
   b. These agents are most active during mitosis at **metaphase,** blocking chromosomal migration and cell division.
   c. **Resistance** is often accounted for by increased levels of the ***MDR1* gene product *P*-glycoprotein** that transports drugs out of the cell.
2. ***Selected drugs***
   a. **Vinblastine (Velban, Velsar)**
      (1) Vinblastine is administered IV. Although a marker for its therapeutic effect, **bone marrow suppression with leukopenia** is the dose-limiting toxicity; other adverse effects include **neurologic toxicity,** nausea and vomiting, alopecia, and ulceration from subcutaneous extravasation.
      (2) Vinblastine is used in combination with **bleomycin** and **cisplatin** for **metastatic testicular tumors (the PVB regimen).** However, **etoposide** or **ifosfamide** have supplanted its

use. It also is used for various lymphomas, including **Hodgkin disease (the ABVD regimen),** and several solid tumors.

b. **Vincristine (Oncovin, Vincasar)**
   (1) Vincristine is administered IV; it is **less toxic** to bone marrow than **vinblastine. Peripheral neuropathies** are the dose-limiting toxicities. This agent may also cause severe constipation and alopecia.
   (2) Vincristine is used in combination with prednisone to induce remissions in **childhood leukemia.** It is used in several important combinations (e.g., the **MOPP regimen for advanced Hodgkin disease**) as well as for treatment of **non-Hodgkin lymphoma (the CHOP regimen),** rhabdomyosarcoma, and nephroblastoma. Other uses of this agent are being investigated. It is not cross-resistant with **vinblastine.**

c. **Vinorelbine (Navelbine)**
   (1) Vinorelbine can be given **orally.**
   (2) This agent has an **intermediate toxicity** profile relative to vinblastine and vincristine.
   (3) Vinorelbine is used to treat **non–small-cell lung cancer** and **breast and cervical cancer.**

B. Taxanes: paclitaxel (Taxol) and docetaxel (Taxotere)

1. Paclitaxel **stabilizes microtubule formation** to disassembly with **arrest in mitosis.**
2. Paclitaxel shows activity in **ovarian cancer** and in **breast** and **non–small-cell lung cancer,** and **Kaposi sarcoma. Docetaxel** is also used in **androgen-refractory prostate cancer.**
3. This agent is administered **IV.**
4. ***Resistance*** is associated with expression of ***P*-glycoprotein.**
5. **Myelosuppression and peripheral neuropathies** are the dose-limiting toxicities. Paclitaxel also causes **hypersensitivity** specific to the vehicle (50% polyethoxylated castor oil and 50% ethanol) used for its administration. Co-administration of an histamine H_1-receptor antagonist (e.g., diphenhydramine), a histamine H_2-receptor antagonist (e.g., cimetidine), and dexamethasone reduces the incidence of hypersensitivity.

C. Epipodophyllotoxins

1. ***Structure and mechanism of action***
   a. Epipodophyllotoxins are bulky, semisynthetic, multiringed structures derived from the mayapple plant. They block cells at the boundary of the S phase and **prevent entry into the G_2 phase.**
   b. These agents act by forming a ternary complex with **topoisomerase II** and DNA, resulting in **double-stranded DNA breaks.**
2. ***Etoposide (VePesid), teniposide (Vumon)***
   a. These drugs are administered IV. **Leukopenia** is the dose-limiting toxicity.
   b. Etoposide is used for recalcitrant **testicular tumors** and, in combination with cisplatin, for **small-cell lung carcinoma and AML.** Teniposide is used for **ALL.**

D. Antibiotics

1. ***Dactinomycin (actinomycin D) (Cosmegen)***
   a. **Structure and mechanism of action**
      (1) Dactinomycin is a chromophore containing peptides isolated from ***Streptomyces.*** It is one of the most potent cytotoxic agents.
      (2) Dactinomycin **intercalates between adjacent guanosine–cytosine base pairs of the DNA** double helix to form a very stable complex.
      (3) This agent is **phase nonspecific.**
      (4) Dactinomycin strongly **impairs RNA synthesis** and, to a lesser extent, DNA synthesis.
   b. **Pharmacologic properties**
      (1) Dactinomycin is administered by **IV** infusion.
      (2) **Resistance** to this agent is related to the generation of ***P*-glycoprotein,** to increased **glutathione peroxidase** activity, and to decreased activity of **topoisomerase II.**
   c. **Therapeutic uses**
      (1) Dactinomycin is used to treat **rhabdomyosarcoma** and **Wilms tumor in children.** It is also used for **gestational trophoblastic tumor, metastatic testicular carcinoma,** and **Ewing sarcoma.**

(2) This agent has been used in combination with **vincristine** and **cyclophosphamide** for the treatment of solid tumors in children.

d. **Adverse effects. Bone marrow suppression** is the dose-limiting toxicity. Dactinomycin also produces GI disturbances, oral ulcers, and alopecia.

2. ***Doxorubicin (Adriamycin, Doxil), daunorubicin (daunomycin, [Cerubidine]), idarubicin (Idamycin),*** and the analogs of doxorubicin, ***epirubicin (Ellence), valrubium (Valstar), and mitoxantrone (Novantrone)***

a. **Pharmacologic properties**

(1) Doxorubicin, daunorubicin, and idarubicin are **DNA-intercalating agents** that block the **synthesis of DNA and RNA.**

(2) Doxorubicin, daunorubicin, and idarubicin also fragment DNA because of the **inhibition of topoisomerase II** or the **generation of superoxide** anion radicals.

(3) These agents are primarily toxic during the **S phase** of cell cycle.

(4) Doxorubicin, daunorubicin, and idarubicin are all administered **IV.**

(5) Doxorubicin, daunorubicin, and idarubicin produce both **reversible acute and irreversible chronic cardiomyopathies;** the chronic type is related to the cumulative dose of the drug and is the dose-limiting toxicity.

b. **Doxorubicin**

(1) Doxorubicin is one of the most used anticancer agents.

(2) This agent is **myelosuppressive.**

(3) Doxorubicin is used in many standard regimens. It is part of the ABVD regimen (as adriamycin) for **Hodgkin disease,** CHOP regimen (as hydroxydaunomycin) for **non-Hodgkin lymphoma,** CAF regimen (as adriamycin) for **breast carcinoma,** M-VAC regimen for **bladder carcinoma,** and VAD regimen for **multiple myeloma. Other uses** of this agent include leukemias, malignant lymphomas, thyroid malignancies, GI stromal tumors (GIST), ovarian cancer, and small-cell lung cancer, as well as others.

c. **Daunorubicin and idarubicin** are used primarily in the treatment of **acute lymphocytic** and **myelogenous leukemias,** often in combination with cytarabine.

d. **Epirubicin** is used for early stage, as well as metastatic, **breast cancer.**

e. **Valrubicin** is used to treat refractory **urinary bladder cancer.**

f. **Mitoxantrone** is used to treat prostate cancer and **non-Hodgkin lymphoma.**

3. ***Bleomycin (Blenoxane)***

a. **Structure and mechanism of action**

(1) Bleomycin is a mixture of copper-chelating glycopeptides produced by ***Streptomyces verticillus.*** It causes **DNA chain scission and fragmentation.** Cells with chromosomal aberrations accumulate in the G_2 phase of the cell cycle.

(2) Bleomycin is **inactivated by bleomycin hydrolase,** which is found in many tissues—**except skin and lung**—that are major sites of toxicity.

b. **Pharmacologic properties**

(1) Bleomycin is administered **parenterally.** High drug concentrations are found in the **lungs and skin.**

(2) Resistance to bleomycin is mediated by increased levels of hydrolase or increased DNA repair activity.

c. **Therapeutic uses.** Bleomycin is used to treat **testicular carcinoma** (usually in combination with cisplatin and etoposide, or vinblastine and cisplatin, PVB regimen) and **squamous cell carcinomas.** It is also used in combination chemotherapy for **Hodgkin** (ABVD regimen) and **non-Hodgkin lymphomas.**

d. **Adverse effects.** The most serious adverse effect is a cumulative **dose-related pulmonary toxicity** that may be fatal. Bleomycin also causes serious **cutaneous toxicity.** Acute reactions that can be fatal occur in 1% of patients with lymphoma; this reaction consists of the **anaphylactoid-like reactions** of profound hyperthermia, hypotension, and cardiorespiratory collapse.

E. Camptothecins

1. ***Topotecan (Hycamtin)*** is a natural compound derived from *Camptotheca acuminata.* This agent inhibits **topoisomerase I** (an enzyme that allows relaxation and replication of specific regions of supercoiled DNA), thus resulting in **DNA damage.** Topotecan is used for **ovarian cancer** and **small-cell lung cancer.** The main side effect of this drug is **myelosuppression.**

2. ***Irinotecan (Camptosar)*** is another inhibitor of **topoisomerase I**. This agent is used for **metastatic colorectal cancer** in combination with **5-FU and leucovorin.** Toxicity of this drug includes **diarrhea,** which can be severe, and **myelosuppression.**

V. MISCELLANEOUS AGENTS

A. Cisplatin (Platinol) and other platinum compounds

1. ***Structure and mechanism of action***
   a. Cisplatin is a small platinum coordination complex that enters cells by diffusion and active transport. After intracellular replacement of its chloride atoms by water, it acts by **complexing with DNA to form crosslinks.** Adjacent **guanines** are most frequently crosslinked, which leads to the **inhibition of DNA replication and transcription.**
   b. The effect of cisplatin is most prominent during the S phase of the cell cycle.
2. ***Pharmacologic properties.*** Cisplatin is administered **IV.**
3. ***Therapeutic uses.*** Cisplatin is used to treat **testicular tumors** (usually with **bleomycin** and **vinblastine, PVB regimen**), **ovarian carcinomas** (with **doxorubicin**), and **bladder carcinomas.** It is also used for several other carcinomas.
4. ***Adverse effects***
   a. The dose-limiting toxicity of cisplatin is **cumulative damage to the renal tubules** that may be irreversible following high or repeated doses, but which is routinely **prevented by hydration and diuresis** of the patient.
   b. This agent almost always produces **nausea and vomiting.** It is **ototoxic,** with tinnitus and hearing loss, and it also produces **peripheral neuropathy.** Cisplatin is only moderately myelosuppressive.
5. ***Carboplatin (CBDCA, JM-8) (Paraplatin).*** Carboplatin is administered IV for patients with **ovarian cancer,** as well as **non-Hodgkin lymphoma, non–small-cell lung cancer, testicular cancer,** and **transitional cancers of the urinary tract.** This agent has **similar but less severe toxicities** than cisplatin. This dose-limiting toxicity of carboplatin is **myelosuppression.**
6. ***Oxaliplatin*** (Eloxatin) is used for **metastatic colon cancer** in conjunction with **5-FU and leucovorin.** This agent can cause myelosuppression and **peripheral neuropathy.**

B. Procarbazine (Matulane)

1. ***Structure and mechanism of action***
   a. Procarbazine is a substituted hydrazine that needs to be activated metabolically.
   b. Procarbazine produces **chromosomal breaks** and inhibits **DNA, RNA, and protein synthesis.**
2. ***Pharmacologic properties.*** Procarbazine is administered **orally.** It is lipophilic and enters most cells by diffusion; it is **found in the CSF.**
3. ***Therapeutic uses***
   a. Procarbazine is particularly useful in the treatment of **Hodgkin disease** as part of the **MOPP regimen**; it is also active against **non-Hodgkin lymphoma** and **brain tumors.**
   b. Procarbazine has no cross-resistance with other anticancer drugs.
4. ***Adverse effects***
   a. Procarbazine most commonly produces **leukopenia** and **thrombocytopenia,** along with GI disturbances. Myelosuppression is dose dependent.
   b. Procarbazine augments the effects of **sedatives.** It also causes **infertility.**
   c. Procarbazine is a weak **monoamine oxidase inhibitor** that may cause **hypertension,** particularly in the presence of sympathomimetic agents and **food with high tyramine content.**
   d. This agent has a **10% risk of causing acute leukemia.**

C. Hydroxyurea (Hydrea, Droxia)

1. Hydroxyurea inhibits **ribonucleoside diphosphate reductase** (during the S-phase of the cell cycle), which catalyzes the conversion of ribonucleotides to deoxyribonucleotides and is crucial for the **synthesis of DNA.**

2. Hydroxyurea is primarily used in the management of **chronic granulocytic leukemia** and other myeloproliferative disorders. This agent synergizes with radiotherapy.
3. The major adverse effect of hydroxyurea is **hematopoietic depression.**

D. L-asparaginase (Elspar)

1. L-asparaginase is an enzyme that **reduces levels of L-asparaginase,** an amino acid **not synthesized by some tumors,** to **inhibit protein synthesis** and cell division.
2. This agent is **synergistic with methotrexate** when the folic acid analogue is administered prior to L-asparaginase.
3. L-asparaginase is administered **IV or intramuscularly.**
4. This agent is used in **lymphoblastic leukemia** and for the induction of remission in **ALL** (with **vincristine** and **prednisone**).
5. L-asparaginase is **minimally marrow suppressive;** it is toxic to the **liver and pancreas. Hypersensitivity** and anaphylactic shock to the protein may develop. **Hemorrhaging** may occur due to the inhibition of clotting factor synthesis.

E. Bortezomib (Velcade)

1. Bortezomib **inhibits proteosome signaling pathways (NF-KB).** Cancerous cell rely on proteosomes for proliferation as well as metastases.
2. Bortezomib is approved for treatment of **multiple myeloma** in patients who have received at least two prior courses of therapy.
3. GI complaints are the most common side effects of bortezomib, but peripheral neuropathy has also been reported.

F. Biologic agents

1. Biologic response modifiers are compounds that influence how an individual responds to the presence of a neoplasm.
2. Many biologic response modifiers have been produced using recombinant DNA technology, including **tumor necrosis factor, the interferons,** and **the interleukins,** among others.
3. ***Cytokines and cytokine modifiers***
   a. **Interferon alfa-2b (Intron-A)** is approved for treatment of **hairy cell leukemia**, and **Kaposi sarcoma.**
   b. **Interleukin-2 (aldesleukin) (Proleukin)** is approved for metastatic **kidney cancer** and **melanoma.**
   c. **Thalidomide (Thalomid) and lenalidomide (Revlimid)** are **tumor necrosis factor modifiers.** They assist in degradation of THF-α mRNA encoding protein. These agents are used in treatment of **brain tumors, Kaposi sarcoma, multiple myeloma,** and many noncancerous conditions. Thalidomide's most common adverse effects are sedation, constipation, and peripheral neuropathy (30%). **Thalidomide** is also **highly teratogenic. Lenalidomide** is an analog of thalidomide with increased potency and an apparent decreased toxicity.
4. ***Tyrosine kinase inhibitors***
   a. **Imatinib (Gleevec), Dasatinib (Sprycel)**
      (1) Imatinib and dasatinib are **tyrosine kinase inhibitors** that are specific for **Bcr-Abl** oncoprotein (dasatinib also inhibits several other kinases).
      (2) These agents are used for **chronic myelogenous leukemia,** which displays the bcr-abl chromosomal translocation (**Philadelphia chromosome**).
      (3) **Imatinib** has also been used for **GI stromal tumors** (GIST), which express another tyrosine kinase inhibited by Imatinib, **c-kit. Dasatinib** is also used for **ALL.**
      (4) These are oral agents, and their main toxicities are **edema** and nausea and vomiting.
   b. **Gefitinib (Iressa)**
      (1) Gefitinib is an inhibitor of **epidermal growth factor receptor tyrosine kinase** that is overexpressed in many cancers.
      (2) It is approved for use in **non–small-cell lung cancer** where it is generally used with **gemcitabine and cisplatin.**
      (3) Side effects of this oral agent include **severe diarrhea** and **acne** and other skin abnormalities.

c. **Erlotinib (Tarceva)**
   (1) Erlotinib is another inhibitor of **epidermal growth factor receptor tyrosine kinase.**
   (2) This agent is used for **non–small-cell lung cancer** in patients who have failed at least one trial of prior chemotherapy, and **advanced pancreatic cancer.**
   (3) **Rash, diarrhea,** and **cough** are common side effects of this oral agent.

5. ***Monoclonal antibodies (MABs)***
   a. **Rituximab (Rituxan)**
      (1) Rituximab is a chimeric (human/mouse) **antibody to IgG** that binds to **CD20 antigen on B cells.** This antigen is overexpressed on B cells of non-Hodgkin lymphoma tissues. The net effect of this interaction is **cell lysis,** possibly secondary to antibody-dependent cytotoxicity or complement cytotoxicity.
      (2) This agent is used for relapsed **non-Hodgkin lymphoma** (R-CHOP regimen). It is also used for **mantle cell lymphoma.**
      (3) Dermatologic and GI side effects are most common; however, neutropenia has been reported.
   b. **Trastuzumab (Herceptin)**
      (1) Trastuzumab is a humanized **IgG antibody** against the **epidermal growth factor receptor, HER2/neu,** which is overexpressed in 25%–30% of breast cancers. Expression of this protein is associated with **decreased survival due to more aggressive disease.** The net effect is the **arrest of the cell cycle** via antibody-mediated cytotoxicity.
      (2) This agent is used in **HER2/neu-positive metastatic breast cancers** in combination with **paclitaxel.** It is also used after the first-line therapy has failed.
      (3) Diarrhea and hematologic effects are most common.
   c. **Cetuximab (Erbitux)**
      (1) Cetuximab is a chimeric human–mouse **IgG antibody to epidermal growth factor receptor (EGFR).** Its mechanism of action differs from that of **imatinib** in that cetuximab actually **blocks the receptor.** The action of this drug results in **inhibition of cancer cell growth** and **induction of apoptosis. Overexpression** of EGFR in colorectal cancer is associated with **decreased survival** and overall poor prognosis.
      (2) Cetuximab is currently approved for **EGFR-expressing metastatic colon cancer** alone or in combination with **irinotecan.**
      (3) The most common effect is rash that may be severe.
   d. **Bevacizumab (Avastin)**
      (1) Bevacizumab is the first humanized **IgG directed against human vascular endothelial growth factor (VEGF) interaction with its receptors (VEGFR1, VEGFR2),** which are involved in **angiogenesis,** an important process in cancer proliferation and metastasis.
      (2) This agent is approved for **metastatic colon cancer in combination with 5-FU.**
      (3) Toxicities are mainly dermatologic and GI, but can include proteinuria, hypertension, and congestive heart failure. Reports implicate this agent in rare cases of **bowel perforation.**

VI. STEROID HORMONE AGONISTS AND ANTAGONISTS AND RELATED DRUGS

General properties of steroid hormones and their antagonists are covered in Chapter 10. Their use in malignancy is considered here.

A. **Use in neoplasia.** Use of these agents in neoplasia is predicated on the **presence of steroid hormone receptors in target cells** and on the ability of the hormone to stimulate or inhibit cell growth. In the former case, hormonal antagonists are used; in the latter, hormonal agonists.

B. **Adrenocorticosteroids (e.g., prednisone, hydroxycortisone, dexamethasone)**
   1. Adrenocorticosteroids are **lymphocytic and antimitotic agents.**

2. Adrenocorticosteroids can be administered orally. They are useful in **acute leukemia** in children, **malignant lymphoma**, and both **Hodgkin and non-Hodgkin lymphoma** (CHOP and MOPP regimens).
3. Adrenocorticosteroids have significant systemic effects, and long-term use is not recommended.

C. Mitotane (*o,p*′-DDD) (Lysodren)

1. Mitotane is an oral agent specific for the treatment of **inoperable adrenocortical carcinoma.**
2. Mitotane **inhibits glucocorticoid biosynthesis** and selectively causes atrophy of the tumors within zona reticularis and fasciulata by an unknown mechanism.
3. Nausea, vomiting, lethargy, and dermatitis are common side effects. **CNS depression** is the dose-limiting toxicity.

D. Progestins are useful in the management of **endometrial hyperplasia and carcinoma** and as second-line therapy for metastatic hormone-dependent breast cancer. **Megestrol (Megace)** is an example. This agent is also useful to stimulate appetite in patients with cancer and AIDS-related **cachexia.**

E. Estrogens

1. Estrogens inhibit the effects of endogenous androgens and androgen-dependent metastatic **prostatic carcinoma.** Rarely, estrogens are used for **palliative purposes in metastatic breast cancer. Diethylstilbestrol** is usually the agent of choice.
2. Estrogens are more effective when combined with **orchiectomy.**
3. **Cardiac and cerebrovascular complications** and **carcinoma of breast, endometrium, and ovary** are potential adverse effects.

F. SERMS: Tamoxifen (Nolvadex), Toremifene (Fareston), Raloxifen (Evista)

1. The SERMS (**selective estrogen receptor modulators**) are drugs that have estrogen receptor agonist or antagonist properties depending on the target tissue. In the breast, tamoxifen and toremifene and raloxifen are estrogen antagonists.
2. These agents inhibit estrogen-dependent cellular proliferation and may increase the production of the growth inhibitor TGF-β (transforming growth factor-beta)
3. These agents are administered orally and reach **steady-state in 4–6 weeks.**
4. Tamoxifen and toremifene are used in postmenopausal women with or recovering from **metastatic breast cancer.** They are effective in patients who have **estrogen receptor–positive** tumors. They have no effect in ER-negative tumors. Recommended treatment duration is 5 years.
5. Tamoxifen is also used as **adjunctive therapy to oophorectomy and to leuprolide or goserelin** (see below) in premenopausal women with estrogen receptor-positive tumors.
6. Tamoxifen and raloxifen are used as **prophylactic** agents in women at high risk for breast cancer.
7. Moderate nausea, vomiting, and **hot flashes** are the major adverse effects of tamoxifen; **endometrial cancer and thrombosis** are potential adverse effects of long-term therapy.

G. Pure antiestrogens, Fulvestrant (Faslodex)

Fulvestrant is a pure anti-estrogen; it has no agonist activity in any tissue. It is approved for use in hormone **receptor positive metastatic breast cancer in postmenopausal women** with disease progression following antiestrogen therapy

H. Gonadotropin-releasing hormone analogues: leuprolide (Lupron), triptorelin (Trelstar), and goserelin (Zoladex)

1. These agents are peptides that, on long-term administration, **inhibit luteinizing hormone (LH) and follicle-stimulating hormone (FSH) secretion** from the pituitary and reduce the circulating levels of gonadotropins, and consequently estrogen and testosterone. Use of these agents results in **castration** levels of testosterone in men and **postmenopausal levels of estrogen** in women.

2. These agents are effective in **prostatic carcinoma and in estrogen-positive breast cancer.**
3. **Initial administration** of these agents, before pituitary-receptor desensitization occurs, may result in **increased LH and FSH release,** with a transitory increase in testosterone and an **exacerbation of disease.** Leuprolide and goserelin are often administered with antiandrogen **flutamide** (Eulexin) or **bicalutamide** (Casodex), which **block the translocation of androgen receptors to the nucleus** and thereby prevent testosterone action.

I. **Aromatase inhibitors: Anastrozole (Arimidex), Letrozole (Femara), Exemestane (Aromasin), Aminoglutethimide (Cytadren)**

1. The American Society of Clinical Oncology recommends that that every postmenopausal woman with ER-positive breast cancer receive adjuvant aromatase inhibitor therapy.
2. ***Anastrozole*** and ***letrozole*** are reversible aromatase inhibitors that have no effect on synthesis of steroids other than estrogens. They are used as an adjunct for **postmenopausal women with ER-positive early breast cancer,** women with breast cancer who have progressed on tamoxifen, and as first-line treatment of ER-positive or ER-unknown **advanced local breast cancer.** Anastozole is approved for use in women who have received 2–3 years of tamoxifen and are switching to anastrazole for a total of 5 years of adjunct therapy. Recent studies have shown that anastrozole offers advantage over tamoxifen in these circumstances. An adverse effect of these drugs is **hot flashes and vasomotor symptoms.** Long-term effects include **osteopenia** and **osteoporosis. Alendronate** is a useful adjunct for both drugs.
3. ***Exemestane*** inhibits aromatase irreversibly. This agent is used for **postmenopausal women with breast cancer** who have progressed on tamoxifen. It is also approved for up to 5 years of use for women switching from tamoxifen. Exemestane does not exhibit cross-resistance with other aromatase inhibitors. Side-effect profile includes **hot flashes** and fatigue.
4. ***Aminoglutethimide*** inhibits **corticosteroid synthesis** as well as the enzyme aromatase, which aids in conversion of androstenedione to estrone. This agent is used in treatment of **metastatic receptor-positive breast cancer** (both estrogen and progestin receptors); it has also been used in **prostate cancer. Hydrocortisone** has to be administered at the same time **to prevent adrenal insufficiency.** This agent is oral but its lack of specificity has reduced its overall use.
5. All of the above agents are **thrombolemic** but with a reduced incidence compared to tamoxifen.

J. **Androgen antagonists: flutamide (Eulexin), bicalutamide (Casodex), nilutamide (Nilandron)**

1. ***Flutamide and bicalutamide*** are competitive antagonists of the androgen receptor; nilutamide is an irreversible inhibitor of the androgen receptor.
2. These agents are used in combination **with either chemical or surgical castration** for the treatment of prostate cancer.
3. ***Adverse effects*** are due to decreased androgen activity and include fatigue, **loss of libido, and impotence**. Other adverse effects are decreased hepatic function and GI disturbances.

VII. ADJUNCT AGENTS

A. **Leucovorin** (folinic acid, [Fusilev]) is a form of folate that is used to "**rescue**" patients from **methotrexate toxicity** (Fig. 12-3) as well as in combination regimens with 5-FU.

B. **Filgrastim (Neupogen)** and **pegfilgastim** (Neulasta) are recombinant human granulocyte colony–stimulating hormone (G-CSF) agents that **increase neutrophil production** and are used for prophylaxis and treatment of chemotherapy-induced **neutropenia.**

C. **Sargramostim (Leukine),** a recombinant human granulocyte/macrophage colony– stimulating hormone (GM-CSF), is used to **assist graft recovery** in patients undergoing bone marrow transplantation.

D. **Epoetin alfa (Epogen)** and **darbepoetin alfa (Aranesp)** are used in **anemia** caused by chemotherapy or renal failure. They are analogs of erythropoietin.

E. **Allopurinol (Zyloprim, Alloprim)** is a purine analog. It **inhibits xanthine oxidase** and is frequently used during chemotherapy to **prevent acute tumor cell lysis** that results in severe hyperuricemia and nephrotoxicity.

F. **Oprelvekin (Neumega)** is a recombinant **interleukin** that is indicated for chemotherapy-induced **thrombocytopenia** as well as for prophylaxis of this potentially dangerous complication.

G. **Amifostine (Ethyol)** is a **cytoprotective agent** that is dephosphorylated to active free thiol, which then acts as a **scavenger of free radicals.** It is used to **reduce renal toxicity** associated with **cisplatin** therapy. It is also used to **reduce xerostoma** in patients undergoing irradiation of head and neck regions.

DRUG SUMMARY TABLE

Alkylating Agents
Mechlorethamine (Mustargen)
Cyclophosphamide (Cytoxan)
Ifosfamide (Ifex)
Melphalan (Alkeran)
Chlorambucil (Leukeran)
Busulfan (Myleran)
Carmustine (BiCNU, Gliadel)
Lomustine (CeeNU)
Streptozocin (Zanosar)
Thiotepa (Thioplex)
Dacarbazine
Temozolomide (Temodar)

Antimetabolites
Methotrexate (Trexall)
Pemetrexed (Alimta)
Cytarabine (Cytosar-U)
Fluorouracil (Adrucil)
6-Mercaptopurine (Purinethol)
6-Thioguanine
Cladribine (Leustatin)
Fludarabine (Fludara)
Tretinoin (Vesanoid)

Natural Products
Vinblastine (Velban)
Vincristine (Oncovin)
Vinorelbine (Navelbine)
Paclitaxel (Taxol)
Docetaxel (Taxotere)
Etoposide (Vepesid)
Teniposide (Vumon)
Dactinomycin (Cosmegen)
Doxorubicin (Adriamycin, Doxil)
Daunorubicin (Cerubidine)
Idarubicin (Idamycin)
Epirubicin (Ellence)
Valrubicin (Valstar)
Mitoxantrone (Novantrone)
Bleomycin (Blenoxane)
Topotecan (Hycamtin)
Irinotecan (Camptosar)

Miscellaneous Agents
Cisplatin (Platinol)
Carboplatin (Paraplatin)
Oxaliplatin (Eloxatin)
Procarbazine (Matulane)
Hydroxyurea (Hydrea, Droxia)
l-Asparaginase (Elspar)
Interferon alfa-2b (Intron A)
Aldesleukin (Proleukin)
Thalidomide (Thalomid)
Lenalidomide (Revlimid)
Imatinib (Gleevec)
Dasatinib (Sprycel)
Gefitinib (Iressa)
Erlotinib (Tarceva)
Bortezomib (Velcade)
Rituximab (Rituxan)
Trastuzumab (Herceptin)
Bevacizumab (Avastin)

Steroid Hormones and Antagonists
Mitotane (Lysodren)
Megestrol (Megace)
Diethylstilbestrol
Tamoxifen (Nolvadex)
Toremifene (Fareston)
Raloxifen (Evista)
Fulvestrant (Faslodex)
Leuprolide (Lupron)
Triptorelin (Trelstar)
Goserelin (Zoladex)
Anastrozole (Arimidex)
Letrozole (Femara)
Exemestane (Aromasin)
Aminoglutethimide (Cytadren)
Flutamide (Eulexin)
Bicalutamide (Casodex)
Nilutamide (Nilandron)

Adjunct Agents
Leucovorin (Fusilev)
Filgrastrim (Neupogen)
Pegfilgrastim (Neulasta)
Sargramostim (Leukine)
Epoetin alfa (Epogen/Procrit)
Darbepoetin alfa (Aranesp)
Allopurinol (Alloprim, Zyloprim)
Oprelvekin (Neumega)
Amifostine (Ethyol)

Review Test for Chapter 12

Directions: Each of the numbered items or incomplete statements in this section is followed by answers or by completions of the statement. Select the ONE lettered answer or completion that is BEST in each case.

1. A second-year medical student finds a few hours a week to work in a cancer research laboratory. Her project involves testing various chemotherapy agents (including adriamycin, etoposide, and VP-16) on colon cancer lines established from patient biopsies. She performs Northern blot analysis on multiply resistant cell lines and is likely to find increased expression of what gene?

(A) *bcr-abl*
(B) *EGFR*
(C) *MDR*
(D) *HER2*
(E) *HGPRT*

2. A 25-year-old man presents with recurrent bouts of hypoglycemia with mental status changes that are rapidly reversed by eating. He is not diabetic, and his serum levels of insulin are markedly elevated. His C-peptide levels are also elevated. You begin treating the patient for a presumed insulinoma with which of the following agents?

(A) Cyclophosphamide
(B) Melphalan
(C) Carmustine
(D) Thiotepa
(E) Streptozocin

3. A 73-year-old woman with breast cancer and history of congestive heart failure is placed on a chemotherapy regimen that includes the use of methotrexate (MTX) after her mastectomy. This agent's activity is related to its ability to do what?

(A) Carbamylate intracellular macromolecules
(B) Indirectly inhibit DNA synthesis
(C) Block chromosomal migration and cell differentiation
(D) Complex with DNA to form crosslinks
(E) Inhibit estrogen-dependent tumor growth

4. A 53-year-old man presents with changes in bowel frequency and pencil-thin stools with occasional bright red blood in the stool. A further work-up, including computed tomography (CT) scanning of the chest, abdomen, and pelvis, demonstrates lesions consistent with metastasis in the liver. His therapy will likely include which of the following chemotherapeutic agents?

(A) Carmustine
(B) Fluorouracil
(C) Leuprolide
(D) Temozolamide
(E) Tamoxifen

5. A 53-year-old woman with breast cancer undergoes a breast-conserving lumpectomy and lymph node biopsy. The pathology report returns with mention of cancer cells in two of eight lymph nodes removed. Following radiation therapy, chemotherapy is started that includes the use of paclitaxel. Which side effect is the patient likely to complain of?

(A) Blood in the urine
(B) Easy bruising
(C) Hot flashes
(D) Shortness of breath
(E) Numbness and tingling

6. A 74-year-old man with a 100-pack/year history of smoking is evaluated for hemoptysis. A computed tomography (CT) scan of the chest shows numerous pulmonary nodules. A nodule on the pleural surface is selected for CT-guided biopsy by the interventional radiologist. The biopsy report is small-cell carcinoma of the lung, and chemotherapy containing etoposide is started. This drug works by

(A) Inhibiting topoisomerase II
(B) Inhibiting dihydrofolate reductase
(C) Alkylating double-stranded DNA
(D) Stabilizing microtubules, with resultant mitotic arrest
(E) Causing DNA chain scission and fragmentation

7. A 56-year-old woman with metastatic breast cancer is started on chemotherapy. Her initial treatment will include both cyclophosphamide and doxorubicin. Careful attention is required because of doxorubicin's well-documented toxicity, which is

(A) Hemorrhagic cystitis
(B) Acne
(C) Peripheral neuropathy
(D) Hot flashes
(E) Cardiomyopathy

8. A world-class cyclist was diagnosed with metastatic testicular cancer with lesions in both his lung and brain. He forgoes the standard treatment for his condition because he learns one of the drugs typically used for his condition could ultimately compromise his pulmonary function. Which of the following is included in the standard regimen and is associated with his feared complication?

(A) Cisplatin
(B) Busulfan
(C) Aminoglutethimide
(D) Bleomycin
(E) Cyclophosphamide

9. A 35-year-old otherwise healthy man presents with fullness in the inguinal region with swelling of the ipsilateral leg. A computed tomography (CT) scan demonstrates several confluent enlarged lymph nodes. Biopsy specimens demonstrate malignant $CD20^+$ B cells. A diagnosis of diffuse B-cell lymphoma is made. Which of the following biologics will likely be given to the patient?

(A) Traztuzumab
(B) Rituxan
(C) Dactinomycin
(D) l-Asparaginase
(E) Interferon-α

10. A 17-year-old girl sees her physician for swollen lymph nodes in the supraclavicular region. A core biopsy demonstrates Reed-Sternberg cells and fibrotic bands, a finding characteristic of nodular sclerosis Hodgkin disease. Which of the following combined regimens might be used in this patient?

(A) CHOP
(B) CMF
(C) FOLFOX
(D) BEP
(E) ABVD

11. A 63-year-old postmenopausal woman is diagnosed with early stage breast cancer, which is initially managed by partial mastectomy and radiation therapy. Her tumor was positive for expression of estrogen receptors. Which agent would you recommend to this patient to prevent relapse?

(A) Leuprolide
(B) Hydroxyurea
(C) Anastrozole
(D) Carboplatin
(E) Goserelin

12. A 56-year-old man complains of fatigue and malaise. On physical examination he has significant splenomegaly. His white blood cell count is dramatically elevated, and the physician suspects leukemia. Chromosomal studies indicate a (9:22) translocation, the Philadelphia chromosome, confirming the diagnosis of chronic myelocytic leukemia (CML). Which of the following might be used in his treatment?

(A) Anastrozole
(B) Rituximab
(C) Imatinib
(D) Gefitinib
(E) Amifostine

13. A 37-year-old man presents with changes in bowel habits for the last several months. He complains of small stool caliber along with occasional blood in his stools. Colonoscopy reveals the diagnosis of colon adenocarcinoma. Further work-up demonstrates that there are metastatic lesions in his liver. The oncologist recommends the use of becacizamab. This agent

(A) Inhibits cell cycle progression
(B) Induces differentiation of cells
(C) Blocks signaling by EGFR
(D) Inhibits angiogenesis
(E) Inhibits HER2/neu signaling

14. A 54-year-old woman complains of headaches, nausea, and vomiting. A computed tomography (CT) scan of the head reveals a large mass in the frontal lobe. She underwent surgery to remove the mass, which was shown to be a glioblastoma multiforme (GBM). In addition to receiving radiation, which agent should be given?

(A) Thalidomide
(B) Cisplatin
(C) Thioguanine
(D) Temozolomide
(E) Mercaptopurine

15. A 63-year-old African-American man with a history of prostate cancer had his prostate removed 10 years ago. His prostate-specific antigen levels have begun to rise again, and he complains of back pain, suggesting metastatic disease. A computed tomography (CT) scan demonstrates enlarged paraaortic lymph nodes and osteoblastic lesions of his lumbar spine. Therapy with which agent should be started?

(A) Anastrozole
(B) Leuprolide
(C) Tamoxifen
(D) Mitotane
(E) Prednisone

16. A 56-year-old woman with a significant smoking history was diagnosed with small-cell lung cancer 2 years ago and was successfully treated. Now on follow-up computed tomography (CT) scan there are several new pulmonary nodules, and the oncologist elects to begin second-line chemotherapy with a DNA topoisomerase I inhibitor. Which of the following is such an agent?

(A) Ciprofloxacin
(B) Etoposide
(C) Vinorelbine
(D) Teniposide
(E) Irinotecan

17. A 42-year-old premenopausal woman recently underwent partial mastectomy and radiation therapy for a small tumor in her breast. There were no lymph nodes involved, and the tumor was estrogen-receptor positive. The oncologist explains that there is little advantage to adding systemic chemotherapy in such an early-stage cancer but does recommend that the patient take tamoxifen. Which of the following is a concerning side effect of tamoxifen?

(A) Thromboembolism
(B) Bowel perforation
(C) Aplastic anemia
(D) Myelosuppression
(E) Hypotension

Answers and Explanations

1. **The answer is C.** Gene amplification of the multidrug resistance *(MDR1)* gene is found in many tumors and confers resistance to many chemotherapy agents. *MDR1* encodes a transport protein that actively pumps various chemotherapy agents out of the cell. Although *bcr-abl, EGFR,* and *HER2* may be overexpressed in tumors, they don't necessarily confer resistance to chemotherapy. *HGPRT* is overexpressed in some tumors, but it only confers resistance to methotrexate.

2. **The answer is E.** Streptozocin is toxic to β cells of the islets of Langerhans in the pancreas and is therefore used in the treatment of insulinomas. Melphalan is a derivative of nitrogen mustard used to treat multiple myeloma, melanoma, and carcinoma of the ovary. Carmustine is a drug used to treat neoplasms of the brain, as it has excellent central nervous system (CNS) penetration. Thiotepa is used in the treatment of bladder cancer.

3. **The answer is B.** Methotrexate inhibits the enzyme dihydrofolate reductase, which ultimately decreases the availability of thymidylate to produce DNA. Nitrosureas can carbamylate intracellular molecules. Vinca alkaloids such as vinblastine block chromosomal migration and cellular differentiation. Cisplatin works primarily by complexing with DNA to form crosslinks. Agents like tamoxifen inhibit estrogen-dependent tumor growth.

4. **The answer is B.** Fluorouracil is an important agent in cases of metastatic colon cancer and is part of the FOLFOX regimen. Carmustine is used in the treatment of brain tumors, as is temozolomide. Leuprolide is used to treat hormone-sensitive prostate cancer, and tamoxifen is used to treat breast cancer.

5. **The answer is E.** Paclitaxel is often used in the treatment of breast as well as ovarian and lung cancer. Its main toxicity is myelosuppression and peripheral neuropathy that usually manifests as numbness and tingling in the distal extremities. Blood in the urine can indicate hemorrhagic cystitis, a complication of cyclophosphamide use. Easy bruising can result from mechlorethamine use. Hot flashes are a common complaint in patients using tamoxifen. Shortness of breath can result from pulmonary fibrosis secondary to busulfan or bleomycin use.

6. **The answer is A.** Etoposide is used in the treatment of small-cell lung carcinomas as well as testicular tumors. Its mechanism of action is related to its ability to inhibit topoisomerase II. Methotrexate inhibits dihydrofolate reductase. Alkylating agents include mechlorethamine, cyclophosphamide, and ifosfamide. Paclitaxel and docetaxel stabilize microtubules and thereby disrupt mitosis. Bleomycin causes DNA chain scission and fragmentation.

7. **The answer is E.** Doxorubicin is associated with dose-limiting cardiomyopathy. Before using this agent, a thorough cardiac evaluation is required, including an echocardiogram or nuclear medicine scan of the heart. Hemorrhagic cystitis is a complication of cyclophosphamide, prevented by coadministration of MESNA. Acne is a side effect of prednisone and EGFR inhibitors. Peripheral neuropathy is a result of taxanes such as paclitaxel. Hot flashes often accompany tamoxifen use.

8. **The answer is D.** Bleomycin is included in the treatment of metastatic testicular neoplasms and can cause pulmonary fibrosis. Busulfan can also cause pulmonary fibrosis; however, it is not used in the treatment of testicular neoplasms. Cisplatin is highly emetogenic and can cause nephrotoxicity as well as ototoxicity. Aminoglutethimide is an inhibitor of steroid synthesis used in Cushing syndrome as well as some cases of breast cancer. Cyclophosphamide can cause hemorrhagic cystitis.

9. **The answer is B.** Rituxan is used in conjunction with cyclophosphamide, Hydroxydaunomycin (doxorubicin), Oncovin (vincristine), and prednisone (R-CHOP), one of the regimens for

non-Hodgkin lymphoma. Traztuzumab is used for HER2$^+$ breast cancer. Dactinomycin is a protein synthesis inhibitor used to treat such pediatric tumors as rhabdomyosarcoma and Wilms tumor. l-Asparaginase is a recombinant enzyme used to treat leukemias. Lastly, interferon-α can be used to treat hairy cell leukemia.

10. The answer is E. ABVD is a treatment regimen used for Hodgkin disease and includes adriamycin, bleomycin, vinblastine, and dacarbazine. CHOP is used for Hodgkin disease. CMF, or cyclophosphamide, methotrexate, and fluorouracil, is used for breast cancer. FOLFOX, a regimen that uses fluorouracil, oxaliplatin, and leucovorin, is used in the treatment of colon cancer. BEP (bleomycin, etoposide, and platinum [cisplatin]) is used in the management of metastatic testicular neoplasms.

11. The answer is C. Anastrozole is an aromatase inhibitor used to inhibit estrogen synthesis in the adrenal gland, a principle source in postmenopausal women. Hydroxyurea is used in the treatment of some leukemias as well as myeloproliferative disorders. Leuprolide and goserelin are GNRH antagonists used to treat prostate cancer. Carboplatin is used in the treatment of ovarian cancers and others.

12. The answer is C. Imatinib is an orally active small molecule inhibitor of the oncogenic bcr-abl kinase produced as a result of the Philadelphia chromosome, used to treat CML. It also inhibits the c-Kit receptor and can be used in GI stromal tumors (GISTs). Anastrozole is used in the management of breast cancer. Rituximab is an antibody used in the treatment of non-Hodgkin lymphoma. Gefitinib is an orally active small-molecule inhibitor of the EGF receptor used in the treatment of some lung cancers. Amifostine is used as a radioprotectant with or without cisplatin.

13. The answer is D. Bevacizumab is a monoclonal antibody to vascular endothelial growth factor (VEGF). VEGF is required to provide angiogenesis to a growing tumor, and this antibody prevents this process. Many traditional chemotherapy agents inhibit cell cycle progression at various check points. Isotretinoin is capable of inducing differentiation in some leukemias. There are several agents now available to inhibit EGFR signaling, including gifitinib, cetuximab, and erlotinib. Trastuzumab is also a monoclonal antibody, but it inhibits HER2/neu signaling.

14. The answer is D. Temozolomide is an orally active alkylating agent related to dacarbazine used along with radiation for the treatment of glioblastoma multiforme and other high-grade astrocytomas. Thalidomide is used in the treatment of multiple myeloma. Thioguanine and mercaptopurine are purine analogues that are used primarily in acute lymphoblastic leukemia. Cisplatin is also often used with radiation in tumors of the lung, head, and neck.

15. The answer is B. Leuprolide is used to treat metastatic prostate cancer by decreasing the secretion of luteinizing hormone (LH) and follicle-stimulating hormone (FSH) from the pituitary, leading to decreased testosterone, used by the tumor cells to grow. Anastrozole is used in breast cancer in postmenopausal women to decrease estrogen levels. Tamoxifen is also used in breast cancer to inhibit estrogen-mediated gene transcription. Mitotane is used in the treatment of inoperable adrenocortical carcinomas. Prednisone is used in the treatment of leukemias and lymphomas.

16. The answer is E. Irinotecan and topotecan are two antineoplastic agents that inhibit DNA topoisomerase I. Etoposide and teniposide are epipodophyllotoxins that inhibit DNA topoisomerase II. Ciprofloxacin is an antibiotic that inhibits bacterial DNA topoisomerase I. Vinorelbine is a vinca alkaloid that disrupts microtubule assembly.

17. The answer is A. Patients with estrogen receptor-positive tumors benefit from tamoxifen adjunct treatment. It, however, carries a risk of thromboembolism as well as the potential to develop endometrial cancer. Becazumab has been associated with the risk of bowel perforation. Many traditional chemotherapeutic agents are associated with myelosuppression, and in fact, that is the mechanism for the effects against leukemias. The antibiotic chloramphenicol has been associated with both myelosuppression and aplastic anemia. Many of the therapeutic monoclonal antibodies can cause infusional hypotension.

chapter 13

Toxicology

I. PRINCIPLES AND TERMINOLOGY

A. **Toxicology** is concerned with the deleterious effects of physical and chemical agents (including drugs) in humans (Table 13-1). Toxicity refers to the ability of an agent to cause injury; hazard refers to the likelihood of injury.

1. ***Occupational toxicology*** is concerned with chemicals encountered in the workplace (there are over 100,000 in commercial use). For many of these agents (air pollutants and solvents), **threshold limit values** (TLVs) are defined in either parts per million (ppm) or milligrams per cubic meter (mg/m^3) (Table 13-2). These limits are either time-weighted averages (TLV-TWA; i.e., concentrations for a workday or workweek); short-term exposure limits (TLV-STEL), which reflect the maximum concentration that should not be exceeded in a 15-minute interval; or ceilings (TLV-C), which are the concentrations to which a worker should never be exposed.
2. ***Environmental toxicology*** is concerned with substances encountered in food, air, water, and soil; some chemicals that enter the food chain are defined in terms of their **acceptable daily intake (ADI),** the level at which they are considered safe even if taken daily. **Ecotoxicology** is concerned with the toxic effects of physical and chemical agents on populations and organisms in a defined ecosystem.

B. **The dose–response relationship** implies that higher doses of a drug or toxicant in an individual result in a graded response and that higher doses in a population result in a larger percentage of individuals responding to the agent (quantal dose–response). The most commonly used index of toxicity for drugs used therapeutically is the **therapeutic index** (TI), which is defined as the ratio of the dose of drug that produces a toxic effect (TD_{50}) or a lethal effect (LD_{50}) to the dose that produces a therapeutic effect (ED_{50}) in 50% of the population as determined from quantal dose–response curves for toxicity and therapeutic effect.

C. **Risk and hazard.** Risk is defined as the expected frequency of occurrence of unwanted effects of a physical or chemical agent. Ratios of benefits to risks influence the acceptability of compounds. Hazard is defined as the ability of a toxicant to cause harm in a specific setting; it relates to the amount of a physical or chemical agent to which an individual will be exposed.

D. **NOEL** (no-observable-effect level) is defined as the **highest dose of a chemical that does not produce an observable effect in humans.** This value, based on animal studies, is used for chemicals for which a full dose–response curve for toxicity in humans is unknown or unattainable. The ADI of a chemical according to the World Health Organization (WHO) is the "daily intake of a chemical, which during the entire lifetime appears to be without appreciable risk on the basis of all known facts at that time." ADI values are calculated from NOELs and certain other "uncertainty" factors, including estimated differences in human and animal sensitivity to the toxic agent.

table 13-1 Acute and Evident Changes in the Poisoned Patient and Possible Causes

Changes	Causes
Cardiorespiratory abnormalities	
Hypertension, tachycardia	Amphetamines, cocaine, phencyclidine (PCP), nicotine, antimuscarinic drugs
Hypotension, bradycardia	Opioids, clonidine, β-receptor blocking agents, sedative-hypnotics
Hypotension, tachycardia	Tricyclic antidepressants, phenothiazines, theophylline
Rapid respiration	Sympathomimetics (including amphetamines, salicylates), carbon monoxide, any toxin that produces metabolic acidosis (including alcohol)
Hyperthermia	Sympathomimetics, salicylates, antimuscarinics, most drugs that induce seizures or rigidity
Hypothermia	Alcohol, phenothiazines, sedatives
Central nervous system effects	
Nystagmus, dysarthria, ataxia	Phenytoin, alcohol, sedatives
Rigidity, muscular hypertension	Phencyclidine, haloperidol, sympathomimetics
Seizures	Tricyclic antidepressants, theophylline, isoniazid, phenothiazines
Flaccid coma	Opioids and sedative–hypnotics
Hallucinations	LSD, poisonous plants (nightshade, jimsonweed)
Gastrointestinal changes	
Ileus	Antimuscarinics, narcotics, sedatives
Cramping, diarrhea, increased bowel sounds	Organophosphates, arsenic, iron, theophylline, *Amanita phalloides*
Nausea, vomiting	*Amanita phalloides*
Visual disturbances	
Miosis (constriction)	Clonidine, opioids, phenothiazines, cholinesterase inhibitors (including organophosphate insecticides)
Mydriasis (dilation)	Amphetamines, cocaine, LSD, antimuscarinics (including atropine)
Nystagmus	Phenytoin, alcohol, sedatives (including barbiturates), phencyclidine
Ptosis, ophthalmoplegia	Botulism
Skin changes	
Flushed, hot, dry skin	Antimuscarinics (including atropine)
Excessive sweating	Nicotine, sympathomimetics, organophosphates
Cyanosis	Drugs that induce hypoxemia or methemoglobinemia
Icterus	Hepatic damage from acetaminophen or *Amanita phalloides*
Mouth and taste alterations	Caustic substances
Burns	Garlicky breath: arsenic, organophosphates
Odors	Bitter almond breath; cyanide
	Rotten egg odor: hydrogen sulfide
	Pear-like odor: chloral hydrate
	Chemical smell: alcohol, hydrocarbon solvents, paraldehyde, gasoline, ammonia
Green tongue	Vanadium
Metallic taste	Lead, cadmium

E. **Duration of exposure is used to classify toxic response.**
   1. ***Acute exposure*** resulting in a toxic reaction represents a single exposure or multiple exposures over 1–2 days.
   2. ***Chronic exposure*** resulting in a toxic reaction represents multiple exposures over longer periods of time.
   3. ***Delayed toxicity*** represents the appearance of a toxic effect after a delayed interval following exposure.

F. **Route of exposure** can determine the extent of toxicity and outcome (e.g., **anthrax** exposure).

G. Most toxicants to which humans are exposed (e.g., **heavy metals**) cause toxic effects directly, including binding to functional groups on proteins containing O, S, and N atoms. In other

table 13-2 Threshold Limit Values for Selected Air Pollutants and Solvents

	TLV (ppm)	
	TWA	*STEL*
Air Pollutant		
Carbon monoxide	25	–
Nitrogen dioxide	3	5
Ozone	0.05	–
Sulfur dioxide	2	5
Solvent		
Benzene	0.5	2.5
Carbon tetrachloride	5	10
Chloroform	10	–
Toluene	50	–

instances, in a process referred to as **toxication** (or bioactivation), a substance may be converted in the body to the chemical form that is directly toxic or participates in reactions that generate other highly reactive toxic species, such as **superoxide anion (O_2^-)** and **hydroxyl (OH) free radicals** and **hydrogen peroxide (H_2O_2)**, which can cause DNA, protein, and cell membrane damage and loss of function.

H. Endogenous **glutathione** plays a central role in detoxication of these reactive species either directly, or coupled to **superoxide dismutase** and **glutathione peroxidase** (Fig. 13-1). Superoxide dismutase coupled to **catalase** is also involved in detoxication pathways (Fig. 13-1). Endogenous **metallothionine** offers some limited protection from metal toxicity.

II. AIR POLLUTANTS

A. General characteristics

1. Air pollutants enter the body primarily through inhalation and are either absorbed into the blood (e.g., gases) or eliminated by the lungs (e.g., particulates). Five major agents account for 98% of known air pollutants (see below). Ozone is also of special concern in certain geographic locations.
2. Air pollutants are characterized as either **reducing types** (sulfur oxides) or **oxidizing types** (nitrogen oxides, hydrocarbons, and photochemical oxidants).

B. Carbon monoxide (CO)

1. ***Properties and mechanism of action***
   a. Carbon monoxide is a colorless, odorless, nonirritating gas produced from the incomplete combustion of organic matter. It is the **most frequent cause of death from poisoning** (see Table 13-2 for threshold limit values).
   b. Carbon monoxide competes for and **combines with the oxygen-binding site of hemoglobin to form carboxyhemoglobin,** resulting in a functional anemia. The binding affinity of carbon monoxide for hemoglobin is 220 times higher than that of oxygen itself. Carboxyhemoglobin also interferes with the dissociation in tissues of the remaining oxyhemoglobin.
   c. Carbon monoxide also binds to cellular respiratory cytochromes.
   d. CO concentrations of 0.1% (1,000 ppm) in air will result in 50% carboxyhemoglobinemia. **Smokers** may routinely exceed normal carboxyhemoglobin levels of 1% by up to 10 times.
2. ***Poisoning and treatment***
   a. CO intoxication (>15% carboxyhemoglobin) results in **progressive hypoxia.** Symptoms include headache, dizziness, nausea, vomiting, syncope, seizures, and at carboxyhemoglobin concentrations above 40%, a cherry-red appearance and coma.

b. Chronic low-level exposure may be harmful to the cardiovascular system. Populations at special risk include smokers with ischemic heart disease or anemia, the elderly, and the developing fetus.

c. **Treatment** includes removal from the source of CO, maintenance of respiration, and administration of oxygen. Hyperbaric oxygen may be required in severe poisoning.

C. Sulfur dioxide (SO_2)

1. *Properties and mechanism of action*

a. Sulfur dioxide is a colorless, irritant gas produced by the combustion of sulfur-containing fuels (see Table 13-2 for threshold limit values).

b. Sulfur dioxide is converted to some extent in the atmosphere to **sulfuric acid** (H_2SO_4), which has irritant effects similar to those of sulfur dioxide.

2. *Poisoning and treatment*

a. At low levels (5 ppm), SO_2 has irritant effects on exposed membranes (eyes, mucous membranes, skin, and upper respiratory tract with bronchoconstriction). Asthmatics are more susceptible. **Delayed pulmonary edema** may be observed after severe exposure.

b. SO_2 poisoning is treated by therapeutic interventions that reduce irritation of the respiratory tract.

D. Nitrogen dioxide (NO_2)

1. *Properties and mechanism of action*

a. Nitrogen dioxide is an irritant brown gas produced in fires and from decaying silage. It also is produced from a reaction of nitrogen oxide (from auto exhaust) with O_2 (see Table 13-2 for threshold limit values).

b. Nitrogen dioxide causes the degeneration of alveolar type I cells, with rupture of alveolar capillary endothelium.

2. *Poisoning and treatment*

a. Acute symptoms include irritation of eyes and nose, coughing, dyspnea, and chest pain.

b. Severe exposure may in 1–2 hours result in **pulmonary edema** that may subside and then recur more than 2 weeks later. Chronic low-level exposure also may result in pulmonary edema.

c. NO_2 poisoning is treated with therapeutic interventions that reduce pulmonary irritation and edema.

E. Ozone (O_3)

1. *Properties and mechanism of action*

a. Ozone is an irritating, naturally occurring bluish gas found in high levels in polluted air and around high-voltage equipment (see Table 13-2 for threshold limit values).

b. Ozone is formed by a complex series of reactions involving NO_2 absorption of ultraviolet light with the generation of free oxygen.

c. Ozone causes functional pulmonary changes similar to those with NO_2. Toxicity may result from free radical formation.

2. *Poisoning and treatment*

a. Ozone irritates mucous membranes and can cause decreased pulmonary compliance, pulmonary edema, and increased sensitivity to bronchoconstrictors. Chronic exposure may cause decreased respiratory reserve, bronchitis, and pulmonary fibrosis.

b. Treatment is similar to that used in NO_2 poisoning.

F. Hydrocarbons

1. Hydrocarbons are oxidized by sunlight and by incomplete combustion to short-lived aldehydes such as **formaldehyde** and **acrolein;** aldehydes are also found in, and can be released from, certain construction materials.

2. Hydrocarbons irritate the mucous membranes of the respiratory tract and eyes, producing a response similar to that seen with SO_2 exposure.

G. Particulates

1. Inhalation of particulates can lead to **pneumoconiosis,** most commonly caused by **silicates (silicosis)** or **asbestos (asbestosis). Bronchial cancer** and **mesothelioma** are associated with asbestos exposure, particularly in conjunction with cigarette smoking.
2. Particulates adsorb other toxins, such as polycyclic aromatic hydrocarbons, and deliver them to the respiratory tract.
3. Particulates also increase susceptibility to pulmonary dysfunction and disease. They may yield fibrotic masses in the lungs that develop over years of exposure.

III. SOLVENTS

A. Aliphatic and halogenated aliphatic hydrocarbons

1. Aliphatic and halogenated aliphatic hydrocarbons include fuels and industrial solvents such as ***n*-hexane, gasoline, kerosene, carbon tetrachloride, chloroform,** and **tetrachloroethylene** (see Table 13-2 for threshold limit values).
2. These agents are central nervous system (CNS) depressants and cause neurologic, liver, and kidney damage. Cardiotoxicity is also possible.
3. ***Polyneuropathy*** from cytoskeletal disruption predominates with ***n*-hexane** poisoning. **Neural effects,** such as memory loss and peripheral neuropathy, predominate with **chloroform** and **tetrachloroethylene** exposure. **Chloroform** also causes **nephrotoxicity.**
4. ***Hepatotoxicity*** (delayed) and **renal toxicity** are common with **carbon tetrachloride** poisoning. **Carcinogenicity** has been associated with **chloroform, carbon tetrachloride,** and **tetrachloroethylene.** All of these effects may be mediated by free radical interaction with cellular lipids and proteins.
5. ***Chloroform*** can sensitize the heart to **arrhythmias.**
6. Aspiration with chemical pneumonitis and pulmonary edema is common.
7. ***Treatment*** is primarily supportive and is oriented to the organ systems involved.

B. Aromatic hydrocarbons

1. ***Benzene.*** Of this class of solvents, benzene poisoning is **most common; CNS depression is the major acute effect.** Chronic exposure can result in severe bone marrow depression, resulting in aplastic anemia and other blood dyscrasias. Low-level benzene exposure has been linked to leukemia. No specific treatment is available for benzene poisoning.
2. ***Toluene*** depresses the CNS. It can cause fatigue and ataxia at relatively low levels (800 ppm), and loss of consciousness at high levels (10,000 ppm).

C. Polychlorinated biphenyls (PCBs)

1. PCBs are stable, highly lipophilic agents that were used industrially before 1977 but still persist in the environment.
2. Dermatologic disorders, reproductive dysfunction, and carcinogenic effects linked to PCBs may be largely due to other contaminating polychlorinated agents such as the **dioxin,** 2,3,7,8-tetrachlorodibenzo-p-dioxin (**TCDD**).

IV. INSECTICIDES AND HERBICIDES

A. Organophosphorus insecticides

1. ***Properties and mechanism of action***
   a. Organophosphorus insecticides include **parathion, malathion,** and **diazinon.**
   b. As insecticides, these agents are preferred over chlorinated hydrocarbons because they do not persist in the environment. However, the potential for acute toxicity is higher.

c. Organophosphorus insecticides are characterized by their ability to **phosphorylate the active esteratic site of acetylcholinesterase (AChE).** Toxic effects result from acetylcholine (ACh) accumulation (see Chapter 2).
d. These agents are well absorbed through the skin and via the respiratory and gastrointestinal (GI) tracts.
e. Some other organophosphate insecticide compounds (e.g., **triorthocresyl phosphate**) also phosphorylate a "neuropathy target esterase," which results in **delayed neurotoxicity** with sensory and motor disturbances of the limbs.

2. ***Treatment of poisoning***
   a. Assisted respiration and decontamination are needed as soon as possible to prevent the irreversible inhibition ("aging") of AChE, which involves strengthening of the phosphorus-enzyme bond.
   b. **Atropine** reverses all muscarinic effects but does not reverse neuromuscular activation or paralysis.
   c. **Pralidoxime** (2-PAM) (Protopam) reactivates AChE, particularly at the neuromuscular junction. It often is used as an adjunct to **atropine** (may reverse some toxic effects); however, it is most effective in **parathion** poisoning.

B. Carbamate insecticides

1. Carbamate insecticides include, among others, **carbaryl, carbofuran, isolan,** and **pyramat.**
2. These agents are characterized by their ability to **inhibit AChE by carbamoylation.**
3. Carbamate insecticides produce toxic effects similar to those of the phosphorus-containing insecticides. Generally, the toxic effects of carbamate compounds are less severe than those of the organophosphorus agents because carbamoylation is rapidly reversible.
4. ***Pralidoxime*** therapy is not an effective antidote because it does not interact with carbamylated acetylcholinesterase.

C. Chlorinated hydrocarbon insecticides

1. Chlorinated hydrocarbons include **dichlorodiphenyltrichloroethane (DDT)** and its derivatives; **benzene hexachlorides,** including **lindane;** cyclodienes such as **dieldrin** and **chlordane;** and **toxaphenes.**
2. These agents are absorbed through the skin, lungs, and GI tract to varying degrees.
3. Chlorinated hydrocarbons persist in the environment after application. The use of chlorinated hydrocarbons is limited in many countries.
4. These agents **inactivate the sodium channel of excitable membranes,** resulting in repetitive neuronal firing with **paresthesias, tremor,** or **seizures.** No specific treatment for poisoning with chlorinated hydrocarbons exists.

D. Botanical insecticides

1. ***Nicotine*** stimulates nicotinic receptors and results in membrane depolarization. Poisoning is characterized by salivation, vomiting, muscle weakness, seizures, and respiratory arrest; it can be treated with anticonvulsants and agents for symptomatic relief (see Chapters 2 and 5).
2. ***Pyrethrum,*** a common household insecticide, is toxic only at high levels. Allergic manifestations are the most common adverse effect.
3. ***Rotenone*** poisoning is rare in humans and generally results in GI disturbances that are treated symptomatically.

E. E. Herbicides

1. ***Paraquat***
   a. Paraquat causes acute GI irritation with bloody stools, followed by delayed respiratory distress and the development of **congestive hemorrhagic pulmonary edema,** which is thought to be caused by superoxide radical formation and subsequent cell membrane disruption. Death may ensue several weeks after ingestion.
   b. Treatment consists of prompt gastric lavage; administration of cathartics and adsorbents benefits some victims.
2. ***2,4-Dichlorophenoxyacetic acid (2,4-D) and related compounds*** cause neuromuscular paralysis and coma. Long-term toxic effects are rare. Dioxin contaminants may be responsible for some of the toxic effects that have been observed (e.g., in "Agent Orange").

V. FUMIGANTS AND RODENTICIDES

A. Cyanide

1. Cyanide possesses a high affinity for ferric iron; it **reacts with iron and cytochrome oxidase** in mitochondria to inhibit cellular respiration, thereby blocking oxygen use.
2. ***Poisoning***
   a. Cyanide is absorbed from all routes (except alkali salts, which are toxic only when ingested).
   b. Cyanide causes transient CNS stimulation followed by **hypoxic seizures** and death.
   c. Cyanide poisoning is signaled by bright red venous blood and a characteristic **odor of bitter almonds.**
3. ***Treatment***
   a. Treatment must be immediate with administration of 100% oxygen.
   b. **Amyl or sodium nitrite,** which oxidizes hemoglobin and produces methemoglobin, which effectively competes for cyanide ion, can also be administered.
   c. **Sodium thiosulfate** can be administered to accelerate the conversion of cyanide to nontoxic thiocyanate by mitochondrial rhodanase (sulfurtransferase).

B. Warfarin

1. Warfarin is one of the most frequently used rodenticides; it also is used as an anticoagulant.
2. Warfarin antagonizes the action of vitamin K in the synthesis of clotting factors.
3. This agent induces bleeding and hemorrhagic conditions on repeated ingestion of high doses; these effects can be reversed with **phytonadione (vitamin K_1).**

C. Strychnine

1. Strychnine competitively **blocks the postjunctional glycine inhibition of neuronal activity,** resulting in CNS excitation and seizures, including dramatic and violent contractions of voluntary muscle. Death is by **respiratory paralysis.**
2. Poisoning must be treated immediately; treatment includes support of respiration, and **diazepam** administration to prevent seizures.

D. Thallium

1. Acute thallium poisoning results in GI irritation, motor paralysis, and respiratory arrest.
2. Chronic exposure to thallium results in hair loss (alopecia) and reddening of the skin. Liver, kidney, and brain damage with prominent neurologic symptoms and encephalopathy can occur.
3. Treatment includes the administration of oral **ferric ferrocyanide (Prussian blue),** which binds thallium in the GI tract and increases its fecal excretion. Hemodialysis and forced diuresis are also used.

VI. HEAVY METAL POISONING AND MANAGEMENT

A. Lead

1. ***Inorganic lead poisoning***
   a. Historically, paint and gasoline were major sources of lead exposure and still can be found in the environment. Other sources of inorganic lead include "home crafts" such as pottery and jewelry making.
   b. Inorganic metallic lead oxides and salts are slowly absorbed through all routes except the skin. Organic lead compounds are also well absorbed across the skin. The GI route is the most common route of exposure in nonindustrial settings (children absorb a higher fraction than adults); the respiratory route is more common for industrial exposure.
   c. Inorganic lead binds to hemoglobin in erythrocytes, with the remainder distributing to soft tissues such as the brain and kidney. Through redistribution, it later accumulates in bone, where its elimination half-life is 20–30 years.
   d. Chronic exposure results in the **inhibition of δ-aminolevulinic acid dehydratase** and a block in the conversion of δ-aminolevulinic acid to porphobilinogen (see Fig. 13-1). This leads to

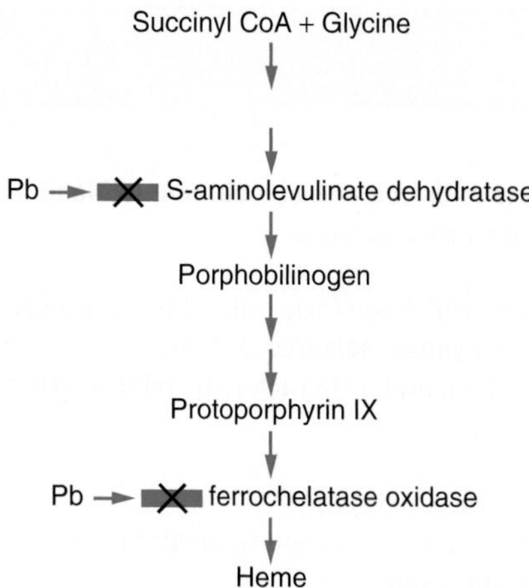

FIGURE 13-1. Inhibition of heme synthesis by lead (Pb).

anemia. Ferrochelatase is also inhibited, resulting in the accumulation of protoporphyrin IX. Lead also increases erythrocyte fragility.

e. **CNS effects** (lead encephalopathy) are common after chronic exposure to lead, particularly in children, for whom no threshold level has been established. Early signs of poisoning include vertigo, ataxia, headache, restlessness, and irritability; **wristdrop** is a common sign of **peripheral neuropathy.** Projectile vomiting, delirium, and seizures may occur with the progression of encephalopathy with lead concentrations >100 μg/dL. Mental deterioration with lowered IQ and behavioral abnormalities may be a consequence of childhood exposure.

f. GI upset, including epigastric distress, is also seen, particularly in adults. Constipation and a metallic taste are early signs of exposure to lead. Intestinal spasm with severe pain (lead colic) may become evident in advanced stages of poisoning. Renal fibrosis may also occur with chronic exposure. Lead also may increase spontaneous abortion. It is associated with altered production of sperm.

2. ***Organic lead poisoning***

a. Organic lead poisoning is increasingly rare due to phased elimination of tetraethyl and tetramethyl lead (antiknock components in gasoline). Both agents are highly volatile and are absorbed through the skin and respiratory tract, often from sniffing gasoline.

b. **Acute CNS abnormalities** (hallucinations, headaches, and insomnia) are generally seen.

3. ***Treatment***

a. Treatment requires the termination of exposure and supportive care.

b. **Chelation therapy:** Severe exposures are generally treated with **calcium disodium EDTA** (ethylenediamine tetraacetic acid versenate) or **dimercaprol** (BAL); less severe cases may be treated with **penicillamine** (Cuprimine, Depen).

B. Arsenic

1. ***Inorganic arsenic***

a. **Properties and mechanism of action**

(1) Inorganic arsenic can be found in coal and metal ores, herbicides, seafood, and drinking water.

(2) Inorganic arsenic is absorbed through the GI tract and lungs.

(3) Trivalent forms (arsenites) of inorganic arsenic are more toxic than the pentavalent forms (arsenates).

(4) **Arsenites inhibit sulfhydryl enzymes** (pyruvate dehydrogenase/glycolysis is especially sensitive), resulting in damage to the epithelial lining of the GI and respiratory tracts and damage to tissues of the nervous system, liver, bone marrow, and skin.

(5) **Arsenates uncouple mitochondrial oxidative phosphorylation by "substituting" for inorganic phosphate.**

b. **Acute poisoning**

(1) Symptoms include severe nausea, vomiting, abdominal pain, laryngitis, and bronchitis; capillary damage with dehydration and shock may occur. Diarrhea is characterized as **"rice-water stools."** There is often a garlicky breath odor.

(2) Initial episodes of arsenic poisoning may be fatal; if the individual survives, bone marrow depression, severe neuropathy, and encephalopathy may occur.

c. **Chronic poisoning**

(1) Chronic poisoning may result in weight loss due to GI irritation; perforation of the nasal septum; hair loss; sensory neuropathy; depression of bone marrow function; and kidney and liver damage. The skin often appears pale and milky ("milk and roses" complexion) because of anemia and vasodilation. Skin pigmentation, hyperkeratosis of the palms and soles, and white lines over the nails may be observed after prolonged exposure.

(2) Inorganic arsenicals have been implicated in cancers of the respiratory system.

d. **Treatment** is primarily supportive after acute poisoning and involves emesis, gastric lavage, rehydration, and restoration of electrolyte imbalance. Chelation therapy with **dimercaprol** (BAL) or its analogue, **unithol,** is indicated in severe cases. **Succimer**, another derivative of dimercaprol, may also be used.

2. ***Organic arsenicals and treatment***

a. Organic arsenicals are excreted more readily and are less toxic than inorganic forms; poisoning is rare.

b. **Arsine gas** (AsH_3) poisoning may occur in industrial settings. The effects are **severe hemolysis** and subsequent renal failure; symptoms include jaundice, dark urine, and severe abdominal pain.

c. Treatment includes **transfusion** and **hemodialysis** for renal failure. Chelation therapy is ineffective.

C. Mercury

1. ***Inorganic mercury***

a. **Properties and mechanism of action**

(1) Inorganic mercury occurs as a potential hazard primarily because of occupational or industrial exposure. The major source of poisoning is by consumption of contaminated food.

(2) **Elemental mercury (Hg)** is poorly absorbed by the GI tract but is volatile and can be absorbed by the lungs. Hg itself causes CNS effects; the ionized form, $\mathbf{Hg^{2+}}$, accumulates in the kidneys and causes damage in the proximal tubules by combining with sulfhydryl enzymes.

(3) **Mercuric chloride ($HgCl_2$)** is well absorbed by the GI tract and is toxic.

(4) **Mercurous chloride (HgCl)** is also absorbed by the GI tract but is less toxic than $HgCl_2$.

b. **Acute poisoning and treatment**

(1) **Mercury vapor** poisoning produces chest pain, shortness of breath, nausea, vomiting, and a metallic taste. Chemical pneumonitis and gingivostomatitis may also occur. Muscle tremor and psychopathology can develop.

(2) **Inorganic mercury salts**

(a) Inorganic mercury salts cause hemorrhagic gastroenteritis producing intense pain and vomiting. Hypovolemic shock may also occur.

(b) **Renal tubular necrosis** is the most prevalent and serious systemic toxicity.

c. **Treatment** involves removal from exposure, supportive care, and chelation therapy with **dimercaprol, unithol,** or **succimer.** Hemodialysis may be necessary.

d. **Chronic poisoning**

(1) **Mercury vapor** poisoning may lead to a **fine tremor** of the limbs that may progress to choreiform movements, and **neuropsychiatric symptoms** that may include insomnia, fatigue, anorexia, and memory loss, as well as changes in mood and affect. **Gingivostomatitis** is also common. Erethism (a combination of excessive perspiration and blushing) may also occur. Excessive salivation and gingivitis are often present.

(2) **Inorganic mercury salts.** Renal injury predominates. Erythema of extremities (**acrodynia**) is often coupled with anorexia, tachycardia, and GI disturbances.

2. ***Organic mercurials (methylmercury)***
   a. Organic mercurials are found in seed dressings and fungicides.
   b. Organic mercurials can be absorbed from the GI tract and often distribute to the CNS, where they exert their toxic effects, including paresthesias, ataxia, and hearing impairment. **Visual disturbances** often predominate.
   c. Exposure of the fetus to methylmercury in utero may result in mental retardation and a syndrome resembling cerebral palsy.
   d. Treatment is primarily supportive.

D. **Iron** (see Chapter 7)

E. **Metal-chelating agents**

1. ***General properties***
   a. Metal-chelating agents usually contain two or more electronegative groups that form stable coordinate-covalent complexes with cationic metals that can then be excreted from the body. The greater the number of metal–ligand bonds, the more stable the complex and the greater the efficiency of the chelator.
   b. These agents contain functional groups such as -OH, -SH, and -NH, which compete for metal binding with similar groups on cell proteins. Their effects are generally greater when administered soon after exposure.
2. ***EDTA (ethylenediamine tetraacetic acid)***
   a. EDTA is an efficient chelator of many transition metals. Because it can also chelate body calcium, **EDTA** is administered intramuscularly or by intravenous (IV) infusion as the **disodium salt of calcium.**
   b. EDTA is rapidly excreted by glomerular filtration.
   c. This agent is used primarily in treatment of **lead poisoning.**
   d. EDTA is nephrotoxic, particularly of renal tubules, at high doses. Maintenance of urine flow and short-term treatment can minimize this effect.
3. ***Dimercaprol*** (BAL)
   a. Dimercaprol is an oily, foul-smelling liquid administered intramuscularly as a 10% solution in peanut oil.
   b. Dimercaprol interacts with metals, reactivating or preventing the inactivation of cellular sulfhydryl-containing enzymes. **Dimercaprol** is most effective if administered immediately following exposure.
   c. This agent is useful in **arsenic, inorganic mercury,** and **organic mercury** poisoning (and lead poisoning). It may redistribute arsenic and mercury to the CNS and is, therefore, not recommended for treatment of chronic poisoning with these agents.
   d. The adverse effects of dimercaprol include tachycardia, hypertension, gastric irritation, and pain at the injection site.
   e. **Succimer** (Chemax) is a derivative of dimercaprol that can be taken orally and is approved for use in children to treat **lead poisoning.** It does not mobilize other essential metals to any appreciable extent. The adverse effects of succimer are generally minor and include nausea, vomiting, and anorexia. A rash indicating hypersensitivity may require the termination of therapy. It is also used to treat **arsenic** and **mercury** poisoning.
   f. **Unithol** (Dimaval) is another analogue of dimercaprol over which it has advantages (few adverse effects) for treatment of **mercury, arsenic,** and **lead** poisoning.
4. ***Penicillamine*** (Cuprimine, Depen)
   a. Penicillamine is a derivative of **penicillin** that is well absorbed from the GI tract.
   b. This agent is used primarily to chelate excess copper in individuals with **Wilson disease.**
   c. Penicillamine is also used for **copper and mercury poisoning** and as an adjunct for the treatment of lead and arsenic poisoning.
   d. Allergic reactions and rare **bone marrow toxicity** and **renal toxicity** are the major adverse effects.
5. ***Deferoxamine*** (Desferal), Desferasirox (Exjade)
   a. Deferoxamine is a specific **iron-chelating agent** that on parenteral administration binds with ferric ions to form ferrioxamine; it also binds to ferrous ions. Deferoxamine can also

remove iron from ferritin and hemosiderin outside bone marrow, but it does not capture iron from hemoglobin, cytochromes, or myoglobin.

b. Rapid IV infusion of deferoxamine may result in hypotensive shock due to the release of histamine. It may also be administered intramuscularly.

c. Deferoxamine is metabolized by plasma enzymes and excreted by the kidney, turning urine red.

d. Deferoxamine may cause allergic reactions and rare **neurotoxicity** or **renal toxicity.** Deferoxamine therapy is contraindicated in patients with renal disease or renal failure.

e. Desferasirox is an oral iron chelator approved for treatment of **iron overload.**

VII. DRUG POISONING

A. General management of the poisoned patient (see Table 13-1)

1. Observe vital signs.
2. Obtain history.
3. Perform a toxicologically oriented physical examination.

B. Symptoms

1. More than a million cases of acute poisoning occur each year in the United States, many in children and adolescents.
2. The symptoms of most drug and chemical poisonings are extensions of their pharmacologic properties. Common causes of death include CNS depression with respiratory arrest, seizures, cardiovascular abnormalities with severe hypotension and arrhythmias, cellular hypoxia, and hypothermia.

C. Treatment. Measures to support vital functions, slow drug absorption, and promote excretion are generally sufficient for treatment. If available, specific antidotes can also be used.

1. ***Vital function support***

   a. In the presence of severe CNS depression, it is important to clear the **airway** and maintain adequate **breathing** and **circulation** (**ABC**). Comatose patients may die as a result of airway obstruction, respiratory arrest, or aspiration of gastric contents into the tracheobronchial tube.

   b. Other important supportive measures include maintaining electrolyte balance and maintaining vascular fluid volume with IV **dextrose infusion.**

2. ***Drug absorption***

   a. Drug absorption may be slowed or prevented by decontamination of the skin. Induction of vomiting with **ipecac** orally is no longer recommended for routine use at home, and is contraindicated in children under 6 years. Its use is also limited in the emergency room in favor of activated charcoal.

   b. Emesis is **contraindicated** if corrosives have been ingested (reflux may perforate the stomach or esophagus), petroleum distillates have been ingested (may induce chemical pneumonia if aspirated), the patient is comatose or delirious and may aspirate gastric contents, or CNS stimulants have been ingested (may induce seizure activity with stimulation of emesis).

   (1) Gastric lavage is performed only when the airway is protected by an endotracheal tube.

   (2) Chemical adsorption with activated charcoal

   (a) Activated charcoal will bind many toxins and drugs, including **salicylates, acetaminophen,** and **antidepressants.**

   (b) This procedure can be used in combination with gastric lavage.

   (3) Cathartics are used occasionally to speed removal of toxins from the GI tract. **Sorbitol** is a recommended agent in the absence of heart failure. **Magnesium sulfate** can be used in the absence of renal failure.

3. ***Promotion of elimination*** may be achieved by the following:

a. **Chemically enhancing urinary excretion.** Urinary excretion can be enhanced by the administration of agents such as **sodium bicarbonate,** which raises urinary pH and decreases renal reabsorption of certain organic acids such as aspirin and phenobarbital.

b. **Hemodialysis** is an efficient way to remove certain low molecular weight, water-soluble toxins and restore electrolyte balance. **Salicylate, methanol, ethanol, ethylene glycol, paraquat,** and **lithium** poisonings are effectively treated this way; hemoperfusion may enhance the whole-body clearance of some agents (**carbamazepine, phenobarbital, phenytoin**). Drugs and poisons with large volumes of distribution are not effectively removed by dialysis.

4. ***Antidotes*** (see respective agents) are available for some poisons and should be used when a specific toxin is identified. Some examples include **naloxone, acetylcysteine, physostigmine, metal chelators** (see above), **atropine, pralidoxime,** and **ethanol**.

DRUG SUMMARY TABLE

Deferasirox (Exjade)
Deferoxamine (Desferal)
Dimercaprol (BAL)
EDTA (ethylenediamine tetraacetic acid) (calcium disodium versenate)
Penicillamine (Cuprimine, Depen)
Pralidoxime (Protopam)
Succimer (Chemet)
Unithol (Dimaval)

Review Test for Chapter 13

Directions: Each of the numbered items or incomplete statements in this section is followed by answers or by completions of the statement. Select the ONE lettered answer or completion that is BEST in each case.

1. What treatment would be appropriate in a 3-year-old boy with a dramatically elevated blood level of lead?

(A) Pyridoxine
(B) Glucagon
(C) Digibind
(D) Calcium disodium EDTA
(E) Deferoxamine

2. A 56-year-old chronic alcoholic is brought to the emergency room with altered mental status and complains of not being able to see. He reports running out of "whiskey" and ingesting wood alcohol (methanol). His laboratory test results demonstrate a severe anion gap and acute renal failure. Which of the following would be appropriate therapy?

(A) Hyperbaric oxygen
(B) Fomepizole
(C) Lidocaine
(D) Ethylene glycol
(E) Methylene blue

3. An 18-year-old man is brought to the emergency room by his friends because he "passed out." His friends tell the physician that they were at a party and the patient drank a couple of beers and took several Valium (diazepam). On examination the patient is unresponsive, with decreased respirations (8 per minute). What would be an appropriate treatment?

(A) Flumazenil
(B) Ethyl alcohol
(C) Dextrose
(D) Strychnine
(E) Carbon tetrachloride

4. A 23-year-old known heroin addict is brought to the emergency room for unresponsiveness. On examination he is found to have pin-point pupils and respiratory depression. His fingerstick glucose measurement is normal. What is the most appropriate agent to administer at this point?

(A) Insulin
(B) Naloxone
(C) Dimercaprol
(D) Penicillamine
(E) Atropine

5. A 2-year-old child is brought to the emergency room because he recently ingested numerous "iron pills" his mother was taking for her anemia. The child now has severe abdominal pain, bloody diarrhea, nausea, and vomiting. His serum iron is dramatically elevated. What should be given to treat this toxicity?

(A) Activated charcoal
(B) Phlebotomy
(C) Mercury vapor
(D) Deferoxamine
(E) Succimer

6. Which of the following is a sensitive indicator of lead toxicity?

(A) Wristdrop
(B) "Rice-water" stools
(C) "Milk and roses" complexion
(D) Odor of bitter almonds

7. Central nervous system (CNS) disturbances and depression are a major toxic effect of

(A) Ionic mercury (Hg^{2+})
(B) Trivalent arsenic
(C) Pentavalent arsenic
(D) Elemental mercury

8. Which of the following toxic agents would pose a problem with dermal exposure?

(A) Inorganic arsenic
(B) Organophosphate insecticides
(C) Inorganic lead
(D) Cadmium

9. Which of the following is the most common result of benzene poisoning?

(A) Central nervous system (CNS) depression
(B) Stimulation of red blood cell production
(C) Delayed hepatotoxicity
(D) Cardiotoxicity

10. Atropine can be used effectively as an antidote to poisoning by which toxic agent?

(A) Parathion
(B) Carbaryl
(C) Methanol
(D) Chlorophenothane (DDT)

Answers and Explanations

1. **The answer is D.** Calcium disodium EDTA is a chelator used in the treatment of inorganic lead poisoning. The drug is given intravenously for several days along with dimercaprol. Deferoxamine is used in cases of iron toxicity. Pyridoxine is used in a toxicology setting to reverse seizures due to isoniazid overdose. Digibind is a Fab fragment antibody used in cases of Digoxin toxicity. Glucagon can be used to treat β blocker toxicity.

2. **The answer is B.** Fomepizole is an inhibitor of alcohol dehydrogenase, which might otherwise convert methanol to formic acid, which is the true toxin in such cases causing blindness and renal failure. Ethylene glycol (antifreeze) can cause similar toxicity and is also treated with fomepizole. Hyperbaric oxygen is used in the treatment of carbon monoxide poisoning. Lidocaine can be used to help manage arrhythmias in the case of digoxin toxicity. Methylene blue is used in the treatment of methemoglobinemia.

3. **The answer is A.** Flumazenil is a benzodiazepine antagonist used in the management of such overdoses. Ethyl alcohol can be used to treat ingestion of both methanol and ethylene glycol; however, such use often results in ethanol intoxication, and fomepizole is preferred as it does not cause the same effects. Dextrose is an effective treatment for altered mental status due to hypoglycemia in a diabetic patient. Strychnine is a rat poison that can cause seizures when ingested, which are managed by giving diazepam. Carbon tetrachloride is an industrial solvent that can cause fatty liver and kidney damage.

4. **The answer is B.** Given the patient's history and clinical findings, he is likely to be experiencing opioid overdose. The drug of choice in such a scenario is naloxone, an opioid-receptor antagonist. Insulin is used to treat hyperglycemia, which is less likely to cause altered mental status than is hypoglycemia. Dimercaprol is a chelator used in many cases of heavy metal toxicity (i.e., lead). Penicillamine is used in the treatment of copper toxicity, as in Wilson disease. Atropine is used to treat cholinergic toxicity, which can cause miosis, although an unlikely cause in this clinical presentation.

5. **The answer is D.** Deferoxamine is an iron chelator that is given systemically to bind iron and promote its excretion. Activated charcoal, good for the absorption of numerous toxic ingestions, is ineffective in this case as it does not bind iron. Phlebotomy is a treatment for iron overload in such conditions as hereditary hemochromatosis. Succimer is an orally available substance related to dimercaprol, used for lead toxicity. Mercury vapor is toxic and its ingestion is treated with dimercaprol or penicillamine.

6. **The answer is A.** The most common neurologic manifestation of lead poisoning is peripheral neuropathy, a common sign of which is wristdrop. Lead poisoning also affects the hematopoietic system as a result of inhibition of δ-aminolevulinic acid dehydratase (and ferrochelatase). In children, lead poisoning may be manifested by encephalopathy.

7. **The answer is D.** The central nervous system (CNS) is the major target organ for elemental mercury. Ionic Hg^{2+} predominantly affects the renal system.

8. **The answer is B.** In contrast to the organophosphate insecticides, inorganic forms of arsenic, lead, and cadmium are poorly absorbed through the skin.

9. **The answer is A.** The major acute effect of benzene poisoning is central nervous system (CNS) depression. Chronic exposure may lead to bone marrow depression.

10. **The answer is A.** If administered early in poisoning, atropine reverses the muscarinic cholinoceptor effects of organophosphate insecticides such as parathion, which inhibit acetylcholinesterase (AChE). Pralidoxime (2-PAM) is often used as an adjunct to atropine. Inhibition of AChE by carbamate insecticides such as carbaryl is reversed spontaneously. The toxicity of methanol and chlorophenothane (DDT) is unrelated to acetylcholine action.

Comprehensive Examination

Directions: Each of the numbered items or incomplete statements in this section is followed by answers or by completions of the statement. Select the ONE lettered answer or completion that is BEST in each case.

1. A 17-year-old male patient was placed on carbamazepine therapy by his neurologist to control newly developed seizures of unknown etiology. The patient was also recently given a macrolide antibiotic by his family physician for a presumed "walking pneumonia." Halfway through his antibiotic course, the patient again developed seizures. What could account for this new seizure activity?

(A) Inhibition of the cytochrome P-450 monooxygenase system
(B) Induction of the cytochrome P-450 monooxygenase system
(C) Impairment of renal excretion of the antiseizure medication
(D) Induction of glucuronyl transferase activity in the liver
(E) Reduction in the amount of nicotinamide adenine dinucleotide phosphate (NADPH)

2. A 21-year-old man sustains multiple blunt traumas after being beaten with a baseball bat by a gang. Aside from his fractures, a serum creatine kinase measurement is dramatically elevated and the trauma team is worried as the myoglobinuria caused by the trauma can cause kidney failure. They immediately begin to administer bicarbonate to alkalinize the urine. How does this serve to decrease myoglobin levels?

(A) Increasing glomerular filtration
(B) Promoting renal tubular secretion
(C) Inhibiting renal tubular reabsorption
(D) Increasing hepatic first-pass metabolism
(E) Inducing the P-450 system

3. Which of the following correctly describes the formula for a loading dose?

(A) Loading dose = (desired plasma concentration of drug) × (clearance)
(B) Loading dose = (clearance) × (plasma drug concentration)
(C) Loading dose = (0.693) × (volume of distribution)/(clearance)
(D) Loading dose = (amount of drug administered)/(initial plasma concentration)
(E) Loading dose = (desired plasma concentration of the drug) × (volume of distribution)

4. A 32-year-old HIV-positive man follows up with an infectious disease (ID) specialist in the clinic. The results of his recent blood work suggest that the virus has become resistant to multiple nucleoside reverse transcriptase inhibitors. The ID specialist decides to include in the treatment a nonnucleoside inhibitor (nevirapine), which works by binding to a site near the active site on the reverse transcriptase. Nevirapine is an example of what?

(A) Full agonist
(B) Reversible competitive antagonist
(C) Partial agonist
(D) Noncompetitive antagonist
(E) Irreversible competitive antagonist

5. Which of the following drugs is a selective α-adrenergic receptor agonist that is available over the counter?

(A) Epinephrine
(B) Phenylephrine
(C) Isoproterenol
(D) Norepinephrine
(E) Phentolamine

6. Pilocarpine is what type of pharmacologic agent?

(A) Indirect muscarinic agonist
(B) α_2-Adrenergic agonist
(C) Carbonic anhydrase inhibitor
(D) β-Adrenergic antagonist
(E) Direct-acting muscarinic agonist

7. Which of the following is a short-acting acetylcholinesterase inhibitor?

(A) Pyridostigmine
(B) Bethanechol
(C) Edrophonium

(D) Scopolamine
(E) Methantheline

8. Dantrolene

(A) Inhibits calcium release from the sarcoplasmic reticulum
(B) Functions as a $GABA_B$ receptor agonist
(C) Facilitates GABA activity in the central nervous system (CNS)
(D) Reactivates acetylcholinesterase
(E) Competitively inhibits the effects of acetylcholine

9. A 63-year-old man with a history of multiple myocardial infarctions is admitted for shortness of breath. A diagnosis of congestive heart failure is made on clinical grounds, and a cardiologist orders a positive inotropic agent for his heart failure. He is also concerned about maintaining perfusion to the kidneys, so an agent that increases renal blood flow is also desirable. Which of the following agents produces both of these effects?

(A) Epinephrine
(B) Dopamine
(C) Isoproterenol
(D) Terbutaline

10. Clonidine works by

(A) Activating β_1-adrenergic receptors
(B) Activating α_1-adrenergic receptors
(C) Activating β_2-adrenergic receptors
(D) Activating α_2-adrenergic receptors
(E) Blocking β-adrenergic receptors

11. A 23-year-old woman presents with hypertension, anxiety, and palpitations. Her thyroid-stimulating hormone levels are normal, but she has increased levels of urinary catecholamines. She is referred to an endocrine surgeon after a computed tomography (CT) scan shows a unilateral pheochromocytoma. The surgeon should start therapy with which of the following agents prior to removing the lesion?

(A) Dopamine
(B) Phentolamine
(C) Pancuronium
(D) Pseudoephedrine
(E) Isoproterenol

12. A 45-year-old man with a history remarkable for both asthma and angina now has a kidney stone stuck in his right ureter. The urologist needs to perform cystoscopy, but the anesthesiologist is concerned about using a β-blocker during surgery to control the patient's blood pressure in light of his history of asthma. Ultimately, it is decide to use an ultra-short acting β-blocker and closely monitor both his blood pressure and respiratory status. Which of the following is best to use in this situation?

(A) Atenolol
(B) Norepinephrine
(C) Albuterol
(D) Pseudoephedrine
(E) Esmolol

13. A neurosurgeon decides to start a patient on a diuretic that works by altering the diffusion of water relative to sodium (an osmotic diuretic), which is helpful in reducing cerebral edema. Which agent did the physician likely prescribe?

(A) Furosemide
(B) Hydrochlorothiazide
(C) Spironolactone
(D) Acetazolamide
(E) Mannitol

14. Which of the following would be useful in treating nocturnal enuresis?

(A) Mannitol
(B) Indomethacin
(C) Furosemide
(D) Vasopressin
(E) Probenecid

15. Vasopressin

(A) Reduces ADH levels
(B) Increases permeability of the collecting duct
(C) Inserts aquaporins into the plasma membrane of collecting duct cells
(D) Increases diffusion of sodium
(E) Reduces production of prostaglandins

16. A 45-year-old man with a 60-pack/year history of smoking presents to his primary care provider with loss of appetite, nausea, vomiting, and muscle weakness. A chest computed tomography (CT) scan reveals enlarged hilar lymph nodes and a suspicious mass in the left hilar region. A presumptive diagnosis of lung cancer is made. Laboratory results reveal low levels of sodium, which in this setting has likely contributed to the syndrome of inappropriate ADH secretion. Which medication might be helpful for this patient's symptoms?

(A) Clofibrate
(B) Demeclocycline
(C) Allopurinol
(D) Acetazolamide
(E) Furosemide

17. Which of the following drugs inhibits xanthine oxidase?

(A) Colchicine
(B) Indomethacin
(C) Probenecid
(D) Clofibrate
(E) Allopurinol

18. Which of the following is a common adverse effect of quinidine?

(A) Cinchonism
(B) Lupuslike syndrome
(C) Seizures
(D) Constipation
(E) Pulmonary fibrosis

19. What is the mechanism of action of β-blockers in heart disease?

(A) Prolongation of AV conduction
(B) Activation of the sympathetic system
(C) Promotion of automaticity
(D) Increase in heart rate
(E) Arteriolar vasodilation

20. Which of the following would be useful in the management of arrhythmia due to Wolf-Parkinson-White syndrome?

(A) Digoxin
(B) Lidocaine
(C) Amiodarone
(D) Adenosine
(E) Atropine

21. Which of the following inhibit HMG-CoA reductase?

(A) Nicotinic acid
(B) Rosuvastatin
(C) Ezetimibe
(D) Cholestyramine
(E) Gemfibrozil

22. Which of the following would be a good option to help a patient fall asleep with minimal "hangover"?

(A) Secobarbital
(B) Zolpidem
(C) Chlordiazepoxide
(D) Flumazenil
(E) Buspirone

23. Which of the following is a good choice to treat newly diagnosed generalized anxiety disorder (GAD) in a patient who is a truck driver?

(A) Alprazolam
(B) Triazolam
(C) Buspirone
(D) Trazodone
(E) Thiopental

24. A 57-year-old man with a strong family history of Parkinson disease sees a neurologist for an evaluation. On examination, the neurologist notes a slight pill-rolling tremor and subtle gait abnormalities. He begins treatment with levodopa, along with the addition of carbidopa. How does carbidopa work in this setting?

(A) Restores dopamine levels in the substantia nigra
(B) Inhibits monoamine oxidase (MAO)
(C) Inhibits catechol-*O*-methyltransferase (COMT)
(D) Functions as a dopamine agonist
(E) Inhibits the metabolism of levodopa outside the central nervous system (CNS)

25. The patient in the previous question returns to see his neurologist 3 years later. At this time the patient's symptoms have progressed, and he now has marked bradykinesia and a profound shuffling gait. In an attempt to prevent further deterioration, the neurologist prescribes a catechol-*O*-methyltransferase (COMT) inhibitor on top of the patient's levodopa and carbidopa. Which agent below is likely to have been added?

(A) Entacapone
(B) Selegiline
(C) Ropinirole
(D) Amantadine
(E) Benztropine

26. Which of the following is a noncompetitive NMDA receptor inhibitor that can be used to treat Alzheimer disease?

(A) Memantine
(B) Donepezil
(C) Tacrine
(D) Tolcapone
(E) Pramipexole

27. A 43-year-old high-profile attorney sees a psychiatrist with expertise in addiction medicine. He explains that he has recently received his third drunk driving citation and fears losing his license to practice unless he stops drinking altogether. He says he "just can't stop" once he starts. He tells the physician that he doesn't have time to attend Alcoholics Anonymous and "wants a pill." The physician explains that there is something that might work if the patient is truly serious. What agent is the physician considering?

(A) Lorazepam
(B) Flumazenil
(C) Naloxone
(D) Disulfiram
(E) Carbamazepine

28. A nonstimulant agent that can be used to treat attention-deficit/hyperactivity disorder (ADHD) is

(A) Methylphenidate
(B) Caffeine
(C) Dextroamphetamine
(D) Atomoxetine
(E) Modafinil

29. Which of the following can be used to treat a 22-year-old with a recent diagnosis of schizophrenia?

(A) Baclofen
(B) Haloperidol
(C) Chloral hydrate
(D) Phenobarbital
(E) Imipramine

30. Soon after drug administration, the patient in the above question begins making odd faces with spastic movements of his neck. Which of the following should be administered to treat these dystonic reactions?

(A) Fluphenazine
(B) Bromocriptine
(C) Dantrolene
(D) Prolactin
(E) Benztropine

31. Which of the following is a potential side effect of clozapine?

(A) Cholestatic jaundice
(B) QT prolongation
(C) Agranulocytosis
(D) Photosensitivity
(E) Galactorrhea

32. Risperidone works primarily through inhibition of receptors for

(A) Dopamine
(B) Serotonin
(C) Histamine
(D) Acetylcholine
(E) Norepinephrine

33. A 7-year-old boy is brought to the neurologist by his mother. She states that the boy's teacher says there are times in class when he stares "into space" and smacks his lips. In the office the boy has one such episode while having an electroencephalogram (EEG), which demonstrates a 3-per-second spike and wave tracing. Which drug is the best for this condition?

(A) Phenytoin
(B) Carbamazepine
(C) Prednisone
(D) Lorazepam
(E) Ethosuximide

34. Which of the following is a complication of phenytoin use?

(A) Hepatotoxicity
(B) Gingival hyperplasia
(C) Thrombocytopenia
(D) Aplastic anemia
(E) Stevens-Johnson syndrome

35. Tiagabine works by

(A) Inhibiting GABA uptake by inhibiting the GABA transporter
(B) Increasing GABA by stimulating its release from neurons
(C) Increasing GABA-stimulated chloride channel opening
(D) Prolonging GABA-induced channel opening
(E) Blocking T-type calcium channels

36. Which of the following agents is approved for treatment of diabetic neuropathy?

(A) Phenytoin
(B) Carbamazepine
(C) Acetazolamide
(D) Valproic acid
(E) Gabapentin

37. A 5-year-old boy is brought to the emergency room by his parents after they found him with an empty bottle of aspirin. They are not sure how many tablets the boy consumed.

On examination, the child is hyperpneic and lethargic. While the emergent treatment is started, a sample is drawn for an arterial blood determination. What pattern is most likely to be indicated by the arterial blood gas values?

(A) Mixed metabolic alkalosis and respiratory alkalosis
(B) Mixed respiratory alkalosis and metabolic acidosis
(C) Mixed respiratory acidosis and metabolic acidosis
(D) Mixed respiratory acidosis and metabolic alkalosis
(E) Mixed metabolic acidosis and metabolic alkalosis

38. Which of the following is an antineoplastic agent that has been shown to help patients with rheumatoid arthritis?

(A) Valdecoxib
(B) Ketorolac
(C) Methotrexate
(D) Entocort
(E) Auranofin

39. Which of the following is true regarding infliximab?

(A) It is a recombinant antibody to TNF-α
(B) It is a humanized antibody to TNF-α
(C) It is a fusion protein that binds to TNF-α receptor
(D) It is a recombinant protein resembling IL-1
(E) It is a recombinant protein composed of a portion of LFA-3

40. Which of the following is useful in an acute gout attack?

(A) Probenecid
(B) Sulfinpyrazone
(C) Allopurinol
(D) Colchicine
(E) Celecoxib

41. What is the mechanism of action of tacrolimus?

(A) It increases transport to the nucleus of the transcription factor NF-AT
(B) It stimulates apoptosis of some lymphoid lineages
(C) It decreases the activity of calcineurin
(D) It inhibits mTOR, which in turn delays the G_1–S transition
(E) It inhibits proliferation of promyelocytes

42. Which of the following is an alkylating agent that may cause hemorrhagic cystitis and cardiomyopathy?

(A) Azathioprine
(B) Cyclosporine
(C) Tacrolimus
(D) Cyclophosphamide
(E) Basiliximab

43. Your resident asks you what the mechanism of action of tPA is. What is your answer?

(A) It inhibits platelet aggregation
(B) It increases antithrombin activity
(C) It impairs fibrin polymerization
(D) It blocks GPIIa/IIIb
(E) It activates plasminogen bound to fibrin

44. Which of the following is an antidote for iron overdose?

(A) Protamine
(B) Deferoxamine
(C) Vitamin K
(D) Fresh frozen plasma
(E) Charcoal

45. Which of the following medications would provide the best relief from episodic attacks of Ménière disease?

(A) Furosemide
(B) Ondansetron
(C) Diazepam
(D) Emetrol
(E) Dronabinol

46. A 56-year-old woman with severe rheumatoid arthritis returns to see her rheumatologist. She had been referred to a gastroenterologist, who had found multiple gastric ulcers on esophagogastroduodenoscopy. She is reluctant to give up the use of NSAIDs and afraid of the potential cardiovascular toxicity of COX-2 inhibitor. At this point, what would be reasonable for the rheumatologist to prescribe?

(A) Omeprazole
(B) Lansoprazole
(C) Nizatidine
(D) Metronidazole
(E) Misoprostol

47. A 29-year-old man who recently immigrated to the United States sees his physician for a burning sensation in his epigastrium. He is referred to a gastroenterologist, who performs esophagogastroduodenoscopy with biopsy that demonstrates ulcers with the presence of *Helicobacter pylori.* Use of which of the following regimens would provide the most effective and shortest treatment?

(A) Pepto Bismol, clarithromycin, amoxicillin, and omeprazole
(B) Pepto Bismol, metronidazole, tetracycline, and ranitidine
(C) Clarithromycin, metronidazole, and omeprazole
(D) Clarithromycin, amoxicillin, and omeprazole
(E) Pepto Bismol, metronidazole, and amoxicillin

48. An 83-year-old man with multiple medical problems develops worsening constipation during his hospitalization for lower extremity cellulitis. The hospitalist decides to start giving a laxative. Which of the following is an appropriate choice and why?

(A) Psyllium, because it is a bulk-forming laxative good for chronic constipation
(B) An osmotic agent, such as senna, which is administered rectally
(C) A stool softener such as lactulose administered rectally
(D) A stool softener such as methylcellulose that inhibits water reabsorption
(E) A salt-containing osmotic agent such as docusate, useful in preventing constipation

49. A 35-year-old intravenous drug abuser in a methadone maintenance program is admitted to the hospital for a work-up of suspected pulmonary tuberculosis. While in the hospital, he complains of diarrhea and cramping. After stool studies return with a negative result, you decide to begin an antidiarrheal. Which of the following is a good choice for this patient?

(A) Kaolin
(B) Codeine
(C) Diphenoxylate
(D) Loperamide
(E) Propantheline

50. Which of the following would be an appropriate treatment to begin in a patient with Crohn disease?

(A) Glucocorticoids
(B) Sulfasalazine
(C) Bismuth subsalicylate
(D) Octreotide
(E) Loperamide

51. The above patient returns for follow-up, and she still complains of bloody diarrhea, fever, and weight loss. The gastroenterologist has placed her on a trial of steroids, and yet she still complains of her symptoms. The gastroenterologist could consider using which of the following agents?

(A) Infalyte
(B) Opium tincture
(C) Mesalamine
(D) Infliximab
(E) Diphenoxylate

52. Adverse effects seen with high blood levels of theophylline include

(A) Seizures
(B) Arrhythmias
(C) Nervousness
(D) Nausea and vomiting
(E) All of the above

53. A 62-year-old male alcoholic being treated for non-insulin-dependent diabetes mellitus comes to the emergency department with a 1-hour history of nausea, vomiting, headache, hypotension, and profuse sweating. What is the most likely causative agent?

(A) Clomiphene
(B) Glyburide
(C) Chlorpropamide
(D) Nandrolone
(E) Vasopressin

54. An 81-year-old man with a history of coronary artery disease and a recent diagnosis of hypothyroidism presents to the emergency department with an acute myocardial infarction. What is the most likely causative agent?

(A) Medroxyprogesterone
(B) Levothyroxine
(C) Thiocyanate
(D) Flutamide
(E) Diethylstilbestrol (DES)

55. A 32-year-old woman being treated for an acute exacerbation of lupus erythematosus complains of pain on eating. What is the most likely causative agent?

(A) Oxytocin
(B) Androlone
(C) Vasopressin
(D) Prednisone
(E) Clomiphene

56. It is likely that the acquisition of antibiotic resistance in gram-negative bacilli such as vancomycin is a result of

(A) Spontaneous mutation
(B) Transformation
(C) Transduction
(D) Conjugation
(E) Transposition

57. A 30-year-old patient is undergoing chemotherapy for Hodgkin disease and develops a fever, prompting an admission by his oncologist. He is found to have a severely decreased white blood cell count, and therapy is started with several antibiotics for febrile neutropenia. Assuming his regimen contains imipenem, which of the following must also be administered?

(A) Probenecid
(B) Clavulanic acid
(C) Sulbactam
(D) Cycloserine
(E) Cilastatin

58. A 17-year-old boy presents with right lower quadrant pain with guarding and rebound. A computed tomography (CT) scan demonstrates appendicitis, and he is taken to the operating room. What would be a good antibiotic to administer prophylactically before the surgery?

(A) Cefazolin
(B) Cefoxitin
(C) Ceftriaxone
(D) Aztreonam
(E) Oxacillin

59. A 23-year-old woman, who is 23 weeks pregnant, develops a bladder infection due to *Pseudomonas* spp. She has a documented allergy to penicillin. What is the best choice of treatment given the patient's history and condition?

(A) Cefoxitin
(B) Aztreonam
(C) Imipenem
(D) Piperacillin
(E) Ciprofloxacin

60. A 37-year-old alcoholic is recovering in the hospital from pneumonia due to *Haemophilus influenzae*. His treatment included the use of intravenous antibiotics. The nurse calls you to evaluate the patient as he returned from a visit from his "buddy" outside. The nurse tells you he smells like alcohol and he is flush, warm, and uncomfortable. You suspect a disulfiram-like reaction. What antibiotic was he likely treated with?

(A) Vancomycin
(B) Bacitracin
(C) Chloramphenicol
(D) Isoniazid
(E) Cefamandole

61. Which of the following can occur in an adult patient treated with chloramphenicol?

(A) Gray baby syndrome
(B) Bone marrow suppression
(C) Disulfiram-like reaction
(D) Nephrotoxicity
(E) Ototoxicity

62. A 32-year-old man complains of a persistent, dry cough for several days with a mild fever and fatigue. The family physician suspects a diagnosis of "walking pneumonia" on clinical grounds, presumably due to *Mycoplasma pneumoniae.* Which of the following groups of antibiotics would be effective?

(A) Penicillins
(B) Cephalosporins
(C) Vancomycin
(D) Chloramphenicol
(E) Macrolides

63. Which of the following is a side effect of clindamycin?

(A) Dizziness
(B) Bruising
(C) Difficulty hearing
(D) Diarrhea
(E) Tendon pain

64. An 18-year-old African-American army recruit with a history of G-6-PDH deficiency is to be stationed in Somalia. During his tour of duty he develops a cyclic fever, malaise, and weakness. A thin blood smear shows malarial organisms within red blood cells. Which antimalarial is likely to exacerbate the hemolysis, given his enzyme deficiency?

(A) Chloroquine
(B) Pyrimethamine
(C) Doxycycline
(D) Primaquine
(E) Sulfasalazine

65. A 54-year-old diabetic woman was seen in the emergency room 3 weeks ago with complaints of swelling, warmth, and pain in her foot. She was diagnosed with cellulitis and sent home on a 10-day course of an oral first-generation cephalosporin. She returns with severe diarrhea, and *Clostridium difficile* is suspected. What is the initial treatment for this condition?

(A) Clindamycin
(B) Metronidazole
(C) Ciprofloxacin
(D) Neomycin
(E) Silver sulfadiazine

66. A 37-year-old woman recently had a large soft tissue sarcoma surgically resected from her retroperitoneum. She is to receive both radiation and chemotherapy, with cyclophosphamide as part of her chemotherapy. Which agent should be given in conjunction with this drug?

(A) MESNA
(B) Allopurinol
(C) Leucovorin
(D) Cilastatin
(E) MOPP

67. A 54-year-old woman is undergoing an experimental high-dose regimen with adriamycin and cyclophosphamide for breast cancer. As this treatment is particularly myelosuppressive, the oncologist is worried that her white blood cell count will drop dangerously low, making her susceptible to opportunistic infections. In addition to the chemotherapy, what is the oncologist likely to administer to prevent neutropenia?

(A) Epoetin alfa
(B) Filgrastim
(C) Interferon alfa-2b
(D) Oprelvekin
(E) Amifostine

68. Trastuzumab works by

(A) Inhibiting the oncoprotein bcr-abl
(B) Blocking estrogen-mediated gene transcription
(C) Preventing phosphorylation of a receptor tyrosine kinase
(D) Targeting cells for destruction by antibody-mediated cellular cytotoxicity (ADCC)
(E) Reducing circulating levels of tumor necrosis factor (TNF)

69. Which of the following might be considered for treatment of acute myelocytic anemia (M3 variant)?

(A) Cisplatin
(B) Lomustine
(C) Tretinoin
(D) Fluorouracil
(E) Streptozocin

70. Chromosomal studies in a 56-year-old man indicate a (9:22) translocation, the Philadelphia chromosome, confirming the diagnosis of chronic myelocytic leukemia (CML). Which of the following might be used in his treatment?

(A) Anastrozole
(B) Rituximab
(C) Imatinib
(D) Gefitinib
(E) Amifostine

71. Which agent can be used to treat hairy cell leukemia?

(A) Interferon alfa-2b
(B) Interleukin-2
(C) All-*trans*-retinoic acid
(D) Rituximab
(E) Daunorubicin

72. A 63-year-old woman develops metastatic colon cancer. The pathologist confirms that a biopsy specimen retrieved from a recent colonoscopy demonstrates that the tumor overexpresses epidermal growth factor receptor (EGFR). The oncologist decides to add a monoclonal antibody to EGFR to her treatment. Which of the following would be added?

(A) Rituximab
(B) Erlotinib
(C) Gefitinib
(D) Cetuximab
(E) Traztuzamab

73. Which of the following should be considered to treat an acetaminophen overdose in a 17-year-old girl?

(A) Trientine
(B) Sorbitol
(C) N-acetylcysteine
(D) Ipecac
(E) Diazepam

74. Organophosphate poisoning is treated with

(A) Pralidoxime
(B) Parathion
(C) Amyl nitrate
(D) Bethanechol
(E) Nicotine

75. What should be given to correct coagulopathy due to an overdose of warfarin in a 73-year-old man?

(A) Aminocaproic acid
(B) Vitamin K
(C) Heparin
(D) Vitamin D
(E) Oprelvekin

Answers and Explanations

1. **The answer is B.** Both carbamazepine and macrolide antibiotics are known inducers of the cytochrome P-450 system. Thus, it is likely that the original therapeutic levels of antiseizure medicine were decreased to nontherapeutic levels when the metabolism of the drug was increased with the addition of the antibiotic. Some common drugs that inhibit P-450 include cimetidine, chloramphenicol, and disulfiram. Impaired renal excretion results in increased, not decreased, levels of drugs. The induction of glucuronyl transferase is a possible drug interaction, although less likely in this case. The P-450 system requires nicotinamide adenine dinucleotide phosphate (NADPH); therefore, a deficiency would result in decreased, not increased, activity by the system.

2. **The answer is C.** Alterations in urinary pH alters renal reabsorption of substances. In this case, alkalinization traps filtered myoglobin in the urine so that it cannot be reabsorbed, which leads to decreased levels in the serum. The other mechanisms such as increasing glomerular filtration and promoting tubular secretion are other potential ways to alter plasma drug/metabolite levels. Myoglobin is not hepatically metabolized; therefore, hepatic or P-450 metabolism would not alter myoglobin levels.

3. **The answer is E.** Loading dose = (desired plasma concentration of the drug) × (volume of distribution). The formula for the maintenance dose, once the loading dose is given, = (desired plasma concentration of drug) × (clearance). The elimination rate = (clearance) × (plasma drug concentration). The half-life of a drug = (amount of drug administered)/(initial plasma concentration). And lastly, the volume of distribution = (amount of drug administered)/(initial plasma concentration).

4. **The answer is D.** By definition, drugs that do not bind to the active site, such as nonnucleotide reverse transcriptase inhibitors, are noncompetitive antagonists. They function by causing changes in the active site so that it can not bind its native substrate. Agonists are drugs that elicit the same activity as the endogenous substrate, whereas partial agonists only induce some of the activities of the endogenous substrate. Competitive inhibitors, like nucleoside reverse transcriptase inhibitors, can be either reversible or irreversible.

5. **The answer is B.** Phenylephrine is a selective α_1-adrenoreceptor agonist that causes nasal vasoconstriction, which results in decreased nasal secretion. Epinephrine is the most potent of the adrenergic receptor agonists, followed by norepinephrine. Isoproterenol is the weakest antagonist. But the previous three agents also bind β-adrenergic receptors and are not available over the counter. Phentolamine is just the opposite, an α_1-adrenergic antagonist.

6. **The answer is E.** Pilocarpine is a direct-acting muscarinic agonist used in the management of acute narrow-angle glaucoma, often with an indirect-acting muscarinic agonist like physostigmine. Carbonic anhydrase inhibiters (e.g., acetazolamide), β-adrenoreceptor agonists, and even α_2-adrenoreceptor agonists can be used in the treatment of glaucoma.

7. **The answer is C.** In myasthenia gravis, autoantibodies develop to nicotinic acetylcholine receptors, causing impaired neuromuscular dysfunction that results in muscular fatigue. This fatigue can be treated with acetylcholinesterase inhibitors. Edrophonium is the shortest-acting agent in this class and used to diagnosis this disorder, with such weakness immediately corrected with its use. Pyridostigmine is a longer-acting agent used in the treatment of the disease. Bethanecol is a direct-acting muscarinic cholinergic agonist, whereas both scopolamine and methantheline are both muscarinic-receptor antagonists.

8. **The answer is A.** Dantrolene is used in the treatment of malignant hyperthermia and works by inhibiting the release of calcium from the sarcoplasmic reticulum. Baclofen, an antispasmatic

used in the treatment of multiple sclerosis, inhibits synaptic transmission as a $GABA_B$-receptor agonist. Benzodiazepines function to facilitate GABA activity in the central nervous system (CNS) and spinal cord. Pradoxime reactivates acetylcholinesterase. Nondepolarizing neuromuscular junction blockers such as atracurium competitively inhibit the effects of acetylcholine.

9. **The answer is B.** Dopamine is useful in the management of congestive heart failure, as it has both positive inotropic effects on the heart and preserves blood flow to the kidneys. Epinephrine and isoproterenol increase cardiac contractility while decreasing peripheral resistance. Albuterol is a β_1 agonist used in the management of asthma, and terbutaline is another β agonist used to suppress labor, in the event of threatened labor of a premature fetus.

10. **The answer is D.** Clonidine activates prejunctional α_2-adrenergic receptors in the central nervous system (CNS) to reduce sympathetic tone, thereby decreasing blood pressure. Activation of α_1-adrenergic receptors increases blood pressure, which is useful for the treatment of hypotension. β_1-adrenoreceptor agonists are used primarily for increasing heart rate and contractility. β_2-adrenergic agonists are used to dilate airways in the management of asthma. β-adrenoreceptor antagonists are used in the treatment of angina and hypertension.

11. **The answer is B.** An α-adrenoreceptor antagonist such as phentolamine is indicated for the treatment of pheochromocytomas in the preoperative state as well as if the tumor is inoperable. β-blockers are then used systemically, following effective α blockade, to prevent the cardiac effects of excessive catecholamines. Pseudoephedrine is an α-adrenoreceptor antagonist available over the counter to relieve nasal discharge. There is no role for adrenergic receptor agonists such as dopamine or isoproterenol or for that matter nondepolarizing muscle relaxants such as pancuronium.

12. **The answer is E.** Esmolol is an ultrashort acting β_1 antagonist that is relatively specific for the heart; however, the short half-life of this drug should allow the anesthesiologist to fine tune the delivery and readily reverse the effects should there be problems with respiration. Atenolol is a much longer acting agent that would not provide such control. Norepinephrine would actually adversely affect the patient's angina, as it is stimulatory to the heart. Albuterol is a β agonist used in the treatment of asthma. Pseudoephedrine is an over-the-counter α agonist used in cold formula preparations.

13. **The answer is E.** Mannitol is an osmotic diuretic frequently used in management of cerebral edema caused by various insults. This agent works by altering the diffusion of water relative to sodium by "binding" the water, with a resultant reduction of sodium reabsorption. Furosemide and hydrochlorothiazide act by directly altering reabsorption of sodium in various parts of the nephron. Spironolactone antagonizes mineralocorticoid receptor. Acetazolamide inhibits carbonic anhydrase.

14. **The answer is D.** Vasopressin can be tried in cases of recalcitrant nocturnal enuresis. Mannitol is most commonly used in management of cerebral edema. Indomethacin can occasionally be used as an antidiuretic agent in diabetic patients. Furosemide is used in congestive heart failure. Probenecid is used to treat gout.

15. **The answer is C.** Vasopressin causes specific water channels termed aquaporins II to be inserted into the plasma membrane of the luminal surface of the medullary collecting ducts. This directly affects permeability of the collecting duct. Under the conditions of dehydration, as is the case with this patient, the ADH levels increase. Increasing diffusion of sodium represents the mechanism of action of osmotic diuretics. Production of prostaglandins is reduced with the use of agents such as indomethacin.

16. **The answer is B.** Demeclocycline is an ADH antagonist and as such is useful in treatment of SIADH, which is commonly seen in patients with lung cancer. Clofibrate increases the release of ADH centrally. Allopurinol, acetazolamide, and furosemide do not affect actions of ADH to an appreciable degree.

17. **The answer is E.** Allopurinol is a xanthine oxidase inhibitor and is most commonly used in treatment of gout. It is not used for acute attacks, but rather for prevention of recurrent episodes. Colchicine may be used for an acute episode, as well as in long-term therapy;

however, it has a high incidence of side effects. Indomethacin is useful for symptomatic treatment of gout. Probenecid is also useful for prophylaxis of gout; however, it is not a xanthine oxidase inhibitor. This agent inhibits secretion of organic acids. Clofibrate is used in treatment of hypercholesterolemia.

18. **The answer is A.** Cinchonism, or ringing in the ears and dizziness, is common after quinidine use. Lupus-like syndrome can be observed after the use of procainamide. Seizures may occur with lidocaine use. Diarrhea can occur with the use of quinidine, not constipation. Pulmonary fibrosis is a long-term complication of amiodarone use.

19. **The answer is A.** Beta-adrenoreceptor antagonists prolong AV conduction. They reduce sympathetic stimulation. These agents depress automaticity. Beta-blockers decrease heart rate and can cause arteriolar vasoconstriction.

20. **The answer is D.** Adenosine, a class V antiarrhythmic, is used for the treatment of paroxysmal supraventricular tachycardias, including those of Wolf-Parkinson-White syndrome. Digoxin and amiodarone can be used for management of atrial fibrillation. Lidocaine is used in treatment of many arrhythmias. Atropine is used for bradyarrhythmias.

21. **The answer is B.** Rosuvastatin is an HMG-CoA reductase inhibitor. Nicotinic acid inhibits the process of esterification of fatty acids, thereby reducing plasma triglyceride levels. Ezetimibe reduces cholesterol absorption. Cholestyramine can bind bile acids and prevents their enterohepatic circulation. Gemfibrozil reduces hepatic synthesis of cholesterol.

22. **The answer is B.** Zolpidem has actions similar to those of benzodiazepines, although it is structurally unrelated. It is used as a hypnotic and anxiolytic with minimal abuse potential. Barbiturates such as secobarbital are rarely used because of their lethality on overdose. Chlordiazepoxide is a long-acting benzodiazepine, whereas most hypnotics are short-acting benzodiazepines. Flumazenil is a benzodiazepine receptor antagonist that will not reverse the effects of zolpidem. Buspirone is not used as a hypnotic and has little sedative effect.

23. **The answer is C.** Buspirone is a partial serotonin 5-HT_{1A}-receptor agonist that has efficacy comparable to that of benzodiazepines for the treatment of anxiety, but is significantly less sedating. Alprazolam is an intermediate-acting benzodiazepine used in the treatment of generalized anxiety disorder (GAD) but still has some sedation, which would be undesirable in this situation. Triazolam is a short-acting benzodiazepine, and trazodone is a heterocyclic antidepressant, both used to induce sleep. Thiopental is a barbiturate sometimes used to induce anesthesia.

24. **The answer is E.** Carbidopa, unlike levodopa, does not penetrate the central nervous system (CNS); it does inhibit levodopa's metabolism in the gut, allowing lower doses of levodopa and decreased side effects. Levodopa is a precursor to dopamine and can help restore levels of dopamine in the substantia nigra. Monoamine oxidase inhibitors should be used with caution along with levodopa, as this can lead to a hypertensive crisis. Bromocriptine is a dopamine agonist used in the treatment of Parkinson disease. Catechol-*O*-methyltransferase (COMT) inhibitors are yet another class of agents used in the treatment of Parkinson disease.

25. **The answer is A.** Levodopa is metabolized, in part by catechol-*O*-methyltransferase (COMT); therefore, an inhibitor such as entacapone is an adjunct treatment for patients on levodopa. It does however increase the side effects including diarrhea, postural hypotension, nausea, and hallucinations. Selegiline is a monoamine oxidase inhibitor (MAOI) used in the treatment of Parkinson disease. Ropinirole is a nonergot dopamine agonist used in early Parkinson disease that may decrease the need for levodopa in later stages of the disease. Amantadine has an effect on the rigidity of the disease as well as the bradykinesia, although it has no effect on the tremor. Benztropine is muscarinic cholinoceptor antagonist used as an adjunct drug in Parkinson disease.

26. **The answer is A.** Memantine is an NMDA-receptor inhibitor that is well tolerated and shown to slow the rate of cognitive decline in Alzheimer patients. Donepezil and tacrine are acetylcholinesterase inhibitors, which have shown similar activities. Tolcapone is a catechol-*O*-methyltransferase (COMT) inhibitor rarely used in Parkinson disease because of the possibility of hepatic

necrosis. Pramipexole is used as a dopamine receptor agonist in the management of Parkinson disease.

27. **The answer is D.** Disulfiram is an inhibitor of aldehyde dehydrogenase, which blocks the breakdown of acetaldehyde to acetate during the metabolism of alcohol. The buildup of acetaldehyde results in flushing, tachycardia, hypertension, and nausea to invoke a conditioned response to avoid alcohol ingestion. Lorazepam is useful in the prevention of seizures as a result of alcohol withdrawal, whereas carbamazepine is used should they develop. Flumazenil is used for benzodiazepine overdose and naloxone for opioid overdose.

28. **The answer is D.** Atomoxetine is a nonstimulant drug used in the management of attention-deficit/hyperactivity disorder (ADHD) that works by inhibiting norepinephrine reuptake. The stimulate agents used for the treatment of ADHD include methylphenidate and dextroamphetamine and work by inhibiting dopamine reuptake. Caffeine is a stimulant in many beverages, which may have some role in the management of some headaches. Modafinil is a newer agent used in the treatment of narcolepsy.

29. **The answer is B.** Haloperidol is an antipsychotic agent used in acute psychotic attacks and for the treatment of schizophrenia. It is a dopamine-receptor antagonist that acts predominately at the dopamine D_2 receptor. Baclofen is a $GABA_B$ receptor antagonist that is used in the treatment of spinal cord injuries. Choral hydrate is a hypnotic agent that works similarly to ethanol. Phenobarbital is a barbiturate used in the treatment of seizures and as an anesthetic. Imipra-amine is a tricyclic antidepressant and is not used in schizophrenia.

30. **The answer is E.** Acute dystonias are a complication of antipsychotics that work primarily through dopamine D_2 receptors and therefore have a high incidence of extrapyramidal effects. Haloperidol and agents such as fluphenazine are the most likely offenders. Such reactions are best managed with an anticholinergic agent such as benztropine. Another complication of haloperidol is the neuroleptic malignant syndrome, which is treated with a dopamine agonist receptor and dantrolene. Hyperprolactinemia with galactorrhea is common with agents that block dopamine's actions, as dopamine normally represses prolactin release.

31. **The answer is C.** Agranulocytosis occurs more frequently with clozapine than with other agents, requiring routine blood tests. It is the only agent that improves the negative symptoms of schizophrenia. Cholestatic jaundice and photosensitivity are common with chlorpromazine. Galactorrhea is a side effect of older high-potency agents that block dopamine. QT prolongation is a complication of agents such as thioridazine and ziprasidone.

32. **The answer is B.** The unique affinities of various antipsychotics result in their unique activities and their unique side effects. Risperidone is an atypical antipsychotic that works by blocking the $5\text{-}HT_{2A}$ serotonin receptor. The older high-potency antipsychotics inhibit dopamine receptors. Agents such as clozapine inhibit histamine receptors. Atropine is an antagonist at cholinergic receptors.

33. **The answer is E.** Ethosuximide is the drug of choice for absence seizures in children. Valproic acid has more side effects and therefore is a second-line drug. Prednisone is used in infantile seizures. Phenytoin and carbamazepine can be used in partial seizures or in tonic-clonic seizures. Lorazepam is often used in the treatment of status epilepticus.

34. **The answer is B.** Gingival hyperplasia is a unique side effect of phenytoin, which can be partially avoided by meticulous oral hygiene. Several anticonvulsants can cause hepatotoxicity, including valproic acid. Aplastic anemia is a rare, but a potential complication of carbamazepine, ethosuximide. Valproic acid is also associated with thrombocytopenia. Ethosuximide has been associated with a severe form of erythema multiforme, the Steven-Johnson syndrome.

35. **The answer is A.** Tiagabine is an anticonvulsant used in conjunction with drugs such as phenytoin. Its mechanism is related to its ability to inhibit GABA transport into the cell, thereby decreasing GABA uptake. Gabapentin works by stimulating the release of GABA from neurons. Benzodiazepines function to increase GABA-stimulated chloride channel opening, whereas

barbiturates prolong GABA- induced chloride channel opening. Ethosuximide works by blocking T-type calcium channels.

36. **The answer is E.** Many antiseizure drugs find applications for other diseases. Gabapentin is approved for the treatment of diabetic nephropathy, an unfortunate consequence in this patient's presentation. Phenytoin is also used for the treatment of arrhythmias. Carbamazepine is used in the management of trigeminal neuralgia. Acetazolamide, sometimes used as a treatment for absence seizure control, is used in the treatment of glaucoma. Valproic acid can be used in the prophylaxis of migraine headaches.

37. **The answer is B.** Salicylate toxicity initially increases the medullary response to carbon dioxide, with resulting hyperventilation and respiratory alkalosis. Increases in lactic acid and ketone body formation result in a metabolic acidosis. All other choices are incorrect in this particular setting. Treatment includes correction of acid–base disturbances, replacement of electrolytes and fluids, cooling, alkalinization of urine, and forced diuresis.

38. **The answer is C.** From the presented list, only methotrexate is known to be an antineoplastic agent. This medication has been used successfully in rheumatoid arthritis and other rheumatologic conditions. Celecoxib is a COX-2 inhibitor. Ketorolac is a powerful analgesic used for multiple autoimmune conditions. Entocort is a glucocorticoid that can be used in some arthritides. Auranofin is a gold compound that is rarely used anymore.

39. **The answer is A.** Infliximab is a recombinant antibody to TNF-α; it has been successfully used in the treatment of Crohn disease, rheumatoid arthritis, and some other autoimmune conditions. Adalimumab, an agent also used for rheumatoid arthritis, is a humanized antibody to TNF-α. Etanercept, a subcutaneous agent approved for treatment of rheumatoid arthritis, is a fusion protein that binds to TNF-α receptor. Anakinra, an IL-1 blocker also used for rheumatoid arthritis, is a recombinant protein resembling IL-1. Alefacept, an agent used for psoriasis, is a recombinant protein composed of a portion of LFA-3.

40. **The answer is D.** Colchicine is often used to treat an acute gouty attack. Probenecid and sulfinpyrazone reduce urate levels by preventing reabsorption of uric acid. These agents are used for chronic gout. Allopurinol is a xanthine oxidase inhibitor; it is also used for treatment of chronic gout. Celecoxib is the only COX-2 inhibitor on the market.

41. **The answer is C.** Tacrolimus decreases the activity of calcineurin, which leads to a decrease in nuclear NF-AT and the transcription of T-cell-specific lymphokines and early T-cell activation. Inhibiting transport to the nucleus of the transcription factor NF-AT refers to mechanism of action of cyclosporine. Stimulating apoptosis of some lymphoid lineages refers to glucocorticoids. Inhibiting mTOR, which in turn delays the G_1–S transition, represents the mechanism of action of sirolimus. Inhibiting proliferation of promyelocytes refers to azathioprine.

42. **The answer is D.** Cyclophosphamide has been successfully used for treatment of lupus nephritis; however, it does carry significant morbidity associated with its use. Azathioprine works by suppressing T-cell activity. Cyclosporine inhibits T-helper cell activation. Tacrolimus inhibits transcription of T-cell-specific lymphokines. Baciliximab is a monoclonal antibody against CD-25 used to reduce the incidence and severity of renal transplant rejection.

43. **The answer is E.** As the name suggests, tPA activates plasminogen bound to plasmin, thereby acting as a thrombolytic. Inhibiting platelet aggregation refers to clopidogrel and ticlopidine. Increasing antithrombin activity refers to heparin and its analogues. Impairing fibrin polymerization refers to dextran. Finally, blocking GPIIa/IIIb refers to abciximab.

44. **The answer is B.** Deferoxamine is an iron-chelating agent and as such can be given in cases of iron supplement overdose. Protamine is an antidote for heparin. Vitamin K and fresh frozen plasma are given for coumarin reversal. Charcoal is an agent sometimes used for gastric lavage.

45. **The answer is C.** Diazepam and lorazepam are very effective at treating the vertigo associated with Ménière disease. Loop diuretics, such as furosemide, can precipitate vertigo secondary to volume depletion and resultant orthostatic hypotension. Ondansetron is a powerful antiemetic.

Emetrol is an over-the-counter antiemetic for infants. Dronabinol, a synthetic cannibinoid, has been used for weight loss.

46. The answer is E. Misoprostol is approved for use in patients taking nonsteriodal anti-inflammatory drugs (NSAIDs), both to decrease acid production and to increase bicarbonate and mucous production. Both omeprazole and lansoprazole are proton inhibitors that would not increase the protective mucus and bicarbonate. Nizatidine is an H_2-blocker that would also do nothing to increase the production of protective prostaglandins. Metronidazole is an antibiotic used to treat *Helicobacter pylori.*

47. The answer is A. Pepto Bismol, clarithromycin and amoxicillin, and omeprazole can be used for 7 days to eradicate *Helicobacter pylori* associated with peptic ulcer disease (metronidazole and tetracycline are additional choices for antibiotics). Pepto Bismol, metronidazole, and amoxicillin were the original triple therapy. The use of a proton pump inhibitor is usually preferred to an H_2-blocker. Regimens containing clarithromycin are used for cases of resistance to metronidazole.

48. The answer is A. Psyllium and methylcellulose are bulk-forming agents good for chronic constipation. The osmotic agent lactulose is given orally. Stool softeners such as docusate are useful in preventing constipation. Salt-containing osmotic agents such as magnesium sulfate are good for acute evacuation of the bowels. Senna is an irritant agent that stimulates intestinal motility.

49. The answer is D. Loperamide would be a good choice in this patient as it effectively controls diarrhea. Both codeine and diphenoxylate are opioids with abuse potential, especially in patients with abusive histories. Diphenoxylate is available in combination with atropine to reduce the potential for abuse. Anticholinergic agents such as propantheline prevent cramping but have little effect on diarrhea. Kaolin is good for absorbing toxins from the intestines.

50. The answer is A. Glucocorticoids are used in the management of moderate cases of Crohn disease. 5-Amino salicylic acid (5-ASA) compounds such as sulfasalazine are used in mild cases of ulcerative colitis. Octreotide is used for diarrhea secondary to increased release of gastrointestinal hormones. Bismuth subsalicylate and loperamide can be used in the treatment of uncomplicated diarrhea.

51. The answer is D. Infliximab is a monoclonal antibody approved for the treatment of refractory Crohn disease when mesalamine or steroids fail. Infalyte is an oral rehydration solution used in cases of childhood diarrhea. Opium tincture and diphenoxylate are opioid preparations for uncomplicated diarrhea.

52. The answer is E. Theophylline is associated with all of the reactions listed. They usually occur at elevated blood levels, generally accepted as greater than 20 μg/dL. However, adverse drug reactions may occur at any blood level.

53. The answer is C. A disulfiram-like reaction may be seen in non-insulin-dependent diabetics treated with chlorpropamide, an oral hypoglycemic, when used in combination with alcohol.

54. The answer is B. Elderly patients with subclinical hypothyroidism are at risk for arrhythmias, angina, or myocardial infarction if they have underlying cardiovascular disease when they begin treatment with thyroid hormones such as levothyroxine. These potential adverse effects occur because of increased cardiovascular workload as well as the direct effect of thyroid hormone on the heart.

55. The answer is D. Prednisone, a steroid commonly used to treat exacerbations of lupus erythematosus, can cause peptic ulcer disease due to the inhibition of the prostaglandins that normally protect the mucosa.

56. The answer is D. Conjugation is the principal mechanism for the acquisition of antibiotic resistance among enterobacteria and involves the transfer of resistance transfer factors on plasmids through sex pili. The other mechanisms for gene transfer, including random mutation, transformation, transduction, and transposition are not as common among these organisms.

57. **The answer is E.** Cilastatin must be given with imipenem. It is an inhibitor of renal dehydropeptidase, which normally would degrade imipenem. Probenecid increases penicillin concentrations by blocking their excretion by the kidney. Both clavulanic acid and sulbactam are penicillinase inhibitors used to increase the spectrum against penicillinase-producing species. Cycloserine is a second-line agent for gram-negative organisms and tuberculosis.

58. **The answer is A.** Cefazolin, a first-generation cephalosporin, is often used for surgical prophylaxis because it has activity against most gram-positive and some gram-negative organisms. Second-generation agents (cefoxitin) and third-generation agents (ceftriaxone) are not used because they have less gram-positive coverage. Aztreonam lacks activity against anaerobes and gram-positive organisms. Oxacillin is primarily active against staphylococci.

59. **The answer is B.** Aztreonam is active against *Pseudomonas* spp., appears to be safe during pregnancy, and does not show cross-hypersensitivity with penicillins. Piperacillin, cefoxitin, and imipenem all have some overlap in penicillin-allergic patients. Although ciprofloxacin is good in nonpregnant patients, it is absolutely contraindicated in pregnancy.

60. **The answer is E.** Cefamandole, a cephalosporin, is known to precipitate a disulfiram-like reaction. Bacitracin is not used intravenously, only topically. Chloramphenicol is associated with bone marrow suppression. Vancomycin can be associated with flush on infusion. Isoniazid is an antituberculoid antibiotic.

61. **The answer is B.** Bone marrow suppression results in pancytopenia in treated patients, which in rare cases can lead to aplastic anemia. Gray baby syndrome is associated with chloramphenicol use in infants. Disulfiram-like reactions can occur with some cephalosporins. Aminoglycosides and vancomycin can result in nephrotoxicity and ototoxicity.

62. **The answer is E.** Macrolides such as azithromycin or clarithromycin are the agents of choice for the treatment of mycoplasmal diseases. As mycoplasma have no cell wall, drugs such as penicillins, cephalosporins, or vancomycin are ineffective. Chloramphenicol is relatively toxic and reserved for select infections.

63. **The answer is D.** Diarrhea due to pseudomembranous colitis with *Clostridium difficile* overgrowth is common with many broad-spectrum antibiotics, especially clindamycin. Bruising can occur with some cephalosporins. Dizziness is common with tetracyclines such as minocycline. Ototoxicity can result in hearing loss with vancomycin and aminoglycosides. Tendon pain is possible due to the cartilage toxicity associated with fluoroquinolones.

64. **The answer is D.** Primaquine is associated with intravascular hemolysis or methemoglobinuria in G-6-PDH deficiency patients, as it causes oxidative damage to hemoglobin. Chloroquine and pyrimethamine do not cause hemolysis, although they are often used with sulfa drugs, which can cause hemolysis in such patients. Chloroquine rarely causes hemolysis, and doxycycline is not known to cause problems in G-6-PDH deficiency.

65. **The answer is B.** Metronidazole is the preferred treatment for *Clostridium difficile* colitis, which probably resulted from the patient's use of a broad-spectrum antibiotic for her initial infection. Vancomycin is considered in the treatment of *Clostridium difficile* colitis in refractory cases. Clindamycin use is often associated with *Clostridium difficile* colitis. Ciprofloxacin can be used for the treatment of diverticulitis, but not colitis. Neomycin is used to sterilize the bowel, which is not the goal in this case. Silver sulfadiazine is used to treat skin infections in burn patients.

66. **The answer is A.** MESNA is often given with cyclophosphamide and ifosfamide to help detoxify metabolic products that can cause hemorrhagic cystitis. Allopurinol is given with chemotherapy agents such as busulfan to reduce renal precipitation of urate. Leucovorin is given to rescue patients in the case of methotrexate toxicity. Cilastatin is an inhibitor of imipenem degradation. MOPP is a multidrug regimen (mechlorethamine, Oncovin (vincristine), procarbazine, and prednisone) used in the treatment of Hodgkin disease.

67. **The answer is B.** Filgrastim is a recombinant form of granulocyte colony-stimulating factor (G-CSF) given to prevent chemotherapy-induced neutropenia. Epoetin alfa is commonly used to prevent anemia while on chemotherapy. Oprelvekin is an agent used to help treat

chemotherapy-induced thrombocytopenia. Interferon alfa-2b is used in the management of specific leukemias and lymphomas. Amifostine is given to patients receiving radiation to the head and neck to preserve salivary function.

68. The answer is C. Trastuzumab is an antibody to the extracellular domain of the receptor tyrosine kinase HER2/neu. In some breast cancers, HER2/neu is expressed in high levels leading to autophosphorylation in the absence of ligand binding. Trastuzumab blocks such signaling. Imatinib is used in chronic myelogenous leukemia and inhibits bcr-abl. Tamoxifen functions by inhibiting estrogen-mediated gene transcription. Rituximab targets $CD20^+$ cells in B-cell lymphomas for ADCC. Thalidomide works in part by inhibiting TNF production.

69. The answer is C. Tretinoin is all-*trans*-retinoic acid and produces remission by inducing differentiation in the M3 variant of acute myelogenous leukemia (AML), characterized by aberrant expression of a retinoic receptor-α gene. Cisplatin is often used in the treatment of cancers of the lung, head, and neck. Lomustine has good central nervous system (CNS) penetration and is used in brain tumors. Fluorouracil is also used in multiple tumors including those of the breast and colon. Lastly, streptozocin is used in the treatment of insulinomas.

70. The answer is C. Imatinib is an orally active small molecule inhibitor of the oncogenic bcr-abl kinase produced as a result of the Philadelphia chromosome, used to treat chronic myelogenous leukemia. It also inhibits the c-Kit receptor and can be used in gastrointestinal stromal tumors (GISTs). Anastrozole is used in the management of breast cancer. Rituximab is an antibody used in the treatment of non-Hodgkin lymphoma. Gefitinib is an orally active small molecule inhibitor of the EGF receptor, used in the treatment of some lung cancer. Amifostine is used as a radio-protectant, with or without cisplatin.

71. The answer is A. Interferon alfa-2b is used for the treatment of hairy cell leukemia, chronic myeloid leukemia, Kaposi sarcoma, and lymphomas. Interleukin-2 is used in the treatment of metastatic renal cell carcinoma. All-*trans*-retinoic acid is used to induce remission in M3 acute myelogenous leukemia (AML). Rituximab is used to treat $CD20^+$ non-Hodgkin lymphoma. Daunorubicin is an antibiotic-type compound used in the treatment of some leukemias and lymphomas.

72. The answer is D. Cetuximab inhibits the EGF receptor by binding to the extracellular domain of the receptor. Other EGFR signaling inhibitors include erlotinib and gefinitib, although both of these molecules are orally active and penetrate the cell to perturb EGFR signaling from within the cell. Rituximab and Traztuzamab are both antibodies as well, but are used in the treatment of non-Hodgkin lymphoma and breast cancer, respectively.

73. The answer is C. N-acetylcysteine is used in the case of acetaminophen toxicity. It provides sulfhydryl groups for the regeneration of glutathione stores in the body. Trientine is a copper-chelating agent sometimes used in Wilson disease. Sorbitol is used as a cathartic to help remove toxins from the gastrointestinal tract. Ipecac has been used to induce emesis in cases of toxic ingestions. Diazepam can be used to prevent seizures when strychnine is ingested.

74. The answer is A. Pralidoxime reactivates acetylcholinesterase to reverse the effects of exposure to organophosphates, of which parathion is actually an example. Amyl nitrate can be used in cases of ingestion of the cytochrome oxidase inhibitor cyanide. Bethanechol is a direct-acting muscarinic cholinoceptor agonist used to treat urinary retention and overdose and can result in symptoms similar to organophosphate poisoning. Nicotine is sometimes found in insecticides and can cause vomiting, weakness, seizures, and respiratory arrest.

75. The answer is B. Warfarin is an orally active inhibitor of vitamin K-dependent carboxylation of various clotting factors. In the event of supratherapeutic doses of warfarin, the anticoagulation can be reversed by giving vitamin K. Heparin is an intravenous preparation that is also an anticoagulation agent. Aminocaproic acid inhibits plasminogen activation and is used in the treatment of hemophilia. Vitamin D is used in cases of its deficiency or in the treatment of osteoporosis. Oprelvekin is a recombinant form of interleukin-11 that stimulates platelet production and does not affect the clotting factors.

Index

Page numbers in *italics* denote figures; those followed by "t" denote boxes; Q denotes questions; E denotes explanations

A

E

N

O

Q

R

U

V